Textbook of Contraception, Sexual and Reproductive Health

Textbook of Contraception, Sexual and Reproductive Health

Edited by

Johannes Bitzer
University Women's Hospital, Basel, Switzerland

Tahir A. Mahmood
Victoria Hospital, Kirkcaldy, UK

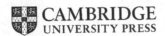

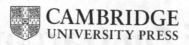

Shaftesbury Road, Cambridge CB2 8EA, United Kingdom

One Liberty Plaza, 20th Floor, New York, NY 10006, USA

477 Williamstown Road, Port Melbourne, VIC 3207, Australia

314–321, 3rd Floor, Plot 3, Splendor Forum, Jasola District Centre, New Delhi – 110025, India

103 Penang Road, #05–06/07, Visioncrest Commercial, Singapore 238467

Cambridge University Press is part of Cambridge University Press & Assessment, a department of the University of Cambridge.

We share the University's mission to contribute to society through the pursuit of education, learning and research at the highest international levels of excellence.

www.cambridge.org
Information on this title: www.cambridge.org/9781108958622

DOI: 10.1017/9781108961097

First published 2024

A catalogue record for this publication is available from the British Library.

A Cataloging-in-Publication data record for this book is available from the Library of Congress.

ISBN 978-1-108-95862-2 Paperback

....

Every effort has been made in preparing this book to provide accurate and up-to-date information that is in accord with accepted standards and practice at the time of publication. Although case histories are drawn from actual cases, every effort has been made to disguise the identities of the individuals involved. Nevertheless, the authors, editors, and publishers can make no warranties that the information contained herein is totally free from error, not least because clinical standards are constantly changing through research and regulation. The authors, editors, and publishers therefore disclaim all liability for direct or consequential damages resulting from the use of material contained in this book. Readers are strongly advised to pay careful attention to information provided by the manufacturer of any drugs or equipment that they plan to use.

Contents

About the Authors   viii
List of Contributors   ix

Section 1 Sexual and Reproductive Health and Rights, Public Health Aspects and Prevention in Sexual and Reproductive Healthcare

1 **Sexual and Reproductive Health and Rights**   1
Chiara Benedetto

2 **European Laws on Sexual and Reproductive Health and the Different Policies regarding Access to Sexual and Reproductive Healthcare**   8
Teresa A. Bombas

3 **The Main Threats to Sexual and Reproductive Health and the Principal Components of Good Sexual and Reproductive Healthcare**   15
Johannes Bitzer

4 **The Principles and Roles of Sexuality Education**   23
Evert Ketting

5 **Sexual Reproductive Health: Public Health Aspects**   28
Tahir A. Mahmood and Johannes Bitzer

6 **General Principles of Preventive Medicine in Sexual and Reproductive Healthcare**   38
Johannes Bitzer

7 **Screening in Sexual and Reproductive Healthcare**   46
Rolf Kirschner, Harald Moi, Gilbert G. G. Donders

8 **Reproductive Life Plan and Preconception Care, Including Vaccination**   49
Kai Haldre

Section 2 Sexual and Reproductive Healthcare

Section 2A Sexual and Reproductive Healthcare: Contraception

9 **The Reproductive Endocrinology of Contraception**   61
Sven O. Skouby and Kresten Rubeck Petersen

10 **Evidence-Based Clinical Practice in Contraceptive Counselling and Care**   71
Sarah Sultana Grixti, Olivia Anne Cassar, and Charles Savona-Ventura

11 **Combined Hormonal Contraception**   77
Gabriele S. Merki-Feld and Frans J. M. E. Roumen

12 **Progestogen-Only Contraception**   88
Frans J. M. E. Roumen, Gabriele S. Merki-Feld and Katarina Sedlecky

13 **Nonhormonal Contraception**   97
Kristina Gemzell-Danielsson, Juan Acuna and Helena Kopp Kallner

14 **Permanent Methods of Contraception in Women**   109
Omar Thanoon, Chu Chin Lim, and Tahir A. Mahmood

15 **Emergency Contraception**   114
Sharon T. Cameron

16 **Management of Issues Associated with Female Contraceptives: Bleeding**   118
Katarina Sedlecky and Johannes Bitzer

v

17 **Management of Issues Associated with Female Contraceptives: Mood** 123
Johannes Bitzer

18 **Management of Issues Associated with Female Contraceptives: Sexuality** 126
Johannes Bitzer

19 **Management of Issues Associated with Female Contraceptives: Drug–Drug Interactions** 131
Katarina Sedlecky, Gabriele S. Merki-Feld and Frans J. M. E. Roumen

20 **Contraception in Women with Cancer** 140
Anne Gompel

21 **Contraception in Women with Benign Breast Disease and Benign Uterine and Ovarian Conditions** 146
Giovanni Grandi, Maria Chiara Del Savio, and Fabio Facchinetti

22 **Contraception in Women with Cardiovascular Conditions** 154
Angelo Cagnacci, Claudia Massarotti, Laura Gabbi, and Anjeza Xholli

23 **Contraception in Women with Metabolic Conditions** 159
Angelo Cagnacci, Anna Biasioli, Claudia Massarotti, Laura Gabbi, Anjeza Xholli

24 **Contraceptive Choices for Women with HIV Infection** 165
Katarina Sedlecky, Gabriele S. Merki-Feld and Frans J. M. E. Roumen

25 **Contraception in Women with Neurological Conditions** 170
Gabriele S. Merki-Feld, Frans J. M. E. Roumen and Katarina Sedlecky

26 **Contraception in Women with Psychiatric Conditions** 174
Gabriele S. Merki-Feld, Frans J. M. E. Roumen and Katarina Sedlecky

27 **Contraception in Disabled Women** 178
Johannes Bitzer

28 **Contraception in Women with Immunosuppressive Diseases** 183
Charles Savona-Ventura, Alison Fava, and Judith-Marie Mifsud

29 **Contraception in Women with Lupus Autoimmune Diseases** 187
Parivakkam S. Arunakumari and Charlotte Gatenby

30 **Contraception in Women with Chronic Kidney Disease** 192
Jean-Jacques Ries and Johannes Bitzer

31 **Contraception in Women with Diabetes** 196
Parivakkam S. Arunakumari and Charlotte Gatenby

32 **Contraception in Women with Thyroid Dysfunction** 200
Christina I. Messini, George Anifandis, Alexandros Daponte and Ioannis E. Messinis

33 **Contraception in Women with Polycystic Ovary Syndrome** 204
Christina I. Messini, George Anifandis, Alexandros Daponte, Ioannis E. Messinis

34 **Contraception in Women with Special Needs: Life-Course Approach** 208
Johannes Bitzer

35 **Male Contraception** 217
Gideon A. Sartorius and Yacov Reisman

Section 2B Sexual and Reproductive Healthcare: Termination of Pregnancy

36 **Termination of Pregnancy: Overview** 223
John J. Reynolds-Wright, Sharon T. Cameron

37 **Termination of Pregnancy: Medical Methods** 229
John J. Reynolds-Wright, Sharon T. Cameron

38 **Termination of Pregnancy: Surgical Methods** 233
Barbara Salje, Michelle Cooper

39 **Termination of Pregnancy at Different Gestational Phases** 239
John J. Reynolds, Sharon T. Cameron

40 **Post-abortion Care** 243
Dominique Baker, Chu Chin Lim, Tahir Mahmood

Section 2C Sexual and Reproductive Healthcare: Infertility

41 **Infertility** 249
Ioannis E. Messinis, Christina I. Messini,
George Anifandis, Alexandros Daponte

42 **Hormones and Female Sexuality** 256
Elisa Maseroli, Linda Vignozzi

Section 2D Sexually Transmitted Infections

43 **Vulvovaginitis** 267
Gilbert G. G. Donders, Werner Mendling,
Francesco de Seta, Henry J. C. de Vries

44 **Sexually Transmitted Genital Infections: HPV, Tricho, Herpes, Chlamydia** 274
Gilbert G. G. Donders, Henry J. C. de Vries

45 **Sexually Transmitted Genital Infections: Syphilis, Gonorrhoea, Hepatitis, HIV** 280
Brigitte Maria Frey Tirri

Section 3 Sexual Healthcare

Section 3A Sexual Dysfunction and Counselling

46 **Sexual Counselling: General Principles** 289
Johannes Bitzer

47 **Disorders of Desire, Arousal and Orgasm in the Female** 294
Rossella E. Nappi, Lara Tiranini and Giulia Stincardini

48 **Sexual Pain Disorders in the Female** 300
Francesca Tripodi

49 **Vulvodynia** 311
Leonardo Micheletti, Gianluigi Radici, Chiara Benedetto

50 **Disorders of Desire, Arousal and Orgasm in the Male** 317
Yacov Reisman

Section 3B Sexual Healthcare along the Life Course

51 **Life-Course Approach to Sexual Health** 333
Johannes Bitzer

52 **Sexual Violence** 340
Johannes Bitzer

53 **Sexual and Reproductive Healthcare for LGBTI*** 347
Johannes Bitzer

Section 4 Sexual and Reproductive Health Indicators and Policies

54 **Indicators of Sexual and Reproductive Health and Their Relevance to Policy Development** 353
Charlotte Gatenby, Sambit Mukhopadhyay

55 **Health Systems for Sexual and Reproductive Health** 358
Charlotte Gatenby, Sambit Mukhopadhyay and Tahir A. Mahmood

56 **Prevention and Health Promotion in Sexual and Reproductive Health** 365
Susan Brechin, Mark Steven, Helena Young

Index 371

About the Authors

Johannes Bitzer Professor Emeritus, MD
Former Chairman and Professor Emeritus of the Department of Obstetrics and Gynaecology at the University Hospitals of the University of Basel. Former Head of the Division of Psychosomatic and Psychosocial Obstetrics and Gynaecology at the University of Basel. Past President of the European Society of Contraception, Past President of the International Society of Psychosomatic Obstetrics and Gynaecology and member of several international executive and advisory boards in family planning, sexology and menopause. Past member of the Executive Committee of the European Board and College of Obstetrics and Gynaecology (EBCOG) and Director of knowledge-based assessment on the education committee of EBCOG. Treasurer and representative of EBCOG at the Multidisciplinary Joint Committee of Sexual Medicine. Formerly a member of the Board of Trustees of the International Menopause Society, Chair of the Education Committee and Board member of the European Menopause and Andropause Society. Director of the Diploma of Advanced Studies in Sexual Medicine at the Advanced Study Centre of the University of Basel. Editor-in-Chief of the European Journal of Contraception and Reproductive Health Care and Associate Editor of the Journal of Sexual Medicine.

During his specialisation in obstetrics and gynaecology he was trained in behavioural sciences and psychotherapy. His research and practical interests are in contraceptive and menopause counselling as well as menopausal therapies and contraceptive technology, epidemiology, sexual and reproductive health and the interface between obstetrics/gynaecology and psychology/psychiatry, which includes infertility counselling, psycho-oncology and a life-course approach in SRH care.

He has more than 200 peer-reviewed publications, has edited 3 books, written 45 book chapters and given more than 350 invited lectures and workshops.

Tahir Mahmood CBE, MD, FRCPI, FFRSH, MBA, FACOG, FRCPE, FEBCOG, FRCOG Consultant Gynaecologist, Victoria Hospital, Kirkcaldy, and Spire Murrayfield Hospital, Edinburgh, Scotland. He served as Vice President Standards, Royal College of Obstetricians and Gynaecologists (2007–10), was President of the European Board and College of Obstetrics and Gynaecology (EBCOG, 2014–17), President of Edinburgh Obstetrical Society (2012–14) and President of the Northern Obstetrical and Gynaecological Society of Scotland (1999–2011). He was National Lead for Heavy Menstrual Bleeding Audit in England and Wales (2010–15), and Member of FIGO Hyperglycaemia in Pregnancy Working Group (2014–16). He is currently International UNFPA Consultant for the EECA Region, Chair of the EBCOG Standards of Care and Position Statements Group, Chair of the Quality Assurance Committee of the EBCOG Standing Committee of Fellowship Examination, and Life Trustee of the Lindsay Stewart R&D Foundation of the Royal College of Obstetricians and Gynaecologists. In the recent past, he has held honorary Senior Clinical Lectureships at the Universities of Edinburgh, Dundee and St. Andrews in Scotland. He has edited 15 manuscripts and has published more than 200 research papers, 50 chapters and has delivered more than 200 lectures by invitation. He was appointed as Commander of the Order of the British Empire (CBE) in the New Year's Honours list in 2012.

Contributors

Juan Acuna MD MSC FACOG
Assistant Dean for Research
Chair, Department of Epidemiology and Public Health
Associate Professor Obstetrics and Gynecology, Genetics and Epidemiology
Khalifa University of Science and Technology, College of Medicine and Health Sciences, Abu Dhabi, United Arab Emirates

George Anifandis MD PhD
Associate Professor of Embryology
Department of Obstetrics and Gynaecology, University of Thessaly, School of Health Sciences, Faculty of Medicine, Larissa, Greece

Parivakkam S. Arunakumari MD FRCOG MFFP
Department of Obstetrics and Gynaecology, Norfolk and Norwich University Hospital, Norwich, UK

Dominique Baker
Department of Obstetrics & Gynaecology, Victoria Hospital, Kirkcaldy, UK

Chiara Benedetto MD PhD FCNGOF FEBCOG FRCOG FACOG
Department of Obstetrics and Gynaecology, University of Turin S. Anna Hospital, Turin, Italy
Johannes Bitzer MD PhD FFRSH (Hon)
Division of Psychosomatic Obstetrics and Gynaecology, University Women's Hospital, Basel, Switzerland

Anna Biasioli
Department of Maternal and Child Health, University-Hospital of Udine, Udine, Italy

Teresa A. Bombas MD
Coimbra University Hospital Centre, Coimbra, Portugal

Susan Brechin FRCOG MD FFSRH FHEA MIPM ILM
Fife Health and Social Care Partnership, Whyteman Brae Hospital, Kirkcaldy, UK

Angelo Cagnacci MD PhD
Clinic of Obstetrics and Gynaecology, DINOGMI, IRCCS-Ospedale San Martino, Genoa, Italy

Sharon T. Cameron MD FRCOG MFSRH
Chalmers Sexual and Reproductive Health Service, Edinburgh, UK

Olivia Anne Cassar MD MRCOG MSc
Department of Obstetrics and Gynaecology, University of Malta, Msida, Malta

Maria Chiara Del Savio
Department of Medical and Surgical Sciences for Mother, Child and Adult, University of Modena and Reggio Emilia, Azienda, Modena, Italy

Michelle Cooper MRCOG MFSRH
Chalmers Sexual and Reproductive Health Service, Edinburgh, UK

Alexandros Daponte MD Dr Med FCOG
Professor of Obstetrics and Gynaecology
Department of Obstetrics and Gynaecology, University of Thessaly, School of Health Sciences, Faculty of Medicine, Larissa, Greece

Francesco de Seta
Department of Medical Sciences, University of Trieste, Trieste, Italy; Institute for Maternal and Child Health, Istituto di Ricovero e Cura a Carattere Scientifico (IRCCS), Burlo Garofolo, Trieste, Italy

Henry J. C. de Vries
Department of Dermatology, Amsterdam University Medical Centers (UMC), Academic Medical Center at the University of Amsterdam, Amsterdam, The Netherlands
Amsterdam Institute for Infection and Immunology, Infectious Diseases, Amsterdam University Medical Centers (UMC), Amsterdam, The Netherlands
Department of Infectious Diseases, Public Health Service Amsterdam, Center for Sexual Health, Amsterdam, The Netherlands

Gilbert G. G. Donders MD PhD
Gynaecology and Obstetrics Regional Hospital,
H Hart, Tienen, Belgium

Fabio Facchinetti
Department of Medical and Surgical Sciences for
Mother, Child and Adult, University of
Modena and Reggio Emilia, Azienda,
Modena, Italy

Alison Fava MD MRCS MRCOG PhD
Department of Obstetrics and Gynaecology,
University of Malta, Msida,
Malta

Brigitte Maria Frey Tirri MD
Baselland Women's Clinic, Baselland Cantonal
Hospital, Liestal, Switzerland

Laura Gabbi
Clinic of Obstetrics and Gynaecology,
DINOGMI, IRCCS-Ospedale San Martino,
Genoa, Italy

**Charlotte Gatenby MBCHB MFSRH PGCME
DIPM**
SRH Subspecialty Training Fellow
Norfolk and Norwich University Hospital NHS Trust
Norwich, United Kingdom

Kristina Gemzell-Danielsson MD PhD
Department of Women's and Children's
Health, Karolinska University Hospital,
Stockholm, Sweden

Anne Gompel MD PhD
Department of Gynaecology, Paris Descartes
University, Paris, France

Giovanni Grandi
Department of Medical and Surgical Sciences for
Mother, Child and Adult, University of Modena and
Reggio Emilia Modena, Italy

Kai Haldre MD PhD
Gynaecologist Centre for Infertility Treatment East
Tallinn Central Hospital Women's Clinic Tallinn,
Estonia

Helena Kopp Kallner MD PhD
Karolinska University Hospital, Stockholm,
Sweden

**Evert Ketting LRCPSI LM MD MHA FEBCOG FECSM
FRCOG**
International SRHR Consultant, Zeist, Netherlands

Rolf S. Kirschner MD MHA
Oslo University Hospital, Oslo, Norway

Chu Chin Lim FRCOG
Department of Women and Child Health, Victoria
Hospital, Kirkcaldy, UK

**Tahir A. Mahmood CBE MD FRCPI MBA FACOG
FRCPE FEBCOG FRCOG**
Department of Gynaecology, Victoria Hospital,
Kirkcaldy, Scotland and Spire Murrayfield Hospital,
Edinburgh, UK

Elisa Maseroli
Andrology, Women's Endocrinology and Gender
Incongruence Unit, Azienda Ospedaliero-
Universitaria Careggi, Florence, Italy

Claudia Massarotti
Clinic of Obstetrics and Gynaecology, DINOGMI,
IRCCS-Ospedale San Martino, Genoa, Italy

Louise Melvin BSc MBBS FFSRH
Consultant in Sexual & Reproductive Health and
Interim Clinical Lead for NHS GGC Gender Service
Sandyford Sexual Health Service, Glasgow, UK

Werner Mendling
German Centre for Infections in Gynecology and
Obstetrics at Landesfrauenklinik, Helios University
Hospital Wuppertal, Wuppertal, Germany

Gabriele S. Merki-Feld
Senior Gynecologist and Lecturer
Clinic for Reproductive Endocrinology
University Hospital Zürich
Department of Reproductive Endocrinology,
University of Zurich Hospital, Zurich, Switzerland

Christina I. Messini MD PhD
Assistant Professor of Obstetrics and Gynaecology
Department of Obstetrics and Gynaecology,
University of Thessaly, School of Health Sciences,
Faculty of Medicine, Larissa, Greece

Ioannis E. Messinis MD PhD FRCOG
Department of Obstetrics and Gynaecology,
University of Thessaly, Larissa, Greece

Leonardo Micheletti MD
Department of Gynaecology and Obstetrics,
University of Turin, Turin, Italy

Judith-Marie Mifsud MD Dip in Sexual &
Reproductive Medicine MSc EFOG-EBCOG
Department of Obstetrics and Gynaecology,
University of Malta, Msida, Malta

Harald Moi MD PhD
Specialist in Dermatology and Venereology,
Professor Emeritus, University of Oslo, Oslo,
Norway
Oslo University Hospital, Oslo, Norway

Sambit Mukhopadhyay MD DNB MMedSci
FRCOG
Department of Obstetrics and Gynaecology,
Norfolk and Norwich University Hospital,
Norwich, UK

Rossella E. Nappi MD PhD MBA
Department of Obstetrics and Gynaecology, IRCCS
San Matteo Polyclinic, University of Pavia,
Pavia, Italy

Gianluigi Radici
Department of Surgical Sciences, University of
Torino, Torino, Italy

Kresten Rubeck Petersen MD DMSc
Department of Obstetrics and Gynaecology,
Hvidovre Hospital, Hvidovre, Denmark

Yacov Reisman MD PhD FECSM ECPS
Urologist and Certified Sexologist
Flare-Health, Amsterdam, Netherlands
Reuth Rehabilitation Hospital, Tel Aviv, Israel

John J. Reynolds-Wright
MRC Centre for Reproductive Health, University of
Edinburgh, Edinburgh, UK; Chalmers Centre, NHS
Lothian, Edinburgh, UK

Jean-Jacques Ries
Senior Consultant, Obstetrician Gynecologist
Department Obstetrics and Gynecology
University Hospital Basel, Basel, Switzerland

Frans J. M. E. Roumen MD PhD
Zuyderland Medical Centre, Heerle, Netherlands

Barbara Salje
Obstetrics and Gynaecology, NHS Tayside,
Dundee, UK

Gideon A. Sartorius
University Women's Hospital, Basel,
Switzerland

Prof. Charles Savona-Ventura MD DScMed FRCOG
AccCOG FRCPI FRCP Edin
Professor and Head of Department of Obstetrics &
Gynaecology
Director Centre of Traditional Chinese Medicine &
Culture
University of Malta
Department of Obstetrics and Gynaecology,
Mater Dei Hospital, Msida, Malta

Katarina Sedlecky
Family Planning Centre, Institute for
Mother and Child Health Care, Belgrade,
Serbia

Sven O. Skouby MD DMSc
Endocrinological and Reproductive Unit,
Department of Obstetrics and Gynaecology,
Herlev University Hospital,
Copenhagen, Denmark

Mark Steven
Team Leader, Sexual Health & Blood Borne Viruses
(SHBBV) Development Team, NHS Fife, Scotland,
UK

Giulia Stincardini
Department of Obstetrics and Gynaecology, IRCCS
San Matteo Polyclinic, University of Pavia,
Pavia, Italy

Sarah Sultana Grixti MD MRCP (UK) MSc MRCOG
Department of Obstetrics and Gynaecology,
University of Malta, Msida, Malta

Omar Thanoon FRCOG JBOG
Department of Obstetrics and Gynaecology,
Victoria Hospital, Kirkcaldy, UK

Lara Tiranini
Department of Obstetrics and Gynaecology,
IRCCS San Matteo Polyclinic, University of Pavia,
Pavia, Italy

Francesca Tripodi Psychotherapist, Sexologist, ECPS
Institute of Clinical Sexology, Rome, Italy
International Online Sexology Supervisors (IOSS)

Linda Vignozzi MD
Division of Women's Endocrinology and Gender
Incongruence, University of Florence Careggi
Hospital, Florence, Italy

Anjeza Xholli
Clinic of Obstetrics and Gynaecology,
DINOGMI, IRCCS-Ospedale San Martino, Genoa,
Italy

Helena Young
Sexual and Reproductive Health Speciality Trainee,
NHS Greater Glasgow and Clyde,
Scotland, UK

Section 1

Sexual and Reproductive Health and Rights, Public Health Aspects and Prevention in Sexual and Reproductive Healthcare

Chapter

1

Sexual and Reproductive Health and Rights

Chiara Benedetto

Introduction

Sexual and reproductive health (SRH) has been defined as:

a state of complete physical, mental and social well-being and not merely the absence of disease or infirmity, in all matters relating to the reproductive system and to its functions and processes. Reproductive health therefore implies that people are able to have a satisfying and safe sex life and that they have the capability to reproduce and the freedom to decide if, when and how often to do so. Implicit in this last condition are the right of men and women to be informed and to have access to safe, effective, affordable and acceptable methods of family planning, as well as other methods of their choice for regulation of fertility which are not against the law and the right of access to appropriate health-care services that will enable women to go safely through pregnancy and childbirth and provide couples with the best chance of having a healthy infant. [1]

Reproductive health encompasses being able to control one's fertility through access to contraception and abortion, being free from sexually transmitted infections (STIs), sexual dysfunction and sequelae related to sexual violence or female genital mutilation. It also includes the possibility of safe sexual experiences free of coercion, discrimination and/or violence. Although the recognition of SRH as an essential component of human rights dates back to the second half of the twentieth century, the full achievement of these rights remains elusive for many [2]. This is why universal access to reproductive health is included in the 2030 United Nations Agenda for Sustainable Development Goals (SDG), specifically in SDGs 3, 5 and 16 (see Figure 1.1) [3].

Family Planning

Family planning is recognized as a fundamental human right and plays a pivotal role in gender equality and girls' and women's empowerment, reducing poverty and achieving sustainable development. High-quality contraceptive services are essential to assist women in exercising their right to have children by choice and to decide freely and responsibly on the number and spacing of their children. Access to family planning services and education is also pivotal to improving prevention of sexually transmitted infections, including HIV.

> **Worldwide Figures**
>
> Out of 1.1 billion women worldwide in the reproductive age range (15–49 years) who need family planning services, 190 million had an unmet need for contraception in 2019 [4].

The growing use of contraceptive methods has led to improvements in health-related outcomes such as the reduction in undesired and high-risk pregnancies and in maternal and infant mortality [5]. Indeed, increased contraception use has reduced the maternal mortality rate by 26% over the past decade. Reducing the number of pregnancies also reduces childbirth complications and mortality due to unsafe abortion practices and dangers associated with high parities. Moreover, the use of contraceptives by young girls and boys increases the chances of receiving proper education and finishing school, with consequent positive effects on women's status and economic outcomes [6].

Therefore, the right to family planning education, information and services is pivotal to children's health and reproductive choice and it is central to women's SRH and empowerment. States must eliminate all legal, financial, social and institutional barriers that hamper access to comprehensive, quality, child- and youth-friendly SRH services and should implement programs to guarantee access to a full range of family planning services and contraceptives.

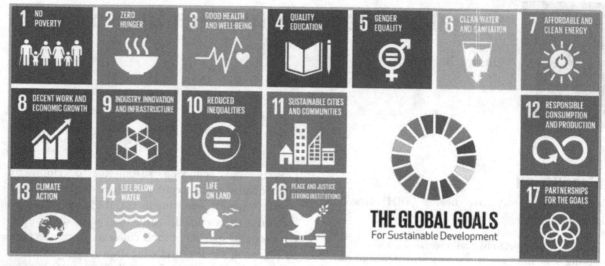

Figure 1.1 The 2030 United Nations Agenda for Sustainable Development Goals

Sexuality and Reproductive Information and Education

Sexuality and reproductive information and education should be universally available to all women and men to enable them to exercise and fulfil their SRH and rights. Sexuality education is defined as:

> Learning about the cognitive, emotional, social, interactive and physical aspects of sexuality. Sexuality education starts early in childhood and progresses through adolescence and adulthood. It aims at supporting and protecting sexual development. It gradually equips and empowers children and young people with information, skills and positive values to understand and enjoy their sexuality, have safe and fulfilling relationships and take responsibility for their own and other people's sexual health and well-being.

Worldwide Figures

Only 34% of young people have comprehensive correct knowledge about HIV prevention and transmission [7].

Sexuality information and education have various positive and lifelong effects on the health and well-being of young people. Indeed, the introduction of national sexuality education programs in several countries has been shown to increase the use of contraception, to delay the initiation of sexual intercourse and to reduce the number of sexual partners, the incidence of STIs and the number of teenage and unplanned pregnancies as well as the number of abortions. Moreover, good-quality sexuality education empowers young people to develop stronger and more meaningful relationships, thus contributing to the prevention of gender-based violence [8]. This is why access to sexuality and reproductive education is protected, which require governments around the world to guarantee the overall protection of health, well-being and dignity and specifically to guarantee the provision of unbiased and accurate sexuality education.

Access to Safe Abortion

Access to safe abortion is a complex determinant of girls' and women's health. Although it is a fundamental human right protected under numerous international and regional human rights treaties and national-level constitutions, it remains inaccessible, unavailable, illegal or permitted under very limited circumstances in 40% of countries worldwide. Moreover, even in countries where abortion is legal, there may be barriers to accessing safe abortion services such as restrictive laws, poor availability of resources, high costs of service, social stigma, conscientious objection of healthcare providers and unnecessary requirements (such as mandatory delays or counseling, misleading information, the need for family members' or a husband's authorization). These barriers contribute to increasing the number of girls and women who turn to unsafe abortion [9]. Unsafe abortion is defined as a procedure to terminate a pregnancy, practiced by individuals without the necessary training or using outdated or damaging methods or carried out in settings without meeting minimal medical standards.

Worldwide Figures

One out of three to four pregnancies ends in an induced abortion. Each year unsafe abortion is responsible for 4.7–13.2% of maternal deaths [10].

Unsafe abortion may lead to serious complications such as hemorrhage, sepsis, peritonitis, trauma to the gynecological and/or abdominal organs and reproductive tract infections, as well as permanent disability, including infertility [11]. Barriers to services and the laws that prohibit safe abortion expose girls and women to serious health risks, violating their rights to bodily integrity and to life itself. Sexuality and reproductive education, accessible contraception, training of abortion providers and access to legal abortion contribute to the prevention of unsafe abortion.

Maternal Healthcare

Maternal, perinatal and neonatal health matters to every person, society and country and should be considered pivotal from the point of view of human rights and well-being. Maternal health is the health of women during pregnancy, childbirth and the postpartum period.

Worldwide Figures

- More than 810 women die due to pregnancy and childbirth every day.
- Approximately 90% of maternal deaths occur in low- and lower-middle-income countries.
- The maternal mortality ratio dropped by about 38% between 2000 and 2017.
- Births attended by skilled health personnel increased from 58% in 1990 to 81% in 2019 [12].

The causes of maternal death may be directly related to childbirth such as obstetric complications during pregnancy, delivery or postpartum (e.g., hemorrhage, hypertension and sepsis) or indirectly related to childbirth, including existing health conditions during pregnancy or health problems that developed during the pregnancy itself. Interventions aimed at achieving adequate maternal nutrition, improving hygiene practices, antenatal care, emergency obstetric care and postnatal care contribute to the prevention of most maternal deaths [13].

Preconception counseling is a targeted counseling intervention that seeks to prevent specific problems before conception. It is based on three main concepts:

- **Risk assessment**: history of medical, surgical, psychosocial, genetic, nutrition, pharmaceutical and behavioral (e.g., smoking, alcohol and/or drug use) risks and implementation of control measures to remove or reduce them.
- **Health promotion**: optimization of health behavior by improving knowledge and increasing risk awareness, promotion of vaccination policies and of early booking into prenatal/antenatal services.
- **Targeted interventions**: involve preconception supplementation with folic acid and may entail the use of appropriate contraception to delay pregnancy until optimal health is achieved.

Antenatal care, provided by skilled healthcare professionals to pregnant women, tries to ensure the best health conditions, for both mother and child, during pregnancy and childbirth. It may include risk identification, prevention and management of pregnancy-related or concurrent diseases, health education and promotion (Table 1.1).

In 2016, the World Health Organization (WHO) drafted a model of antenatal care that recommends a minimum of eight antenatal contacts: the first up to 12 weeks' gestation (first trimester), two contacts in the second trimester (at 20 and 26 weeks' gestation) and five contacts scheduled at 30, 34, 36, 38 and 40 weeks (in the third trimester). Implementation of this

Table 1.1 Basic interventions recommended for antenatal care

Regular maternal and fetal well-being assessments
Nutritional counseling and physical activity advice
Iron and folic acid supplementation
Daily calcium supplementation in populations with low dietary calcium intake
Screening for major complications in pregnancy (e.g., hypertensive disorders, preeclampsia, asymptomatic bacteriuria, gestational diabetes mellitus)
Investigation as to smoking, alcohol intake and preexisting infectious diseases

Table 1.2 Basic interventions recommended for postnatal care

Identification of postpartum complications (e.g., hemorrhage, preeclampsia or infection)
Identification of maternal mental health problems
Nutritional counseling and hygiene advice
Family planning and contraceptive counseling
Breastfeeding support
Assessment of the newborn

model allows for a decrease in stillbirth risk as compared to models with four or fewer contacts [14].

Postnatal care, provided by healthcare professionals to women and children in the 6–8 weeks after birth, is a continuation of the care given to the woman throughout her pregnancy, labor and birth (Table 1.2). Healthcare professionals should support breastfeeding for its multiple benefits for both child and maternal health [15].

Gender-Based Violence

Gender-based violence is any act of violence inflicted upon an individual because of his or her gender or sexual orientation. The violence may take different forms – physical, sexual or psychological – and it encompasses harmful practices such as child marriage and female genital mutilation. Although boys and men can also be subjected to it, most gender-based violence is inflicted on girls and women.

> **Worldwide Figures**
>
> An estimated 30% of girls and women have experienced physical and/or sexual intimate partner violence and 7% have experienced non-partner sexual violence in their lifetime.

Violence against women is a gross violation of women's human rights and a manifestation of unequal power relations between men and women. Violence can have a range of short- and/or long-term consequences. It can lead to disorders in psychological well-being such as depression, anxiety and post-traumatic stress disorder, suicide, alcohol and drug abuse and/or disabilities. Moreover, girls and women exposed to violence experience SRH problems including undesired pregnancies, adverse maternal and newborn health outcomes and STIs, as well as gynecological complications. Intimate partner

violence during pregnancy can lead to miscarriage, stillbirth, premature birth and/or low-birth-weight babies [16, 17].

The twentieth and twenty-first centuries witnessed an increase in activities to research, raise awareness and advocate for the prevention of all kinds of gender-based violence at both the national and international levels. Most countries have laws that penalize at least some forms of violence, including some violence against girls and women (such as domestic violence or rape) and against children. Unfortunately, numerous countries continue to have inadequate legislation.

Female Genital Mutilation

Female genital mutilation (FGM) is defined as all procedures that involve partial or total removal of the external female genitalia or other injury to the female genital organs for nonmedical reasons. It violates the human rights of girls and women to health, security and physical integrity and to be free from torture and cruel, inhuman and/or degrading treatment, as well as the right to life. Female genital mutilation is often carried out on minors and therefore is also a violation of children's rights. Female genital mutilation is of global concern and is mainly practiced in Africa, the Middle East and Asia, as well as among migrants from these areas living around the world.

> **Worldwide Figures**
>
> - More than 200 million girls and women alive today have been subjected to FGM and more than 3 million girls are estimated to be at risk for FGM annually.
> - About 500,000 European girls and women have undergone genital mutilation and 180,000 are at risk of doing so [18].

Female genital mutilation is associated with a series of short-term (i.e., pain, excessive bleeding, shock, infection, sepsis or even death) and long-term health risks (i.e., chronic pain, decreased sexual enjoyment, psychological consequences and childbirth complications) [19]. In 2012, the United Nations General Assembly passed a resolution banning the practice of FGM. The resolution advocates all necessary measures be taken, including enforcing legislation, raising awareness and allocating sufficient resources to protect girls and women from this form of violence.

Child Marriage

Child marriage refers to any formal marriage or informal union between a child under the age of 18 and an adult or another child. Child marriage violates a range of human rights such as gender equality, freedom from slavery, access to education, freedom of movement, freedom from violence and the right to consensual marriage.

Worldwide Figures

- More than 650 million girls and women alive today were married before 18.
- Twenty-one percent of young women (20–24 years old) were child brides [20].

Child marriage increases the risk of STIs (in particular HIV and HPV) and cervical cancer, of pregnancy-related diseases and complications (i.e., preeclampsia, postpartum hemorrhage, sepsis and obstetric fistula) and of babies with low birth weight, preterm delivery and severe neonatal conditions. Most child brides have a lower level of education and financial independence and a higher risk of social isolation and domestic violence than more educated women who marry as adults [21].

The United Nations and other international agencies declared child marriage a violation of human rights in 1948. A multifaceted approach is required to end child marriage that includes targeted interventions at different levels with appropriate programs to provide families and communities with education and reproductive healthcare services.

Conclusive Remarks: Actions to Be Taken

Advancing SRH and rights requires not only improvements in healthcare services but also social, educational and legislative changes. Integrating human rights into healthcare can help overcome some of the most relevant challenges to SRH on a global scale. Political commitment, at the highest national and international levels, is to be obtained so as to allocate the necessary resources to promote gender equality and improve healthcare services. Indeed, the education of professionals toward a thinking approach wherein SRH and human rights are wholly integrated and girls and women are empowered is pivotal to ramp up this process and produce spin-offs that would benefit individuals and society as a whole.

Empowerment starts from education in the community: social policies should ensure primary education to all girls and boys and include sexuality and reproductive education programs. Education may also be provided in focus groups, at educational meetings or through social media, enabling minorities such as migrants to be correctly informed. Two such examples are the Global Communication Campaign for Women's Health and the WELL! (Women Empowerment Learning Links) Campaign set up by the International Federation of Gynaecology and Obstetrics (FIGO) Women Health and Human Rights (WHHR) Committee, which were run for the general population to raise awareness on hot topics within SRH.

Last but not least, changes in law and policies are to be made in some countries. The FIGO WHHR Committee prepared a handbook entitled *Advocating for Girls' and Women's Health and Human Rights* to provide guidance on how the National Societies of Obstetricians and Gynaecologists can engage in rights-based advocacy to influence Governments to make progress on achieving girls and women's health and rights (Figure 1.2) [22].

References

1. World Health Organization. *Integrating poverty and gender into health programmes: A sourcebook for health professionals. Module* on sexual and reproductive health. Manila: WHO Regional Office for the Western Pacific, 2008. https://apps.who.int/iris/handle/10665/206996.

2. Berro Pizzarossa L. Here to stay: The evolution of sexual and reproductive health and rights in international human rights law. *Laws*. 2018;7:29–35.

3. Rosa W. Transforming our world: The 2030 agenda for sustainable development. In Rosa W (ed.), *A new era in global health*. New York: Springer, 2017, pp. 529–68. bit.ly/40.

4. United Nations Department of Economic and Social Affairs, Population Division. *World fertility and family planning 2020: Highlights*. New York: United Nations Department of Economic and Social Affairs, Population Division (ST/ESA/SER.A/440), 2020.

5. Guttmacher Institute. Family planning can reduce high infant mortality levels. 2016. bit.ly/3DnfUxY.

6. Cleland J, Conde-Agudelo A, Peterson H, Ross J, Tsui A. Contraception and health. *Lancet*. 2012;**380**(9837):149–56. https://doi.org/10.1016/S0140-6736(12)60609-6.

Figure 1.2 Handbook cover page

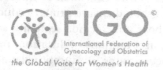

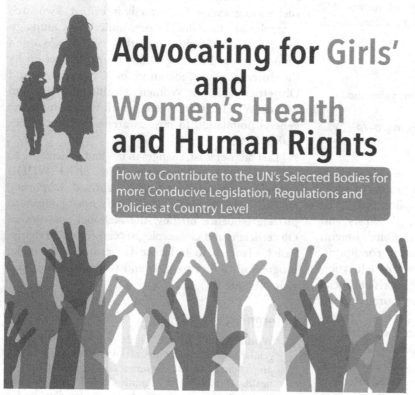

Advocating for Girls' and Women's Health and Human Rights

How to Contribute to the UN's Selected Bodies for more Conducive Legislation, Regulations and Policies at Country Level

Chiara Benedetto

Foreword
Professor CN Purandare

7. United Nations Educational, Scientific and Cultural Organization. *Emerging evidence, lessons and practice in comprehensive sexuality education: A global review 2015.* New York: United Nations Educational, Scientific and Cultural Organization, 2015.

8. European Expert Group on Sexuality Education. Sexuality education: What is it? *Sexuality, Society and Learning.* 2016;**16**(4):427–31 26.

9. Erdman JN, Cook RJ. Decriminalization of abortion: A human rights imperative. *Best Pract Res Clin Obstet Gynaecol.* 2020;**62**:11–24.

10. Say L, Chou D, Gemmill A et al. Global causes of maternal death: A WHO systematic analysis. *Lancet Glob Health.* 2014;**2**(6):e323–e333.

11. Haddad LB, Nour NM. Unsafe abortion: Unnecessary maternal mortality. *Rev Obstet Gynecol.* 2009;**2**(2):122–6.

12. World Health Organization. *Trends in maternal mortality 2000 to 2017: Estimates by WHO, UNICEF, UNFPA, World Bank Group and the United Nations Population Division.* Geneva: World Health Organization, 2019. License: CC BY-NC-SA 3.0 IGO.

13. Maternal Mortality. September 2021. bit.ly/3wz7Wy5.

14. World Health Organization. *WHO recommendations on antenatal care for a positive pregnancy experience.* Geneva: World Health Organization, 2016.

15. World Health Organization, Department of Maternal Child and Adolescent Health. WHO recommendations on postnatal care of the mother and newborn. 2013. www.ncbi.nlm.nih.gov/books/NBK190086.

16. García-Moreno C, Pallitto C, Devries K et al. *Global and regional estimates of violence against women: Prevalence and health effects of intimate partner violence and non-partner sexual violence.* Geneva: World Health Organization, 2013.

17. Altarac M, Strobino D. Abuse during pregnancy and stress because of abuse during pregnancy and birthweight. *J Am Med Womens Assoc 1972.* 2002;**57**(4):208–14.

18. World Health Assembly Resolution on Female Genital Mutilation (WHA61.16). European Institute for Gender Equality. bit.ly/3HF63WY.

19. World Health Organization. Eliminating female genital mutilation. bit.ly/3JkgjVB.

20. United Nations International Children's Emergency Fund. Child marriage UNICEF data. bit.ly/3Y6QRHy.

21. Dahl GB. Early teen marriage and future poverty. *Demography.* 2010;**47**(3):689–718. https://doi.org/10.1353/dem.0.0120.

22. Benedetto C. Advocating for girls' and women's health and human rights. Global Library of Women's Medicine, 2019. bit.ly/3jffvqo

Chapter 2

European Laws on Sexual and Reproductive Health and the Different Policies regarding Access to Sexual and Reproductive Healthcare

Teresa A. Bombas

Introduction

Although all human rights are relevant to sexual reproductive health rights (SRHR), the European Council has identified certain human rights as having key importance. These are the rights to health, to life, to freedom from torture and other ill treatment, to privacy and to equality and non-discrimination [1].

All individuals, regardless of sex, age, gender, sexual orientation, gender identity, socio-economic status, ethnicity, cultural background and legal status, have a right to autonomy and to make decisions governing their bodies and to access services that support that right [2].

According to the World Health Organization (WHO), essential sexual reproductive health (SRH) services must meet public health and human rights standards, including the 'Availability, Accessibility, Acceptability and Quality' framework of the right to health [3, 4]:

- Accurate information and counselling on SRH, including evidence-based, comprehensive sexuality and reproductive health education (CSRE).
- Information, counselling and care related to sexual well-being, function and satisfaction.
- Prevention, detection and management of sexual and gender-based coercion and violence.
- Counselling and services for a range of safe and effective modern contraceptive methods, with a defined minimum number and type of methods, including post-partum and post-abortion contraception.
- Safe and effective antenatal, childbirth and postnatal care, including emergency obstetrics and neonatal care.
- Safe and effective abortion services and care, including treatment of complications of unsafe abortion and incomplete abortion and post-abortion contraception.
- Information and counselling for and prevention, management and treatment of infertility.
- Prevention, detection and treatment of sexually transmitted infections (STIs), including HIV and reproductive tract infections.
- Prevention, detection and management of reproductive tract cancers.

Despite progress having been made on SRHR in Europe, some people in European countries continue to face widespread denials and infringements [1]. In some countries, policies and laws relating to SRHR have been made more restrictive [5]. Harmful gender stereotypes, stigma and social norms continue as well as violence and coercive practices [6].

Specific Areas of Consideration on Sexual Reproductive Health and Care

Access to Contraception

Worldwide, since 1990, as access to contraceptives has increased, the rate of unintended pregnancy has fallen. Progress is not uniform, however. Although nearly 60% of European women of childbearing age use a form of contraception, 35% of pregnancies in Europe are considered unplanned [7].

In Europe, there is an average unmet need for contraception among women aged 15–49 years who are married/in a union of 9% (ranging from 4% in France to 21% in Montenegro) [8]. The European Society of Contraception and Sexual Health and Care (ESC) published the 2019 Position Paper on Sexual and Reproductive Health and Rights [9], which emphasized that '[c]ontraception saves lives, improves health and is highly cost-effective. Availability of contraception must be made more equitable throughout Europe. A wide range of contraceptives must be freely available to women and men, in order to fulfil their reproductive rights.'

Since its debut in 2017, the *European Contraception Policy Atlas*, published by the European Parliamentary Forum for Sexual and Reproductive Rights (EPF) has become an acknowledged tool of reference for information on contraception in Europe. This map scores 46 countries by traffic light colours on access to their access to contraceptive supplies, family planning counselling and online information. The findings show that, for many European countries, ensuring that people have choice over their reproductive lives is not a priority, and these findings reveal a very uneven picture across Europe (Table 2.1). Since its publication, the *Contraception Policy Atlas* has contributed to legislative changes in 9 countries as well as improved online resources in a handful of countries:

- 19 countries (41%) cover contraceptives in their national health system and include LARCs
- 13 countries (28%) cover contraceptives in the national health systems for young people to 25 years old or older

Table 2.1 Tracking government policies on access to contraceptive supplies, family planning counselling and the provision of online information on contraception (2022)

Colours	Countries (Ranking Points Scale)
	Belgium (96.4%), France (90.1%), UK (87.6%), Netherlands (87.0%), Sweden (81.5%), Portugal (78.7%), Germany (75.1%)
	Estonia (74.7%), Norway (71.4%), Iceland (71.3%), Albania (68.1%), Spain (66.0%), Moldova (65.8%), Ireland (65.0%), Malta (63.8%), Finland (63.3%), Austria (62.2%)
	Ukraine (59.8%), Serbia (59.7%), Denmark (59.6%), Croatia (59.3%), Italy (59.3%), Latvia (58.5%), Switzerland (58.3%), Slovenia (57.0%), Bulgaria (56.7%), Kosovo (56.6%), Turkey (55.7%)
	Azerbaijan (54.4%), Romania (54.4%), Armenia (53.9%), Georgia (52.9%), North Macedonia (52.8%), Greece (52.5%), Cyprus (51.4%), Czech Republic (50.8%), Lithuania (50.1%)
	Slovakia (48.1%), Andorra (47.9%), Montenegro (45.7%), Hungary (44.9%), Belarus (44.4%), Bosnia–Herzegovina (44.3%), Russia (42.8%)
	Poland (35.1%)

Source: Adapted from *Contraception Policy Atlas Europe*, 2022 [10]

- 41 countries cover counseling within the national health system 18 countries (39%) provide governmental websites [10].

2022 Highlights on Contraception

- The list of countries with better performance on contraception includes Belgium, France, the United Kingdom, Luxembourg, Sweden, Estonia, the Netherlands, Portugal and Germany.
- Better access to contraception does not negatively influence fertility rates – the top 10 countries have a higher fertility rate than the bottom 10 countries.
- Policy changes to break down financial barriers to contraception have been implemented in Belgium, Bulgaria, Finland, Iceland, the Netherlands, North Macedonia and Spain, particularly for young people and marginalized or vulnerable groups.
- Government policies on access to contraception show encouraging improvements in Albania, Andorra, Finland and Greece; however, Poland shows a deterioration.
- Among the worst-performing states were Hungary, Belarus, Bosnia-Herzegovina, Russia and Poland. Poland proved unable to relinquish its bottom place and was listed in a specially created dark red category this year, following its policy change in 2019 to necessitate prescriptions for emergency contraception (EC) [10, 11].

The WHO Model List of Essential Medicines contains a wide range of contraceptives [12]. One of the main barriers related to access to contraception is their relatively high cost and/or very limited choice. In some European countries, contraceptives are not subsidized under public health insurance schemes and so are available only to the financially privileged. Intrauterine contraception (IUC), pills and condoms are widely used throughout Europe. However, there are wide geographical variations in uptake and barriers to use. It is notable that uptake of both implants and injectables is low, when both these methods are more effective than pills and condoms. So-called first-tier reversible methods (implants and IUC) are not widely available [10, 13].

Following a European Commission 'implementing decision' in 2015, most European countries have deregulated EC pills so that they are available in pharmacies without the need for a prescription. Hungary and Poland are the only countries within the European Union that have not followed the path of deregulation (Poland did deregulate EC for a time but then reversed the decision) [14].

It is important that European countries do not regress on these matters. Governments must make a cost-effective effort to provide accessible, reliable information in order to empower women to make informed decisions about the method most appropriate for them.

Access to Abortion

European Abortion Laws

Since the 1930s, there has been a progressive trend toward liberalization of abortion laws across Europe. The WHO recognizes that in countries with restrictive abortion laws, induced abortion rates are high, the majority of abortions are unsafe, and women's health and lives are frequently put at risk. The WHO estimates that 25 million unsafe abortions take place each year and they often have fatal consequences [15]. 'It is estimated that 89% of the abortions performed in Europe are safe' [16]. The removal of legal restrictions on abortion has shifted clandestine, unsafe procedures to legal and safe ones, resulting in significantly reduced rates of maternal mortality and morbidity [16].

Since 1998, the Center for Reproductive Rights (CRR) has produced *The World Abortion Laws Map*, which is a definitive record of the legal status of abortion in countries across the globe. These laws, which are broken into five categories, fall on a continuum from severe restrictiveness to relative liberality (Table 2.2). According to the CRR, worldwide, 60% of women of reproductive age live in countries that broadly allow abortion and 40% of women live under restrictive laws [17].

Today almost all European countries allow abortion on request or on broad social grounds, at least in the first trimester of pregnancy, and almost all countries also ensure that abortion is legal throughout pregnancy when necessary to protect the health or life of a pregnant individual. A very small minority maintain highly restrictive laws prohibiting abortion in almost all circumstances [19]. 'In the EU, only one Member State does not allow abortion under any circumstances (Malta) and one allows it only under very narrow circumstances with highly restrictive tendencies (Poland)' [17].

The most recent signs of progress on abortion access were:

- Abortion has recently been decriminalized and permitted at a woman's request up to 12 weeks' gestation in Cyprus and up to 14 weeks in the Isle of Man.

- The Republic of Ireland liberalized its abortion law at the end of 2018 and swiftly introduced a primary care–led medical abortion service, alleviating cross-border travel for women after years of hardship. The speed of introduction of the service in Ireland mimicked that in Portugal but the model in Portugal is very different, with providers being almost entirely gynaecologists [17].

- Some European countries' laws set the time limit for abortion on request or broad social grounds between 18 and 24 weeks of pregnancy, whereas many set the limit around the first trimester of pregnancy. All these countries' laws also allow access to abortion care later in pregnancy in specific circumstances, such as where a patient's health or life is at risk. The standard practice across Europe is to not impose time limits on these grounds [26].

'What worries and urges a strong response from the EU is the evident backlash in women's rights, with the right to a safe and legal abortion being one of the key targets in these attacks' [19]. Several databases currently exist that provide information related to country-specific abortion laws and may facilitate better understanding of the legal regulation of abortion. These databases often classify countries as falling on a hierarchical spectrum of access to abortion based on the number and type of grounds under which abortion is permitted. To increase transparency, the Global Abortion Policies Database (GAPD) was launched in 2017 and facilitates the strengthening of knowledge by demonstrating the complexities and nuances of legal texts. The GAPD also contains information related to authorization and service-delivery requirements, conscientious objection, penalties, national SRH indicators, and United Nations (UN) Treaty Monitoring Body concluding observations [19].

Barriers to Access to Abortion

Even when legally available, abortion can be unsafe. There other barriers to access to safe abortion. This leads to the violation of SRHR, but also to inequalities in achieving women's rights across Europe.

Procedural Barriers

In Europe, 18 jurisdictions have waiting periods built into their abortion laws (Table 2.3) [17–20]. There is a wide array of evidence on the emotional harm and

Table 2.2 European abortion laws

Category	Countries
1. Prohibit abortion altogether The laws of the countries in this category do not permit abortion under any circumstances, including when the woman's life or health is at risk.	Andorra, Malta, San Marino
2. To save women's lives The laws of the countries in this category explicitly permit abortion when the woman's life is at risk.	
3. To preserve health The laws of countries in this category permit abortion on the basis of health or therapeutic grounds (The WHO advises that countries permitting abortion on health grounds should interpret 'health' to mean 'a state of complete physical, mental and social well-being and not merely the absence of disease or infirmity').	Israel (R, I, F, +), Liechtenstein (R, PA, +), Monaco (R, I, F, +), Poland (R, I, PA)
4. Broad social or economic grounds These laws are generally interpreted liberally to permit abortion under a broad range of circumstances. These countries often take into account a woman's actual or reasonably foreseeable environment and her social or economic circumstances in considering the potential impact of pregnancy and childbearing.	Finland (R, F, +), Great Britain (F)
5. On request (age limits vary)	Albania, Armenia, Austria, Azerbaijan, Belarus, Belgium, Bosnia–Herzegovina, Bulgaria, Croatia, Cyprus, Czech Republic, Denmark, Estonia, France, Georgia, Germany, Greece, Hungary, Iceland, Italy, Kazakhstan, Kosovo, Latvia, Lithuania, Luxembourg, Macedonia, Moldova, Montenegro, Netherlands, Norway, Portugal, Republic of Ireland, Romania, Russia, Serbia, Slovakia, Slovenia, Spain, Sweden, Switzerland, Turkey, Turkmenistan, Ukraine, Uzbekistan

Source: Adapted from The Abortion Laws Map, Center for Reproductive Rights Current (23 February 2021) including the WHO European countries [17]

Notes: R – abortion permitted in cases of rape; I – abortion permitted in cases of incest; F – abortion permitted in cases of fetal impairment; PA – parental authorization/notification required; + – abortion permitted on additional enumerated grounds relating to such factors as the woman's age or capacity to care for a child

practical difficulties caused by waiting periods for abortion. Reported practical difficulties created by waiting periods include: time off work with associated loss of income, time taken and logistics of traveling, need for childcare and loss of privacy [20]. 'Individualized counseling for the minority who are conflicted when they first attend seems more appropriate than universal requirements that create unnecessary hardships for women, the vast majority of whom have made their decision by the time they present for abortion' [21].

Practical Barriers

Practical barriers such as lack of skilled providers, unaffordability, and lack of information about legal abortion services also undermine access to safe abortion (Table 2.4) [22].

In 2010–14, almost all abortions in developed countries were safe, although a small proportion of less-safe abortions was also seen – notably in Eastern Europe – probably due to the persistence of outdated medical practices such as sharp curettage. The sub-regions with the highest proportions of safe abortions (Northern Europe and North America) also showed the lowest incidence of abortion. Most countries in these two sub-regions have less-restrictive laws on abortion, high contraceptive use, high economic development, high levels of gender equality and well-developed health infrastructures, suggesting that achievement of both low incidence of abortion and high safety in such contexts is possible [16]. National health systems must provide training and access to the WHO-recommended methods [15].

Table 2.3 Jurisdictions in which there are mandatory waiting periods for abortion

Country	Waiting period for abortion (days)
Albania	7
Belgium	6
Germany	3
Hungary	3
Ireland	3
Italy	7
Jersey	7
Kosovo	2
Latvia	3
Luxembourg	3
Montenegro	3
Netherlands	5
North Macedonia	3
Poland	3
Portugal	3
Russia	2–7
Slovakia	2
Spain	3

Table 2.4 Classification of abortion by safety

Safety of abortion care	Considerations
Safe	Provision of information, respect, counselling, provision of medical and/or surgical abortion, recognition and management of complications from unsafe abortion, provision of post-abortion contraception when desired, having in place referral systems for all required higher-level care
Unsafe	Carried out either by a person lacking the necessary skills or in an environment that does not conform to minimal medical standards, or both
Less safe	Done using outdated methods like sharp curettage even if the provider is trained or if women using tablets do not have access to proper information or to a trained person if they need help
Dangerous or least safe	Involves the ingestion of caustic substances or untrained persons use dangerous methods such as insertion of foreign bodies or use of traditional concoctions

Source: Adapted from [16].

[I]n restrictive settings, telemedicine is helping to improve women's access to medical abortion over the internet via not-for-profit organizations such as Women on Web, Women Help Women, and Safe2choose. These organizations provide an online consultation for women and information on how to take the medications, the risks, and the signs that indicate the need to seek medical assistance. [22]

Conscientious Objection

According to the European Parliament's Study on Implications of Conscientious Objection on SRHR, national legislation often allows healthcare professionals to opt out of providing goods and services to which they are morally opposed, including performing abortions or prescribing, selling or advising on contraceptive methods. Moving forward, it should be addressed as denial of medical care rather than as so-called conscientious objection.

A large number of Member States (20+) provide for the right to so-called conscientious objection, which is also recognized by UN instruments and the European Convention on Human Rights. Notably, this is not an absolute right and it should not be used to block access to services to which women are legally entitled.

In practice, this is exactly what happens on a daily basis across the EU – women do not have access to their legally granted right to abortion as the medical staff deny them that medical care, with public hospitals not putting public referral systems in place. This is an evident and multidimensional violation and practical denial of exercising an already achieved legal right [23].

Abortion Stigma

Stigma and the associated secrecy and shame that surround abortion are major factors behind unsafe abortion [23]. Stigma prevents women from seeking help when they suffer a complication after an illegal abortion and this decision to forgo care may lead to death or severe disability. Even in settings where abortion is legal, stigma may result in women delaying an abortion. Stigma also affects providers, who often suffer low morale, lessened prestige and even ostracism for providing this essential service. Moreover, strong criticism may deter qualified healthcare workers and those in training from undertaking abortion care [24]. Strategies to address and lessen abortion stigma within our societies and the healthcare professions are therefore necessary [25]. It is essential that states go beyond reforming restrictive abortion laws to ensure abortion is available in practice to all.

References

1. Council of Europe Commissioner for Human Rights. *Women's sexual and reproductive health and rights in Europe.* Strasbourg: Council of Europe, 2017.

2. World Health Organization. *Action plan for sexual and reproductive health. Towards achieving the 2030 Agenda for Sustainable Development in Europe: Leaving no one behind.* Geneva: World Health Organization, 2016.

3. Starrs AM, Ezeh AC, Barker G et al. Accelerate progress: Sexual and reproductive health and rights for all. Report of the Guttmacher–Lancet Commission. *Lancet.* 2018;**391**:2642–92.

4. World Health Organization and UNDP/UNFPA/WHO/World Bank Special Programme of Research, Development and Research Training in Human Reproduction. *Sexual health and its linkages to reproductive health: An operational approach.* Geneva: World Health Organization, 2017. https://apps .who.int/iris/handle/10665/258738. License: CC BY-NC-SA 3.0 IGO.

5. Policy Department for Citizens' Rights and Constitution al Affairs. *Backlash in gender equality and women's and girls' rights.* Brussels: European Parliament Think Tank, 2018.

6. O'Connell C, Zampas C. The human rights impact of gender stereotyping in the context of reproductive health care. *Int J Gynecol Obstet.* 2019;**144**:116–21.

7. United Nations, Department of Economic and Social Affairs. Population Division. Contraceptive Use by Method 2019: Data Booklet (ST/ESA/SER.A/435). 2019.

8. United Nations. *World family planning highlights.* New York: United Nations Department of Economic and Social Affairs, 2017.

9. Position paper on sexual and reproductive health and rights (Madrid declaration). European Society of Contraception and Reproductive Health. Launched in September 2019 in Madrid at the World Contraception Day event organized by the Sociedad Española de Contracepción (Spanish Society of Contraception). 2019.

10. European Parliamentary Forum. *Contraception atlas.* Brussels: European Parliamentary Forum on Population and Development, 2020. www .contraceptioninfo.eu.

11. Press release (Embargo: 12 November 2020, 14:00 CET). Fourth edition of *Contraception Policy Atlas* launched online with the European Parliament. 2020.

12. World Health Organization. *WHO model lists of essential medicines.* Geneva: World Health Organization, 2017. www.who.int/medicines/publica tions/essentialmedicines/en.

13. United Nations. *World contraceptive use.* New York: United Nations, Department of Economic and Social Affairs Population Division, 2018.

14. European Consortium for Emergency Contraception. *Emergency contraception in Europe: Country-by-country information.* Tirgu Mures: European Consortium for Emergency Contraception, 2018.

15. World Health Organization. *Preventing unsafe abortion.* Geneva: World Health Organization. bit.ly /3HjI4uQ.

16. Ganatra B, Gerdts C, Rossier C et al. Global, regional, and subregional classification of abortions by safety, 2010–14: Estimates from a Bayesian hierarchical model. *Lancet.* 2017;**390**:2372–81.

17. Center for Reproductive Rights. World abortion laws map. 2022. https://maps.reproductiverights.org /worldabortionlaws.

18. Committee on Women's Rights and Gender Equality. Draft report on the situation of sexual and reproductive health and rights in the EU, in the frame of women's health. 5 May 2021 (2019/2165 (INI)).

19. World Health Organization. *Global abortion policies database.* Geneva: World Health Organization. 2018. https://abortion-policies.srhr.org.

20. Rowlands S, Thomas K. Mandatory waiting periods before abortion and sterilization: Theory and practice. *International Journal of Women's Health.* 2020;**12**:577–86.

21. Roberts SCM, Turok DK, Belusa E et al. Do 72-hour waiting periods and two-visit requirements for abortion affect women's certainty? A prospective cohort study. *Women's Health Issues.* 2017;**27**(4):400–6. https://doi.org/10.1016/j.whi.2017.02.009.

22. Cameron S. Recent advances in improving the effectiveness and reducing the complications of abortion

[version 1; peer review: 3 approved]. *F1000Research* 2018, 7(F1000 Faculty Rev):1881. https://doi.org/10 .12688/f1000research.15441.1.

23. European Union. Sexual and reproductive health rights and the implication of conscientious objection. Study commissioned by the Policy Department for Citizens' Rights and Constitutional Affairs at the request of the FEMM Committee. Directorate General for Internal Policies of the Union, PE 604.969, October 2018. bit.ly/3HB1kW5.

24. Hanschmidt F, Linde K, Hilbert A et al. Abortion stigma: A systematic review. *Perspect Sex Reprod Health*. 2016;48(4):169–77.

25. World Health Organization. *Health worker roles in providing safe abortion care and post-abortion contraception*. Geneva: World Health Organization, 2015.

26. Center for Reproductive Rights. *European Abortion Laws: A Comparative Overview*. 2022. New York: Center for Reproductive Rights.

Chapter 3

The Main Threats to Sexual and Reproductive Health and the Principal Components of Good Sexual and Reproductive Healthcare

Johannes Bitzer

Introduction

At the World Conference on Women in Beijing (1995), Reproductive Health was defined as follows: [1]

> Reproductive health implies that, apart from the absence of disease or infirmity, people have the ability to reproduce, to regulate their fertility and to practice and enjoy sexual relationships. It further implies that reproduction is carried to a successful outcome through infant and child survival, growth and healthy development. It finally implies that women go safely through pregnancy and childbirth, that fertility regulation can be achieved without health hazards and that people are safe in having sex.

The World Health Organization (WHO) has expanded the definition: [2, 3]

> Sexual and reproductive health of women within the framework of WHO has been described 'as a state of complete physical, mental and social well-being, and not merely the absence of disease or infirmity, as reproductive health addresses the reproductive processes, functions and system at all stages of life. Reproductive health, therefore, implies that people are able to have a responsible, satisfying and safe sex life and that they have the capability to reproduce and the freedom to decide if, when and how often to do so'.
> ... Implicit in this are the right of men and women to be informed of and to have access to safe, effective, affordable and acceptable methods of fertility regulation of their choice, and the right of access to appropriate health care services that will enable women to go safely through pregnancy and childbirth and provide couples with the best chance of having a healthy infant.

The WHO differentiated the concept of sexual health including sexual well-being :

> Furthermore a central aspect of being human throughout life encompasses sex, gender identities and roles, sexual orientation, eroticism, pleasure, intimacy and reproduction. Sexuality is experienced and expressed in thoughts, fantasies, desires, beliefs, attitudes, values, behaviours, practices, roles and relationships. While sexuality can include all of these dimensions, not all of them are always experienced or expressed. Sexuality is influenced by the interaction of biological, psychological, social, economic, political, cultural, legal, historical, religious and spiritual factors.

Based on these definitions four dimensions can be distinguished:

(a) The dimension of prevention (unwanted pregnancy, sexually transmitted infection (STI), sexual violence).
(b) The dimension of health maintenance and promotion (screening for diseases of the genital organs, risky behaviour).
(c) The dimension of quality of life.
(d) The achievement of goals in life (capacity for enjoying sexuality, safe motherhood etc.).

The Main Threats to Sexual and Reproductive Health

Several publications from different institutions and international organizations have given comprehensive overviews with respect to the different factors which represent a continuous threat to the sexual and reproductive health of women and men [4–7].

Medical Conditions

Apart from diseases and clinical conditions which affect both sexes there are conditions having a more specific impact on women's reproductive and sexual health [5, 6].

Diseases of the Genital Organs

Basically all gynaecological disorders can negatively impact sexual and reproductive health. Benign and malignant diseases of genital organs and endocrine disorders can lead to infertility, pain and sexual dysfunction The focus of sexual and reproductive healthcare lies in the prevention and early detection of these disorders (see Chapter 6).

Pathologies of Pregnancy, Delivery and Postpartum

Maternal and neonatal morbidity and mortality are important markers of sexual and reproductive health which result from the interaction between individual risk and quality of healthcare [5, 6]. Maternal mortality rates between cities, provinces and neighbourhoods, even within the same country, vary considerably.

The estimated maternal mortality ratio is 25 times greater in some countries of the European region than in others, and perinatal mortality is up to 10 times higher. In addition, a 60% higher relative risk of maternal mortality was observed in women of non-Western origin. It is a tragedy that women are dying from preventable causes of death such as haemorrhage, sepsis, anaemia and eclampsia. Globally, more than 45 million women receive inadequate or no antenatal care.

Sexually Transmitted Infections Including Human Immunodeficiency Virus

More than 1 million STIs are acquired every day worldwide [8]. Each year, there are an estimated 357 million new infections with one of four STIs: chlamydia, gonorrhoea, syphilis and trichomoniasis. More than 500 million people are estimated to have genital infection with the herpes simplex virus (HSV). More than 290 million women have a human papillomavirus (HPV) infection.

Sexually transmitted infections such as HSV type 2 and syphilis can increase the risk of human immunodeficiency virus (HIV) acquisition and have serious reproductive health consequences beyond the immediate impact of the infection itself (e.g., infertility or mother-to-child transmission). Globally, 1 million women and girls acquire HIV every year. Drug resistance, especially for gonorrhoea, is a major threat to reducing the impact of STIs worldwide.

Infertility

Until now, there is no consensus on the prevalence of infertility [9, 10]. This is because most data come from individual clinics and their numbers are not representative of the total population of an area or a country. Some studies report an incidence of 10–20% among the reproductive age group.

The unfulfilled wish for a child is a life crisis with very different outcomes. Sometimes it can be overcome by medical interventions and sometimes couples can adapt to the situation and redefine their life plans, but it can also lead to severe mental health problems like depression or post-traumatic stress reaction. Many factors contribute to infertility: STIs and pelvic inflammatory disease, endometriosis, endocrine disorders, male factors, psychosocial stress, anxiety and ambivalence.

Unintended Pregnancies

In 2015–19, there were 121 million unintended pregnancies annually (80% uncertainty interval [UI] 112.8–131.5), corresponding to a global rate of 64 unintended pregnancies (UI 60–70) per 1,000 women aged 15–49 years [11, 12]. Sixty-one per cent (58–63) of unintended pregnancies ended in abortion (totalling 73.3 million abortions annually [66.7–82.0]), corresponding to a global abortion rate of 39 abortions (36–44) per 1,000 women aged 15–49 years.

Being an adolescent mother is a huge societal burden as it restricts the mother's ability to return to school to finish her studies whilst needing to look after her offspring with little societal support. These young women are prone to fall pregnant again with a shorter inter-pregnancy interval and more often suffer from anaemia or other illnesses and have a higher maternal morbidity and mortality risk. With the untimely death of the mother, the surviving children tend to leave school early and female children are more likely to marry and have children at a younger age. The loss of early education together with early marriage and pregnancy thus perpetuates a cycle of poverty and gender inequality for many generations. Globally each year, up to 200 million women have an unmet need for modern contraception.

Unsafe Abortion

Unfortunately, abortion laws are diverse and complex globally and around 25% of women aged 15–44 live in countries where abortion is not legally permitted or is restricted [13, 14]. Such inequality leads to a four times higher unsafe abortion rate in these countries compared with those countries with less-restrictive policies.

It is regrettable that, even in the twenty-first century, despite the availability of safer medical means of abortion, more than 47,000 women and girls die each year from unsafe abortion–related complications. Unsafe abortion remains one of the five main causes of maternal mortality globally, accounting for 13% of maternal deaths. Globally, 25 million unsafe abortions are carried out each year.

Sexual Violence

Violence against women is a violation of human rights and is rooted in gender inequality [15–17]. It is a public health problem and an impediment to sustainable development. Globally, one in three women worldwide have experienced physical and/ or sexual violence by an intimate partner or sexual violence, not including sexual harassment, by any perpetrator. Adolescent girls, young women, women belonging to ethnic and other minorities, transwomen and women with disabilities face a higher risk of different forms of violence. Humanitarian emergencies may exacerbate this and lead to additional forms of violence against women and girls. Globally, 38–50% of murders of women are committed by intimate partners.

Female genital mutilation (FGM) is a special form of sexual violence [18]. It comprises all procedures that involve partial or total removal of the external female genitalia, or other injury to the female genital organs for non-medical reasons. The procedure has no health benefits for girls and women and can cause severe bleeding and problems urinating, cyst formation and infections, as well as complications in childbirth and increased risk of newborn deaths.

More than 200 million girls and women alive today have been subjected to FGM in 30 countries in Africa, the Middle East and Asia where FGM is concentrated. Female genital mutilation is mostly carried out on young girls between infancy and age 15. Female genital mutilation is a violation of the human rights of girls and women.

Another form of (sexual-reproductive) violence against women is forced sterilization without informed consent and against the will of the respective individuals. This is a special problem in vulnerable populations like the disabled [5].

Discrimination against sexual minorities is a global problem including early interventions in intersex individuals not giving them the opportunity to develop their reproductive function. Discrimination and neglect in care for the LGBTIQ* community is another form of social and medical violence [5].

Sexual Dysfunctions

Many health conditions and psychosocial factors can reduce and negatively impact sexual well-being [19–22]. The prevalence rates vary among countries, across age groups and between the sexes. Most studies, however, indicate that sexual problems are frequent but also frequently not reported because of cultural barriers and shame. Disorders of sexual well-being are differentiated into four categories: sexual desire disorder, sexual arousal disorder, orgasmic disorder and sexual pain disorder. There is a strong overlap between these different disorders. If women experience pain during intercourse their desire may disappear. A decreased desire may lead to a diminished response to sexual stimuli and contribute to an arousal and orgasmic disorder.

Another important aspect of sexual dysfunctions is their impact on the relationship with a partner and the family. The factors contributing to these problems include biological and individual psychological factors, as well as intimate relationship issues and the sociocultural environment.

Gaps in Sex Education and Sexual Care for Vulnerable Groups

Comprehensive sexuality and reproductive health education (CSRE) is an age-appropriate, lifelong process which starts from birth [23, 24]. In schools, CSRE is a curriculum-based process of teaching and learning about the cognitive, emotional, physical and social aspects of sexuality [24]. It aims to equip children and young people with knowledge, skills, attitudes and values that will empower them to realize their health, well-being and dignity; develop respectful social and sexual relationships; consider how their choices affect their own well-being and that of others; and understand and ensure the protection of their rights throughout their lives.

Comprehensive sexuality and reproductive health education must be accurate, scientifically sound and culturally sensitive; respect the principle of non-discrimination and promote diversity; address gender norms and promote tolerance and respect [23]. In the majority of countries globally, there is no appropriate CSRE education due to cultural, religious, political and other opposition.

Another gap relates to the absence of sexual and reproductive health services for special groups [5].

- Adolescents needing comprehensive care with a focus on age-adapted information and education (see Chapter 53).
- LGBT communities with their special needs regarding contraception, protection against STIs, support against discrimination (see Chapter 57).
- Migrant populations at high risk of post-traumatic stress disorders, depression or exposure to violence [25].
- Disabled needing contraceptive counselling adapted to the individual impairment and capacity (see Chapter 27).
- Sex workers exposed to STI risk, violence and so forth.

The 'Malignant' Interaction and Self-Intensifying Vicious Circle of the Different Threats

Lack of access to screening and early detection of **malignant** diseases like cervical carcinoma leads to preventable death, infertility and so forth. Lack of access to comprehensive sexual education can contribute to unwanted pregnancies, STIs, sexual dysfunction and so forth. Lack of access to contraception leads to unintended pregnancies with negative medical, obstetrical, neonatal and psychosocial outcomes. These unwanted pregnancies may be accompanied by or be the result of sexual violence and frequently lead to lack of obstetrical and perinatal care with complications for the mother and the baby. Lack of contraceptive protection may lead to unsafe abortion and complications like infections, destruction of genital organs, infertility and sexual dysfunctions.

Infertility may contribute to social discrimination, exposure to violence and sexual dysfunctions. These sexual problems may lead to marital dissatisfaction, violence, promiscuity or STIs, which may again result in infertility with all its consequences. Female genital mutilation can lead to obstetrical complications and ill psychosexual health.

Many women worldwide are unfortunately exposed to this vicious circle with dramatic results for their health over their life course, leading not only to increased mortality but also to a long line of morbidities and suffering. Taking into account these threats to sexual and reproductive health of women, it is important on a national and international level from a public health and political perspective to look into specific indicators which allow an evaluation of the present status and serve as control variables to see the effect of interventions. At the same time, it is important to look at the determinants of the sexual reproductive health (SRH) of individuals and groups to design strategies for improvement

Indicators of Sexual and Reproductive Health

Several indicators have been proposed to allow social scientists, international organizations and national policy makers to get a quantitative overview regarding the status of sexual and reproductive health. These indicators are diagnostic tool and also an instrument to monitor and follow up interventions with respect to specific outcomes.

The WHO proposes this list: [26, 27]

1 Total fertility rate.
2 Contraceptive prevalence.
3 Maternal mortality ratio.
4 Antenatal care coverage.
5 Births attended by skilled health personnel.
6 Availability of basic essential obstetric care.
7 Availability of comprehensive essential obstetric care.
8 Perinatal mortality rate.
9 Prevalence of low birth weight.
10 Prevalence of positive syphilis serology in pregnant women.
11 Prevalence of anaemia in women.
12 Percentage of obstetric and gynaecological admissions owing to abortion.
13 Reported prevalence of women with genital mutilation.
14 Prevalence of infertility in women.
15 Reported incidence of urethritis in men.
16 Prevalence of HIV infection in pregnant women.
17 Knowledge of HIV-related preventive practices.

In this list, different types of data and assessments are included:

1. Demographic data (total fertility rate).
2. Prevalence data (contraception, anaemia, syphilis serology in pregnant women, prevalence of low birth weight, prevalence of women with FGM, prevalence of infertility, prevalence of HIV infection in pregnant women).
3. Rates and ratios (maternal mortality ratio, perinatal mortality rate).
4. Data about services and knowledge (antenatal care coverage, births attended by skilled health

personnel, availability of comprehensive essential obstetric care, knowledge of HIV–related preventive practices).

The Determinants of Sexual and Reproductive Health

The sexual and reproductive health of an individual is the result of macro and micro factors which vary from country to country and from individual to individual. These factors can be described as a pyramid with three levels (see Figure 3.1).

The Political and Socioeconomic Frame

On this level, policies, laws and sociocultural factors have an important general impact on SRH.

Laws, Policies and Human Rights

Discrimination against women regarding sexual activity and choice increases risk of violence and the lack of protective laws exposes women to sexual violence [28]. Restrictive abortion laws increase the risk for women of unsafe abortion [29].

- Sixty-eight countries currently prohibit abortion entirely or permit it only to save a woman's life.
- Sixty countries allow women to decide whether to terminate a pregnancy.

- Fifty-seven countries permit abortion to protect a woman's life and health.
- Fourteen countries permit abortion for socioeconomic motives.
- Thirty-nine per cent of the world's population lives in countries with highly restrictive laws governing abortion.
- Restrictive laws regarding adolescents' choices reduce access to family-planning services.

Sociocultural Factors

Many factors result from a culture of male dominance which have an important impact on the SRH of women. Male dominance contributes to early marriage, which increases health risks of adolescents. The exclusion of women from education leads to adolescent pregnancies with all the complications. The lower social status of women with respect to men exposes them to more violence and risk of marital rape.

The lack of autonomy for women reduces their access to family planning and contraception and the lack of sexual education increases the risk of unplanned pregnancy, sexual violence, and risky behaviour and it excludes women from important information related to their sexual health.

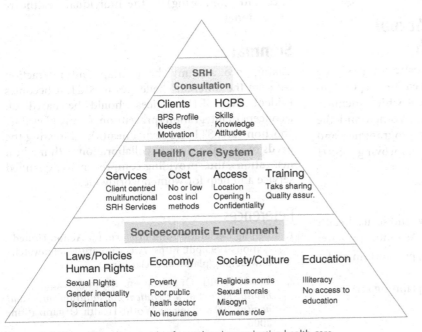

Figure 3.1 The multilevel pyramide of sexual and reproductive health care

Economy

Economic precarity leads to limitations and austerity programmes which in general affect the economically weak such as women in general and young women in particular.

Health Services

These first-level factors have an important influence on the implementation, financing and qualification of health services representing the second level of determinants . Lack of access to comprehensive sexual and reproductive health services and mother and child care leads to increased rates of unplanned pregnancies, undetected STIs and so forth. To implement good-quality services a national health policy has to ensure availability, accessibility, affordability for women and men and well-trained health professionals in evidence-based practice and patient-centred care.

Individual Level

The SRH of an individual is influenced by these aforementioned factors, but individual factors also contribute, such as the genetic profile of the individual, her/his health beliefs, myths and misconceptions and, last, but not least, the motivation leading to a health-preserving and preventive behaviour.

Response to Threats to Sexual and Reproductive Health

Several international programmatic targets and action plans have been developed to respond to these threats. The H4+ initiative – which includes UNAIDS, UNFPA, UNICEF, UN Women and the World Bank – works to develop programmes and defining targets aiming at improving SRH worldwide.

World Health Organization

The five core aspects of reproductive and sexual health adopted by the 57th World Health Assembly [30] are:

1. Improving antenatal, perinatal, postpartum and newborn care.
2. Providing high-quality family-planning services, including infertility services.
3. Eliminating unsafe abortion.
4. Combatting STIs, including HIV, reproductive tract infections, cervical cancer and other gynaecological morbidities.
5. Promoting sexual health.

United Nations Population Fund, Millennium Goals

SRH/FP targets in global, regional and national policies [31, 32]

Goal 3: Good health and well-being

- Target 3.1: Maternal mortality.
- Target 3.3: End epidemics and other communicable diseases.
- Target 3.7: Universal access to SRH, including family planning, education and information and integration in national strategies and programmes.
- Target 3.8: Universal health coverage and access to quality services, medicines and vaccines.

Goal 5: Gender equality

- Target 5.6: Universal access to SRH in line with the International Conference on Population and Development and Beijing Platforms of Action.

These programmes have to address the different levels described earlier in this chapter reaching from advocacy (politicians, media) to health policies (prioritizing SRH, financing, training, quality assurance and monitoring) to the individual healthcare professional.

Summary

Taking into account the overlap and interaction between the different challenges to SRH, it becomes evident that SRH services should be based on a concept of integration (prevention, family planning, abortion care, STI and sexual health), addressing the needs of special groups in collaboration with medical institutions, thus providing comprehensive, qualified service and help for women worldwide.

References

1. Beijing Declaration and Platform for Action United Nations 1995.pdf. https://www.un.org/womenwatch/daw/beijing/platform/declar.htm

2. World Health Organization. *Defining sexual health: Report of a technical consultation on sexual health, 2002*. Geneva: World Health Organization, 2006.

3. Sexual health and its linkages to reproductive health. bit.ly/3HEG7KR.

4. bit.ly/3wElE2M.

5. European Society of Contraception and Reproductive Health. Position paper on sexual and reproductive health and rights (Madrid declaration). 2019. www .escrh.eu.

6. Rowland S. After the Nairobi Summit, how can further progress in sexual and reproductive health and rights be achieved in the Eastern Europe and Central Asia region? *Ezr J Contracept Reprod Health Care.* 2020;**25**(2):95–7.

7. Mahmood T, Bitzer J, Nizard J, Short M. A joint position statement by the European Board and College of Obstetrics and Gynaecology (EBCOG) and the European Society of Contraception and Reproductive Health (ESCRH). The sexual reproductive health of women: Unfinished business in the Eastern Europe and Central Asia region. *Eur J Contracept Reprod Health Care.* 2020;**25**(2):87–94.

8. World Health Organization. *Global incidence and prevalence of selected curable sexually transmitted infections.* Geneva: World Health Organization, 2008.

9. Strickler RC. Factors influencing fertility. In Keye Jr. WR, Chang RJ, Rebar RW, Soules MR (eds.), *Infertility evaluation and treatment.* Philadelphia, PA: W. B. Saunders, 1995, pp. 8–18.

10. National Institute for Health and Care Excellence. *Fertility problems: Assessment and treatment. Clinical guideline 2013.* London: National Institute for Health and Care Excellence, 2013.

11. bit.ly/3HF4GaA.

12. Gipson JD, Koenig MA, Hindin MJ. The effects of unintended pregnancy on infant, child, and parental health: A review of the literature. *Studies in Family Planning.* 2008;**39**(1):18–38.

13. Sedgh G, Bearak J, Singh S et al. Abortion incidence between 1990 and 2014: Global, regional, and subregional levels and trends.*Lancet.* 2016;**388**:258–67.

14. World Health Organization. *Unsafe abortion: Global and regional estimates of incidence of unsafe abortion and associated mortality in 2003.* 5th edition. Geneva: World Health Organization, 2003.

15. García-Moreno C, Pallitto C, Devries K et al. *Global and regional estimates of violence against women: Prevalence and health effects of intimate partner violence and non-partner sexual violence.* Geneva: World Health Organization, 2013.

16. bit.ly/3HkuNT3.

17. Altarac M, Strobino D. Abuse during pregnancy and stress because of abuse during pregnancy and birthweight. *J Am Med Womens Assoc 1972.* 2002;**57**(4):208–14.

18. World Health Assembly Resolution on Female Genital Mutilation (WHA61.16) European Institute for Gender Equality. bit.ly/3HkuNT3.

19. World Health Organization. *The ICD 10 international classifications of mental and behavioral disorders.* Geneva: World Health Organization, 2013.

20. American Psychiatric Association. *Diagnostic and statistical manual of mental disorders.* 5th edition. Washington, DC: American Psychiatric Association, 2013.

21. Mitchell KR, Jones KG, Wellings K et al. Estimating the prevalence of sexual function problems: The impact of morbidity criteria. *Journal of Sex Research.* 2016;**53**(8):955–67.

22. McCabe MP, Sharlip ID, Lewis R et al. Incidence and prevalence of sexual dysfunction in women and men: A consensus statement from the Fourth International Consultation on Sexual Medicine. *JSM.* 2015;**13**(2):144–52.

23. Federal Centre for Health Education and World Health Organization Regional Office for Europe. *Standards for sexuality education in Europe.* Cologne: Federal Centre for Health Education, 2010. bit.ly/3WHsChL.

24. United Nations Population Fund. *UNFPA operational guidance for comprehensive sexuality education: A focus on human rights and gender.* New York: United Nations Population Fund, 2014. bit.ly/40eIsDy.

25. Smith A, LeVoy M, Mahmood T, Mercer C. Migrant women's health issues: Addressing barriers to access to healthcare for migrant women with irregular status. *Entre Nous WHO Europe.* 2016;**85**:18–21.

26. World Health Organization. *Reproductive health indicators: Guidelines for their generation, interpretation and analysis for global monitoring.* Geneva: World Health Organization, 2006.

27. World Health Organization. *Technical consultation on reproductive health indicators: Geneva, 21–22 September 2005. Summary report.* Geneva: World Health Organization, 2007.

28. United Nations Department of Economic and Social Affairs, Population Division. *Reproductive health policies 2014.* New York: United Nations Department of Economic and Social Affairs, Population Division, 2014.

29. Finer N, Fine JB. Abortion law around the world: Progress and pushback. *Am J Public Health*. 2013;**103**(4):585–9.

30. World Health Organization. Fifty-seventh world health assembly: Geneva, 17–22 May 2004. Summary records of committees, reports of committees. 2004. https://apps.who.int/iris/handle/10665/260147.

31. United Nations Population Fund. Achieving the millennium development goals (10). 2003. www.unfpa.org/sites/default/files/pub-pdf/MDGs_pds.pdf.

32. World Health Organization. Millennium development goals. bit.ly/40d1HgJ.

The Principles and Roles of Sexuality Education

Evert Ketting

Historical Development of Sexual Education

Sexual education (SE) started in Sweden in 1955, when it became mandatory in schools. In the 1970s and 1980s, more Western European countries adopted it – first other Scandinavian countries, then other European nations such as Germany (1968) and Austria (1970). In the Netherlands and Switzerland, SE began in the 1970s but was not yet a mandatory subject. The introduction continued during the rest of the century, first in France and the United Kingdom, and from there it spread further. In only a few European countries has SE not yet been introduced in schools.

In Central and Eastern Europe, SE as currently understood was implemented after the fall of communism and some 20–40 years later than in Western Europe. Before that, there had been a few initiatives, but those were mostly "preparation for marriage and family life" programs that did not pay attention to sexuality. In some of these countries, like Estonia [1], SE came soon after the year 2000.

In the United States, SE has always been highly politicized. After the onset of the HIV/AIDS pandemic in the 1980s, the responsible surgeon general, C. Everett Koop, issued a report calling for comprehensive SE and AIDS education in public schools. This resulted in a countermove toward "abstinence-only" education, which was almost the opposite of "comprehensive education." Since then, SE has been a battlefield of moral conservatives versus public health advocates. In actual practice, school SE remained rather marginal. The vast majority of Americans simply feel that SE is the sole responsibility of parents. There is a national sex conference every year that is organized by the National Center for Sex Education in New Jersey [2].

In 2009, school SE became an important topic for United Nations (UN) organizations. In that year, the United Nations Educational, Scientific and Cultural Organization (UNESCO) issued a technical guidance document on SE [3]. The International Planned Parenthood Federation (IPPF), Population Council, and others released a comparable guide [4]. One year later, the German Federal Centre for Health Education (BZgA) published *Standards for Sexual Education in Europe* [5]. Finally, in 2014, the United Nations Population Fund (UNFPA) followed with *Operational Guidance* [6].

What Makes Sexual Education "Comprehensive"?

Nowadays, SE is often referred to as comprehensive sexual education or simply CSE. The reason is basically that this CSE should be clearly distinguished from abstinence-only education. In the United States, the latter approach became very popular in the 1990s, when the federal government and individual states strongly supported it. This approach was also used in developing countries. Abstinence-only education is quite similar to the ABC approach often used in international family-planning programs funded by the United States. The A stands for abstinence, the B stands for be faithful, and the C stands for condom use. In Europe, abstinence-only education never became popular. One of the reasons has been that it does not produce the main intended result of sexual abstinence until marriage [7].

In the renewed second edition of UNESCO's "Technical Guidance on Sexuality Education," a definition is given of comprehensive SE:

> Comprehensive sexuality education (CSE) is a curriculum-based process of teaching and learning about the cognitive, emotional, physical and social aspects of sexuality. It aims to equip children and young people with knowledge, skills, attitudes and values that will empower them to: realize their health, well-being and dignity; develop respectful social and sexual relationships; consider how their choices affect

their own well-being and that of others; and, understand and ensure the protection of their rights throughout their lives. *[8, p. 16]*

In this definition, CSE is limited to lessons in educational institutions. Furthermore, CSE is not simply transfer of knowledge, but also working on (behavioral) skills and on the formation of attitudes and values. The aim is to "empower" pupils – that is, equip them with the responsibility to look after their own sexual well-being and that of others. The renewed "Guidance" presents criteria for *comprehensive* SE, the most important ones being:

1. Scientifically accurate: the content is based on facts and evidence.
2. Incremental: it represents a continuing educational process starting early in life.
3. Age and developmentally appropriate: adapted to the needs and understanding of learners.
4. Curriculum-based: it guides the learning process.
5. Based on human rights: knowledge of sexuality is treated as a human right.
6. Based on gender equality: gender norms and how they influence sexual realities is a focal issue.

This definition and the criteria that determine CSE have become the global norm in SE. A good indication has been that the 2018 renewed second edition of UNESCO's "Guidance," which introduced this definition, was coauthored with five other UN agencies. In a European study published in 2018, it was found that about half of the European countries had CSE programs in schools. All were in Western or Central Europe. Programs that did not sufficiently meet the comprehensiveness criterion were mainly in Southern and Eastern Europe [9].

Methods of Sexual Education

Because the purpose of SE is much wider than the transfer of knowledge, proper delivery requires a variety of teaching methods. This is one of the reasons training of teachers gets a lot of attention [10]. Sexuality can become very personal and private, which requires special precautions. *Standards for Sexuality Education in Europe* [5] mentions eight characteristics that are more or less typical for the methods used in SE:

1. Guaranteeing safety for learners: the privacy and boundaries of learners should be respected. Learners are encouraged to be open, but this does not mean that they have to disclose personal experiences.

2. Active participation of students: student are not passive recipients of SE, but instead have an active role in organizing, delivering, and evaluating lessons. In this way, the program should respond to students' learning needs.

3. Interactive delivery of lessons: the experiences and needs of students should be used as starting points because, in the end, sexual education should be internalized and used by students in their actual behavior.

4. Continuous process: programs should be based on the understanding that the development of sexuality is a lifelong process. In school curricula, certain topics should be repeated at higher educational levels, where they should be dealt with in more detail.

5. Teaching in multi-sectorial settings: sexual education can be, and often is, integrated in different carrying subjects of the curriculum such as health, social orientation, life skills and even religion.

6. Context-oriented: subjects should be linked to the actual social situation and living environment of students. This is where opportunities and threats manifest themselves.

7. Close collaboration with parents and the community: not only schools but also parents (and other educational services in the community) have important roles to play in sexuality education. Ideally, they should complement each other.

8. Gender responsiveness: this is to ensure that different gender needs and concerns are addressed.

Teaching methods applied in SE reflect the pedagogical functions of this education. Its aim is largely to equip learners with knowledge, attitudes and skills that will enable them to deal with their developing sexuality in satisfactory and responsible ways. This is why active involvement of learners is important. Often-used teaching methods include small group discussions, role-plays, various games, group tasks and other interactive methods.

Practical International Documents on Sexual Education

Since 2009, when the first UN publication was released, several publications with standards and guidelines for SE have been published. The first international agency publishing a guide was the IPPF in

2006 [11]. An annotated overview of the most important publications includes:

Standards for Sexuality Education in Europe (*Standards*) [5] was prepared by the European Expert Group on Sexuality Education and released by the German BZgA. This multinational group of specialists was put together in 2008 and was still functioning in 2020. *Standards* has been very influential in the European region, which is partly indicated by its availability in 13 languages. It provides an essential framework for SE for European countries, many of which have quite a long tradition in this field. The latter partly explains why *Standards* differs in several respects from two other important publications on the subject – *It's All One Curriculum* and *International Technical Guidance on Sexuality Education*. Three years after *Standards*, the BZgA released a practical guide explaining the process of creating and introducing an SE curriculum [12].

It's All One Curriculum (International Sexuality and HIV Curriculum Working Group[1], 2009 [13]), was developed under the leadership of the Population Council in collaboration with six other specialized agencies, including the international and regional American IPPF organizations.

International Technical Guidance on Sexuality Education (UNESCO, 2010), was produced by UNESCO and others (widely known as the "UNESCO guidance" [3]). In 2018, a revised new edition was released that adopted the term *comprehensive*, just like *Standards* had done 2 years earlier [8]. This new edition came much closer to *Standards* in several respects. Because of the crucial importance of these three publications, it is useful to highlight some essential similarities and differences.

All three publications have two "parts" (*Standards*), "volumes" (UNESCO guidance), or "books" (Working Group document). The first part basically outlines the background, purposes, concepts, rationale, and basic principles, whereas the second part focuses on learning objectives, age groups, and the content of curricula. They differ in four aspects:

1. *Standards* promotes "holistic SE," meaning that it not only addresses all relevant aspects of sexuality, but it also puts sexuality in a wider perspective of personal and sexual growth and development. In 2016, the term *holistic* was replaced by *comprehensive* so as to avoid confusion. *Standards* basically perceives sexuality as a positive human capacity. The UNESCO guidance has a narrower focus that starts from serious concerns about the HIV/AIDS epidemic. It therefore primarily emphasizes the need to avoid risky sexual contacts, but it also addresses avoiding those risks through safer sex practices. The Working Group document has yet another focus: it attempts to integrate sexuality, gender, HIV/AIDS, and human rights issues into one curriculum.

2. *Standards* address the need for sexuality education for the entire age range from birth onwards. It also differentiates between the learning needs of successive age groups. The UNESCO guidance also does this, but starts at age 5, whereas the Working Group document addresses only the learning needs of adolescents.

3. The UNESCO guidance includes a comprehensive review of studies on the impact of SE in terms of sexual and preventive behavior, which is not included in the other two publications. This review is valuable for advocacy purposes as it clearly demonstrates that most (comprehensive) programs do have beneficial results and that they do not produce adverse effects.

4. Only the Working Group document includes SE lessons – 54 in total – which can be adapted to local conditions for immediate use. In that respect, it is very useful for the practice of SE, whereas the other two publications mainly address the policy and programming levels.

The UNFPA became active in this field in 2014, when it released *Operational Guidance* with a focus on human rights and gender [6]. One year later (2015), this was followed by *The Evaluation of Comprehensive Sexuality Education Programmes* [13]. In 2016, the European Expert Group and the BZgA produced a publication on the same subject [14]. The UNFPA and UNESCO have become two of the most active UN agencies in promoting and supporting SE.

The BZgA in Cologne is by far the most prominent agency in Europe in guiding and supporting SE. It collaborates with the WHO as a center for health education, and it coordinates and supports the work of the European Expert Group on Sexuality Education. The UN agencies just mentioned and the IPPF have members in the Expert Group. Besides this, the BZgA

---

[1] Referred to as the "Working Group document."

supports, if requested, the development of SE in European and Central Asian countries. After releasing *Standards* (2010) and the related "Implementation Guidance" (2013), the BZgA has continued to support research and publication, often with the UNFPA Regional Office for Europe and Central Asia. The most important research publication in the past 5 years, in which the BZgA collaborated with the IPPF European Network, has been the report on "Sexuality Education in Europe and Central Asia" (2018). This report is the first that gives a detailed overview of the realities of SE in this region [12]. Several articles based on this research appeared in scientific journals after 2018.

Topics Addressed in Sexual Education

One question in the European SE study [9] concerned topics discussed in SE programs. Data on these topics were obtained from 19 of the 23 countries.[2] Four others did not respond, mainly because respondents felt they were not sufficiently informed [15]. Respondents were given a list of 15 topics plus two extra open choices. Table 4.1 presents an overview of the results, by order of prominence of each topic, for all countries combined. The total score represents the number of countries where the topic is included in school curricula, plus the extensiveness of dealing with the subject.[3] The results show that human biology is most often dealt with, immediately followed by diseases HIV/AIDS and sexually transmitted infections (STIs). Item 4, "Love, Marriage, and Partnership," probably means that sexuality should preferably be experienced in that particular context. Next come pregnancy, birth, and contraception – the typical family-planning topics. From item 7, "gender roles," on, the topics become more social, psychological, and interactive and less physical and medical. Those are the ones that tend to be included only in comprehensive programs. The strong emphasis international organizations place on sexuality education as a human right is not reflected in the teaching topics in most of the surveyed countries. Finally, the clearly sexpositive issue of sexual pleasure is by far the least commonly discussed topic. This means that sexuality is mainly treated as a problem.

Based on the questionnaire responses, the widest range of topics is addressed in programs that could be

Table 4.1 Topics addressed in sexuality education by rank order*.

No.	Main topics dealt with	Total score
1	Biological aspects and body awareness	66
2	HIV/AIDS	63
3	Sexually transmitted infections (STIs)	58
4	Love, marriage, and partnership	55
5	Pregnancy and birth	50
6	Contraception	50
7	Gender roles	46
8	Mutual consent to sexual activity	40
9	Sexual orientation	35
10	Sexual abuse and violence	32
11	Access to safe abortion	31
12	Online media and sexuality	30
13	Domestic violence	29
14	Human rights and sexuality	25
15	Sexual pleasure	18

* The maximum score is 76 (all countries deal extensively with this topic).

classified as comprehensive. For example, in Sweden, 10 topics were extensively addressed. Non-comprehensive programs tend to be limited to typical medical prevention issues. The results of the same study also show that learners appreciate comprehensive programs much more than non-comprehensive ones.

References

1. Haldre K, Part K, Ketting E. Youth sexual health improvement in Estonia, 1990–2009: The role of sexuality education and youth-friendly services. *Eur J Fam Plann Repr Health Care*. 2012;**17**(5):351–62.

2. For the US Center for Sex Education, see www .sexedcenter.org.

3. United Nations Educational, Scientific and Cultural Organization. *International technical guidance on sexuality education: Volumes I & II*. Paris: United Nations Educational, Scientific and Cultural Organization, 2009. http://unesdoc.unesco.org/image s/0018/001832/183281e.pdf.

4. Population Council/International Sexuality and HIV Curriculum Working Group. *It's all one curriculum*. New York: Population Council/International Sexuality and HIV Curriculum Working Group, 2009. www .popcouncil.org/publications/books/2010_ItsAllOne.

---

[2] Two more countries had already been excluded from this analysis for other reasons.
[3] If the topic is discussed only briefly, the score is 1; if it is discussed extensively, the score is 2.

5. Federal Centre for Health Education and World Health Organization Regional Office for Europe. *Standards for sexuality education in Europe.* Cologne: Federal Centre for Health Education, 2010. bit.ly/40d1HgJ.

6. United Nations Population Fund. *UNFPA operational guidance for comprehensive sexuality education: A focus on human rights and gender.* New York: United Nations Population Fund, 2014. bit.ly/40d1HgJ.

7. Mathematica Policy Research. *Impacts of four title V, section 510 abstinence education programs: Final report.* Princeton, NJ: Mathematica Policy Research, 2007.

8. United Nations Educational, Scientific and Cultural Organization. *International technical guidance on sexuality education: An evidence-informed approach.* 2nd revised edition. Paris: United Nations Educational Scientific and Cultural Organization, 2018. www.unaids.org/sites/default/files/media_asset/ITGSE_en.pdf.

9. Ketting E, Ivanova O. *Sexuality education in Europe and Central Asia: State of the art and recent developments. An overview of 25 countries.* Cologne: Federal Centre for Health Education, 2018. bit.ly/3Rf6j1S.

10. World Health Organization Regional Office for Europe and Federal Centre for Health Education.

Training matters: A framework for core competencies of sexuality educators. Cologne: Federal Centre for Health Education, 2017. bit.ly/3Re3OwI.

11. International Planned Parenthood Federation. *Framework for comprehensive sexuality education.* London: International Planned Parenthood Federation, 2006. bit.ly/3HfPE9S.

12. Federal Centre for Health Education and World Health Organization Regional Office for Europe. *Standards for sexuality education in Europe: Guidance for implementation.* Cologne: Federal Centre for Health Education and World Health Organization Regional Office for Europe, 2013. bit.ly/3HfPE9S.

13. United Nations Population Fund. *The evaluation of comprehensive sexuality education programmes.* New York: United Nations Population Fund, 2015.

14. Ketting E, Friele M, Michielsen K, European Expert Group on Sexuality Education. Evaluation of holistic sexuality education: A European expert group consensus agreement. *Eur J Contracep Repr Health Care.* 2016;**21**(1):68–80.

15. Ketting E, Brockschmidt L, Ivanova O. Investigating the "C" in CSE: Implementation and effectiveness of comprehensive sexuality education in the WHO European region. *Sex Education.* 2020;**10**:12–15. https://doi.org/10.1080/14681811.2020.1766435.

Chapter

5

Sexual Reproductive Health
Public Health Aspects

Tahir A. Mahmood and Johannes Bitzer

Introduction

The World Health Organization (WHO) has defined sexual reproductive health (SRH) as:

> A state of complete physical, mental and social well-being, in all matters relating to the reproductive system. It addresses the reproductive processes, functions and systems at all stages of life. Reproductive health, therefore, implies that people are able to have a responsible, satisfying and safe sex life and that they have the capability to reproduce and the freedom to decide if, when and how often to do so. [1]

> 'Reproductive healthcare is defined as the constellation of methods, techniques and services that contribute to reproductive health and well being by preventing and solving reproductive health problems. It also includes sexual health, the purpose of which is the enhancement of life and personal relations, and not merely counselling and care related to reproduction and sexually transmitted diseases.' Implicit in this are the right of men and women to be informed of and to have access to safe, effective, affordable and acceptable methods of fertility regulation of their choice, and the right of access to appropriate health care services that will enable women to go safely through pregnancy and childbirth and provide couples with the best chance of having a healthy infant. [2]

Reproductive health affects both men and women. Women, however, bear the brunt of reproductive ill heath, not only as a result of their biological status, but also because of a wider social, economic and political disadvantage. There are public health, human rights and economic reasons for investment in reproductive health.

Evolution of Various Components of Sexual Reproductive Health

Since the mid-1990s, the concept of SRH has evolved from provision of contraception to measurement of pregnancy-related morbidity such as rates of abortions and teenage pregnancies and maternal mortality rates, to a broad understanding of the many factors such as gender inequality which can affect SRH. The United Nations International Conference on Population and Development (ICPD) (1994) placed traditional fertility-control programmes with demographic goals with a programme of action (PoA) [3]. These PoAs not only placed the SRH of individuals, particularly women and girls, at their core, but also affirmed SRH, reproductive rights and gender equality as human rights and cornerstones of sustainable development [4].

United Nations International Conference on Population and Development 1994 and Programme of Action

The PoA committed ICPD member states to providing universal access to a core set of health services: education related to sexuality and reproduction, prevention of sexually transmitted infections (STIs), family planning, safe abortion and maternal and newborn care. On the twenty-fifth anniversary of ICPD 1994 (Cairo Declaration), a conference of all stakeholders took place in Nairobi, where it was recognized that outcomes related to SRH have generally improved, but many countries have not been able to meet their targets [5, 6]. Still more commitment at national levels is required to meet the UN sustainable development targets 2030 [4].

While improvements in aggregate SRH outcomes are noteworthy, they conceal considerable inequalities at regional, national and international levels. Often these disparities stem from economic, social, cultural, religious and structural determinants of health. Poverty is a significant determinant of health outcomes, as women living in poverty are disadvantaged compared to their wealthier counterparts. Public health policies are quite often examined through the lens of public health ethics: social justice, contested views of harms and benefits and autonomy [7].

Components of Public Health Policies

Social Justice

The most significant risk factor for women living in poverty is lack of access to education, information, employment and health services, so they are prevented from gaining influence to challenge societal gender-power imbalances. Despite them being at increased risk of unintended pregnancies, their ability to access preventive services is limited. Negative views about sexuality can lead to adverse outcomes for LGBT and survivors of gender-based violence.

Contested Views of Harms and Benefits

Sexuality and reproductive health frequently implicate personal preferences. Sociocultural attitudes and religious beliefs can lead to heated discussions about how to assess competing harms and benefits. Public policies and laws involving adolescent sex education, same-sex marriage and abortion sometimes collide with contested values related to premarital sexual activity and human life itself.

Autonomy

A number of factors can affect autonomy in the SRH context. In order to make informed decisions, individuals must have access to evidence-based information and individuals must be respected as persons to make choices without discrimination. Individuals must have socioeconomic means to access those choices.

Sexual Rights

Sexual rights embrace human rights that are already recognized in national laws, international human rights documents and other consensus statements [8]. They include the right of all individuals, free of coercion, discrimination and violence, to:

- Access the highest attainable standard of sexual health, including SRH services.
- Seek, receive and impart information related to sexuality.
- Receive sexuality education.
- Demand respect for bodily integrity.
- Choose their partner.
- Decide whether to be sexually active.

- Engage in consensual sexual relations.
- Enter a consensual marriage.
- Decide whether and/or when to have children.
- Pursue a satisfying, safe and pleasurable sexual life.

The responsible exercise of human rights requires all individuals to respect the rights of others. To ensure these rights and to promote SRH, the WHO has summarized the SRH services women and men should have access to [9]:

- Accurate information and counselling on SRH, including evidence-based, comprehensive sexuality and reproductive health education (CSRE).
- Information, counselling and care related to sexual well-being, function and satisfaction.
- Prevention, detection and management of sexual and gender-based coercion and violence.
- Counselling and services for a range of safe and effective modern contraceptive methods, with a defined minimum number and type of methods, including postpartum and post-abortion contraception.
- Safe and effective antenatal, childbirth and postnatal care, including emergency obstetrics and neonatal care.
- Safe and effective abortion services and care, including treatment of complications of unsafe or incomplete abortion and post-abortion contraception.
- Information and counselling, prevention, management and treatment of infertility.
- Prevention, detection and treatment of STIs, including HIV and reproductive tract infections.
- Prevention, detection and management of reproductive tract cancers.

Public Health Perspective on Sexual Reproductive Health

The challenge for public health institutions is to devise policies within these constraints to achieve ICPD targets locally, regionally and nationally. Public health work takes account of all the research and the needs of the population and is governed by the following:

- Public health goes beyond the individual and refers to the health status of populations.
- Public health includes investigating the factors which contribute in a negative or positive way to

the health of populations by using the scientific instruments of epidemiology.

- Based on epidemiological data, public health suggests and promotes policies to maintain and improve health.
- Public health develops and investigates the impact of interventions on the health status of populations.

Sexual Reproductive Health Status of Populations

The assessment needs a clear definition of the population studied, a definition and explanation of the indicators measured and correct data collection and statistical analysis. These are mainly prevalence studies such as:

World Health Organization data on various aspects of SRH services provision include the following:

- Prevalence rates data collected nationally.
- Consumer surveys.
- A modified Delphi process involving all stakeholders to define priorities.
- Women's voices/focus groups discussions.

Factors Contributing to Sexual Health of Different Populations

Public health uses the methods of epidemiology to investigate the impact of a large number of factors having an impact on SRH.

Environment (Natural and Socioeconomic)

Examples

- Air quality and male fertility parameters.
- Exposure to substances and their impact on the fertility of women.
- War and sexual violence.
- Poverty and high rates of unintended pregnancies.

Laws and Sociocultural Norms

Examples

- Restrictive laws regarding access to abortion and high rate of unsafe abortion.
- Restrictive laws regarding access to contraceptives and rate of unintended pregnancies.
- Early marriage and risk of violence [2].

- Female genital mutilation and risk of sexual dysfunction [1–4].

Health Systems

Examples

- Low investment in SRH services by governments and rate of unintended pregnancies, STIs incidence and so forth. (There is evidence that every US dollar spent on SRH services has a return on investment estimated to be $120) [10].
- Lack of access to long-acting reversible contraceptives and high rate of unintended pregnancies [11].
- Difficult access to family-planning services and safe abortion.
- Lack of access to safer options such as medical abortion [12].

Education

Examples

- Misconceptions and misinformation about the risk of getting pregnant and high rate of adolescent pregnancies.
- Misconceptions, misinformation and lack of knowledge about sexuality associated with sexual dysfunction.
- Misinformation and lack of knowledge about fertility and infertility.
- High-risk behaviour.
- Adolescent education in sexuality and education about safe sex [13].

Addressing Sexual Reproductive Health Services for Populations with Special Needs

The World Health Organization and the UNFPA recognize following groups of individuals in this category. Both organizations have urged all countries to develop standard operating procedures for individual groups to streamline provision of SRH services to meet their needs.

- Physically impaired.
- LGBT.
- Immigrant populations with no irregular status [14].
- Women once at risk of female genital mutilation [15].
- Women with perinatal mental health issues [16].

- Women at risk of domestic violence [17].
- Women and men with learning disabilities [18].
- Older age [19].
- Sex workers [20].
- Victims of sexual assault.
- Homeless young people.

Sexual Reproductive Health Policy

Based on the data about prevalence and epidemiological studies about contributing factors, public health has the task to influence policy. Public health professionals use different instruments so as to exert this influence.

Environment (Natural and Socioeconomic)

Examples

- Elaborate programmes and develop interventions to reduce environmental risk factors and risk factors at the workplace.
- Engage in collaboration with institutions and governmental bodies to define standards of air quality and quality of nutrition.
- Support initiatives and policies to reduce marginalization and poverty.

Laws, Policy and Sociocultural Norms

Examples

- Give expert and scientific support to laws and policies that can protect individual reproductive rights by collaboration with lawmakers.
- These include:
  o Abortion rights [3–6].
  o Protection against violence and discrimination [4, 5].
  o Age at marriage.
  o Abandonment of legal restrictions regarding provision of contraceptives [1, 2, 4].

Health Systems

Examples

Service Delivery Modelling

Example
Guidelines/protocols for each service

- Open-access services where people can be tested for STIs quickly and confidentially.
- Partner notification guidance.
- National screening programmes for STIs and HIV.
- Locality based integrated one-stop sexual health services for STIs and contraception provision on an individualized basis [21].
- Strategies to promote all methods of contraception including higher use of long-acting reversible contraception in all age groups.
- Early access to abortion.
- Strategies to reduce repeat abortion and unwanted pregnancy immediately after childbirth [22].

Health Workforce

Example
Health sector regulations and professional association guidelines for task sharing

- School educators/nurses trained to provide education about relationships and sex.
- Trained counsellors in SRH able to discuss choices and decisions with women seeking termination of pregnancy in a non-judgemental way.
- Strategies to enhance skills and knowledge transfer from West to East in a global context (European Board and College of Obstetrics and Gynaecology (EBCOG) and United Nations Population Fund (UNFPA) Eastern Europe and Central Asia joint travelling fellowship) [23].

Health Information Systems

Example

- Programme requirements for reporting, monitoring and evaluation.

Medical Products, Vaccines and Technologies

Example
Contraceptive methods that programmes are allowed to provide

- Assessing new technologies such as more recent hormonal methods for male contraception.
- Human papillomavirus (HPV) immunization to reduce the risk of HPV-associated cancers in both female and male populations.

Health Promotion: Online resource: 'My contraception' to choose the right contraception

- Online resource: 'My HIV', developed by the Terrence Higgin Trust, which helps people to manage all aspects of HIV.
- Use of social media in education and health promotion.
- Patient feedback surveys.
- Working with TV personalities, sportspersons and supermodels who can act as ambassadors.

Behavioural Science: Understanding Attitudes Which Can Influence Sexual Health Outcomes: In order to develop local, regional and national SRH policies and services, data should be collected regularly. It is recognized that attitudes within the population continue to change about SRH services provision with ever-changing economic and political environments. Hence collection of data for the followings regularly could influence policymakers.

- Personal beliefs such as perceived risk of catching STI or HIV or of an untimed pregnancy.
- Personal perception of risk associated with certain sexual behaviour, use of alcohol, smoking and drugs.
- Attitude that the use of condoms or hormonal contraception can decrease sexual pleasure.
- Social norms, peer influence, self-esteem and confidence can impact the way people feel and their attitude towards risky activities.
- Relationships within families – whether young people can engage their parents in an open and supportive conversation.
- Religion can be a powerful influence on attitudes around sexuality and relationships.
- Influence of sources of information (media, Internet, school, friends and families) and the reliability of that information.

Financing

Example
While recognizing SRH services provision should remain a priority, it is also acknowledged that all decisions about healthcare should follow the principle of value for money. This is even more important when the financial resources are under huge pressure. Therefore, allocation of resources should be aligned in such a way that it benefits the most vulnerable and those who can least afford to pay. The following link provides an overview of the health sector budget: bit.ly/40ao1aX.

Governance and Leadership
Healthcare systems require that mechanisms are in place for robust monitoring of performance of all SRH services, and that they are meeting their objectives and targets as set out by policy advisors and health commissioners.

Example
Definition of priorities for investment and oversight consistent with sector goals, system requirements and client rights.

Monitoring Success of Programme
It is suggested that data are collected regularly by using a set of outcome indicators as described by various organizations. It may be more useful to use WHO and UNFPA outcome indicators to compare individual country's performance globally and also with its neighbours'. Such comparisons help individual countries to diversify their resources to much-needed neglected services.

Example
- Internationally agreed outcome indicators as defined by the WHO [24] and the UNFPA.
- Standards of care such as that established by the EBCOG [25].
- National Institute for Health and Care Excellence (NICE) quality standards.

Delivering Sexual and Reproductive Healthcare in Practice
Reproductive healthcare encompasses a whole-life approach for all individuals in relation to SRH, pregnancy-related health and health unrelated to pregnancy. It should be supported by and implemented through age-appropriate education. Individuals should have the ability to make informed choices and to exercise freedom of expression.

The services should be user-centred and everyone should be able to access reproductive healthcare when needed. Public health policies should reduce inequalities and improve sexual health outcomes.

Sexual health needs vary according to many factors such as age, gender, sexuality and ethnicity, and some groups are particularly at risk of poor health. While individuals' needs vary, certain core needs are common to everyone.

It should be acknowledged that for every pound spent on contraception, 11 pounds are saved in other healthcare costs [26]. The NICE has produced a review of the effectiveness of various strategies to improve sexual health outcomes [27].

Identifying Target Areas

The EBCOG and the European Society of Contraception and Reproductive Health (ESCRH) published a position statement to mark the twenty-fifth anniversary of ICPD 25 in Nairobi in 2019. The WHO has also published a three-stage process for strengthening policies and programmes for public health departments (see Table 5.1) [28].

In this section, we focus on key areas where sustainable models of care are required to address national and global inequalities in SRH as identified in ICPD 25. Each country faces its own unique public health challenges. Therefore access to local data is important for public health teams to prioritize key areas for a targeted approach that will achieve the best results.

Addressing Unmet Needs for Effective Contraceptive Methods

Up to 50% pregnancies are unplanned in England In order to address this issue, the following targeted strategies have been recommended [21].

- Joined-up SRH services to be provided at multiple sites, open access, no referral required from a general practitioner.
- Working with behavioural scientists to develop tools that would encourage more responsive and preventive behaviour (drug misuse, smoking, alcohol, obesity, mental health and violence).
- Working in partnership with stakeholders to develop local strategies to reduce health inequalities.

Implement strategies for age-sensitive sexuality education in schools delivered by SRH nurses and schoolteachers. It has been reported that the state of implementation of sexual education differs widely between and even within countries [29].

Reducing Teenage and Adolescent Pregnancy Rates and Increasing the Use of Long-Acting Contraceptives As the Main Method of Contraception

Rationale

- Being an adolescent mother is a huge societal burden as it restricts the mother's opportunity to complete her education and attain qualifications for a career.
- Without using a reliable method, these women are at increased risk to fall pregnant again.
- Shorter inter-pregnancy intervals increase maternal morbidity and mortality.
- In countries with restrictive abortion laws, these women may resort to unsafe abortion.
- In the United Kingdom, about a third of women seek an abortion who have had one before.
- Studies in America have reported a significant decline in the teenage pregnancy rate due to improved contraceptive use. There is a serious concern that in the light of the most recent pronouncement by the Supreme Court of the United States, SRH rights may be compromised in some states [38].
- The NICE clinical guideline CG30 has demonstrated that long-acting reversible contraceptives are more cost-effective than condoms and the pill.
- Improve uptake of various options for emergency contraception is effective in reducing the proportion of unplanned pregnancies.
- Post-abortion contraception support services are offered in a range of settings with convenient opening times and appropriately trained staff.

Table 5.1 WHO three-stage process for strengthening policies and programmes

Assessment/ data	Stage 1	Stage 2	Stage 3	output
SRH challenges	Strategic assessment	Developing and testing programme innovations	Scaling up successful interventions	Improved SRH status and programme

Policy and programme strengthening

Adapted from [28]

Addressing Barriers to Healthcare Access for Migrant Women with Irregular Status

Rationale

Humanitarian crises can further compound the risks associated with poor/inadequate SRH service availability. The EBCOG has recently published a position statement to highlight these issues, especially what we have learnt about atrocities committed during the Ukraine–Russia conflict and its effect on the provision of not only SRH services but all healthcare services [39]. Inadequate SRH services have been linked to unintended pregnancies, complications related to unsafe abortions, gender-based violence and an increase in HIV and STIs. Pregnant women and adolescents arriving at international borders are acutely affected by inadequate access to medical care and are also at increased risk of sexual violence. Patient and public involvement is needed to develop national/local strategies for the provision of SRH and STI testing and treatment in culturally sensitive environments. Complimentary services should be provided for well women and children such as educational interventions, immunization programmes, cancer screening and guidance in general health services.

Addressing Restrictive Abortion Laws

Rationale

Within Eastern Europe and Central Asia, 67% of women of reproductive age are using some form of modern or traditional contraception, albeit the use of unreliable traditional methods remains popular in several countries, hence a higher incidence of untimed and unwanted pregnancies. Because of restrictive abortion laws in some countries or lack of availability of safer methods of abortion, more than 47,000 women and girls die each year from unsafe abortion–related complications [5]. Barriers to access to safer abortion increase the risk of illegal abortion–related complications like sepsis and maternal morbidity and mortality. Provision of effective contraception and condom use skills, STI prevention education, sexual self-efficacy and SRH curriculums have reported improved outcomes [30].

Reducing Overall (Unsafe/Safe) Abortion Rates

Rationale

Within the United Kingdom, the abortion rate of 33 per 1,000 for women aged 20 has remained largely unchanged since 2001. Teenage pregnancy is associated with overt, low aspirations and not participating in education, employment or training. Teenage parents are at greater risk of poor mental health. Improved outcomes have been reported due to early access to post-coital contraception and medical abortions in non-judgemental environments, effective contraception and condom use skills, STI prevention education, sexual self-efficacy and SRH curriculums in schools.

Tackling the Epidemic of Sexually Transmitted Diseases in the Wider Population

Rationale

There is evidence that reducing the number of sexual partners and avoiding overlapping relationships can reduce the risk of contracting STIs. This information should be conveyed through sex education programmes. Rates of infectious syphilis are rising significantly again. Gonorrhoea is becoming more difficult to treat and it can quickly develop resistance to drugs. Chlamydia remains quite prevalent and often has no symptoms. It has been suggested that all sexually active people be tested annually or with each change of partner as a routine part of primary care. Within the United Kingdom, an incremental rise in STI rates has been noted among the 25–49 age group and accounts for 46% of all diagnosed STIs [21]. Although STI rates in people older than 50 account for 3% of all STIs, a rising trend has been noted in that age group as well.

Tackling Sexually Transmitted Infections, Especially HIV, among High-Risk Groups

Rationale

In England in 2011, one person was diagnosed with HIV every 30 minutes. Almost half of the adults newly diagnosed with HIV were diagnosed after the point at which they should have started treatment. Late diagnosis of

HIV is more common in older age groups compared with younger age groups. Within England, a significant proportion of STI diagnoses among gay and bisexual men continues to be in younger age groups: 34% of genital warts, 24% of gonorrhoea, 22% of genital herpes and chlamydia and 13% of syphilis cases in those aged younger than 24. Untreated STIs facilitate HIV transmission by increasing HIV infectiousness and susceptibility. Certain types of HPV are linked with cervical (women) and other oral and genital cancers (men). Policy advisors should implement gender-neutral HPV vaccination for young adults [31]. High rates of STIs and HIV persist in individuals not accessing services. Future service delivery frameworks should invest in promotion of prevention strategies [32].

Develop a Diverse and Multi-skilled Workforce

Rationale

Safe, efficient, cost-effective and high-quality care relies on the right mix of skills. Local services should have a multidisciplinary sexual health workforce where their skills can be used to the best effect appropriate for their skills and assigned role [4, 5]. Local area workforce modelling should include specialists, general practitioners, practice nurses, pharmacists, schoolteachers and college tutors. Arrangements should be in place for continuing professional development for all members of the local SRH team.

Tackling Sexual and Gender-Based Violence

Rationale

Violence against women is a violation of human rights, and prevention of female genital mutilation should be a priority [33]. Physical or sexual violence is usually perpetuated by an intimate partner. Adolescent girls, young women, women belonging to ethnic and other minorities, trans women and women with disabilities face a higher risk of different forms of violence. Humanitarian emergencies may exacerbate additional violence against women and girls. Gender equality should be promoted through legislation. Effective strategies should be put in place to achieve the ICPD 25 target of 'zero sexual and gender based violence, including zero child, early and forced marriage, as well as zero female genital mutilation' [34]. Healthcare providers should develop referral pathways for victims of gender-based violence in a sensitive manner irrespective of the cause of the clinic appointment.

Working on a Comprehensive Life-Course Approach to Women's Health

Rationale

The ICPD 25 stated that infant mortality rates and mortality rates for children under 5 years old remain stubbornly high in middle- and low-resourced countries [35, 36]. A wide gulf remains across the globe as regards maternal morbidity and mortality rates. It is regrettable that women are dying from preventable causes such as haemorrhage, sepsis, anaemia and eclampsia. Cervical cancer screening and treatment organization in most middle- and low-income countries require urgent attention. Lack of access to infertility treatment, menstrual symptoms management, access to hormonal treatment and post-reproductive health issues are linked to poor health outcomes.

Summary

Reproductive health implies that people can have a responsible, satisfying health reproductive system, a safer sex life and freedom to access safe and effective methods of contraception. Both men and women also have access to appropriate healthcare services. Individuals face inequalities in reproductive health services. The ICPD 25 has committed all governments to meet the Sustainable Development Goals by 2030. Public health has an important role to play in achieving those targets so no one is left behind [37].

References

1. World Health Organization. *Defining sexual health: Report of a technical consultation on sexual health, 2002.* Geneva: World Health Organization, 2006.

2. World Health Organization. *Sexual health and its linkages to reproductive health.* Geneva: World Health Organization, 2006. bit.ly/40ao1aX.

3. United Nations. *Programme of action: Report of the International Conference on Population and Development, Cairo. A/CONF.171/13/Rev.1.* New York: United Nations Secretariat, 1994.

4. United Nations. *Transforming our world: The 2030 agenda for sustainable development. A/RES/70/1.* New York: United Nations, 2015. bit.ly/3DorfO9.

5. Mahmood T, Bitzer J, Nizard J, Short M, on behalf of the European Board and College of Obstetrics and

Gynaecology and the European Society of Contraception and Reproductive Health. The sexual reproductive health of women: Unfinished business in the Eastern Europe and Central Asia Region. *European Journal of Obstetrics & Gynaecology and Reproductive Biology*. 2020;247:246–53.

6. Mahmood T, Bitzer J. Accelerating progress in sexual and reproductive health and rights in Eastern Europe and Central Asia: Reflecting on ICPD 25 Nairobi summit. *European Journal of Obstetrics & Gynaecology and Reproductive Biology*. 2020;247:254–6.

7. Beauchamp DE, Steinbock B. (eds.). *New ethics for the public's health*. New York: Oxford University Press, 1999.

8. International Planned Parenthood Federation. *Sexual and reproductive health and rights: A crucial agenda for the post-2015 framework*. London: International Planned Parenthood Federation, 2014. www.ippf.org /sites/default/files/report_for_web.pdf.

9. World Health Organization. *Action plan for sexual and reproductive health: Towards achieving the 2030 agenda for sustainable development in Europe. Leaving no one behind*. Geneva: World Health Organization, 2006. bit.ly/3HEVBOX.

10. World Health Organization. *Every woman, every child: The global strategy for women's, children's and adolescents' health 2016–2030*. Geneva: World Health Organization, 2006.EEEC_GSUpdate_Full_E N_2017_value%20for%20money.pdf.

11. Mahmood T, Benedetto C. EBCOG position statement: Call for action for the prevention of unintended pregnancies by promoting wider use of long acting reversible contraceptives. November 27, 2015. bit.ly/3Y9cg2S.

12. European Board and College of Obstetrics and Gynaecology. EBCOG position paper on medical abortion. November 27, 2015. www.ebcog.org/publi cations/tag/medical%20abortion.

13. Cameron S, Cooper M, Kerr Y, Mahmood T. EBCOG position statement: Public health role of sexual health and relationships education. *European Journal of Obstetrics and Gynaecology and Reproductive Biology*. 2019;234:223–4.

14. Smith A, Levoy M, Mahmood T, Mercer C. Migrant women's health issues: Addressing barriers to access to healthcare for migrant women with irregular status. *Entre Nous WHO Europe*. 2016;85:18–21.

15. World Health Organization. *Classification of female genital mutilation*.Geneva: World Health Organization, 1997. www.who.int.

16. Mahmood T, Mercer C, Tschudin S et al. Perinatal mental health: Bridging the gaps in policy and practice. *Entre Nous WHO Europe*. 2016;85:22–3.

17. Aston G, Bewley S. Abortion and domestic violence. *Obstetrician and Gynaecologist*. 2009;11:163–8.

18. Boycott-Garnett R, Tattersall J, Dunn J. *Final report: Talking about sex and relationships: The views of young people with learning disabilities*. Project Report. Leeds: CHANGE, 2010.

19. Rees M, Lambrinoudaki I, Bitzer J, Mahmood T. Joint opinion paper 'Aging and Sexuality' by the European Board and College of Obstetrics and Gynaecology and the European Menopause and Andropause Society(EMAS). *European Journal of Obstetrics and Gynaecology and Reproductive Biology*. 2018;220:132–4.

20. Sex workers and sexual health: Projects responding to needs. UK Network of Sex Work Projects, 2009.

21. Department of Health. A framework for sexual health improvement in England. 2013. www.dh.gsi.gov.uk /mandate.

22. Cameron ST, Berugoda N, Johnstone A, Glasier A. Assessment of a fast track referral service for intrauterine contraception following early medical abortion. *Journal of Family Planning and Reproductive Healthcare*. 2012;38(3):175–8.

23. Mahmood T, Khomasuridze T. Improving standards of care in sexual and reproductive health in Eastern Europe and Central Asia: A joint initiative of the UNFPA EECA Region and EBCOG. *Entre Nous WHO Europe*. 2015;83:26–7.

24. World Health Organization. *WHO report on global sexually transmitted infection surveillance*. Geneva: World Health Organization, 2018. bit.ly/3jlHjcG.

25. Mahmood T. *EBCOG standards of care for women's health in Europe: Gynaecological services*. Brussels: European Board and College of Obstetrics and Gynaecology, 2014. www.ebcog.org.

26. McGuire A, Hughes D. *The economics of family planning services, 1995. Long-acting reversible contraception: The effective and appropriate use of long-acting reversible contraception (CG30)*. London: National Institute for Health and Care Excellence, 2005.

27. National Institute for Health and Care Excellence. *NICE impact sexual health*. London: National Institute for Health and Care Excellence, 2019. www .nice.org.uk.

28. World Health Organization. *The WHO strategic approach to strengthening sexual and reproductive health policies and programmes*. Geneva: World Health Organization, 2007. www.who.int.

29. Ketting E, Ivanova O. *Sexuality education in Europe and central Asia: State of the art and recent developments. An overview of 25 countries*. Cologne: Federal Centre for Health Education,2018. BzgA_IP PFEN_ComrehensiveStudyReport_online.pdf.

30. Desrosiers A, Betancourt T, Kergoat Y et al. A systematic review of sexual and reproductive health interventions for young people in humanitarian and lower-and middle-income country settings. *BMC Public Health.* 2020;**20**(666):1–27. https://doi.org/10.1186/s12889-020-08818-y.

31. Verheijen RHM, Mahmood T, Donders G, Redman CWE. EBCOG position statement: Gender neutral HPV vaccination for young adults. *European Journal of Obstetrics and Gynaecology and Reproductive Biology.* 2020;**246**:187–9. https://doi.org/10.1016/j.ejogrb.2020.01.016.

32. Sonnenberg P, Clifton S, Beddows S et al. Prevalence, risk factors, and uptake of interventions for sexually transmitted infections in Britain: Findings from the National Surveys of Sexual Attitudes and Lifestyles(Natsal). *Lancet.* 2013;**382**:1795–1806. https://dx.doi.org/10.1016/s0140-6736(13)61947-9.

33. European Board and College of Obstetrics and Gynaecology. EBCOG position statement on female genital mutilation. *European Journal of Obstetrics and Gynaecology and Reproductive Biology.* 2017;**214**:192–3. https://dx.doi.org/10.1016/j.ejogrb.2017.04.019.

34. Santhya KG, Jejeebhoy SJ. Sexual and reproductive health and rights of adolescent girls: Evidence from low-and middle-income countries. *Global Public Health: An International Journal for Research, Policy and Practice.* 2015;**10**(2):189–221.

35. United Nations Population Fund. *Sexual and reproductive health and rights: An essential element of universal health coverage, background document for the Nairobi summit on ICP25. Accelerating the promise.* New York: United Nations Population Fund, 2019. bit.ly/3HH2zmT.

36. ICPD 25. Key trends in the UNECE region. 2019. www.unece.org/index.php?id=51520&L=0.

37. WHO Europe. *Action plan for sexual and reproductive health: Towards achieving the 2030 agenda for sustainable development in Europe. Leaving no one behind.* Copenhagen: WHO Europe, 2016. WHO/Europe | Home.

38. Louwen F, Mukhopadhyay S, Mahmood T et al. The United States Supreme Court ruling and women's reproductive rights: A position statement issued by The European Board and College of Obstetrics and Gynaecology (EBCOG). *European Journal of Obstetrics and Gynecology.* 2022;**279**:130–1.

39. Savona-Ventura C, Mahmood T, Mukhopadhyay S et al. The consequences of armed conflict on the health of women and newborn and sexual reproductive health: A position statement by the European Board and College of Obstetrics and Gynaecology (EBCOG). *European Journal of Obstetrics & Gynecology and Reproductive Biology.* 2022;**274**:80–2.

General Principles of Preventive Medicine in Sexual and Reproductive Healthcare

Johannes Bitzer

Introduction

Prevention in medicine describes an activity designed to protect a person against an undesired health outcome. Different types of prevention can thereby be differentiated [1].

- Primary prevention – intervening before health effects occur through measures such as providing vaccinations, altering risky behaviours (poor eating habits, tobacco use) and banning substances known to be associated with a disease or health condition.
- Secondary prevention – screening to identify diseases in the earliest stages, before the onset of signs and symptoms, through measures such as mammography and regular blood pressure testing.
- Tertiary prevention – managing disease post diagnosis to slow or stop disease progression through measures such as operations, drug therapy, chemotherapy, rehabilitation and screening for complications.

Prevention in the field of sexual and reproductive health (SRH) is based on two major concepts [2–4].

One concept is the biopsychosocial approach. This approach takes into account that SRH is influenced and impacted by medical and psychosocial factors which can be grouped into three major categories: physical health (body), mental health (mind, psyche) and social health (environment or life circumstances).

This means that SRH preventive interventions are not limited to medical approaches but include also interventions targeting the behaviour of women and men (behavioural medicine and psychology) as well as interventions on a social and sociocultural level (public health, health policies, advocacy). This approach also implies collaboration among healthcare professionals with different backgrounds and specialties.

The second concept is the life-course approach to women's health. The life-course approach considers an individual's entire progress throughout life to explain certain outcomes. The outcomes depend on the interaction of multiple protective and risk factors throughout people's lives. The life-course approach to health examines how biological (including genetics), social and behavioural factors throughout life and across generations act independently, cumulatively and interactively to influence health outcomes. In the following chapters different targets for prevention in SRH are summarized along the three levels of prevention from a biopsychosocial perspective, integrating the stressors and resources along an individual's life course.

Targets of Prevention in Sexual and Reproductive Healthcare

Prevention of Unintended Pregnancies

To protect women against unwanted pregnancies different strategies have been described which can be subdivided into three different levels of prevention.

Primary Prevention

- Comprehensive sexual education [5, 6]. Comprehensive sexual education aims at helping adolescents to understand and develop their individual sexuality by teaching and learning about the cognitive, emotional, physical and social aspects of sexuality. It aims to equip children and young people with knowledge, skills, attitudes and values that will empower them to realize their health, well-being and dignity; develop respectful social and sexual relationships; consider how their choices affect their own well-being and that of others; and understand and ensure the protection of their rights throughout their lives (see also Chapter 4). This enforces the aspects of self-determination regarding when and with whom the individual wants to have a sexual encounter or relationship.

- Contraception (see also Chapters 9, 10) [7, 8]. A large number of contraceptive methods are available (hormonal and non-hormonal, short-acting and long-acting) with different profiles regarding efficacy, health risks, side effects and additional benefits that allow healthcare providers to tailor the available methods to individuals' needs. Long-acting reversible contraceptives have proven to be the most effective methods for protection and can be used across the different life phases, including adolescence and pre-menopause (see Chapter 10). This preventive strategy depends on the availability and accessibility of services and contraceptive counselling, which should follow the principles of patient-centred communication and shared decision-making.

Secondary Prevention

- Early detection of pregnancy. A precondition for early detection is easy access to pregnancy tests without discrimination.
- Safe termination of pregnancy [9–11]. Safe abortion is at the centre of secondary prevention. This implies legalization of termination of pregnancy based on the pregnant woman's decision (sexual and reproductive rights), the availability of and access to medical abortion and safe surgical abortion, and post-abortion contraceptive counselling and care (see Chapter 36).

Tertiary Prevention

- Access to regular pregnancy control and treatment for complications [12, 13]. Unintended pregnancies have been shown to be at higher risk of pregnancy and birth complications as well as postpartum disorders including dysfunctions of the mother–child relationship. The preventive strategy includes regular visits and early detection of medical and psychological complications in the postpartum period for the mother as well as the child.

Prevention and Treatment of Sexually Transmitted Infections, Including HIV

The implications for women of sexually transmitted infections and HIV are described in Chapter 3.

Primary Prevention

- Safer sex practices. The principles of safer sex include knowledge about risks, regular use of condoms, communication among partners and post-exposure prophylaxis for HIV and STIs [14–18]. When used consistently and correctly, male latex condoms are highly effective in preventing the sexual transmission of HIV, chlamydia gonorrhoea, human papillomavirus (HPV), genital herpes, hepatitis B, syphilis and cancroid.
- Vaccination. The HPV vaccine, bivalent, quadrivalent or nonavalent, is recommended routinely for females aged 11 and 12 years and can be administered beginning at 9 years of age [19, 20]. The HBV vaccination series is recommended for all adolescents and young adults who have not previously received the hepatitis B vaccine. The HAV vaccination series should be offered to adolescents and young adults who have not previously received the HAV vaccine series [18]. See also later in this chapter.

Secondary Prevention

- Early detection of infections [17, 18]. This strategy depends on regular check-ups with proactive asking about risks and screening. The main element of this strategy is the regular integration of taking sexual histories into the clinical practice [18]. The main questions in sexual history are:

Do you have sex with men, women or both?

In the past 2 months, how many partners have you had sex with?

In the past 12 months, how many partners have you had sex with?

Is it possible that any of your sex partners in the past 12 months had sex with someone else while they were still in a sexual relationship with you?

What do you do to protect yourself from STIs and HIV?

Have you ever had an STI?

Have any of your partners had an STI?

Additional questions to identify HIV and viral hepatitis risk include:

Have you or any of your partners ever injected drugs?

Have your or any of your partners exchanged money or drugs for sex?

Do I need to know anything else about your sexual practices?

- Measures to prevent spread [15]. Partner tracing is a central element in limiting the spread of STIs. It involves identifying, testing and treating sexual contacts/partners of an individual (index patient) diagnosed with one or more STIs. This should be undertaken by appropriately trained staff. The aim is to prevent reinfection in the index patient, treat undiagnosed infection(s) in sexual contact(s), reduce the burden of infection(s) in the community and reduce new infection rates by interrupting the chain of transmission.

There are different types of contact tracing:

- Index referral – the index patient informs contact(s).
- Provider referral – the clinical service informs all contacts, maintaining the confidentiality and anonymity of the index patient. This is usually done when the index patient does not wish to inform sexual contact(s).
- Conditional referral – the index attempts to inform contacts within a certain time limit, failing which the clinical service takes on the responsibility.

Tertiary Prevention

Early and effective treatment to avoid complications and spread of disease (see Chapter 45).

Prevention of Cervical Cancer

Cervical cancer is an example of the effectiveness of preventive actions (see Chapter 7) [19–21].

Primary Prevention

- Safer sex. Understanding cervical carcinoma as a sexually transmitted viral infection, the general recommendations mentioned earlier in this chapter apply, including the use of condoms, which reduces the risk of HPV infection by up to 80%.
- Vaccination. After having found that HPV 6, 11, 16, 18, 31, 33, 45, 52 and 58 are responsible in total for about 90% of all cervical cancers in Europe, the HPV vaccine, bivalent, quadrivalent or nonavalent is recommended routinely for females aged 11 and 12 years and can be administered beginning at 9 years of age. The vaccination is also recommended for females aged 13–26 years who have not yet

received all doses or completed the vaccine series. The fact that these viruses affect boys also, increasing the risk of developing genital and oral cancer that boys can transmit to girls, the quadrivalent or nonavalent HPV vaccine is recommended routinely for males aged 11 and 12 years and also can be administered beginning at 9 years of age. The realization of the vaccination programme differs across countries.

Secondary Prevention

Screening. There is a long-standing tradition in gynaecology of early detection of cervical dysplasia and early cancerous lesions by cytology and, more recently, by HPV testing, either separately or combined. There is still some controversy and different countries have different guidelines, taking into account that HPV testing shows higher sensitivity (> 95%) than cervical cytology in women older than 30 years. The high negative predictive value (> 98%) offers good security, but low positive predictive value (< 10%) makes it a poor screening tool in younger women younger than 30 years due to high rates of HPV infection at these ages.

Tertiary Prevention

Effective treatment to prevent recurrence and metastatic disease includes colposcopic examination and cervical conization procedures with follow-up visits.

Prevention of Unsafe Abortion with Complications

See also Chapter 3 [9–11, 22].

Primary Prevention

Primary prevention includes sexual education and qualified contraceptive counselling and care, including the provision of long-acting reversible contraceptives and access to special services for contraception postpartum, post abortion and post termination of pregnancy. Another primary prevention strategy focuses on the fight for sexual and reproductive rights of women.

Secondary Prevention

The basic strategy is early detection of an unwanted pregnancy with easy access to services. This includes the provision of services ensuring respectful and non-judgemental treatment without discrimination towards unmarried women or any other groups.

Tertiary Prevention

This includes the fight for abortion rights, access to medical abortion and, where necessary, safe surgical abortion procedures.

Prevention of Sexual Dysfunctions

The pathogenesis of sexual dysfunctions is multifactorial, including biological and psychosocial factors [23–25]. The consequences range from impairment of sexual well-being and quality of life of individuals to relationship difficulties, conflicts and breakup of families and other psychosocial consequences like poverty and violence.

Primary Prevention

- Sexual education (see earlier in this chapter). Comprehensive sexual education includes two main components: protection of sexual health by contraception, prevention of STIs and early detection of disease; and promotion of sexual well-being by providing information about the physiology and psychology of the human sexual response and how to make sexuality pleasurable and enjoyable. Education also informs about the medical and psychosocial factors which may contribute to the impairment of sexual well-being.

Secondary Prevention

- Taking a sexual history. In the medical consultation doctors should be proactively asking about sexual health and well-being by integrating sexual history into the general medical history (see later in this chapter). Visits in the context of contraception, pregnancy, post partum and in pre- and post-menopause provide an opportunity for women, men and couples to seek information and to talk about their sexual well-being in a respectful way. Counselling to women, men and couples should be based on the principles of:
  - Empathic listening to provide emotional relief.
  - Information and education in language adapted to the individual patient.
  - Dispelling myths and misconceptions and empowering patients by helping them to understand the factors contributing to their problem.

Tertiary Prevention

Access to qualified care for women, men and couples suffering from sexual dysfunctions:

- By helping patients to talk about their problem (see section in this chapter on basic counselling).
- By establishing a diagnosis.
- By understanding the factors which contribute to the problem.
  - Biological, psychological, interpersonal and social factors.
  - Past, triggering and problem-maintaining factors.
  - By informing patients about possible solutions (medical, psychological, physical) and finding the best individual therapy by a process of shared decision-making.

Prevention of Sexual Violence

Sexual violence is a worldwide pandemic with disastrous consequences for the individual victims and society as a whole (see Chapter 52) [26].

Primary Prevention

- Sexual education in schools. Comprehensive sexual education includes normative statements about the equality of women and men relating to self-determination and autonomy. It includes the freedom of choice and protection against coercion and transgression of limits.
- Community work. Communities define cultural values and rules regarding sexuality with definitions of the roles of women and men and definition of what is allowed and forbidden in sexuality and behavioural norms. Some of these traditions facilitate or even legitimize acts of violence against women. To prevent this it is important and necessary to collaborate with community leaders to discuss the impact of these rules on the health of women and girls and to look for solutions.
- Advocacy (political, legal). Beyond cultural traditions are legal frameworks which do not prevent violence but give men superiority and power over women and limit women's rights and freedoms. It is important to create liaisons with politicians, political parties and authorities to achieve necessary changes.

Secondary Prevention

- Early detection of sexual violence. A cornerstone of secondary prevention is taking a sexual history which includes questions about experiences of coercion and violence, taking into account that most sexual violence comes from the intimate partner. The interview can be structured according to Centers for Disease Control (CDC) guidance, including the following questions:

  ○ Do you have a history of unwanted sexual experiences?
  ○ [If patient is confused] Have you ever been forced or coerced to have sex/sexual activity against your will, either as a child or as an adult?
  ○ If yes, does anything about that experience impact your current sexuality?
  ○ If yes, does anything about that experience make seeing a healthcare provider or having a physical examination (if applicable) difficult? If so, I'd like to hear about this so we can work together more easily.

- Another important part of this strategy is support for women and men who are insecure about sexual orientation/gender identity.

  ○ Do you feel you are getting support and acceptance of your sexual orientation/gender identity from your family and friends?
  ○ Are you experiencing any harassment or violence – at home, at work, or in your community – due to your sexual orientation or gender identity?

- Being aware of risk constellations. In screening for victims of violence different symptoms may be indicative like depression, chronic pain, injuries or sexual dysfunction. It is not only physical violence like rape but also other forms of violence like mobbing, insulting behaviour and taking advantage of superiority in the workplace which may result in traumatization of the girl or the woman.

Tertiary Prevention

- Care for victims (see Chapter 52). Victims of sexual violence need easy access to medical and psychological care as well as legal protection and follow up support. Medical care includes physical examination, looking for injuries to the body in general and to the genital organs, screening for infections, emergency contraception and post-exposure prophylaxis to HIV and STIs. Psychological care includes counselling, diagnosis and treatment of post-traumatic stress disorder and an offer to follow up later. This includes also empathic help during the processes of assessment of findings (i.e. gynaecological examination), contact with the police and legal follow-up.

Prevention of Infertility

Infertility can affect physical, mental and social health and lead to life crisis, chronic stress disease, problems with one's identity and relationship difficulties [27].

Primary Prevention

- School. Primary prevention starts already at school with comprehensive sexual education, including information and education about the physiology of reproduction and the life-course changes of fertility as well as the risk factors contributing to infertility.
- Prevention of STIs. Screening for risky behaviour which may compromise the fertility of the individual in the short or long term.
- Family planning. Family-planning consultations should go beyond contraceptive counselling and care and integrate a reproductive life plan, taking into account the changes in fertility along the life course and ageing.

Secondary Prevention

The focus is on the detection and treatment of STIs and pelvic inflammatory disease (PID), which may lead to tubal and uterine pathology resulting in infertility. A second focus is the detection and treatment of endocrine disorders like polycystic ovary syndrome, thyroid dysfunction, diabetes, ovarian dysfunction, and of endometriosis.

Tertiary Prevention

Tertiary prevention focuses on three strategies. One is the advanced reproductive technology which allows patients to overcome the fertility consequences of diseases and helps couples to reach their reproductive aims. The second is helping couples in their wish to adopt a child. The third preventive strategy focuses on those patients and couples who are and will not be able to fulfil their wish. These individuals and couples need help to cope with infertility and reduce the risk of mental health problems and relationship difficulties.

Prevention of Pregnancy and Mother and Child Morbidity and Mortality

Reduction of mother and child morbidity and mortality is one of the major targets of sexual and reproductive healthcare.

Primary Prevention

Pre-conception care (see Chapter 8) [28]. There is a long list of tests and intervention to reduce the risk of maternal and child morbidity and mortality. The precondition for this type of prevention is access to pre-conception care as a routine and as a right. The most important parts are summarized in what follows.

- Folic acid supplements reduce the occurrence of neural tube defects.
- Rubella immunization provides protective sero-positivity and prevents congenital rubella syndrome.
- HIV/AIDS screening allows for timely treatment. Pregnancies can be better planned.
- Hepatitis B vaccination prevents transmission to infants in utero and eliminates the risk to women of hepatic failure, liver carcinoma, cirrhosis and death.
- Diabetes management reduces the threefold increase in birth defects among infants of women with type 1 and type 2 diabetes.
- Hypothyroidism management protects proper neurological development through adjusting the dosage of levothyroxine early in pregnancy.
- Maternal phenylketonuria (PKU) management prevents mental retardation in infants born to mothers with PKU through a low-phenylalanine diet before conception and throughout pregnancy.
- Obesity control reduces the risks of neural tube defects, preterm birth, diabetes, C-section, hypertension and thromboembolic disease.
- Screening for and management of STIs reduces the risk of ectopic pregnancy, infertility, PID, and chronic pelvic pain. It also reduces the risk of fetal death or physical and developmental disabilities, including mental retardation and blindness.
- Fetal alcohol syndrome (FAS) and other alcohol-related birth defects can be prevented.

- Some anti-epileptic drugs are known teratogens. Changing to a less teratogenic treatment regimen reduces harmful exposure.
- Accutane use in pregnancy results in miscarriage and birth defects – avoiding pregnancy or ceasing Accutane use before conception eliminates harmful exposure.
- Oral anticoagulants like Warfarin are teratogens; such medications can be switched before pregnancy.
- Quitting smoking before pregnancy can prevent smoking-associated adverse outcomes, including preterm birth and low birth weight.

Secondary Prevention

The severity of obstetrical complications can be reduced by the early detection of pregnancy complications according to international guidelines regarding premature birth, hypertensive disease, eclampsia, bleeding [29]. Ultrasound and genetic testing, including molecular markers, enlarge the possibilities of early detection not only of fetal morbidity, but also of placental abnormalities threatening the life of the mother. There is also a need to take care of the psychosocial consequences of maternal and fetal morbidities, which may lead to long-term mental health problems for the mother and create difficulties in the relationship with the newborn.

Tertiary Prevention

Obstetrics as a specialty has made enormous scientific and technological progress in the medical treatment of pregnancy and birth complications, leading to a dramatic decrease of mother and child long-term morbidity and mortality in many countries. At the same time an important gap remains between countries. Women and their newborns are still very vulnerable and under-protected with respect to these essential needs and rights.

Prevention of Lifestyle-Associated Sexual and Reproductive Health Risks

Certain important factors are known to have a negative impact on health in general but at the same time impact SRH indirectly in a negative way [4, 30]. These are the so-called lifestyle factors – obesity, smoking, lack of exercise, drugs and chronic stress. In each encounter between a healthcare professional and a patient, the opportunity of addressing these issues and health behavioural counselling should be used.

Primary, Secondary and Tertiary Prevention

Prevention is based on information and empowerment already starting at school, but it is also a persistent task along the life course. Based on the concept of a continuous cognitive and behavioural process women and men are guided through the different stages of change described in the model of motivational interviewing [30]. Another source of help comes from psychological interventions like cognitive behavioural therapy, mindfulness and meditation, designed to help patients to cope with stress and avoid the development of a chronic stress disease with all its consequences [31].

Summary

Prevention in SRH includes education across the lifespan, continuous support regarding health-maintaining behaviour, easy access to high-quality care regarding the prevention of occurrence, early detection and management of complications. Primary, secondary and tertiary preventive strategies range from unintended pregnancies to STIs, from unsafe abortions to sexual dysfunctions, from sexual violence to infertility, from general mother and child morbidity and mortality to lifestyle-related risks. These strategies need close collaboration of different specialists with the aim to create integrative services covering these challenges.

References

1. CDC prevention guidelines. bit.ly/3DqpTCF.

2. World Health Organization. *Defining sexual health: Report of a technical consultation on sexual health, 2002.* Geneva: World Health Organization, 2006.

3. World Health Organization and UNDP/UNFPA/ UNICEF/WHO/World Bank Special Programme of Research, Development and Research Training in Human Reproduction. *Sexual health and its linkages to reproductive health: An operational approach.* Geneva: World Health Organization, 2017. https://apps .who.int/iris/handle/10665/258738.

4. Health matters: A life course approach. bit.ly/3JorAED.

5. Federal Centre for Health Education and World Health Organization Regional Office for Europe. *Standards for sexuality education in Europe: Federal Centre for Health Education.* Cologne: Federal Centre for Health Education and World Health Organization Regional Office for Europe, 2010. bit.ly/3JorAED.

6. United Nations Population Fund. *UNFPA operational guidance for comprehensive sexuality education: A focus on human rights and gender.* New York: United Nations Population Fund, 2014. bit.ly/3JorAED.

7. World Health Organization. *Medical eligibility criteria for contraceptive use.* Geneva: World Health Organization, 2015. bit.ly/3kTOzNk.

8. bit.ly/3kTOzNk.

9. World Health Organization. *Safe abortion: Technical and policy guidance for health systems.* 2nd edition. Geneva: World Health Organization, 2012.

10. National Institute for Health and Care Excellence. *National Institute for Health and Care Excellence guideline: Abortion care.* London: National Institute for Health and Care Excellence, 2019.

11. bit.ly/3kTOzNk.

12. World Health Organization. *Reproductive health strategy to accelerate progress towards the attainment of international development goals and targets: Global strategy adopted by the 57th World Health Assembly.* Geneva: World Health Organization, 2004.

13. World Health Organization. *WHO recommendations on postnatal care of the mother and newborn.* Geneva: World Health Organization, 2014. bit.ly/3HDkmv6.

14. Centers for Disease Control and Prevention, Workowski KA, Berman SM. Sexually transmitted diseases treatment guidelines, 2006. *MMWR Recomm Rep.* 2006;**55**:1–94.

15. World Health Organization. *Global health sector strategy on sexually transmitted infections, 2016–2021.* Geneva: World Health Organization, 2016. bit.ly /3JpUJPM.

16. Centers for Disease Control and Prevention, National Center for HIV/AIDS, Viral Hepatitis, STD, and TB Prevention. *2006 disease profile.* Atlanta, GA: Centers for Disease Control and Prevention, 2008, pp. 1–61. bit.ly/3HDkzhS.

17. www.cdc.gov/std/treatment/sexualhistory.pdf.

18. World Health Organization. Brief sexuality-related communication: Recommendations for a public health approach. bit.ly/3Y7XsS4.

19. bit.ly/3Y4jgOq.

20. Lei J, Ploner A, Elfström KM et al. HPV vaccination and the risk of invasive cervical cancer. *N Engl J Med.* 2020;**383**:1340–8.

21. World Health Organization. Cervical cancer screening.

22. World Health Organization. Preventing unsafe abortion. September 2020.

23. Laumann EO, Glasser DB, Neves RC et al. A population-based survey of sexual activity, sexual problems and associated help-seeking behavior patterns in mature adults in the United States of America. *Int J Impot Res.* 2009;**21**:171–8.

24. McCool ME, Apfelbacher C, Brandstetter S et al. Diagnosing and treating female sexual dysfunction: A survey of the perspectives of obstetricians and gynecologists. *Sex Health.* 2016;**13**:234–40.

25. Ribeiro S, Alarcao V, Simoes R et al. General practitioners' procedures for sexual history taking and treating sexual dysfunction in primary care. *J Sex Med.* 2014;**11**:386–93.

26. World Health Organization. *Health care for women subjected to intimate partner violence or sexual violence: A clinical handbook.* Geneva: World Health Organization, 2014. bit.ly/3XZ7PaQ.

27. National Institute for Health and Care Excellence. *Fertility problems: Assessment and treatment. Clinical guideline 2013.* London: National Institute for Health and Care Excellence, 2013.

28. bit.ly/3kQzKLN.

29. bit.ly/3Ri74XS.

30. Miller WR, Rollnick S. *Motivational interviewing: Helping people change.* New York: Guilford Press, 2013.

31. Kabat Zinn J. *Full catastrophe living: Using the wisdom of your body and mind to face stress, pain, and illness.* New York: Bantam Books, 2013.

Screening in Sexual and Reproductive Healthcare

Rolf Kirschner, Harald Moi, Gilbert G. G. Donders

Introduction

The World Health Organization (WHO) defines screening as the presumptive identification of unrecognized disease in an apparently healthy, asymptomatic population by means of tests, examinations or other procedures that can be applied rapidly and easily to the target population. When applied to sexual and reproductive healthcare, screening entails a routine of clinical, bacteriological, virological, microscopic and other special assessments to asymptomatic individuals of both genders.

Clinical Screening

Relating to sexual and reproductive health, a routine clinical examination should be performed. This would be natural to do when performing the scheduled screening tests for cervical cytology. The examination of the female is by a routine macroscopic gynaecological exam of the vulva, vagina, cervix, uterus and adnexae. The vulva should be checked specifically for signs of dermatological diseases – for example, lichen sclerosus and lichen planus, as well as for signs of vulvodynia. If increased cervical or vaginal discharge is observed, tests relating to diseases of the vagina and cervix may be taken and are described later in this chapter. A bimanual palpation of the uterus and adnexae should be performed to assess for pathology that may need further investigation. An examination of the breasts should be done as well as informing about self-examination at regular intervals.

If a sexually transmitted infection (STI) is suspected or diagnosed, the male partner(s) should be notified and examined. The examination of the male partner should consist of inspection of the penis, including retraction of the foreskin, where relevant tests may then be made from the urethral orifice and first void urine. The scrotum should be inspected as well as the size and shape of both the testes and epididymis.

Screening for Cervical Intraepithelial Neoplasia

Most countries today have an organized program for regular screening, starting from the age of 21–25 years, including intervals of 3 years, until the age of 65–69. In Europe, regular screening with cervical cytology alone is recommended from age 25 every 3 years up to 35 years. It is important that screening is not started at an earlier age than 25 years, as nonclinical changes may be noted, leading to unnecessary worries, controls and treatments that may be harmful. High-risk human papilloma virus (hrHPV) testing should not be performed in women younger than 30 years of age, because many transient HPV infections without clinical relevance occur in young women. In women age 30–35 years, HPV testing is optional. From age 35 to age 65–69 years, screening every 3 years with cervical cytology alone, every 5 years with hrHPV testing alone or every 5 years with hrHPV testing in combination with cytology is recommended. The US Preventive Services Task Force (USPSTF) recommends screening every 3 years with cervical cytology alone in women aged 21–29 years, after which the programs are identical.

Fluid-based cytology is recommended, using specially designed brushes and vials containing a transport preservative. Fluid-based cytology can be used in the laboratory for cytology, HPV testing or both. It is important that the specific method of taking the test is followed.

The sexual and reproductive health (SRH) screener must assess that a proper test has been performed inside the program and, if not, or in cases where clinical inspection has revealed changes that should be further elicited, a fresh smear should be taken and followed up. A new option in the design of cervical screening programs, when HPV primary screening is considered, is the use of self-collected samples; this may simplify logistics and enable new strategies for outreach to women to increase participation in organized screening programs.

Assessment of Human Papilloma Virus Vaccination

Since the first vaccines against HPV were introduced primarily for 11–12-year-old girls, many countries have introduced vaccination programs for both sexes. The nonavalent vaccine is now the most frequently used and recent scientific results show the value regarding SRH [1].

There are two HPV-vaccines marketed, a bivalent (Cervarix), approved in 2008, and a quadrivalent (Gardasil), approved in 2007, later substituted with a nonavalent (Gardasil 9). Gardasil 9 protects against 90% of hrHPV and, in addition, against HPV 6 and HPV 11, which causes visible genital warts. Cervarix protects against HPV 16 and HPV 18, which causes 70% of cervical cancers, but, through cross-reactivity against other hrHPV types, the protection against high-grade cervical dysplasia may reach 90%, similar to Gardasil 9.

Screening for Sexually Transmitted Infections

Facilitating present-day screening, the following STIs can be detected by polymerase chain reaction (PCR) techniques, allowing simultaneous detection of *Neisseria gonorrhoeae*, *Chlamydia trachomatis* and *Trichomonas vaginalis* using similar techniques on the same sample. Screening for *Mycoplasma hominis* and *Ureaplasma urealyticum* should be avoided.

Screening for *Neisseria gonorrhoeae* in asymptomatic women should be considered as follows [2]:

a) Age below 25 years with new or multiple recent sexual partners.
b) When finding vaginal or cervical discharge with risk factors for STIs – that is, a person younger than 30 years and with new sexual contact in the past year, or more than one partner in the past year.
c) Persons diagnosed with any other STI.
d) If a sexual partner has an STI.
e) Any intrauterine interventions or manipulations in areas or populations of high gonorrhea prevalence.

Screening for chlamydia in asymptomatic women should be considered as follows [3]:

a) Age younger than 25 years with a new sexual contact in the past year or more than one partner in the past year.
b) Persons diagnosed with other STIs.
c) Sexual contact with persons with an STI or pelvic inflammatory disease (PID).
d) In preparation for a termination of pregnancy or any planned intrauterine interventions or manipulations.

In a screening setting, a first-void urine specimen can be used, but in case of symptoms or clinical suspicion, a cervical swab provides superior sensitivity to urine. If a mucopurulent cervicitis is observed, a nucleid acid amplification test (NAAT) for chlamydia and gonorrhea should be taken, preferably from the cervix, urethra and/or anus. If available, a NAAT *Mycoplasma genitalium* from cervix should also be taken. Screening for *Mycoplasma genitalium* should not be performed in asymptomatic women, except [4]:

a) Sexual contact with persons with an STI or PID, in particular, contact with persons infected with *M. genitalium*.
b) Before termination of pregnancy.
c) When finding mucopurulent cervicitis with risk factors for STI – that is, a person with age younger than 30 years and a new sexual partner.

Screening for HIV and syphilis should be offered to anyone who

a) Had unwanted or unforeseen unprotected sex.
b) Has a new sex partner.
c) Had sex with a person whose sex life is unknown, is bisexual or is known to have had multiple recent sex partners.

Other Screening Recommendations

If the patient during the past year has been hospitalized in a country with high prevalence of multi-resistant *Staphylococcus aureus* (MRSA), a test for MRSA from the nose, tonsillae and perineum is recommended.

Screening for vaginitis in asymptomatic women is not recommended. However, if obvious discharge is observed that is not recognized by the patient, the patient could be offered further investigation. A pH of the vaginal discharge should be taken. If pH is greater than 4.5, a whiff test and phase contrast microscopy of the vaginal discharge should be performed in order to diagnose bacterial vaginosis, aerobic vaginitis and trichomoniasis. For general policies, however, it has never been established that screening for these conditions in asymptomatic non-pregnant women makes any difference. Still, it becomes clear that such conditions with abnormal vaginal microflora predispose to more rapid development of cervical cancer in HPV-infected women, as well as decreasing fertility and contributing to the burden of a low-quality sex life of many women. Given the important health challenges incorporated in abnormal vaginal microflora as a risk factor, therefore, it could become the object of a future screening tool that needs to be introduced as soon as broad screening and proper treatment options become available.

As a proxy, especially in pregnancy, pH can be used to assess such vaginal health risks. In pregnancy, it is established that bacterial vaginosis and trichomoniasis, as well as aerobic vaginitis, increase the risk of preterm delivery, preterm rupture of the membranes, chorioamnionitis and preterm birth, but as the proper treatment regimens to prevent such complications are not yet fully elucidated, routine screen-and-treat policies for abnormal vaginal flora have not been installed or recommended [5].

Screening by Microscopy of Vaginal Fluid

Screening techniques should promote health, be accessible, lead to a treatment option and be affordable for a community. Microscopy of vaginal fluid could be taken into account for this, as the technique is cheap and easy to access and could promote health by discovering women with asymptomatic bacterial vaginosis, aerobic vaginitis and trichomoniasis [6]. Numerous complications are linked to bacterial vaginosis and aerobic vaginitis – for example, an increased prevalence of chlamydia cervicitis and HPV infection of the cervix. Bacterial vaginosis also has been associated with other STIs like trichomoniasis, PID and HIV, and hence is in itself increasingly considered a sexually transmissible condition.

The recognition of both conditions is easy when microscopy of vaginal fluid is done. In bacterial vaginosis, easily recognizable granular anaerobic microbes have taken over the normal lactobacillary microflora, typically without eliciting an immune response or leucocyte reaction. In aerobic vaginitis, on the other hand, either an infectious component like small bacilli with an inflammatory component (increased leucocytes, toxic leucocytes) or an atrophic component (parabasal epithelial cells) are present in variable degrees. In cases of suspected aerobic vaginitis, cultures can serve as a back-up confirmation but never replace proper microscopy. Screening women with vaginal bacterial culture is not an advisable technique and may lead to maltreatment and preventable antibiotic resistance. If *Trichomonas* infection is suspected in case of negative microscopy, a PCR is indicated.

References

1. Lei J, Ploner A, Elfström KM et al. HPV vaccination and the risk of invasive cervical cancer. *N Engl J Med.* 2020;383:1340–8.

2. Unemo M, Ross J, Serwin AB et al. European guideline for the diagnosis and treatment of gonorrhoea in adults. *Int J STD AIDS.* 2020;29:956462420949126. https://doi .org/10.1177/0956462420949126.

3. Lanjouw E, Ouburg S, de Vries HJ et al. European guideline on the management of chlamydia trachomatis infections. *Int J STD AIDS.* 2016;27:333–48.

4. Jensen JS, Cusini M, Gomberg M, Moi H. European guideline on mycoplasma genitalium infections. *J Eur Acad Dermatol Venereol.* 2016;30:1650–6.

5. Donders GGG. Management of abnormal vaginal flora as a risk factor for preterm birth. In Morrison JC (ed.), *Preterm birth: Mother and child.* London: InTech, 2012. bit.ly/3wF54Qb.

6. Donders G. Diagnosis and management of bacterial vaginosis and other types of abnormal vaginal bacterial flora: A review. *Obstet Gynecol Surv.* 2010;65(7):462–73.

Reproductive Life Plan and Preconception Care, Including Vaccination

Kai Haldre

Preconception Health

During the past decades increasing epidemiological, clinical and basic science research, including both human and animal studies in vitro and in vivo, have been carried out to understand better the role of single parameters of parental health in the health of the offspring and through generations. Research has aimed to define the most vulnerable periods of development in early life and the possible pathways by which unfavorable milieu during fragile growth phases might affect health in adult life. There is a convincing amount of evidence that parental nutritional conditions and environmental stressors during gametogenesis and first days and weeks of embryo development can increase the risk of hypertension, obesity, type 2 diabetes, atopic conditions, some cancers, neurological impairment and mental health problems in adulthood [1–5]. Both human and animal studies have been carried out to show how future mothers' diet, body composition, metabolism and stress before and during conception and early embryonic development determines the diseases in their children's future life and how these effects might last over several generations [1, 2, 4–9].

However, increasing an amount of data has also become available to show how future fathers' ill health, especially over-nutrition, has a long-lasting role in the health of their children and grandchildren [1, 2, 10]. A recent systematic review and meta-regression analysis [11] of trends in sperm quality in samples collected between 1973 and 2011 showed that, during only these four decades, there was a 52.4% decline in sperm concentration and a 59.3% decline in total sperm count among an unselected group of men from North America, Europe and Australia. This analysis did not investigate the causes of the observed declines; at the same time it is known that sperm count is associated with several lifestyle and environmental influences in adult life like the possible effect of pollution with endocrine disrupting chemicals and pesticides, over-nutrition and obesity [1, 10]. Poor sperm count in adulthood has been associated with prenatal exposure to maternal smoking during critical periods in male fetus development. Poor sperm count in turn is associated with overall mortality and morbidity among men [10].

Paternal obesity affects both seminal plasma composition and sperm cells (DNA integrity, epigenome, RNA). Research has shown possible pathways how both these factors can alter the metabolic phenotype of the offspring [10]. The World Health Organization (WHO) has estimated that globally, during the past four decades between 1975 and 2016, the proportion of overweight and obese people has increased three times [12].

Developmental Origin of Health and Disease Concept

The Dutch Famine Study was one of the most influential studies to show that human embryos and fetuses are vulnerable to maternal condition, and that the consequences for future health depend on the timing of the stressor [4, 5, 7, 9, 13]. In 1944–5, before the end of German occupation, there was a 5-month period of extreme food shortage in the western part of the Netherlands. Even in these extreme circumstances women conceived (or were already pregnant). It was possible to keep antenatal records of mothers and birth records of children. This allowed scientists decades later to study the adult health of this birth cohort after exposure to their mothers' severe under-nutrition during different stages of gestation [5, 13]. The authors showed that fetuses exposed to malnutrition in late gestation had impaired glucose tolerance 50 years later. Those exposed to the mother's hunger in early gestation had a threefold increase in coronary heart disease, a higher atherogenic lipid profile and obesity and the proportion of people with self-reported poor health was higher [5]. In addition to other studies, it was shown also here that low birth weight and raised blood pressure in adult life were linked [5]. Low birth weight was associated with the famine to which the fetuses were exposed in mid- and late gestation. Babies exposed in early gestation were heavier than those in the control group (not exposed to famine) [5].

East German endocrinologist Günter Dörner proposed the concept (and coined the term) of fetal programming in the 1970s [4]. Another prominent visionary thinker was an outstanding epidemiologist named David Barker (1938–2013) from the United Kingdom; thus the concept of the developmental origins of health and disease (DOHaD), or fetal programming of adult disease, is also widely known as the Barker hypothesis [4, 14, 15]. His ideas inspired researchers in many countries [14, 15].

The evolutionary explanation of the DOHaD concept is based on the evidence of developmental plasticity [4, 16, 17]. Evolutionary plasticity is defined as "the ability of the genotype to produce different phenotypes in response to different environments" in order to have the best chance of survival [16]. Evolved traits that were once advantageous can become maladaptive due to (unexpected) changes in the environment – this is the concept of evolutionary mismatch that explains the conflict with the postnatal environment and diseases later in life [16, 17]. The maximal plasticity occurs during the periconception period and the period of fetal development.

Epigenetic and metabolic reprogramming in very early development and cell division is thought to be one of the major pathways in DOHaD leading to adult disease. Epigenetic mechanisms regulate gene activity without affecting the genetic constitution. The DNA methylation and changes in histone structure are the main epigenetic mechanisms that control imprinting [18]. These are central to cellular differentiation and developmental plasticity [4]. Imprinting takes place in genes that are essential for embryonic growth, placental function and postnatal behavior [18]. Epigenetic inheritance mechanisms ensure cellular memory systems [9]. Another possible important pathway, which affects early division of cells and placenta function, seems to be the effect of inflammation and oxidative stress [1, 9].

Fleming and coauthors published in their 2018 review in the *Lancet* Series 2 ("Origins of Lifetime Health around the Time of Conception: Causes and Consequences") the following figure that gives a comprehensive overview of how different peri-implantation stressors may lead to adult disease (see Figure 8.1) [1].

Additionally, it has been suggested that responses to stressors during peri-implantation period and placental development are sex-specific [16]. It has been shown that sex differences in cell metabolism, epigenetics and gene expression start from the blastocyst stage (5–6 days after conception) [16]. Genes encoded in sex chromosomes seem to have dosage effects on extra-gonadal development, thus affecting the severity of preimplantation stressors on long-term (sex-specific) alterations of the offspring [16].

In 2003 the DOHaD pioneers started the International Society for Developmental Origins of Health and Disease (https://dohadsoc.org). The aim of the society is to promote research into the fetal and developmental origins of disease involving scientists from many backgrounds. Besides other activities the society started to publish the *Journal of Developmental Origins of Health and Disease* in 2010 (https://dohadsoc.org/journal-of-dohad).

Preconception Period

From the perspective of the intervention needed, the preconception period can be defined in several ways [2, 3, 17]. For example, it might take 2 years for an obese person to reach normal weight and instill healthy eating habits (e.g., to eat 5 portions/400 grams of vegetables and fruits per day). In the case of low levels of folate concentrations this might be corrected with folic acid supplementation in the 3 months before conception. Alcohol and smoking can be stopped when the future parents come to the decision of having a baby [2, 3]. However, the reality is that a lot of pregnancies are not planned but still wished. Thus, a healthy lifestyle from the very beginning and throughout life, prevention of communicable and noncommunicable diseases and supporting women during their pregnancies is the basis of the life-course approach to preconception care and a reproductive life plan.

It has been shown that interventions to improve the future child's health that were started only during pregnancy, like micronutrient supplementation or weight correction, had very modest or no expected effect on the progeny [2]. The life-course approach says that the best scenario would be a continuum of healthy habits and improved nutrition in children,

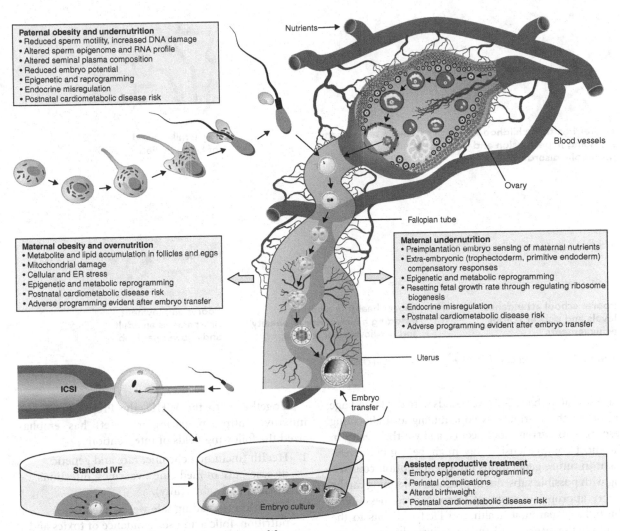

Paternal obesity and undernutrition
- Reduced sperm motility, increased DNA damage
- Altered sperm epigenome and RNA profile
- Altered seminal plasma composition
- Reduced embryo potential
- Epigenetic and reprogramming
- Endocrine misregulation
- Postnatal cardiometabolic disease risk

Nutrients

Blood vessels

Ovary

Fallopian tube

Maternal obesity and overnutrition
- Metabolite and lipid accumulation in follicles and eggs
- Mitochondrial damage
- Cellular and ER stress
- Epigenetic and metabolic reprogramming
- Postnatal cardiometabolic disease risk
- Adverse programming evident after embryo transfer

Maternal undernutrition
- Preimplantation embryo sensing of maternal nutrients
- Extra-embryonic (trophectoderm, primitive endoderm) compensatory responses
- Epigenetic and metabolic reprogramming
- Resetting fetal growth rate through regulating ribosome biogenesis
- Endocrine misregulation
- Postnatal cardiometabolic disease risk
- Adverse programming evident after embryo transfer

Uterus

ICSI

Embryo transfer

Standard IVF

Embryo culture

Assisted reproductive treatment
- Embryo epigenetic reprogramming
- Perinatal complications
- Altered birthweight
- Postnatal cardiometabolic disease risk

Figure 8.1 Peri-implantation stressors and adult disease [1]

adolescents and young people [1, 8, 17, 18]. The role of parents and caretakers and the school environment in selecting a menu and encouraging healthy eating habits in children cannot be overestimated here. A typical diet in high-income countries – high intake of refined sugars, refined grains, high-fat dairy and red meat – leads very often to obesity and there might be at the same time lack of several important nutrients like magnesium, iodine, calcium and vitamins D, A and E [2, 18]. During the past 40 years the number of school-aged obese children and adolescents has increased more than 10 times. Most rapid growth has been noted in low- and middle-income countries [24]. Thus the WHO has highlighted that childhood and adolescent obesity is one of the major health

challenges of the twenty-first century, affecting every country in the world and leading to poorer physical and mental health [19].

The WHO has invited countries all over the world to include immediate action in their public health programs to deal with the increase of obese children [19]. Obesity and overweight in childhood may lead to very different unfavorable consequences (see Figure 8.2) [19].

At the same time, in 2017 it was estimated that globally still more children and adolescents suffered from under-nutrition, being moderately or severely underweight. Under-nutrition takes place also in high-income countries, especially among women and men who suffer from eating disorders. In 2018 it

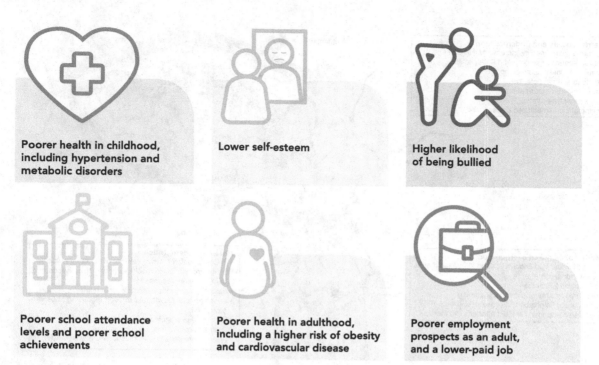

Figure 8.2 Consequences of obesity and overweight in childhood [19]

was estimated that 15–24-year-olds were the largest age cohort in the world, thus contributing and allocating resources to current adolescents' and youths' health in the most comprehensive way might be a good investment in future generations [8]. Contraception counseling with possible subsequent pregnancy planning can be a very appropriate moment to create awareness about the links of parental health and lifestyle habits to the health of the future child and/or existing children and to motivate people to undertake measures on personal level where needed.

Preconception Healthcare: Concepts and Definitions

The WHO has defined preconception care as follows [18]:

> Preconception care is the provision of biomedical, behavioral and social health interventions to women and couples before conception occurs, aimed at improving their health status, and reducing behaviors and individual and environmental factors that could contribute to poor maternal and child health outcomes. Its ultimate aim is improved maternal and child health outcomes, in both the short and long term. [18]

Together with the WHO, the Preparing of Life initiative (https://preparingforlife.net) has emphasized the following fields of intervention:

1 **Health** (including chronic, rare and genetic diseases, use of medicines, vaccines, infectious diseases and subfertility).
2 **Nutrition** (including safe water, adequate nutrition, folic acid use, avoidance of toxics and hygiene).
3 **Lifestyle** (age at pregnancy, inter-pregnancy interval, smoking, alcohol, drugs, violence and female genital mutilation).
4 **Environment** (environmental health and working conditions).

The WHO preconception care package includes timely diagnosis and treatment of communicable diseases like sexually transmitted infections and HIV and timely vaccination against rubella, tetanus and hepatitis B; addressing mental health problems; providing genetic counseling where needed; creating awareness of and providing services for victims of inter-partner violence; preventing and treating complications of female genital mutilation; introducing action to prevent too early, too rapid and unwanted pregnancies [18]. Age-appropriate and comprehensive mandatory sexuality education plays a key role in many areas of the WHO preconception care package, including prevention of inter-partner violence and creating fertility awareness.

In 2018 the United Nations Educational, Scientific and Cultural Organization (UNESCO) published its updated *International Technical Guidance on Sexuality Education* (bit.ly/3WSAInL). Examples of evidence-based interventions in preconception care are described in the WHO preconception care policy brief (bit.ly/3X LxyDS). Specialists in obstetrics and gynecology, sexual medicine, genitourinary medicine, sexually transmitted infections and sexology are in a good position to include elements of this broad view on preconception health-care into their everyday work.

Nutrition

One major focus of the DOHaD concept has been the effect of parents' under- and over-nutrition on adult health, especially on cardiovascular and metabolic noncommunicable diseases of their progeny [2, 4, 5, 8–10, 13, 17]. Every essential micronutrient has its role in human cell metabolism, especially during critical periods of respective tissue or organ development. For example, it is well known that lack of folic acid and vitamin B12 before and during pregnancy can lead to malformations (especially neural tube defects [NTDs]) in the offspring. Mothers and children

exclusively on a vegan diet may lack the needed vitamin B12, iodine, iron, calcium, omega-3 fatty acids and proteins. Advice on how to avoid these deficiencies in vegans can be found on the UK National Health Service website (www.who.int/mediacentre/fa ctsheets/fs394/en). The WHO has defined healthy diet principles in its Fact Sheet 394 from August 2018 [20]. According to the WHO, a healthy diet is based on the following facts (see Figure 8.3) [20]:

The WHO healthy diet advice for adults can be implemented globally, taking into consideration local food availability and eating and cooking traditions (see Figure 8.4) [20].

The first 2 years of a child's life are crucial in many ways. This is the vulnerable time in development when appropriate nutrition ensures healthy growth (including reducing the risk of becoming overweight or obese) and improves cognitive development [20]. According to the WHO, advice on a healthy diet for infants and children is similar to that for adults. At the same time, however, the WHO highlights the following [20]:

- Infants should be exclusively breastfed during the first 6 months of life.
- Infants should be continuously breastfed until 2 years of age and beyond.
- From 6 months of age, breast milk should be complemented with a variety of adequate, safe and

---

Key Facts

- A healthy diet helps to protect against malnutrition in all its forms, as well as noncommunicable diseases (NCDs) such as diabetes, heart disease, stroke and cancer.

- Unhealthy diet and lack of physical activity are leading global risks to health.

- Healthy dietary practices start early in life – breastfeeding fosters healthy growth and improves cognitive development, and may have longer-term health benefits such as reducing the risk of becoming overweight or obese and developing NCDs later in life.

- Energy intake (calories) should be in balance with energy expenditure. To avoid unhealthy weight gain, total fat should not exceed 30% of total energy intake [1–3]. Intake of saturated fats should be less than 10% of total energy intake, and intake of trans fats less than 1% of total energy intake, with a shift in fat consumption away from saturated fats and trans fats to unsaturated fats [3] and toward the goal of eliminating industrially produced trans fats [4–6].

- Limiting intake of free sugars to less than 10% of total energy intake [2, 7] is part of a healthy diet. A further reduction to less than 5% of total energy intake is suggested for additional health benefits [7].

- Keeping salt intake to less than 5 g per day (equivalent to sodium intake of less than 2 g per day) helps prevent hypertension and reduces the risk of heart disease and stroke in the adult population [8].

- WHO member states have agreed to reduce the global population's intake of salt by 30% by 2025; they have also agreed to halt the rise in diabetes and obesity in adults and adolescents as well as in childhood overweight by 2025 [9, 10].

Figure 8.3 The WHO healthy diet principles [20]

For Adults

A Healthy Diet Includes the Following

- Fruits, vegetables, legumes (e.g., lentils and beans), nuts and whole grains (e.g. unprocessed maize, millet, oats, wheat and brown rice).

- At least 400 g (i.e., five portions of fruits and vegetables per day [2], excluding potatoes, sweet potatoes, cassava and other starchy roots.

- Less than 10% of total energy intake from free sugar [2, 7], which is equivalent to 50 g (or about 12 level teaspoons) for a person of healthy body weight consuming about 2,000 calories per day, but ideally is less than 5% of total energy intake for additional health benefits [7]. Free sugars are all sugars added to foods or drinks by the manufacturer, cook or consumer, as well as sugars naturally present in honey syrups, fruit juices and fruit juice concentrates.

- Less than 30% of total energy intake from fats [1–3]. Unsaturated fats (found in fish, avocado and nuts, and in sunflower, soybean, canola and olive oils) are preferable to saturated fats (found in fatty meat, butter, palm and coconut oil, cream, cheese, ghee and lard) and trans fats of all kinds, including industrially produced trans fats (found in baked and fried foods and prepackaged snacks and foods such as frozen pizza, pies, cookies, biscuits, wafers and cooking oils and spreads) and ruminant trans fats (found in meat and dairy foods from ruminant animals such as cows, sheep, goats and camels). It is suggested that the intake of saturated fats be reduced to less than 10% of total energy intake and trans fats to less than 1% of total energy intake [5]. In particular, industrially produced trans fats are not part of a healthy diet and should be avoided [4, 6].

- Less than 5 g of salt (equivalent to about one teaspoon) intake per day [8]. Salt should be iodized.

Figure 8.4 The WHO healthy diet advice for adults can be implemented globally [20]

nutrient-dense foods. Salt and sugar should not be added.

Further reading: World Health Organization. Healthy Diet – Fact sheet No. 394. 2018 (www.who.int /publications/m/item/healthy-diet-factsheet394).

Anemia, Folic Acid, Vitamin B12

It has been estimated that anemia prevalence is similar in the United States, Canada and Northern Europe – around 4% for men and 8% for women [21]. Globally iron deficiency might affect 30–50% of pregnant women, including women in high-income countries [2]. Pregnant adolescents have remarkably increased iron requirements for their own growth and the growth of the fetus; they might have less access to antenatal care [22]. According to the WHO, anemia can be diagnosed in premenopausal females when their hemoglobin level is less than 12 grams per deciliter (g/dl) [21].

Folate is naturally found in leafy vegetables, egg yolks, legumes, some citric fruits and liver. Folic acid is a synthetic compound used in fortified staples or as a supplement. Naturally occurring folate has lower bioavailability than folic acid. The most common causes of macrocytic anemia are deficiency of folate and vitamin B12 [23]. Folate status can be influenced by several unfavorable factors: enzyme methylenetetrahydrofolate reductase (MTHFR) 677CàT gene polymorphism; physiological status like age, pregnancy and lactation; biological factors like coexisting vitamin B6 and B12 status; homocysteine levels; comorbidities like malaria; limited intake of folate sources with food and low socioeconomic status [23]. Assessment of serum folate and red blood cell folate concentrations is useful for monitoring folate status. Globally, it is witnessed and scientifically proven that fortification of staple foods with folic acid is associated with remarkable decrease in NTDs [23].

The WHO has summarized the following nutrition-related health problems, problem behaviors and risk factors that contribute to maternal and childhood mortality and morbidity and that are important in the context of preconception care (see Figure 8.5) [18].

Thyroid Disease, Iodine Supplementation

Iodine is essential for thyroid hormone production. Regionally daily dietary consumption can vary widely since iodine is derived from everyday food. It has been advised that supplementary oral intake of 150 μg of iodine (potassium iodide) should be started around 3 months before planning pregnancy [24]. Women who are on levothyroxine treatment do not need supplemental iodine [24].

Health problems/ problem behaviors/ risk factors	Contribution to maternal mortality and morbidity	Contribution to childhood mortality and morbidity
Folic acid insufficiency		Neural tube defects, other birth defects
Iron-deficiency anemia	Maternal morbidities and mortality	Child mortality, low birth weight, preterm birth, low child cognition (intelligence quotient)
Maternal underweight, often combined with low stature	Complications during pregnancy and delivery, nutrient deficiencies (potentially resulting in obstetric complications)	Preterm birth, low birth weight, stillbirth, type 2 diabetes and cardiovascular disease in later life
Maternal overweight and obesity	Preexisting type 2 diabetes, hypertensive disease of pregnancy, gestational diabetes, hypertensive and thromboembolic disorders, postpartum hemorrhage and anemia, caesarean delivery, induction of labor, instrumental delivery, shoulder dystocia	Birth defects, neural tube defects, preterm delivery, stillbirth, macrosomia
Untreated diabetes mellitus (type 2 and gestational)	Type 2 diabetes, spontaneous abortion, worsening of existing microvascular complications, urinary tract and other infections, preterm labor, obstetric trauma, caesarean section, hypertension, preeclampsia, gestational diabetes mellitus, obstetric trauma, caesarean section, preeclampsia	Birth defects, stillbirth, macrosomia with shoulder dystocia/nerve palsy if delivered vaginally, hypoglycemia after birth, type 2 diabetes in later life
Iodine		Abortion, stillbirth, mental retardation, cretinism, increased neonatal/infant mortality, goiter, hypothyroidism
Calcium	Maternal eclampsia, preeclampsia	

Figure 8.5 The WHO has summarized nutrition-related health problems that are important in preconception care [18]

Normal thyroid function is essential for healthy pregnancy; both hypo- and hyperthyroidism are associated with adverse obstetrical and fetal outcomes [24, 25]. It has been estimated that the prevalence rate of hypothyroidism is 2–3%, hyperthyroidism 0.1–0.4% and thyroid autoimmunity up to 17% [24, 25]. Although being common conditions, according to the extensive American Thyroid Association (ATA) guidelines from 2017, there is insufficient evidence to recommend for or against universal screening for thyroid disease (thyroid-stimulating hormone (TSH) and/or thyroid autoimmunity) before or in early pregnancy [24].

The ATA guidelines advise that all women seeking pregnancy should undergo clinical evaluation. Testing for serum TSH is recommended when any of the following risk factors are found [24]:

1. A history of hypothyroidism/hyperthyroidism or current symptoms/signs of thyroid dysfunction.
2. Known thyroid antibody positivity or presence of a goiter.
3. History of head or neck radiation or prior thyroid surgery.
4. Age older than 30 years.
5. Type 1 diabetes or other autoimmune disorders.
6. History of pregnancy loss, preterm delivery or infertility.
7. Multiple prior pregnancies (≥ 2).
8. Family history of autoimmune thyroid disease or thyroid dysfunction.
9. Morbid obesity (BMI ≥ 40 kg/m^2).
10. Use of amiodarone or lithium, or recent administration of iodinated radiologic contrast.

11. Residing in an area of known moderate-to-severe iodine insufficiency.

Mental Health

In the framework of preconception care, mental health issues are as important as healthy nutrition. Mental health is interlinked with damaging lifestyles like smoking and psychoactive substance abuse, eating disorders leading to under- or overnutrition, teenage pregnancies, unwanted pregnancies and contracting a sexually transmitted infection. Maternal mental health disorders are associated with adverse obstetric, neonatal and childhood physical and mental health outcomes [8]. Interpersonal violence and violence experienced in childhood very often lead to mental health problems. Thus the WHO preconception care package includes the following interventions [18]:

Assessing psychosocial problems

- Providing educational and psychosocial counseling before and during pregnancy.
- Counseling, treating and managing depression in women planning pregnancy and other women of childbearing age.
- Strengthening community networks and promoting women's empowerment.
- Improving access to education for women of childbearing age.
- Reducing economic insecurity of women of childbearing age.

Tobacco and Psychoactive Substance Use

There is a lot of evidence of the unfavorable effects of alcohol consumption and smoking during pregnancy. Fetal alcohol syndrome is associated with lifelong disability. Smoking is associated with higher risk of infertility and preterm births and can affect male fetuses' fertility in the future [2, 10, 18]. The WHO has proposed the following list of actions [18]:

- Screening of women and girls for substance and tobacco use.
- Providing brief tobacco cessation advice, pharmacotherapy (including nicotine replacement therapy, if available) and intensive behavioral counseling services.
- Treating substance use disorders, including pharmacological and psychological interventions.

- Providing family-planning assistance for families with substance use disorders (including postpartum and between pregnancies).
- Establishing prevention programs to reduce substance use in adolescents.

Vaccine-Preventable Diseases

Common sense says that it is good to be healthy before and during pregnancy and to remain in good shape after delivery as well. Thus vaccination contributes largely to better maternal and child health as a good means to prevent all diseases where vaccines are efficient and available.

Rubella Vaccination

All non-pregnant women of reproductive age who are not already vaccinated or who are seronegative for rubella should receive one dose of rubella-containing vaccine (RCV) [26]. One dose of RCV is $\geq$ 95% effective. The RCV should not be given to people with active tuberculosis or severe immunodeficiency. Rubella vaccination should be avoided during pregnancy because of the theoretical risk of teratogenicity. It is advisable to avoid getting pregnant during the month after vaccination. However, vaccination is not an indication for terminating the pregnancy [26]. According to the WHO, rubella vaccination can be done no sooner than 3 months after receiving blood products. It is advisable to avoid administration of blood products for 2 weeks after vaccination. All health workers should be vaccinated with RCV.

Tetanus Vaccination

Birth-associated tetanus follows unhygienic deliveries and abortions when the woman has not been vaccinated. Neonatal tetanus occurs after usage of contaminated instruments to cut the umbilical cord or dirty materials to cover the umbilical stump. Lifelong protection can be achieved with six doses – three primary doses during childhood and three boosters during adolescence – of tetanus-toxoid-containing vaccine (TTCV) through the routine childhood immunization schedule [27]. Immunity is antibody-mediated and depends on the ability of tetanus-specific antibodies to neutralize tetanospasmin. Use of TTCV combinations with diphtheria toxoid is strongly encouraged by the WHO [27]. Newborns can be protected from birth-associated tetanus by maternal tetanus immunization that leads to specific IgG antibody production and generally highly efficient trans-placental transfer of the antibodies to the developing fetus [27].

Pregnant women for whom vaccination history is not clear should receive at least two doses of TTCV with an interval of 4 weeks between the doses and the second dose at least 2 weeks before delivery [27]. A third dose should be given at least 6 months later to ensure protection for a minimum of 5 years. In order to ensure lifelong protection a fourth and fifth dose should be given at intervals of at least 1 year or during subsequent pregnancies [27].

Hepatitis B Vaccination

Safe and effective vaccines against hepatitis B have been available since 1982. According to the WHO, in 2015 global coverage with three doses of hepatitis B vaccine during infancy reached 84% [28]. A primary three-dose series induces protective antibody concentrations in more than 95% of healthy infants, children and young adults. For delayed schedules, including for children, adolescents and adults, three doses are recommended, with the second dose administered at least 1 month later and the third dose 6 months after the first [28].

Human Papilloma Virus Vaccination

Immunization of girls before their sexual debut is considered to be the best prevention measure for cervical cancer and precancerous lesions; thus the WHO has emphasized that HPV vaccines should be included in national immunization programs. All three licensed HPV vaccines – bivalent, quadrivalent and nonavalent – have excellent safety, efficacy and effectiveness profiles [29]. Population-level analysis of the prevention of adverse pregnancy outcomes after 8 years of a national HPV vaccination program was carried out in Australia [30]. This analysis showed that reduction in preterm births and small-for-gestational-age infants took place where maternal vaccination coverage reached 60–80% [30].

References

1. Fleming TP, Watkins AJ, Velazquez MA et al. Origins of lifetime health around the time of conception: Causes and consequences. *Lancet.* 2018;**391**:1842–52.

2. Stephenson J, Heslehurst N, Hall J et al. Before the beginning: Nutrition and lifestyle in the preconception period and its importance for future health. *Lancet.* 2018;**391**:1830–41.

3. Campaigning for preconception health. *Lancet.* 2018;**391**(10132):1749–1864.

4. Gluckman PD, Hanson MA, Buklijas T. A conceptual framework for the developmental origins of health and disease. *J Dev Orig Health Dis.* 2010;**1**:6–18.

5. Painter RC, Roseboom TJ, Bleker OP. Prenatal exposure to the Dutch famine and disease in later life: An overview. *Reprod Toxicol.* 2005;**20**:345–52.

6. Sharpe RM. Programmed for sex: Nutrition–reproduction relationships from an inter-generational perspective. *Reproduction.* 2018;**155**:S1–S16.

7. Fleming TP, Velazquez MA, Eckert JJ. Embryos, DOHaD and David Barker. *J Dev Orig Health Dis.* 2015;**6**:377–83.

8. Patton GC, Olsson CA, Skirbekk V et al. Adolescence and the next generation. *Nature.* 2018;**554**:458–66.

9. Rando OJ, Simmons RA. I'm eating for two: Parental dietary effects on offspring metabolism. *Cell.* 2015;**161**:93–105.

10. Fleming TP. The remarkable legacy of a father's diet on the health of his offspring. *Proc Natl Acad Sci USA.* 2018;**115**:9827–9.

11. Levine H, Jørgensen N, Martino-Andrade A et al. Temporal trends in sperm count: A systematic review and meta-regression analysis. *Hum Reprod Update.* 2017;**23**:646–59.

12. World Health Organization. Obesity and overweight. 2020. bit.ly/3wF9GpC.

13. Lumey LH, Stein AD, Kahn HS et al. Cohort profile: The Dutch Hunger Winter families study. *Int J Epidemiol.* 2007;**36**:1196–1204.

14. Olsen J. David Barker (1938–2013): A giant in reproductive epidemiology. *Acta Obstet Gynecol Scand.* 2014;**93**:1077–80.

15. Cooper C. David Barker (1938–2013). *Nature.* 2013;**502**:304–10.

16. Pérez-Cerezales S, Ramos-Ibeas P, Rizos D et al. Early sex-dependent differences in response to environmental stress. *Reproduction.* 2018;**155**:R39–R51.

17. Barker M, Dombrowski SU, Colbourn T et al. Intervention strategies to improve nutrition and health behaviours before conception. *Lancet.* 2018;**391**:1853–64.

18. World Health Organization. Meeting to develop a global consensus on preconception care to reduce maternal and childhood mortality and morbidity: World Health Organization Headquarters, Geneva, 6–7 February 2012: Meeting report. bit.ly/3ReygqK.

19. World Health Organization. *Taking action on childhood obesity report.* Geneva: World Health Organization, 2018. bit.ly/40bHeZI.

20. World Health Organization. Healthy diet: Fact sheet No. 394. 2018. www.who.int/mediacentre/factsheets/fs394/en.

21. Freeman AM, Rai M, Morando DW. Anemia screening. In *StatPearls*. Treasure Island, FL: StatPearls, 2020. www.ncbi.nlm.nih.gov/books/NBK499905.

22. World Health Organization. Global nutrition targets 2025.Anaemia policy brief. https://apps.who.int/iris/handle/10665/148556.

23. World Health Organization. *Serum and red blood cell folate concentrations for assessing folate status in populations: Vitamin and mineral nutrition information system*. Geneva: World Health Organization, 2015. bit.ly/3RijjUz.

24. Alexander EK, Pearce EN, Brent G et al. Guidelines of the American Thyroid Association for the diagnosis and management of thyroid disease during pregnancy and the postpartum. *Thyroid*. 2017;27:315–89.

25. De Leo S, Pearce EN. Autoimmune thyroid disease during pregnancy. *Lancet Diabetes Endocrinol*. 2018;6:575–86.

26. World Health Organization. Summary of key points from WHO position paper on rubella vaccines. July 2020. bit.ly/3HfiKWZ.

27. Tetanus vaccines: WHO position paper. February 2017. *Wkly Epidemiol Rec*. 2017;92:53–76.

28. Hepatitis B vaccines: WHO position paper. July 2017. *Wkly Epidemiol Rec*. 2017;92:369–92.

29. Human papillomavirus vaccines: WHO position paper. May 2017. *Wkly Epidemiol Rec*. 2017;92:241–68.

30. Yuill S, Egger S, Smith M et al. Has human papillomavirus (HPV) vaccination prevented adverse pregnancy outcomes? Population-level analysis after 8 years of a national HPV vaccination program in Australia. *J Infect Dis*. 2020;222:499–508.

The Reproductive Endocrinology of Contraception

9

Sven O. Skouby and Kresten Rubeck Petersen

Introduction

The provision of quality reproductive health services and education, access to reliable and safe contraception, and safe abortion services and post-abortion care, are important to empower women to achieve their goals and ambitions, avoid unwanted pregnancy and ensure any pregnancy occurs at the right time for them. The introduction of the first oral contraceptive pill in 1960 sparked a movement to put women in control of their sexual and reproductive health through the use of effective modern methods of contraception. A number of technological developments and advances in the understanding of hormones between the 1930s and 1950s made the first steps toward a hormonal contraception possible; understanding of the effects of steroid hormones was advanced, progesterone was characterized, and the first synthetic progestin (norethindrone/ norethisterone) was developed.

Since then, reproductive technology has advanced our understanding of the benefits and potential side effects of traditional oral hormonal products, first and foremost venous thrombotic events. A wide variety of present and possible future endocrinological contraceptive methods have become available [1]. This has enabled women to choose the method that is right for them in different reproductive life phases and making management of common gynecological conditions safer and more cost-effective.

The Hypothalamic-Pituitary-Ovarian Axis

Ovarian maturation and its exquisite cyclic function during the reproductive lifespan fully rely on the coordinate action of the neurohormonal elements of the hypothalamic-pituitary-ovarian (HPO) axis. Therefore, insight into the physiology of the reproductive tract is fundamental for understanding the reproductive endocrinology of current hormonal contraception and paves the way for clinical applications of future refinements via biologic and pharmacologic manipulation of the female reproductive process to control fertility.

The decapeptide gonadotropin-releasing hormone (GnRH) is released in a pulsatile manner to the hypothalamic-hypophyseal portal circulation to reach the anterior pituitary, where GnRH pulses act on gonadotropes, to elicit the secretion of both gonadotropins, luteinized hormone (LH) and the follicular-stimulating hormone (FSH). These, in turn, are released to the systemic circulation to reach the ovary, where, acting in concert on different cellular components, they promote ovarian maturation and production and release of the oocyte, as well as the secretion of sex steroids and other gonadal hormones of peptidergic nature (Figures 9.1–9.3).

Various studies have greatly clarified the interrelationship of the HPO. It is now well established that GnRH must reach the anterior pituitary in episodic pulses approximately every 90 minutes to elicit a normal response. The secreted GnRH has a very short half-life (2–4 minutes), allowing for a rapid decay of the stimulus. The diverse external and internal factors regulating GnRH do so through a complex network of neurotransmitters and neuropeptides in the central nervous system (CNS) and hypothalamus.

In humans, inactivating mutations of two of these neuropeptides, kisspeptin and neurokinin B, or their cognate receptors results in a failure to progress through puberty and in adult infertility, highlighting the crucial role of these neuro peptides in GnRH neuron activation. Dysregulation of GnRH pulsatility is to a varying degree implicated in well-known reproductive pathologies such as polycystic ovary syndrome (PCOS) and hypothalamic amenorrhea [2]. Identification and synthesis of GnRH and its analogues have prompted the use of these agents for suppression of endogenous FSH and LH before follicle stimulation in in vitro follicular (IVF) therapy.

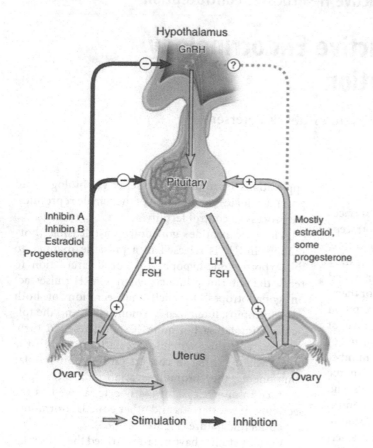

Figure 9.1 The reproductive cycle requires interactions (complex feedback mechanisms) between the hypothalamus, pituitary, and ovaries as indicated in this simplified diagram. CNS: central nervous system; GNRH: gonadotropin-releasing hormone; FSH: follicle-stimulating hormone; LH: luteinizing hormone

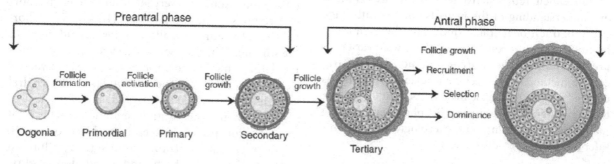

Figure 9.2 Follicular development (adapted from [23])

Continued administration of GnRH agonists leads to an initial phase of stimulation of pituitary gonadotropin release, followed by a shut down of pituitary gonadotropin release, resulting in transient chemical castration. Receptor-binding studies have shown that the effect is owing to a decrease in the number of GnRH receptors on the pituitary gonadotropes, not to an alteration in the affinity of the receptors to GnRH. However, large numbers of reports on experimental and clinical studies have documented that both agonistic and antagonistic GnRH peptides are potent inhibitors of the reproductive process as now adapted as routine in assisted reproductive therapy (ART).

Triggered by the experience from ART, extensive clinical studies have been performed to test the

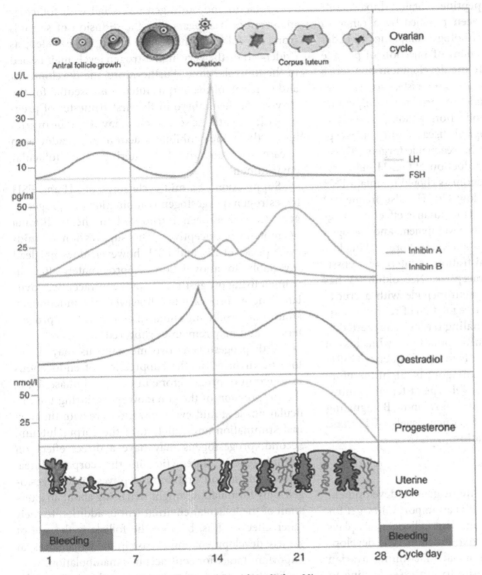

Figure 9.3 The ovarian and uterine cycles (adapted from [24], p. 80)

contraceptive potential of GnRH agonists with a variety of dosage regimens. There appears to be a great deal of individual variation to a given dose of these agents. With daily therapy at sufficiently high doses, complete ovarian inhibition, anovulation, and amenorrhea can be obtained. With progressively lower doses, lesser effects, characterized by oligo-ovulation and a clinical syndrome similar to abnormal uterine bleeding, may be observed – that is, the clinical spectrum of induced ovarian insufficiency produced by these agonistic peptides depending on dosage and duration of use may range from total

amenorrhea approximating castration to infrequent periods, to acyclic bleeding, to intermittent and unpredictable ovulation, to anovulation.

Therefore, use of GnRH analogues for contraception has so far been disappointing. Moreover, complete FSH and LH suppression, although effective for providing contraception, is associated with a hypoestrogenic state, which leads to unacceptable vasomotor symptoms, vaginal atrophy, and loss of bone mineral density.

In contrast to GnRH-agonists, GnRH-antagonists induce a direct block of GnRH receptor with a rapid decrease in LH and FSH, preventing LH surge. The development of non-peptide, orally bioavailable GnRH antagonists has been pursued by a range of pharmaceutical or biotechnology companies in order to overcome the requirement of injection of peptide antagonists. Thus, despite the development of a series of smallmolecule GnRH antagonists, so far, no attempts have been made to produce non-peptide agonists for clinical application although sex steroid–dependent gynecological diseases and contraceptive possibilities seem to be reachable targets [3].

Although unproven, reduction of GnRH pulse frequency by kisspeptin antagonists should maintain FSH levels (still favored by a low GnRH pulse frequency) while reducing LH levels. This putative effect of antagonists would allow follicle development and estrogen production but inhibit ovulation, therefore making kisspeptin antagonist administration an interesting possibility as a female contraceptive. Neurokinin B has emerged as also a novel neuropeptide with a crucial role in the neuroendocrine regulation of reproduction.

Loss of kisspeptin signaling has been suggested to lead to a major loss of GnRH pulsatility, while loss of neurokinin B signaling leads to low-frequency GnRH pulsatility. Neurokinin B antagonists might therefore also have potential as a novel type of female contraception, as disruption of neurokinin B signaling maintains FSH levels but reduces levels of LH and potentially prevents ovulation [4].

Ovary

Because the ovary is the site of gamete development and release in the female, it is an important target for contraceptive manipulation. The follicogenesis plays a central role in reproductive function. The development of a healthy and normal functioning ovarian follicle is in fact prerequisite to processes leading to ovulation and conception. The ovarian follicle is actively involved in the process of steroidogenesis and biosynthesis of a number of proteins and peptides such as inhibin and activin.

Prostaglandins, which are involved in ovulation, are also found in follicular fluid of preovulatory follicles after an LH surge. Potential intra-ovarian intercellular communication may take place by paracrine or autocrine action. The dominant preovulatory follicle has a precise hormonal milieu. It is conceivable that a disturbance of this environment might lead to follicular atresia or anovulation. Follicular fluid is rich in steroid hormones and the steroid concentration in follicular fluid greatly exceeds that in blood.

Prolactin and androgen levels fall with follicular maturation. It appears that the diffusion of steroids from the follicular fluid into blood is restricted, as evidenced by the very high estrogen levels maintained in the follicular fluid. Furthermore, the development and function of the corpus luteum is essential for the survival of the embryo in the first trimester of pregnancy [5]. Synthetic sex steroids may affect the ovaries indirectly by their inhibitory action on gonadotropin release or directly by altering the follicular environment.

Suppression of a mid-cycle surge of LH and FSH by, estrogen–progestogen combinations or progestogens alone has been introduced in the traditional hormonal contraceptives. The suppression of mid-cycle peaks of LH and FSH, however, does not lead invariably to anovulation. Approximately 40% of women using progestin-only oral contraceptives ovulate. These corpora lutea, however, are functionally abnormal, producing subnormal amounts of progesterone, and may remain unruptured.

With progestogens two mechanisms may therefore be involved in the suppression of endogenous production of progesterone in the luteal phase. First, the suppression of the gonadotropins during the follicular phase at mid-cycle may interfere with the normal stimulation and function of the corpus luteum. Second, progestogens may have a direct effect on steroidogenesis (luteolytic) in the corpora lutea. Both combination oral contraceptives and progestogen-only formulations might well bring about an alteration of the follicular environment in addition to their other effects. Thus, because the follicle is the site of gamete development and release in the female, it is an important target for contraceptive manipulation.

Furthermore, the development and function of the corpus luteum are essential for the survival of the conceptus in the first trimester of pregnancy. Suppression of a mid-cycle surge of LH and FSH by estrogens, estrogen–progestogen combination, or progestogens alone has already been alluded to. Corpora lutea have been found in the majority (85%) of women receiving small daily doses of progestogens. These corpora lutea, however, are functionally abnormal, producing subnormal amounts of progesterone.

In recent years, much research has been devoted to the identification and possible function of nonsteroidal ovarian factors. These substances play an important role in modulating intra-ovarian function and in fine-tuning gonadotropin action. Among putative intra-ovarian regulators, several have received considerable attention and may conceivably be a target for fertility regulation. Insulin-like growth factor-I (IGF-I) is a polypeptide involved in amplification of gonadotropin hormonal action. Recent information indicates that IGF-I, which is produced by granulosa cells, binds to the interstitial cells that are not a site of IGF-I gene expression but are endowed with receptors. Thus, it appears that IGF-I may engage in intra-compartmental communication in the interest of coordinated follicular development [3].

Contraceptive Implications

Primordial follicle activation, the first step of folliculogenesis, is independent of gonadotropins or steroids. It has been shown that anti-Müllerian hormone (AMH) can completely block primordial follicle activation, representing a unique mechanism of contraception that spares the pool of quiescent primordial follicles (ovarian reserve). The dominant preovulatory follicle has a precise hormonal milieu. It is conceivable that a disturbance of this environment might lead to follicular atresia or anovulation.

Both combination oral contraceptives and progestogen-only formulations might well bring about an alteration of the follicular environment in addition to their other effects. Follistatin injected into several animal species has been shown to prevent FSH secretion and follicular growth. Similarly, inadequate formation or maintenance of corpora lutea might result from local overproduction of luteinization inhibition factor. Currently, the factors influencing the control of synthesis and release of follicular peptide are not well understood, but considerable efforts are being made to obtain such information [6].

As already mentioned, the ovarian GnRH receptors may be considered an excellent potential target for contraception. The GnRH and its agonists may affect the ovarian function in two different ways [1]. Chronic stimulation of pituitary gonadotropes by potent GnRH agonists may cause cellular desensitization with a subsequent decrease in circulating gonadotropins [2]. The GnRH may directly suppress ovarian steroidogenesis, ovulation, and corpus luteum function. Similarly, the GnRH antagonists can block pituitary gonadotropin secretion. Thus, timed administration of GnRH agonists or antagonists can block ovulation, follicular development, or corpus luteum function, depending on the phase of the cycle when the drug is administered

Interference with Corpus Luteum Function

Corpus luteum function is essential for implantation of the conceptus and its further development in the first 8 weeks of gestation. Thereafter, the hormonal burden for the maintenance of pregnancy is shifted to the placenta. Disruption of luteal function may prevent implantation. After implantation, induction of luteolysis is likely to cause an arrest of fetal development and abortion. Studies in experimental animals and in humans have shown that GnRH analogues may exert luteolytic activity. For example, administration of GnRH agonists to Rhesus monkeys 3–5 days post ovulation has been found to cause a significant shortening of the luteal phase and a decrease in serum progesterone values. Administration of human chorionic gonadotropins (hCGs) prevented the shortening of the luteal phase in animals treated with the analogue. In rats, administration of GnRH antagonists interferes with pregnancy. In monkeys, however, initial attempts to alter early pregnancy with GnRH antagonists have not been successful. In humans as well, GnRH analogues induce luteolysis when given 5–8 days after the LH peak. The early corpus luteum seems to be refractory to luteolytic activity of the agonists [3].

Interference with Follicular Rupture

The precise sequence of events leading to follicular rupture and extrusion of oocytes has not been clarified. In several animal species, including human primates, prostaglandin $F_{2\alpha}$ and prostaglandin E2 may play an important role. Prostaglandin synthetase inhibitors such as indomethacin and ibuprofen have been shown to prevent follicular rupture and ovulation after hCG administration, while the ovaries continue to undergo luteinization.

Furthermore, prostaglandins have luteolytic activity, so their administration in the early luteal phase may interfere with the function of corpus luteum and prevent survival of the conceptus. Vascular endothelial growth factor (VEGF) and angiopoietin are involved in angiogenesis. Angiogenesis is crucial for follicular growth and corpus luteum function. Antagonists to these two factors, when injected into the preovulatory follicle of primates, suppressed ovulation and luteinization in monkeys.

Fallopian Tubes

Oviducts have several major functions in human reproduction: transporting spermatozoa to the site of fertilization, picking up the ovum, and transporting the conceptus to the uterus. Additionally, the fallopian tubes are the sites of fertilization and cleavage, and tubal secretion may be important for nutrition and development of the embryo. Interference with any of these functions might provide contraception. Surgical interruption of the tubes is one of the most widely used techniques of permanent sterilization.

Delivery of pharmacologically active agents or sclerosing substances to occlude the fallopian tube has many attractive features Unfortunately, all are in an experimental stage, and none have undergone extensive clinical trials. The current need is to integrate the delivery system with a safe, effective agent that consistently produces tubal closure. The tubal fluid, composed of serum transudate and specific secretion containing some unique proteins, is regulated quantitatively and qualitatively by ovarian sex steroids.

The tubal mucosa is made of ciliated and nonciliated secretory cells. Nonciliated cells are responsible for tubal secretion, whereas ciliated cells are believed to be involved in gamete transport. The function of these cells is also regulated by estrogen and progesterone. Finally, tubal contractions are known to be important in facilitating the mixing of tubal contents, helping to denude the ovum, promoting fertilization by increasing egg–sperm contact, and regulating egg transport [7].

Nonsteroidal agents, such as gonadotropins, prostaglandins, and other drugs influencing the contraction of smooth muscles can also alter egg transport and the action of the ampullary, isthmic, and uterotubal junctions. These compounds may accelerate or impede the rate of egg transport. If inhibition or modification of tubal cilia beat and/or tubal motility result in an effective contraceptive is still an open question [8].

Endometrium

In the normal ovulatory cycle the endometrium responds to fluctuations in plasma levels of estradiol and progesterone by characteristic morphological changes. If conception does not occur, the corpus luteum degenerates, resulting in a rapid decline in the levels of estradiol and progesterone. This leads to a local inflammatory process in the endometrium with an influx of leucocytes followed by an increase of cytokines, proteases, and chemochines. Subsequently, the interstitial supporting collagen breaks down, which in turn impairs the local blood supply, leading to

thrombosis and loss of endometrial integrity, and the endometrium is shed as menstruation.

After menstruation, the endometrium proliferates as a result of the estrogen produced in the granulosa cells of the growing follicle. The number of estrogen receptors increases, numerous mitoses can be observed, and the individual cell increases in size, as does the nuclear–cytoplasmic ratio. The endometrial glands grow rapidly and become tortuous and the endometrial thickness increases up to 10 fold in 12–14 days along with the preovulatory increase in estradiol.

After ovulation, progesterone secreted from the corpus luteum inhibits the proliferation and initiates a gradual transformation of the endometrium, which makes it suitable for implantation. The stroma gets edematous and the glandular cells accumulate glycogen and other substances in secretory granulae, which is secreted into the glandular lumina, giving the endometrium a characteristic "secretory" histological appearance. Simultaneously, the endometrial arterioles undergo endothelial proliferation and develop a coiling appearance resulting in the formation of the spiral arterioles, which are essential for nourishing the trophoblastic tissue after implantation [9, 10]. The effects of exogenous sex steroids on the endometrium depends on the type of hormonal compound, its dose, and duration of use. The net result tend to transform the endometrium into a state that impairs implantation [11].

Cervix

As the endometrium, the cervical mucus is subjected to changes in the hormonal levels during the ovulatory cycle. The preovulatory rise in estrogen alters the composition and structure of the cervical mucus, making it thin and watery with the characteristic properties of ferning (crystal formation) and spinnbarkeit (stretchability). These changes make the cervical canal readily permeable for spermatozoas, but when progesterone increase after ovulation, the mucus become thick and viscous and the sperm is unable to pass [12].

The inhibiting effect on sperm migration of progestogens is utilized in hormonal contraception and all progestogens have similar effects on the cervical mucus which contributes to their contraceptive effect even if the primary effect may be linked to their ability to inhibit ovulation Women using the progestogen-only pill (POP) and the levonorgestrel-releasing IUD may have ovulatory cycles and these methods exert their primary contraceptive effect in the cervical canal.

Only a few studies have thoroughly examined the effects of POPs on cervical mucus but 2 hours after intake there seems to be a sharp decline in sperm penetration. This effect disappears after 22–24 hours where normal penetration is restored. These findings underlie the recommendation of pill intake as close to 24-hour interval as possible and that a pill taken more than 3 hours late should be considered missed. The effect on cervical mucus in IUD users seem to be fully established after 3–5 days after insertion and there seems to no difference in the effects of the IUDs containing different doses of levonorgestrel [13].

New Knowledge of Hormonal Contraception

Combined Oral Hormonal Contraceptives

Combined oral contraceptives (COCs) are currently used by about 100 million women worldwide. According to United Nations (UN) statistics produced in 2003 (www.un.org/esa/population/publications/contraception), about 48% of women of fertile age in Western Europe were using oral contraceptives while in Japan, where COCs were licensed in 1999, only 1% of women are currently using the pill. Two remarkable changes have occurred over the past four decades. First, there has been a significant reduction in the estrogen component, which is generally ethinyl estradiol.

Second, there have been attempts to find new, safe progestins with various affinities to progesterone, estrogen, androgen and mineralocorticoid receptors. The main goal has been to increase the safety of COCs, particularly by decreasing the risk of venous thromboembolism (VTE). Combined oral contraceptives are well-known inhibitors of the HPO axis [14]. Repeated cyclic administration of mestranol, the 3-methyl ether of ethinyl estradiol, has been shown to suppress both FSH and LH plasma levels.

Inhibition of pituitary gonadotropins is effected at the level of hypothalamus and pituitary. Ethinyl estradiol (50 µg/day), given from day 5 through day 24 of the cycle, causes an abolition of the mid-cycle surge of serum FSH and LH. In sufficient doses, estrogen–progestogen COCs suppress plasma FSH and LH while eliminating the mid-cycle surge. The difference between follicular- and luteal-phase levels of FSH and LH is usually preserved. When administered together, estrogen–progestogen combination has synergistic effects on the HPO axis and can provide effective contraception with as little as 20 µg of ethinyl estradiol or less when combined with progestins in doses two to times as high as required for inhibition of ovulation.

A significant issue with lower doses of ethinyl estradiol is the formation of ovarian cysts owing to less suppression of FSH. The true incidence and clinical impact of this finding is unknown. The endometrial effects of COCs with low doses of ethinyl estradiol and various type of progestogens are primarily linked to the progestogen. During the first cycles of use, the proliferation and maturation of the glandular cells are inhibited and the glands become straight or slightly coiled with increased amount of stroma between them. After prolonged use both the glands and the stroma become atrophic, the secretion of the glands stops and the vessels become thin and dilated and fail to develop the features of spiral arterioles. The progestogens typically used in combined hormonal contraception do not seem to have distinct individual histological features [15].

Patches

The transdermal combined estrogen/progestin contraceptive patch (Ortho Evra/Evra) was approved by the FDA for use in the United States in 2002. The patch is 20 cm^2 (4 5 cm) and delivers 20 mg/ day of ethinyl estradiol (EE) and 150 mg/day of norelgestromin (a biologically active metabolite of norgestimate). The dosing is one patch weekly for 3 consecutive weeks followed by a patch-free week. The patch may be applied to the buttock, abdomen, upper outer arm, or upper torso, excluding the breasts. Mean serum concentrations of hormone are not affected by heat, humidity, exercise, or cold-water immersion. The observed contraceptive failure was 0.7 per 100 woman-years (95% confidence interval [CI], 0.31–1.10), but was higher in women with body weight higher than 90 kg. The transdermal contraceptive is well tolerated and has a side-effect profile similar to COCs. Even though the patch releases less ethinyl estradiol than the pill daily, the area under the curve for ethinyl estradiol concentration over 3 weeks was 71% higher than while taking the pill [16].

Intravaginal Rings

A combined estrogen/progestin contraceptive vaginal ring (CVR) (NuvaRing; Organon USA, Roseland, NJ) w as approved by the FDA for use in the United States in 2001. This contraceptive device consists of a flexible ring made of ethylene vinyl acetate copolymer with an outer ring diameter of 54 mm and a cross-sectional diameter of 4 mm. The vaginal ring releases approximately 120 mg of etonogestrel (a biologically active metabolite of desogestrel) and 15 mg of EE per day [9].

The CVR is used for 3 weeks continuously followed by a 1-week, ring-free period to allow for regular menstrual bleeding. The advantage for the user is that the CVR is not fitted. The Population Council has developed a ring that releases 15 mg of ethinyl estradiol and 150 mg of nestosterone daily. It is effective for more than a year and should be kept in place for 3 weeks, then removed for 1 week and then reinserted again for 3 weeks. Thus, this ring would eventually be much more cost-effective than NuvaRing [17].

Progestogens

The suppressive effect of progestogens alone on FSH and LH release depends on the type and dosage of the steroid used. Progestins used for contraception are derived from either one of two parent compounds, namely progesterone and testosterone. Neither of the parent compounds is efficacious for contraceptive use. Progesterone is poorly absorbed and undergoes extensive hepatic metabolism during the first pass. Even micronized progesterone, which has become available in recent years, is not well absorbed. Instead, progestins structurally related to progesterone and testosterone have proved efficacious for oral contraception. Two important progestins structurally related to testosterone are norethisterone and levonorgestrel. These 19-norprogestins have served as substrates for the synthesis of other contraceptive steroids. Progestins structurally related to norethisterone include norethynodrel, lynestrenol, norethindrone acetate, and ethynodiol diacetate.

Three derivatives of levonorgestrel represent a more recent group of orally active progestins; these include desogestrel, norgestimate, and gestodene. In the 1990s, these progestins were classified as third-generation progestins, which is a confusing classification. It is based mainly on the historical development and may be appropriate for 19-nortestosterone derivatives like desogestrel and gestodene. Also norgestimate has been included in that group, although it is metabolized to norgestrel.

Instead, some old progestins like cyproterone acetate and newer progestins like dienogest and drospirenone are compounds with different molecular structures, and should not be considered 'third-generation progestins/COCs' [18].

Progestogens in low doses (e.g., levonorgestrel 30 mcg or norethisterone 300 mgd daily) have the cervical mucus as the primary target for the contraceptive effect and ovulation is usually intact. The compounds may, however, effect the endometrium and during short-term use the changes are mainly seen in the secretory phase where the glands may not develop properly and the stroma lack the normal edematous appearance. In long-term use, the endometrium become more atrophic. The endometrial effects of POPs that suppress ovulation (e.g., desogestrel 75 mcg taken continuously) are more pronounced, resulting in atrophy with long-term use.

Long-Acting Contraceptive Steroids

These methods comprise a subdermal inserted implant (Nextplanon) and a subcutaneous or intramuscular injection (Depo-Provera). The implant is a rod 4 cm long and 2 mm in diameter containing etonorgestrel, the active metabolite of desogestrel, which is released at a rate of 0.06 mg/day falling to 0.03 mg/day during the second and third year. It is approved for 3-year use. The progestogen depot contains medroxyprogesterone acetate in a dose of 150 mg (intramuscular) or 104 mg (subcutaneous). Both injections are given in 3-month intervals.

The contraceptive effect of the parenterally administered progestogens is primarily due to a blocking of the preovulatory LH-surge, leading to inhibition of ovulation, but both methods have effects on the endometrium and the cervical mucus as well. Both preparations induce amenorrhea in a significant number of users due to the effect on the endometrium [19].

Levonorgestrel-Releasing Intrauterine Devices

The contraceptive effects of these devices are due to the combined effect of a foreign body reaction in the endometrium caused by the device itself and the continuous secretion of levonorgestrel, which the affects the endometrium as well as the cervical mucus. In addition to the effect on the uterus itself, the presence of high local LNG concentration impairs the migration and maturation of the spermatozoas. The common findings in endometrial biopsies from women using the in LNG-IUD releasing 20 mcg/day are glandular atrophy, decidualization, and infiltration of inflammatory cells in the stroma. The changes are more pronounced in endometrium close to the device where the concentration of hormone is expected to be higher. Recently, IUDs with reduced hormonal release (but similar contraceptive efficacy) have been introduced, but it is not known if their effects on the endometrium and sperm function are reduced correspondingly [20].

Progesterone Receptor Modulators

At present two progesterone **receptor modulators** (PRMs) are in clinical use – mifepristone and ulliprstal acetate. During long-term use, they induce a number of changes known as PRM-associated endometrial changes (PAEC), which include cystically dilated glands with features of the proliferative as well as the secretory phase along with abnormal stromal vasculature [21].

Mifepristone is extensively used in medical abortion and not as a contraceptive despite findings of high contraceptive efficacy during continuous use as well as postcoital contraception. In contrast, ulliprstal acetate is in common use as a postcoital contraceptive and both compounds have proven effective by prevention the LH surge when given in the proliferative phase but also when given postovulatory. This is in contrast to the common emergency contraceptive regimen of 1.5 mg levonorgestrel, which is effective only when given preovulatory. It has not been determined how the endometrial effects of PRMs contribute to this effect [22].

Conclusion

There are more contraceptive choices available than ever before. To educate healthcare providers as to the methods available and to inform and educate consumers are cornerstones for successful contraception. Development of new contraceptives for the female depends on a thorough knowledge of the anatomy and physiology of the reproductive tract. Recent advances in our understanding of ovarian endocrinology, coupled with molecular biology and transgenic technology, have enabled identification of several factors that are functionally critical in the regulation of female fertility.

Progress in the area of female reproduction is showing great promise for identifying new contraceptive drug targets that need to be further explored. The development of a nonsteroidal contraception is being vigorously pursued in several laboratories but as yet is still in the preclinical phase. Worldwide, female sterilization is the most widely used method of contraception, as about 30% of families rely on that method. About 20% of women are using an intrauterine device, and slightly less than 20% are using hormonal contraception. About 20% are using nothing.

During almost 60 years of use of COCs, the doses of steroids have decreased remarkably, and although thromboembolic complications are considered rare, about 40 000–50 000 VTEs can still be calculated to occur annually among current users. Thus, despite the developments that improved the safety profile of COCs, adverse metabolic, vascular effects and possible neoplastic effects of COCs remain and therefore necessitate efforts to develop nonsteroidal and nonhormonal, contraceptives progestin-only contraception has retained popularity: POPs and progestin-containing implants, intrauterine devices, injectables, and vaginal rings make it possible to individualize the contraceptive method. In conclusion: while the pharmaceutical development of new contraceptive agents is continuing, sadly with declining resources, the remaining major global challenge is insufficient distribution of available contemporary methods in developing countries.

References

1. DiMarco CS, Speroff L, Glass RH, Kase NG (eds.). *Clinical gynecologic endocrinology and infertility*. 6th edition. Baltimore, MD: Lippincott, Williams & Wilkins, 1999.
2. Moghissi KS. Gonadotropin releasing hormones: Clinical applications in gynecology. *J Reprod Med*. 1990;35(12):1097–1107.
3. Moghissi KS. Vulnerable targets for contraception in the female. *Global Libra Women's Med FIGO*. 2009.
4. Skorupskaite K, George JT, Anderson RA. The kisspeptin–GnRH pathway in human reproductive health and disease. *Hum Reprod Update*. 2014; 20(4):485–500.
5. Adashi EY. Intraovarian peptides: Stimulators and inhibitors of follicular growth and differentiation. *Endocrinol Metab Clin of North Am*. 1992; 21(1):1–17.
6. Chengalvala MV, Meade Jr. EH, Cottom JE et al. Regulation of female fertility and identification of

future contraceptive targets. *Curr Pharm Des*. 2006; **12**(30):3915–28.

7. ES H. Transport of spermatozoa in the female reproductive tract. *Am J Obstet Gynecol*. 1973; **115**(5):703–17.

8. Lyons RA, Saridogan E, Djahanbakhch O. The reproductive significance of human Fallopian tube cilia. *Hum Reprod Update*. 2006;**12**(4):363–72.

9. Deligdisch L. Hormonal pathology of the endometrium. *Mod Pathol*. 2000;**13**(3):285–94.

10. Salamonsen LA. Tissue injury and repair in the female human reproductive tract. *Reproduction*. 2003;**125**(3):301–11.

11. Hickey M, Salamonsen LA. Endometrial structural and inflammatory changes with exogenous progestogens. *Trends in Endocrinology and Metabolism*. 2008;**19**(5):167–74.

12. Han L, Taub R, Jensen JT. Cervical mucus and contraception: What we know and what we don't. *Contraception*. 2017;**96**(5):310–21.

13. Ortiz ME, Croxatto HB. Copper-T intrauterine device and levonorgestrel intrauterine system: Biological bases of their mechanism of action. *Contraception*. 2007;**75**(6 Suppl):S16–30.

14. Erkkola R. Recent advances in hormonal contraception. *Curr Opin Obstet Gynecol*. 2007;**19**(6):547–53.

15. Baird DT, Collins J, Cooke I et al. Ovarian and endometrial function during hormonal contraception. *Hum Reprod*. 2001;**16**(7)1527–35.

16. Burkman RT. Transdermal hormonal contraception: Benefits and risks. *Am J Obstet Gynecol*. 2007; **197**(2):134.e1–6.

17. Brache V, Faundes A. Contraceptive vaginal rings: A review. *Contraception*. 2010;**82**(5):418–27.

18. Sitruk-Ware R, Nath A. The use of newer progestins for contraception. *Contraception*. 2010;**82**(5):410–17.

19. Jacobstein R, Polis CB. Progestin-only contraception: Injectables and implants. *Best Pract Res Clin Obstet Gynaecol*. 2014;**28**(6):795–806.

20. Apter D, Gemzell-Danielsson K, Hauck B, Rosen K, Zurth C. Pharmacokinetics of two low-dose levonorgestrel-releasing intrauterine systems and effects on ovulation rate and cervical function: Pooled analyses of phase II and III studies. *Fertil Steril*. 2014;**101**(6): 1656–62.

21. Wagenfeld A, Saunders PTK, Whitaker L, Critchley HOD. Selective progesterone receptor modulators (SPRMs): Progesterone receptor action, mode of action on the endometrium and treatment options in gynecological therapies. *Expert Opin Ther Targets*. 2016;**20**(9):1045–54.

22. Jadav SP, Parmar DM. Ulipristal acetate: A progesterone receptor modulator for emergency contraception. *J Pharmacol aPharmacother*. 2012; **3**(2):109–11.

23. Araû VR, Gastal MO, Figueiredo JR, Gastal EL. In vitro culture of bovine prenatal follicles: A review. *Reprod. Biol. Endocrinol*. 2014;**12**:78. https://doi.org/10.1186/1477-7827-12-78.

24. Andersen AN, Ernst E, 2011. Gynækologisk Endokrinologi. In Ottesen B, Mogensen O, Forman A (eds.), *Gynækologi*. 4th edition. Copenhagen: Munksgaard Danmark, 2011.

Evidence-Based Clinical Practice in Contraceptive Counselling and Care

Sarah Sultana-Grixti, Olivia Anne Cassar, and Charles Savona-Ventura

Introduction

The provision for access to contraceptive counselling and advice is today considered a basic human right. The 1994 United Nations International Conference on Population and Development (ICPD) held in Cairo emphasized 'the right of men and women to be informed and to have access to safe, effective, affordable and acceptable methods of family planning of their choice'. The guarantee that all individuals, particularly women, have access to available contraceptive information that is of good quality and coercion free opens the path towards gender equality while allowing women to control their life choices and fully participate in their community. The ICPD further reaffirmed that 'the aim of family-planning programmes must be to enable couples and individuals to decide freely and responsibly the number and spacing of their children and to have the information and means to do so and to ensure informed choices and make available a full range of safe and effective methods' [1].

The availability of free access is particularly essential for vulnerable and marginalized groups such and adolescents, people with disabilities, minority communities and women in violent relationships or in conflict/post-conflict regions. Individuals, whatever their circumstances, have a right to be considered equal within society and not be subject to any form of discrimination. These principles underpin the right to access to information and services relating to contraception. Healthcare service providers are therefore obliged to ensure that every individual, whatever the age, has easy access to the full range of contraceptive methods without any imposed legal or informational constraints. Individuals should have the facility to make a free choice based on proper and correct counselling. There should be absolutely no place for any form of coercive practice when information and services for contraceptive advice is being sought [2].

It has been observed that at least one in four women wishing to practise contraception is not using a suitably effective contraceptive method, while 82% of unintended maternities are the result of unmet contraceptive needs. Providing effective access to contraception services would prevent about 22 million unwanted maternities and 25 million terminations of undesired pregnancies. It would also prevent 150,000 maternal deaths annually from complications arising from terminations [2].

Principles of Professional Counselling

The American Counselling Association in 2010 defined professional counselling as 'a professional relationship that empowers diverse individuals, families, and groups to accomplish mental health, wellness, education, and career goals' [3]. The key principle in this definition is empowerment. The counsellor should serve as a medium to assist the individual to come to a self-made well-informed decision or choice. The counsellor, after due assessment of the client, should therefore provide a comprehensive picture of the topic under consideration in an emphatic, warm and supportive environment without allowing personal values and beliefs to influence or in any way coerce the client's decision-making. The consultation should therefore serve to allow clients to confront the issue, assume responsibility and ultimately reach a resolution [4].

Counselling should involve a number of steps leading to the decision-making stage. This stage, depending on the circumstances, can be followed up by an evaluation and re-assessment stage if required. The first stage of the counselling consultation leading to the decision-making stage should follow four steps: (1) Attempt to establish a rapport with the client where the client feels genuinely accepted and free to discuss the issue without feeling in any way judged. (2) Undertake a full assessment of the presenting issues and interrelated factors exploring issues such as medical conditions, interpersonal relationships, family history, financial constraints and religious outlook. (3) Present targeted but unbiased background information relating to the issue in an understandable format outlining the benefits and disadvantages of one course of action in general and in the client's particular identified circumstances. (4) Allow the client to identify the management option most suited to the circumstances.

Counselling is very relevant to a contraceptive-advice seeking consultation. In such a scenario, it is essential to allow the client to feel at ease with the counsellor while allowing the counsellor to learn more about the particular circumstances of the client. Social and medical issues could very well reduce the effectiveness or increase the risks of a contraceptive option – information that needs to be pointed out to the client as part of the background information about contraception. The client can then be assisted to identify the best acceptable contraceptive method suitable for the circumstances.

Potential Effects of Healthcare Provider Attitudes

It is now widely acknowledged that the overall attitude, knowledge and beliefs of the healthcare provider leading the contraception consultation can significantly influence the decision made by the patient receiving the information. This, however, is a difficult area to assess and study. The healthcare professional providing contraceptive advice varies from country to country and from one healthcare setting to another.

The professional status of the healthcare provider leading a contraceptive consultation may range from a healthcare educator or a midwife to a family doctor or even a gynaecologist. The cultural and religious background of the individual leading the consultation may also directly or indirectly influence the way information is imparted.

This provider bias became more visible after a landmark paper in 1992, when Shelton et al. tried to describe the many types of provider bias which can influence how different people present and recommend different methods to different patients [5]. Such intentional or unintentional healthcare provider bias will have a direct effect on which method of contraception the client ultimately chooses but could indirectly lead to a failure to meet the client's needs and preferences.

Several studies have shown that healthcare provider bias is broadly subdivided into client-related and/or method-related factors [6]. These two factors are further influenced by provider-related bias arising from social and cultural norms. These types of bias can be exacerbated by the hierarchical medical model where the belief that the healthcare professional knows better can limit respect for the client and his or her wishes when it comes to making an informed choice [7]. The professional healthcare counsellor must ensure that such biases are eliminated from the consultation.

Client-Related Bias

Client-related bias in a counselling session refers to a situation where the provider imposes unjustified restrictions on the use of certain methods by the clients based on their age, marital status, parity, disabilities, having HIV or seeking permanent methods of contraception. This bias can be intentional, resulting from the counsellor's cultural perceptions – for example, religious beliefs – or unintentional, resulting from the counsellor's level of expertise and knowledge – for example, dealing with specific medical situations.

Most counsellors providing contraception advice, like in every other counselling situation, will tend very often subconsciously to categorize the client sitting across the desk into stereotypes. This can affect communication during the consultation and thus ultimately influence the clinical decisions taken [8]. An example of such a stereotyping bias is the belief that providing contraception to young teenage girls will lead to promiscuity and thus increase the risk of sexually transmitted disease.

This stereotyping may cause the healthcare provider to emphasize advice regarding a particular contraceptive method when the client's needs may actually be better served with another. Such stereotyping may be more prevalent in certain countries where it has been shown to have a potentially significant influence in the provision of contraception, sometimes leading to its denial.

Method-Related Bias

Method-related bias refers to particular perceptions the healthcare counsellor may have towards the different types of contraceptives. These perceptions may be the result of personal experiences or beliefs, inaccurate knowledge or inadequate skills, as well as perceived ease or difficulty in providing a particular method. The commonest method-related bias is the belief that fertility-awareness-based methods of contraception are completely useless and are quickly discarded, if mentioned at all, during the consultation, which concentrates mainly on medical methods of contraception, ignoring the fact that the failure rate of these methods is equivalent to that of spermicides (24.0% vs. 28.0%) [9].

Another common method-related bias relates to the belief that the Cu-IUCD acts primarily as an abortifacient, causing it to be completely shunned by prolife counsellors who ignore the scientific evidence showing that the primary mode of action of the device is to prevent fertilization rather than implantation [10], or that long-term use of the device predisposes to pelvic infection and subsequent infertility and hence should only be used by parous women [11].

In the spirit of providing a comprehensive picture of the topic to allow clients to reach their own decision, the healthcare counsellor should provide information about all the available methods of contraception, outlining fairly and accurately their mode of action, any potential complications associated with their use and the respective failure rates while pointing out any existing medical issues that may increase the client's risks from use (see Table 10.1).

Contraception Counselling

The Bruce Quality of Care Framework has been a guide for the design and delivery of services within the field of contraception [12]. It defines six elements of family planning services that together constitute quality:

Table 10.1 Failure rates of different contraceptives [9]

	Failure rate *
Fertility-awareness based methods	24.0%
Spermicides	28.0%
Barrier methods (male and female condoms, diaphragm, sponge)	12.0–24.0%
Oestrogen–Progestogen contraceptives (oral, patch, vaginal ring, injectable)	9.0%
Progestogen contraceptives (oral, depot)	6.0–9.0%
Etonogestrel implant	0.05%
Levonorgestrel-releasing intrauterine system (LGN-IUS)	0.2%
Copper-bearing intrauterine contraceptive device (Cu-IUCD)	0.8%
Female sterilization	0.5%
Male sterilization	0.15%

* Percentages reflect the number of unintended pregnancies within the first year of typical use.

1. Choice of methods: different people have different needs and demands. Also, people themselves and their preferences change over time. Having the possibility to change method is a cornerstone of a satisfied and continued use of contraceptive methods.
2. The provision of accurate information that is tailor-made to the client's intentions and health.
3. Technical competence: women should not bear the consequences of poor provider technique. The provider requires regular training to make sure that such skills are maintained.
4. Improved interpersonal relations by providers: training in communication skills is essential for providers of care in family planning.
5. Mechanisms that encourage continuity of care should be in place.
6. Appropriate constellation of services that reach beyond conventional concepts in contraception but support women in maintaining their health – for example, diagnosis and treatment of sexually transmitted infections and screening for reproductive coercion and domestic violence.

The WHO adds nine human rights principles to guide family-planning services and providers [13].

1. Non-discrimination. Personal judgments, negative opinions or client related bias should be set aside.
2. Availability of contraceptive information and services. As described earlier, the provider may be prone to method-related bias. Information on any method should not be held back.
3. Accessible information and services. Everyone, including adolescents and people with disabilities, should be able to avail themselves of the services.
4. Acceptable information and services. Information and services should be provided in such a way that is acceptable for the client.
5. Quality. Knowledge and skills should be kept up to date.
6. Informed decision-making.
7. Privacy and confidentiality.
8. Participation. Clients should be asked what they think of the services provided and act on what they said in order to improve care.
9. Accountability: Providers should hold themselves accountable for the care clients are provided and ensuring that their rights are preserved.

Contraceptive Counselling Intervention Types

Many different contraceptive counselling intervention types have been developed for modern contraceptive methods (Table 10.2).

The effectiveness of these individual interventions is still a matter of debate as it very much depends on the setting and the targeted population. Different interventions have different impact on consultation length, which in itself has costs related to human resources. Counselling satisfaction with digital tools alone tends to be low but can greatly decrease provider time when offered prior to the consultation (e.g., in the waiting room). Telephone and video-based interventions have the advantage of providing access to women at a relatively low cost. It can, however, require many attempts to reach a single patient and patients without phones, a change in numbers or software, including smartphone apps or equipment, may make it difficult to reach patients. Counselling interventions during pregnancy, puerperium or in women seeking abortion can reach women who might be unlikely to access healthcare at a later stage. Involving the male partner in counselling can be important when the main contraceptive decision maker is the male. However, partner availability may pose a logistical challenge [14]. The COVID-19 pandemic has had an unforeseen impact on family-planning services. It has surely seen an increased use of digital tools, telephone and video-based interventions. Their role in healthcare and in family-planning counselling is likely to increase.

Communication Issues

Relational communication centres primarily around the establishment of a positive relationship between the healthcare provider or contraception counsellor

Table 10.2 Counselling intervention types

- Paper or digital decision-making tools (e.g., WHO)
- Structured face-to-face counselling
- Telephone counselling
- Video counselling
- Antenatal/immediate post-partum counselling
- Post-partum counselling
- Women undergoing abortion-related counselling
- Systematic counselling outside family-planning services
- Partner counselling
- Community-based interventions

and the patient. Effective relational communication is based on the following key concepts: the development of a feeling of confidence between the counsellor and client, the building up of an impression of trustworthiness of the healthcare professional and shared decision-making. The contraception counsellor has to recognize that contraception is a highly personal decision relating to intimate issues that effect sexuality and future fertility. The healthcare provider may feel conflict between wanting to respect the patient's autonomy in making an informed choice (empowered counselling) and the wish to encourage women to opt for the highly effective methods (directive counselling). Contraception counselling should involve unbiased task-oriented communication providing essential information concerning diagnosis and treatment. This should address issues related to side effects, risks and efficacy of the various contraceptive methods and any particular issues particularly relevant to the client (contingency counselling) (Table 10.3).

Addressing Social Disparities and Prejudices

Any perception of discrimination by the client, irrespective of the counsellor's intentions, will potentially lead to a lack of trust in the healthcare provider and influence decision-making related to suitable contraception choice. The contraception counsellor should adapt and modify the communication approach so that it caters for the needs of different sub-populations and minority groups [8]. Data from ethnic minority groups show that, when compared to Caucasian patients, African-Caribbean were less likely to experience patient-centred communication and to report understanding all that their counsellor had to say, receive less information and experience shorter clinic visits. Such situations may require the involvement of a culturally acceptable translator during the session, though this may raise other communication issues.

An alternative is to supplement the counselling session with patient information leaflets in the language of the client's choice [14]. Adolescent young women also need a targeted unbiased approach to deal with the specific issues related to the choice of contraceptive method. Access to contraceptive information in these young women can be difficult due to social barriers. Digital decision-making tools have a special role to play in this age group as they generally are well versed in the use of technology [15].

Disparities may also be due to geography. People living in remote areas or areas with limited networks

Table 10.3 Communication issues in contraceptive counselling

Side effects and risk	• Essential to promote the concept of informed choice and helps with increasing continuation rates of the contraceptive method chosen.
	○ Provide anticipatory guidance about common issues associated with the method – for example, menstrual changes.
	○ Provide accurate information regarding any concerns the patient may have about any particular method – for example, thrombotic risks.
Efficacy	• Provide information about the failure rates of the chosen contraceptive option/s.
	○ This information must be provided in a way that can be appreciated by the client – for example, stating that 2 out of a 1,000 LNG-IUS users will become pregnant over the course of 1 year is more likely to be understood than simply stating that the LNG-IUS has a failure rate of 0.2%. Alternatively, a visual chart with the information can be made available – for example, WHO tiered counselling [13].
Contingency counselling	• It is essential to identify and address any particular issues the client may have. This may have various facets but may relate to:
	○ financial aspects
	○ provision of emergency measures if the chosen contraceptive option fails or is misused
	○ misconceptions regarding personal fecundity, especially in women who may have had past reproductive health issues
	○ protection afforded by the chosen contraceptive method against sexually transmitted infections – only barrier methods offer protection against them.
	○ issues related to reproductive coercion where the partner tries to maintain control in a relationship through pressure to become pregnant or interference with contraceptive methods. Harm-reduction strategies, such as the use of IUDs, subdermal implants or the depot-injection, may help the woman to remain autonomous and in control of her reproductive function [8].

to central areas may find it difficult to access information and services related to family planning. Solutions to such problems are complex, but even these women have a right to a family-planning service. These women deserve not to be forgotten. Community-based interventions, often by non-governmental organizations, are often necessary in such areas. Decision-making tools, digital or otherwise, may be helpful in areas where it may be difficult to access healthcare professionals.

Practice Guides to Counselling: The GATHER Approach

The GATHER approach to counselling can be used as an aide-memoire to increase patient satisfaction during consultation [16].

- **G-GREET** the client in a welcoming and respectful manner.
- **A-ASK** the client about their contraceptive needs and assess for other health-related issues.
- **T-TELL** them about different contraceptive options and methods.
- **H-HELP** them come to a decision and choose the method best suited to them.
- **E-EXPLAIN** and demonstrate how to use the method. Outline any issues that they might have

with that chosen method and how to deal with such issues.

- **R-RETURN/REFER** A follow-up visit should be scheduled straightaway. Offer information or ways to access information on that chosen method if the client is having issues. Discuss ways the client can contact the service provider in case of emergency. The provider should take the opportunity to assess whether the women needs to be referred to any other services.

Conclusion

Overcoming barriers and biases is key to effective contraception counselling. Such barriers can be overcome by the development of excellent communication skills, addressing social disparities and prejudices during the consultation and using information technology to overcome physical barriers to face-to-face contact.

References

1. International Conference on Population and Development (ICPD). Programme of Action of the International Conference on Population and Development, Cairo, Egypt, 5–13 September 1994, ch. VII, para. 7.2, 7.12, U.N. Doc. A/CONF.171/13/ Rev.1 (1995).

2. Center for Reproductive Rights. *The right to contraceptive information and services for women and adolescents*. New York: Center for Reproductive Rights, 2010.

3. Kaplan DM, Tarvydas VM, Gladding ST. 20/20: A vision for the future of counselling. *Journal of Counseling & Development*. 2014;**92**:366–72.

4. Lambert M, Barley DE. Research summary of the therapeutic relationship and psychotherapy outcome. *Psychotherapy Theory Research & Practice*. 2001;**38**(4):357–61.

5. Shelton JD, Jacobstein RA, Angle MA. Medical barriers to access to family planning. *Lancet*. 1992;**340**(8831):1334–5. https://doi.org/10.1016/0140-6736(92)92505-A. Pmid: 1360046.

6. Solo J, Festin M. Provider bias in family planning services: A review of its meaning and manifestations. Global Health: Science and Practice, September 2019. GHSP-D-19-00130. https://doi.org/10.9745/GHSp-D-19-00130.

7. Calhoun LM, Speizer IS, Rimal R et al. Provider imposed restrictions to clients' access to family planning in urban Uttar Pradesh, India: A mixed methods study. *BMC Health Serv Res*. 2013;**13**(1):532. https://doi.org/10.1186/1472-6963-13-532. Pmid:23465015.

8. Dehlendorf C, Krajewski C, Borrero S. Contraceptive counseling: Best practices to ensure quality communication and enable effective contraceptive use. *Clinical Obstetrics and Gynecology*. 2014;**57**(4):659–73. https://doi.org/10.1097/GRF.0000000000000059.

9. Gavin L, Moskosky S, Carter M et al. Providing quality family planning services: Recommendations of CDC and the U.S. Office of Population Affairs. *Morbidity and Mortality Weekly Report: Recommendations and Reports*. 2014;**63**(4):1–54.

10. Stanford JB, Mikolajczyk RT. Mechanisms of action of intrauterine devices: Update and estimation of postfertilization effects. *Am J Obstet Gynecol*. 2002;**187**:1699–1708.

11. Hubacher D. Intrauterine devices & infection: Review of the literature. *Indian J Med Res*. 2014;**140**(Suppl 1):S53–S57.

12. Bruce J. Fundamental elements of the quality of care: A simple framework. *Studies in Family Planning*. 1990;**21**(2):61–91. https://doi.org/10.2307/19666691.

13. World Health Organization, Department of Reproductive Health and Research and Johns Hopkins Bloomberg School of Public Health/Center for Communication Programs, Knowledge for Health Project. *Family planning: A global handbook for providers (2018 update)*. Geneva: World Health Organization, Department of Reproductive Health and Research and Johns Hopkins Bloomberg School of Public Health/Center for Communication Programs, Knowledge for Health Project, 2018.

14. Cavallaro FL, Benova L, Owolabi OO et al. A systematic review of the effectiveness of counselling strategies for modern contraceptive methods: What works and what doesn't? *BMJ Sex Reprod Health*. 2019;**0**:1–16. Published Online First: 11 December 2019. https://doi.org/10.1136/bmjsrh-2019-200377.

15. Bitzer J, Abalos V, Apter D, Martin R, Black A for Global CARE Group. Targeting factors for change: Contraceptive counselling and care of female adolescents. *European Journal of Contraception and Reproductive Health Care*. 2016;**21**(6):417–30. https://doi.org/10.1080/13625187.2016.1237629.

16. Rinehart W, Rudy S, Drennan M. GATHER guide to counseling. *Popul Rep J*. 1998;**48**:1–31.

Combined Hormonal Contraception

Gabriele S. Merki-Feld and Frans J. M. E. Roumen

Pharmacologic Properties and Metabolic Effects of Contraceptive Hormones

Combined hormonal contraceptives (CHCs) contain a combination of an oestrogen and a progestin. On the European market they are available as a pill, vaginal ring or patch. Researchers recognised decades ago that the oestrogen component in the form of ethinylestradiol (EE) has a significant impact on the coagulation system which causes an increase in the risk of arterial and venous thromboembolic events. To reduce this risk, low-dose CHC have been developed containing ≤ 35 µg of EE. Higher-dose preparations should not be used anymore.

The progestin compounds have also been modified over the decades in order to reduce adverse events and negative impacts on metabolic parameters like glucose and lipid metabolism. Older progestins exert unfavourable adverse events related to their affinity to the androgen receptor. Modern progestins have been developed with minimal androgenic or even anti-androgenic effects (Table 11.1).

The plasma level of EE varies significantly from individual to individual and, to a smaller extent, also within the same individual. This explains why certain adverse events occur in some – but not all – patients. Very low plasma levels might be a problem, for example, in cases of drug–drug interaction or severe obesity.

Mechanism of Action

Combined hormonal contraceptives prevent ovulation and reduce follicular growth by inhibition of gonadotropin secretion. The progestin compound is the main inhibitor of ovulation, produces an endometrium which is not receptive to implantation, thickens the cervical mucus and influences secretion and peristalsis of the tube. The oestrogen compound provides stability of the endometrium and reduces the risk of unscheduled bleeding. Very low-dose pills (EE < 30 µg) are associated with more breakthrough bleeding. Combined hormonal contraceptives are typically used in regimens of 21/7 days or 24/4 days. During the pill-free interval withdrawal bleeding should occur.

Oestrogens in Combined Hormonal Contraceptives

Today CHCs are used with EE, estradiol or estradiol-valerate. Ethinylestradiol is very potent as, related to the 17α-ethinyl-group, this molecule is metabolised very slowly. It can therefore be applied in the very low dose of µg, whereas estradiol is dosed in mg. Upon oral administration EE is absorbed in the upper intestinal tract, which can take from 1 to 2 hours [1]. The fact that EE is so difficult to metabolise means it has a major impact on the liver. It increases the synthesis of certain clotting factors and fibrinolytic factors, sexual-hormone-binding globulin (SHBG), high-density lipoprotein (HDL) cholesterol, very-low-density lipoprotein (VLDL) and angiotensinogen.

The changes in the clotting system increase the probability of developing a blood clot in the venous or arterial system. This risk is modified by the progestin in CHCs and is not lower for CHCs with more natural oestrogen like estradiol and estradiol-valerate. Transvaginal and transdermal applications have the same strong impact on liver proteins [1].

Progestins Typically Used in Combined Hormonal Contraceptives

Progestins in CHCs are used in dosages sufficient for inhibition of ovulation and transformation of the endometrium. Progestins bind with high affinity to progestin receptors, but also to other steroid receptors (Table 11.1). This is the reason they exert a variety of non-gestagenic effects. Those can be used from the clinician to reduce adverse events and/or to optimise

Table 11.1 Progestins used in contraception and their pharmacologic properties

Progestin	Generation	Dose for inhibition of ovulation (mg)	Androgenic activity	Anti-androgenic effect	Anti-mineralo-corticoid effect	Glucocorticoid effect
Derived from Nortestosteron						
Norethisterone	1	0.4	++	−	−	−
Levonorgestrel	2	0.06	+	−	−	−
Norgestimat	3	0.2	(+)	−	−	−
Desogestrel/Etonogestrel	3	0.06	(+)	−	−	−
Gestoden	3	0.04	(+)	−	−	−
Dienogest		1.0	−	+	−	−
Derived from Progesterone						
Medroxyprogesterone acetate		n.a.	(+)	−	−	+
Chlormadino acetate		1.7	−	+	−	+
Cyproterone acetate		1.0	−	++	−	+
Derived from spironolactone						
Drospirenone	4	2.0	−	+	+	−

benefits according to the needs of an individual woman. Oestrogens up-regulate progestin receptors and insofar reinforce the effects of progestins.

Metabolic Effects of Combined Hormonal Contraceptives

Most metabolic effects of CHCs are associated with the strong effect of EE on the liver, of which some are modified from the progestin.

Plasma Lipids

Modern low-dose CHCs with second-, third- or fourth-generation progestins cause minimal, not clinically relevant alterations in triglycerides, HDL and low-density lipoprotein (LDL) cholesterol. It is believed that the oestrogen component of CHCs protects against atherosclerosis. Arterial events are typically thromboembolic events [2]. In women with dyslipidaemia and atherosclerotic plaques CHCs increase the risk of myocardial infarction and therefore are not a first choice [3].

Coagulation System

Oestrogens increase a variety of clotting factors in a dose-dependent manner. Some fibrinolytic factors are increased as well; these changes induce an imbalance in the coagulation system which exposes CHC users to an increased risk of venous thromboembolism (VTE), lung embolism (LE) or a clot in the arterial system (ischemic stroke or myocardial infarction). In young women without risk factors the absolute risk for such an event is very low but increases in a multiplicative way for women with cardiovascular risks. The progestin component modifies the VTE risk [4].

Carbohydrate Metabolism

In contrast to high-dose CHCs, low-dose CHCs do not have a clinically meaningful impact on glucose or insulin plasma levels. The CHCs do not produce diabetes mellitus and may be used by women with well-controlled diabetes mellitus [5].

Endocrine System

Ethinylestradiol induces the formation of SHBG, cortisol-binding globulin (CBG) and thyroid-binding globulin (TBG). Sexual-hormone-binding globulin binds to free testosterone in the plasma. This results in lower levels of free testosterone but not total testosterone. Progestins with androgenic partial effect will to a certain extent antagonise the increase of SHBG.

Cortisol-binding globulin and free cortisol are elevated in CHC users. Total thyroxine is also increased in CHC users, probably as a consequence of the higher levels of TBG, but free thyroxine levels are within the normal range [4].

Clinical Characteristics of Combined Hormonal Contraceptives

Use and Efficacy

Combined hormonal contraceptives are highly efficient if they are used correctly. Most products are applied for 21 days, followed by a 7-day pill-free interval (PFI). Some products with < 30 μg EE are also used in a regimen with 24 days of use with a 4-day PFI. The lower dosages do not have a negative impact on efficacy if the pill is used correctly. They might, however, reduce oestrogen withdrawal symptoms and further reduce the duration of withdrawal bleeding. On the other hand more unscheduled bleeding may occur. Some women might prefer to use their pills in an extended cycle regimen. This is mostly a 63/7 day regimen which may cause more breakthrough bleeding. The impact of a long-term regimen on the risk for breast cancer is not yet known. The combined patch is effective for 1 week. The regimen for use is to apply one 7-day patch weekly for 3 weeks, followed by a patch free week thereafter (21/7 days). The vaginal ring is used for 21 days followed by a break of 7 days (21/7).

The efficacy of CHCs is measured in the Pearl Index (PI), which describes the number of pregnancies in 100 women using this method over 12 months. The PI highly depends on the correct daily use of the pill. Enzyme-inducing drugs might have a negative impact on efficacy. Mostly two PIs are reported – one for correct use and one for typical use. Typical use PIs are mostly much better in European populations than in studies performed in other parts of the world [6]. The combined pill, the vaginal ring and the patch are highly efficient, with a PI of 0.3 (Table 11.2).

Benefits

Combined hormonal contraceptives have a broad range of non-contraceptive benefits (Table 11.3). They can be used to treat women with gynaecologic conditions like dysmenorrhoea, heavy menstrual bleeding, acne and endometriosis. While most CHCs improve dysmenorrhea, formulations containing a progestin with a strong effect on the endometrium, like desogestrel or gestoden,

Table 11.2 Contraceptive failure rates of combined hormonal and other contraceptives [7]

Method	% of women experiencing an unintended pregnancy within first year of use	
	Typical use	Perfect use
No method	85	85
Spermicides	28	18
Condom male	18	2
Diaphragm	12	6
Combined pill	**9**	**0.3**
Evra patch	**9**	**0.3**
NuvaRing	**9**	**0.3**
Progestin-only pill	9	0.7
Depo-Provera	6	0.2
Etonogestrel implant	0.05	0.05
IUD Copper T380Ag*	0.3	0.3
IUD Mirena (LNG)*	0.2	0.2
Female sterilization	0.5	0.5
Male sterilization	0.15	0.1

Table 11.3 Non-contraceptive benefits of combined hormonal contraceptives

LESS

Dysmenorrhoea

Irregular menstrual bleeding

Intensity of menstrual flow/anaemia

Ovarian cysts (≥ 30 mcg EE)

Extrauterine gravidities

Benign breast disease

Acne and hirsutism (CHCs with special progestins)

Premenstrual symptoms (some women)

Endometrial cancer

Ovarian cancer

Colorectal cancer

OTHERS

Maintenance of bone density

Benefit for endometriosis

might have a better impact on endometriosis and heavy menstrual bleeding.

As CHCs are associated with an elevated risk of VTE, it is, however, not recommended any more to use these substances to induce regular cycles or treat dysmenorrhea or acne in women without need for contraception. For endometriosis, a progestin alone would be the first-line treatment in most cases, if no contraception is needed. In women with recurrent ovarian cysts a pill with 30 μg EE will better suppress ovarian activity than lower-dose CHC.

Maintenance of bone density during perimenopause is a benefit but does not outweigh the age-related risk of CHC use during this period. During adolescence CHCs might have a small negative impact on development of peak bone mass. The use of CHCs in anorectic adolescents or low-weight athletes will not increase bone mass if weight does not increase [8]. Low-dose CHCs protect against ovarian, endometrial and colorectal cancers [9, 10]. Fertility returns immediately after stopping CHCs.

Contraindications

Absolute and relative contraindications are listed in Table 11.4. Absolute contraindications include comorbidities, which increase the cardiovascular risk in CHC users, acute liver pathology or hormone-dependent cancer. A family history of cardiovascular events, especially deep VTE, in a young first-degree relative increases significantly the VTE risk. Cardiovascular events in the patient's personal history need to be excluded. Hypertension, severe hyperlipidaemia, obesity and smoking cause long-term arterial plaques and stenosis and thus increase the risk of myocardial infarction and ischemic stroke, especially in women older than 35 years [11].

In comparison with VTE, arterial events are extremely rare, but they are associated with a higher mortality. The risk is very low for young women without contraindications. Relative contraindications do not exclude use of CHCs, but more than one relative contraindication causes a multiplicative risk increase. Smoking and age older than 35 years or obesity and hyperlipidaemia are examples. Medical conditions might require use of medications which accelerate CHC metabolism and thus reduce efficacy. Taking a good medical history before counselling of women with need for contraception is essential (→ Part 3).

Role and Impact of Risk Factors and Special Medical Conditions

Risk of Venous Thrombosis

The incidence of VTE in healthy young women is 2–3/10,000 woman-years. Combined hormonal contraceptives increase this risk two- to fourfold. The VTE varies

Table 11.4 Absolute and relative contraindications of combined hormonal contraceptives

Absolute contraindications

- Positive family history of a thromboembolic event in a first-degree relative.
- Family history of thrombophilia or known thrombophilia of the patient.
- Past history of venous thrombosis, lung embolism, myocardial infarction, ischemic or haemorrhagic stroke.
- Migraine with aura.
- Smoking and age older than 35 years.
- Diabetes with vascular complications.
- Lupus erythematodes with vascular disease.
- Severe hypercholesterolemia or hypertriglyceridemia.
- Liver disease with marked impaired liver function (acute hepatitis, cirrhosis of the liver).
- Hormone-dependent cancer (breast cancer, endometrial cancer).
- More than one relative contraindication can result in an absolute contraindication as risks multiply.
- Hypertension (≥160/100 mmHg).

Relative contraindications

- Overweight (BMI ≥ 25 kg/m^2) and obesity (BMI ≥ 30 kg/m^2).
- Smoking.
- Migraine without aura.
- Age older than 35 years.
- Diabetes.
- Breastfeeding, especially in the first 3 months after delivery.
- Seizure disorders.
- Hyperlipidaemia.
- Thrombophlebitis.
- Gallbladder disease.
- Porphyria.
- Elective surgery.

Table 11.5 Venous thromboembolism risk associated with combined hormonal contraceptives with different progestins

Risk of developing a blood clot (VTE) in a year	
Women not using a CHC pill/ring/patch and not pregnant	2–3 out of 10,000 women
Women using a CHC containing levonorgestrel, norethisterone or norgestimate	5–7 out of 10,000 women
Women using a CHC containing etonogestrel or norelgestromin	6–12 out of 10,000 women
Women using a CHC containing desogestrel, gestodene or drospirenone	9–12 out of 10,000 women
Women using a CHC containing chlormadinone, dienogest or nomegestrol	Not yet known
Pregnancy	48–60 out of 10,000 women

with different types of progestins in CHCs and is lowest in CHCs containing the second-generation progestin levonorgestrel (LNG) [12]. Combined hormonal contraceptives with third- and fourth-generation progestins are associated with a twofold higher risk of VTE in comparison with CHCs containing LNG (Table 11.5 modified from [13]).

The differences in VTE risk between CHCs with different progestins are low (odds ratio 2). In numbers these are three to five events in 10,000 woman-years. Around 1–10% of VTE will cause lung embolism. The European Medical Agency and many country guidelines recommend EE/LNG pills as the first choice for new starters [13]. Dienogest and nomegestrol are progestins in pills containing estradiol and estradiol-valerate. Newer studies indicate that the VTE risk with these pills is not higher than that with pills containing third-generation progestins or drospirenone [12, 14].

Women with cardiovascular risk factors such as those listed among the absolute contraindications can have a 4–20-fold higher risk of VTE, LE, stroke or myocardial infarction and therefore should not use CHCs. The incidence of VTE in CHC users with severe thrombophilia is 430–462 in 10,000 woman-years (RR 40 fold) [15]. The relative risks (RR) are listed in Table 11.6 and more specific information can be found at https://escrh.eu/education/training-improvement-programme/ttt-tool-sessions-eng.

Special Medical Conditions

Positive family history and thrombophilia

- In 29.7% of women with a family history (first-degree relative) of VTE thrombophilia (genetic risk) is diagnosed.
- The classical five thrombophilias are not a typical cause for a positive family history.
- A positive family history is a stronger predictor of VTE than cost-intensive thrombophilia screening.
- Testing women with a positive family history may give false reassurance if the test is negative. They nevertheless will have a markedly increased risk of CHC-related VTE compared to the general population.

Age, smoking, obesity, hypertension

- Age, obesity and smoking are not strong as single risk factor for VTE in young women.

Table 11.6 Venous thromboembolism risk factors and medical conditions

Risk factor	Relative risk (RR) for VTE CHC user vs. nonuser
Family history of VTE [16, 17] : First-degree relative younger than 50 years	RR 2.9
Two relatives, one older than 50 years	RR 4.0
Second-degree relative	RR 1.5–2.3
Thrombophilia in the patient	
Protein C deficiency, protein S deficiency, anti-thrombin III deficiency	RR 10
Pro-thrombin 20210 mutation	RR 3–8
Factor V Leiden mutation	RR 5–10
Obesity	RR 5–10
Heavy smoking	RR 1.5
Age 35–39 years	RR 2
Age younger than 40 years and BMI greater than 30	RR 8–10

Table 11.7 Contraceptive counselling under consideration of the arterial and venous thromboembolism risk in different medical conditions

	Age < 35 years	Age > 35 years
Obesity	Possible	Better not; consider also the VTE risk
Migraine with aura	No	No
Migraine without aura	Possible	No
Hypertension	Possible if BP 140–159/90–99	No
Smoking	Possible	No
Diabetes	Possible if no vascular complication	No
Dyslipidaemia	Possible	No

*Adapted from: Table WHO MEC (www.who.int/publications/i/item/9789241565400)

- However, the multiplicative effect of these risk factors is relevant. Other contraceptive options should be recommended.
- Consider also the arterial risk, which increases mutiplicatively in women ≥ 35 years.

Risk of Cerebral Venous Thrombosis

The incidence of cerebral venous thrombosis (CVT) among young adults is 0.13/10,000 woman-years. The odds ratio (OR) for such an event in CHC users is 5.5. Patients with migraine and thrombophilia are at higher risk. In migraine patients this risk is modified by the frequency of the headache attacks. Typical symptoms include headache, papilledema and epileptic seizure (Table11.7).

Arterial Risks: Myocardial Infarction and Ischemic Stroke

The most relevant risk factors are age older than 35 years, obesity, hypertension, dyslipidaemia and smoking [11]. These conditions induce over time atherosclerotic plaques, which predispose to occlusion. The incidence for myocardial infarction in young women (< 35 years) not using the pill is very low – 0.6/100,000 woman-years. The multiplicative risk with age ≥ 35 years, CHC use and smoking is reflected in the close to 1,000-fold higher incidence of 486 events/100,000 woman-years [18]. Arterial events are associated with higher mortality [11, 19]. Contraceptive options for these women include progestin-only contraceptives, intrauterine devices and male or female sterilization. The risk of ischemic stroke in migraineurs is 5–17 fold that in CHC users and, again, much higher in migraineurs who smoke (OR 34.4) [20, 21].

Age As Risk Factor

Both the risk of a clot in the arteries and VTE have to be considered.

Diabetes and Hypertension

In women younger than 35 years with hypertension CHCs can be used if hypertension is well controlled and if there are no additional risk factors. In all CHC users blood pressure measurements should be performed annually. Combined hormonal contraceptives can be used in young otherwise healthy women with diabetes if there are no vascular complications, no other relative contraindications and diabetes is well controlled.

Liver Disease

Combined hormonal contraceptives should not be used in women with acute liver disease or impaired liver function.

Cancer

Use of CHCs is strongly contraindicated in patients with breast cancer. Combined hormonal contraceptives can be used in women after treatment of cervical cancer. → **Table WHO MEC.**

Obesity

Combined hormonal contraceptives are efficient but associated with a higher risk of VTE (RR two- to fourfold) and arterial events in women aged older than 35 years [22]. There is some concern that, when starting a CHC, the time to reach steady state of the progestin is delayed. Therefore recommendation of additional protection during the first 10 days of CHC use in obese new starters is useful.

Bariatric Surgery

Combined hormonal contraceptives are safe if normal-weight women use them after gastric reduction surgery, including gastric sleeve and band. Associated with reduced efficacy, they cannot be used in women after malabsorptive operations, including gastric bypass. → **Table WHO MEC.** www.who.int/publications/i/item/9789241565400

Breastfeeding

Use of CHCs is not recommended in the first 3 months after delivery for breastfeeding women. Please check **Table WHO MEC** for more recommendations.

Adverse Events

Patients should be informed about potential upcoming adverse events and if such events can be considered harmless or harmful.

Serious Adverse Events

Serious adverse events include VTE, myocardial infarction and stroke, initiation and worsening of migraine, minimal increase in the risk of breast and cervical cancers and major depression. The incidence of cardiovascular events is discussed earlier in this chapter. New starters of CHCs should be informed about the symptoms of VTE and advised to see a doctor if such symptoms occur. Blood pressure should be measured regularly before new prescriptions.

Combined hormonal contraceptives can initiate migraine, increase frequency of migraine and modify a non-aura migraine to a migraine with aura. The latter is associated with a much higher risk of a cerebrovascular insult. In this situation women should switch to another oestrogen-free contraceptive method [23]. Progestin-only contraception has been shown to improve migraine with and without aura [24].

Although CHC are very low dosed today, they cause a very small increase in the risk of breast cancer (BC). In a huge Danish study including women aged 15–49 years the incidence of BC in non-hormonal contraceptive users was 55 cases in 100,000 woman-years, 58 cases in past CHC users and 68 cases in current and previous users. This close to 20% increase in risk has to be discussed in the context of the rarity of such an event in absolute numbers. Thirteen more cases in 100,000 woman-years is a small number. The number of additional cases is higher (n = 21) if CHCs are used for more than 10 years [25]. As the number of pregnancies and the duration of breastfeeding reduce the breast cancer risk, it is not known whether the higher BC risk in long-term CHC users is related to the fact that these women delay their pregnancies and have fewer children than to the hormone exposure. There is some evidence that the LNG-20 IUS and low-dose progestin pills are associated with a similar risk of BC [25].

Combined hormonal contraceptives increase the risk of invasive cervical cancer and intraepithelial neoplasia grade III (CIN 3) [26, 27]. After 5 years of CHC use the risk for cervical cancer has been found to be 1.9–2.0. The risk of developing CIN 3 in a recent Dutch study was 2.7 for CHC users and 1.5 for IUD users. The cervical cancer risk declines after ceasing the hormone and returns after 10 years to that of women who never used the hormone. The pattern of risk was similar in women who tested positive and negative for high-risk papilloma virus. Altogether these numbers are small and should not preclude prescribing a CHC. However, CHC users should have regular PAP smears. The cumulative incidence for cervical cancer after 10-year use of CHC, starting at age 20, is associated with increases from 3.8/1,000 to 4.5/1,000 in more-developed countries and from 7.3/1,000 to 8.3/1,000 in less-developed countries.

During the reproductive years the prevalence of major depression in women is around 14%. Women with depression feel sad, empty and useless and have difficulties functioning in their normal life. The data related to depression and CHC use in previously healthy women are very limited. One study found two additional cases of depression in 10,000 woman-years [28]. Clinical observations indicate that, if hormonal contraception is the source of depression, the mood change occurs typically very soon after initiation of the method. If a woman reports such a relevant change in her mood and no other incident in her life can explain it, CHCs should be stopped immediately and close follow-up provided. Clinical experience is that CHC-induced mood changes resolve within 1.2 weeks after stopping the method.

Harmless Adverse Events

Harmless adverse events include breast tension, headache, nausea, abdominal pain, irritability, changes in libido, unscheduled bleeding, changes in weight and acne. The frequency of these events varies between studies and depends on oestrogen and progestin dose and type (Table 11.1). Progestins with anti-androgenic properties will exert a positive effect on the skin. Harmless side effects occur in 1–15% of CHC new starters and mostly disappear or improve within 3 months. In placebo-controlled trials nausea and breast tension were reported by the same percentage of women in both groups. It makes sense to not change the CHC type too quickly. If adverse events continue and are disturbing, the oestrogen dose or the progestin type in the prescribed CHC can be modified. Vaginal or transdermal application can be an option to improve tolerability. It is important to differentiate between irritability and depression and between simple tension-type headache and migraine.

Unscheduled bleedings in CHC new starters are frequent and harmless. These bleedings – mostly spotting – will in most patients disappear over time. If chlamydia infection has been excluded as a cause of unscheduled bleeding and it has been confirmed that the CHC was used correctly, increasing the oestrogen dose or switching to a progestin which has a strong suppressive effect on endometrial growth may be helpful. In women reporting new headaches or more and stronger headaches, migraine needs to be excluded. Most women might suffer from headaches predominantly in the PFI. A CHC with a lower oestrogen dose or with a shorter PFI, or the vaginal ring, might be an option. Low-dose CHCs do not typically cause weight fluctuation beyond 2 kg. It is not understood why a subgroup of women gains more weight. Weight increase of more than 2 kg was found in around 11% of users [29, 30].

Combined hormonal contraceptives can, similar to the natural cycle, cause changes in mood or irritability. Impacts on mood are not predictable and cannot directly be attributed to a special progestin or oestrogen dose. If these changes are disturbing switching to another progestin is an option. Some women might experience a decrease in libido. This might improve with a less anti-androgenic progestin.

Key Points for Practical Work with the Patient

Although a number of risks are associated with the use of CHCs, only a small subgroup of women will ever experience such events. Taking a thorough patient history will help to avoid such events and understand which benefits of contraceptives can be used in this patient. Such a patient history will include not only the gynaecologic history, but also the general history. It will furthermore aim to understand the reproductive health goals of this individual woman and her personal situation. If risk factors or absolute contraindications are identified suggest progestin-only contraceptives, an intrauterine device or permanent methods for those who do not want any more children. All these methods are also very efficient (Table 11.2). If no other methods are available the risk of CHCs should be balanced against the use of less-effective methods (e.g., a condom) and pregnancy risk.

What to Ask and Check before Prescribing Combined Hormonal Contraceptives

Take a Very Thorough History
General History

Exclude the Following Conditions to Avoid Severe Complications:

1. Previous venous blood clot (venous thrombosis), stroke or heart attack.
2. Thrombogenic mutations in the personal or family history.
3. Migraine with aura.
4. Hypertension (≥ 160/≥ 100 mmHg).
5. Severe liver or gall bladder disease.
6. Systemic lupus erythematodes.
7. Diabetes with vascular complications.
8. Smoking and age older than 35 years.
9. A venous blood clot, stroke or heart attack in any first-degree relative aged ≤ 50 years.
10. Obesity.

Further Issues Important to Address before Balancing Risks and Benefits:

1. Medical conditions.
2. Surgery in the past.
3. Medication (including phytotherapeuticals): consider potential interactions.
4. Psychic and eating disorders.
5. Alcohol, drugs and allergies.
6. Smoking and weight.

Gynaecological History

Most Important Aspects to Optimise Counselling and Use Benefits of Combined Hormonal Contraceptives:

1. Menstrual cycle: interval, duration, intensity of bleeding, symptoms and date of last menstruation.
2. Pregnancies: deliveries, abortions, breastfeeding.
3. Breast, cervical, ovarian and endometrial cancer.
4. Ovarian cysts.
5. Endometriosis.
6. Previous contraceptive methods: tolerability and adherence.
7. Previous use of emergency contraception.
8. Exclude any unclear unscheduled bleeding.

Personal Situation and Reproductive Health Goals

1. Duration of relationship with partner.
2. Plans for motherhood.
3. Need for long-term contraception.
4. Financial issues.
5. Wish for permanent contraception.
6. Protection against sexually transmitted infections.

What to Check before Combined Hormonal Contraceptives Use and What to Check during Annual Follow-Up

As many harmless adverse events will subside during longer use, it makes sense to wait 2–3 months before switching to another CHC or another contraceptive method. A first prescription for 3 months with the option for a follow-up visit to discuss adverse events and questions of the patient is reasonable. In most European countries annual follow-up visits with recheck for risk factors, new medical conditions, drug–drug interactions and blood pressure control are performed before the next prescription. In many regions a PAP smear is performed if the last gynaecologic check was longer ago. Country guidelines differ with regard to the frequency with which a PAP smear is necessary in sexually active women (1–3

years). There is a small increase in the risk of cervical cancer in CHC users. Chlamydia smears are not necessary for a CHC prescription.

Before Prescribing Combined Hormonal Contraceptives

1. Exclude contraindications.
2. Exclude interactions with medications.
3. Check blood pressure.
4. Check size and weight.
5. Perform a pregnancy test (not necessary in women with regular cycles).
6. Perform a PAP smear if possible (exceptions include if women have not yet had intercourse or have no access to this check) and exclude gynaecologic pathology.
7. Offer chlamydia screening (if available) if there is a new partner, if the patient lives in a region with high prevalence or if the woman is at high risk of sexually transmitted infections.
8. Make sure the patient will remember daily pill use. If not the transdermal patch or the vaginal ring might be a better option.
9. Explain how to use the CHC and emphasise the importance of starting the next pack in time and to not extend the hormone-free interval.
10. Explain how efficient the method is if used correctly.
11. Inform about harmless adverse events, especially harmless unscheduled bleeding, during the first months of use.
12. Explain the long-term bleeding pattern of the method.
13. Inform about symptoms of serious adverse events (VTE, pulmonary embolism, migraine, depression) and advise to stop the CHC and to see a doctor as soon as possible in such a situation.
14. Inform what to do if a pill was forgotten, including information about emergency contraception.
15. Inform that CHCs do not protect against sexually transmitted infections.
16. Inform that the pill does not cause infertility and no pill rest is needed.

Missed-Pill Rules

When using missed-pill rules the best option would be to follow the instruction on the leaflet, as the rules are not the same for all types of CHCs. If this is not possible, use the following information:

For effective ovulation inhibition, continuous use and adequate uptake of the pill for at least 7 days is necessary. If one pill is missed or not absorbed due to vomiting within 3 hours of intake, the standard advice is to take the missed pill as soon as possible and take the remaining pills at the usual time, even if it means taking two pills in 1 day. No additional action is needed if the interval between two pills does not exceed 36 hours. If one pill is missed during the first week for 36 hours or longer, back up contraception (e.g., condoms) or avoidance of sexual intercourse should be advised until pills have been taken again for at least 7 consecutive days. Emergency contraception should be considered in case of unprotected intercourse during the preceding 72 hours. If pills were missed in the third week, the best option is to omit the hormone-free interval and start a new pack the next day. Missed-pill rules are published in the World Health Organization's (WHO) selected practice recommendations: bit.ly /3JpGcmZ.

References

1. Sitruk-Ware R, Nath A. Characteristics and metabolic effects of estrogen and progestins contained in oral contraceptive pills. *Best Pract Res Clin Endocrinol Metab*. 2013;**27**(1):13–24.

2. Godsland IF, Crook D, Simpson R et al. The effects of different formulations of oral contraceptive agents on lipid and carbohydrate metabolism. *N Engl J Med*. 1990;**323**(20):1375–81.

3. Dragoman M, Curtis KM, Gaffield ME. Combined hormonal contraceptive use among women with known dyslipidemias: A systematic review of critical safety outcomes. *Contraception*. 2016;**94**(3):280–7.

4. Speroff L. *Clinical gynecologic endocrinology and infertility*. 8th edition. Philadelphia, PA: Lippincott, Williams and Wilkins, 2010.

5. Petersen KR, Skouby SO, Vedel P, Haaber AB. Hormonal contraception in women with IDDM: Influence on glycometabolic control and lipoprotein metabolism. *Diabetes Care*. 1995;**18**(6):800–6.

6. Trussell J, Portman D. The creeping pearl: Why has the rate of contraceptive failure increased in clinical trials of combined hormonal contraceptive pills? *Contraception*. 2013;**88**(5):604–10.

7. European Society for Contraception Teaching and Training tool CHC session. 2019. https://escrheu/ed ucation/training-improvement-programme/tt-tool-sessions-eng.

8. Merki-Feld GS, Bitzer J. Contraception in adolescents with anorexia nervosa: Is there evidence for a negative impact of combined hormonal contraceptives on bone mineral density and the course of the disease?

Eur J Contracept Reprod Health Care. 2020;**25**(3):213–20.

9. Fernandez E, La Vecchia C, Balducci A et al. Oral contraceptives and colorectal cancer risk: A meta-analysis. *Br J Cancer*. 2001;**84**(5):722–7.

10. Iversen L, Sivasubramaniam S, Lee AJ, Fielding S, Hannaford PC. Lifetime cancer risk and combined oral contraceptives: The Royal College of General Practitioners' Oral Contraception Study. *Am J Obstet Gynecol*. 2017;**216**(6):580e581–580e589.

11. Combined hormonal contraceptives (CHCs) and the risk of cardiovascular disease endpoints. CHC-CVD final report 111022v2. 2011.

12. Dragoman MV, Tepper NK, Fu R. A systematic review and meta-analysis of venous thrombosis risk among users of combined oral contraception. *Int J Gynaecol Obstet*. 2018;**141**(3):287–94.

13. VTE risk with CHC. European medical agency. 2013. bit.ly/3DoQFLC.

14. Dinger J, Assmann A, Mohner S, Minh TD. Risk of venous thromboembolism and the use of dienogest- and drospirenone-containing oral contraceptives: Results from a German case-control study. *J Fam Plann Reprod Health Care*. 2010;**36**(3):123–9.

15. Van Vlijmen EF, Wiewel-Verschueren S, Monster TB, Meijer K. Combined oral contraceptives, thrombophilia and the risk of venous thromboembolism: A systematic review and meta-analysis. *J Thromb Haemost*. 2016;**14** (7):1393–1403.

16. Bezemer ID, Van der Meer FJ, Eikenboom JC, Rosendaal FR, Doggen CJ. The value of family history as a risk indicator for venous thrombosis. *Arch Intern Med*. 2009;**169**(6):610–15.

17. Zoller B, Li X, Ohlsson H, Sundquist J, Sundquist K. Age-and sex-specific seasonal variation of venous thromboembolism in patients with and without family history: A nationwide family study in Sweden. *Thromb Haemost*. 2013;**110**(6):1164–71.

18. Acute myocardial infarction and combined oral contraceptives: Results of an international multicentre case-control study. WHO Collaborative Study of Cardiovascular Disease and Steroid Hormone Contraception. *Lancet*. 1997;**349** (9060):1202–9.

19. Lidegaard O, Lokkegaard E, Jensen A, Skovlund CW, Keiding N. Thrombotic stroke and myocardial infarction with hormonal contraception. *N Engl J Med*. 2012;**366**(24):2257–66.

20. Curtis KM, Mohllajee AP, Peterson HB. Use of combined oral contraceptives among women with migraine and nonmigrainous headaches: A systematic review. *Contraception*. 2006;**73**(2):189–94.

21. Tzourio C, Kittner SJ, Bousser MG, Alperovitch A. Migraine and stroke in young women. *Cephalalgia*. 2000;**20**(3):190–9.

22. Merki-Feld GS, Skouby S, Serfaty D. European society of contraception statement on contraception in obese women. *Eur J Contracept Reprod Health Care*. 2015;**20** (1):19–28.

23. Sacco S, Merki-Feld GS, Bitzer J et al. Effect of exogenous estrogens and progestogens on the course of migraine during reproductive age: A consensus statement by the European Headache Federation (EHF) and the European Society of Contraception and Reproductive Health (ESCRH). *J Headache Pain*. 2018;**19**(1):76.

24. Merki-Feld GS, Imthurn B, Langner R, Seifert B, Gantenbein AR. Positive effects of the progestin desogestrel 75 mug on migraine frequency and use of acute medication are sustained over a treatment period of 180 days. *J Headache Pain*. 2015;**16**:522.

25. Morch LS, Skovlund CW, Hannaford PC et al. Contemporary hormonal contraception and the risk of breast cancer. *N Engl J Med*. 2017;**377**(23):2228–39.

26. Loopik DL, IntHout J, Melchers WJG et al. Oral contraceptive and intrauterine device use and the risk of cervical intraepithelial neoplasia grade III or worse: A population-based study. *Eur J Cancer*. 2020;**124**:102–9.

27. International Collaboration of Epidemiological Studies of Cervical Cancer, Appleby P, Beral V et al. Cervical cancer and hormonal contraceptives: Collaborative reanalysis of individual data for 16,573 women with cervical cancer and 35,509 women without cervical cancer from 24 epidemiological studies. *Lancet*. 2007;**370** (9599):1609–21.

28. Skovlund CW, Morch LS, Kessing LV, Lidegaard O. Association of hormonal contraception with depression. *JAMA Psychiatry*. 2016;**73**(11):1154–62.

29. Hani D, Imthurn B, Merki-Feld GS. [Weight gain due to hormonal contraception: Myth or truth?]. *Gynakol Geburtshilfliche Rundsch*. 2009;**49**(2):87–93.

30. Gallo MF, Lopez LM, Grimes DA et al. Combination contraceptives: Effects on weight. *Cochrane Database Syst Rev*. 201;1:CD003987.

Chapter 12

Progestogen-Only Contraception

Frans J. M. E. Roumen, Gabriele S. Merki-Feld and Katarina Sedlecky

Progestogen-Only Contraceptives

Formulations and Delivery Systems

Progestogen-only contraceptives (POCs) contain only a progestogen and no oestrogen. The progestogens used in POCs represent different generations as they have been developed over time. All progestogens have progestogenic, antigonadotropic and antiestrogenic activities. With generation of the progestogen its progestational activity increases and androgenic activity decreases.

A variety of delivery systems is available. Some of them are short-acting such as oral pills; others are intermediate-acting such as injectables or long-acting such as an implant and intra-uterine systems (IUSs). Table 12.1 shows the available POCs according to type of progestogen, molecule they are derived from, activities on other steroid receptors, delivery system and duration of use.

Mode of Action

The mode of action of POCs depends on the dose of progestogen. High doses (depot medroxyprogesterone acetate (DMPA)) inhibit follicle development and subsequent ovulation completely via feedback inhibition of follicle-stimulating hormone and luteinizing hormone, alter the ciliary action in the fallopian tubes, increase the viscosity of cervical mucus – thus interfering with sperm transport – and cause endometrial thinning and atrophy, making implantation less likely. Intermediate doses (DSG pill, DRSP pill, ENG implant) inhibit ovulation effectively but allow follicular development with some oestrogen production, whereas very low doses (NET pill, LNG pill, LNG-IUS) mostly do not inhibit ovulation, but rely for efficacy mainly on their effect on the endometrial level and cervical mucus.

Table 12.1 Characteristics of progestogen-only contraceptives

Progestogen type	Derivative from	Activities on other steroid receptors	Delivery system	Duration of use
Norethisterone (NET)	19-nortestosterone (1st generation)	Mild estrogenic Mild androgenic	Oral pill	Daily
Levonorgestrel (LNG)	19-nortestosterone (2nd generation)	Residual androgenic	Oral pill Intra-uterine system	Daily 3–5 years
Desogestrel (DSG)	19-nortestosterone (3rd generation)	More progestational Less androgenic	Oral pill	Daily
Etonogestrel (ENG)	19-nortestosterone (3rd generation)	More progestational Less androgenic	Subcutaneous implant	3 years
Drospirenone (DRSP)	Spironolactone	Antimineralocorticoid Antiandrogenic	Oral pill	24–4 day regimen
Medroxyprogesterone (DMPA)	17α OH-progesterone	Glucocorticoid Slightly androgenic	Intramuscular or subcutaneous depot injection	3 months

Table 12.2 Percentage of women experiencing an unintended pregnancy during the first year of typical use and the first year of perfect use of a progestogen-only contraceptive [1, 2]

Method	Typical use	Perfect use
Oral pill	9%	0.7%
DMPA injectable	6%	0.2%
LNG-IUS	0.2%	0.2%
Implant	0.05%	0.05%

Contraceptive Efficacy and Return to Fertility

Different delivery options of POC contribute to the variations in perfect and typical use failure rates (Table 12.2). As the effectiveness of oral pills – and, to a lesser degree, of DMPA – depends on users' compliance and adherence to the prescription, their typical use results in higher failure rates than methods that act over a long period independent of any user activity such as the LNG-IUS and the implant. Accidental pregnancies during POC use are more frequently ectopic than with combined oral contraceptive (COC) use. Return to fertility is generally immediate after use of the last pill or removal of the implant and the IUS. For DMPA return to ovulations is delayed until 6–9 months after the last intramuscular or subcutaneous injection.

Indications, Contraindications and Health Benefits

Most POCs are good contraceptive options for nearly all women. They can be used by women with contraindications to combined hormonal contraceptives (CHC) or those with oestrogen-associated adverse events, except for the NET pill as this pill is partly metabolized to estradiol. Progestogen-only contraceptives can be used in breastfeeding women 6 weeks postpartum as they have no negative impact on lactation or negative health outcomes in infants, although long-term studies are only available for the injection [3].

The POC pill, implant and IUS have minimal metabolic effects and are not associated with an increased risk of venous thromboembolism (VTE), arterial thromboembolism (ATE), stroke or acute myocardial infarction. Very limited evidence suggests an increased risk of VTE with DMPA [4]. All POC methods are a possible contraceptive option for smoking women over 35 years of age and for women with medical conditions such as hypertension ($\geq 160/\geq 100$ mmHg), multiple risk factors for arterial

cardiovascular disease and diabetes. For women with strong risk factors on the venous side like thrombophilia and history of VTE or pulmonary embolism (PE), POC pill, implant and IUS can be used if no other method is acceptable or available, as the advantages of using these methods generally outweigh the theoretical or proven risks [5].

The most important contraindications of POCs are acute VTE or PE, unexplained vaginal bleeding, severe liver disease, malignant liver tumours, current or past breast cancer and, for NET and LNG pills, the existence or history of ATE. All POCs reduce dysmenorrhea and have a positive impact on endometriosis-related pelvic pain. The DSG pill has a positive effect on the course of migraine with and without aura in the majority of women. Depot medroxyprogesterone acetate and IUS have additional health benefits such as reduction of heavy menstrual bleeding, protection against iron-deficiency anaemia and inhibition of growth of uterine fibroids; DMPA is also associated with a reduced risk of endometrial cancer and a reduction of sickle cell crises in women with sickle cell anaemia.

Adverse Events and Side Effects

Adverse events differ between POC methods, depending on dose, type of progestogen and route of administration. The most common adverse event of all POCs and the most common reason for early discontinuation is unpredictable, unscheduled uterine spotting or bleeding [6]. This is related to the continuous use of these products and to the low suppression of ovarian activity, which allows the development of unruptured follicle cysts which produce estradiol. These follicle cysts, however, are mostly asymptomatic and harmless and resolve spontaneously. The frequency of unpredictable, unscheduled bleeding decreases over time with all POC methods. It is important to inform women about these changes and to reassure them if they find the bleeding pattern troublesome.

If ultrasound shows an atrophic endometrium, the administration of oestrogens or CHCs will usually stop the unscheduled bleeding with POC (Table 12.3) [7]. However, this is only a temporary solution which is not preferred by most women, and it is not applicable in women with contraindications for oestrogens. Other treatment options for prolonged bleeding include non-steroidal anti-inflammatory drugs (NSAIDs), doxycycline, tranexamic acid, norethisterone or ulipristal acetate (off-label). Clinical experience suggests shortening the interval between injections to

Table 12.3 Treatment options for uterine bleeding irregularities associated with progestogen-only contraceptives [7]

Medication	Daily dosage	Duration of use
Estradiol pill	2 mg	5–7 days
Estradiol patch	50 µg	5–7 days
Monophasic combined hormonal contraceptives	1 pill	21 days
Ibuprofen	2 × 500–800 mg	5 days
Mefenamic acid	2 × 500 mg	5 days
Doxycycline	2 × 100 mg	5 days
Tranexamic acid	2 × 500 mg	5 days
Norethisterone	2 or 3 × 5 mg	21 days/2 or 3 cycles
Ulipristal acetate	1 × 5 mg	5 days

reduce the number of bleeding days and episodes. If the bleeding pattern is unacceptable for the woman a different contraceptive method must be sought.

The incidence of amenorrhoea is also associated with the mode of POC delivery and considered a positive side effect by some women, although for others it may prove unacceptable. According to different studies, it occurs within 1 year in up to 20% of women using the pill, 19–25% of women using the implant, 47–60% of women using the DMPA injection and 35–43% of LNG-IUS users.

Metabolic side effects also depend on dose, type and mode of application of progestogens, and include an initial decrease in bone mineral density (BMD) in DMPA new starters, weight gain predominantly in DMPA or implant users, acne and hair loss due to higher plasma levels of free testosterone as a result of decreased levels of sex-hormone-binding globulin (SHBG) [8]. Mood changes including depression can occur, especially in predisposed women. A minimal but significantly increased risk of breast cancer has been demonstrated in premenopausal users of the LNG-IUS [9]. Depression is a potential adverse effect of the DSG pill and the LNG-IUS, especially in adolescents [10].

Progestogen-Only Pill

Introduction

Progestogen-only pills (POPs), also called mini-pills, were developed in the mid-1960s. Due to the oral intake, POPs undergo extensive hepatic first-pass metabolism before they become active.

Formulations and Dosages

In 2020, four POPs were available in Europe (Table 12.4). In case the window for missed pills – which is different for different pills – is exceeded, additional contraception should be used during the next 7 days [11, 12].

Starting Instructions

Except for the first 7 days of the first pack of the NET pill, no additional contraceptive precautions are needed if started on day 1 of the menstrual cycle, on the day after the last active CHC or another POP method or immediately after a first-trimester abortion. Additional contraception is also not needed when started on day 21 (NET pill, LNG pill) or days 21–28 (DSG pill, DRSP pill) after delivery or second-trimester abortion unless sexual intercourse has already occurred. Additional contraceptive measures are recommended for the first 7 days in case of vomiting within 3 hours after taking the tablet, if started on days 2–5 of the menstrual cycle or, at the latest, on the day after the usual CHC hormone-free interval, or in amenorrhoeic women, presuming that no sexual intercourse took place during the preceding 7 days. If pregnancy cannot be excluded, a pregnancy test should be considered before a patients starts a POP.

Mode of Action

The DSG and DRSP pills inhibit ovulation in up to 97% of cycles, but allow, in comparison with CHCs, more follicular development with some oestrogen production [13]. Occasionally these follicles will develop and not rupture, resulting in ovarian cysts producing high levels of oestrogen which may lead to breast tenderness and breakthrough bleeding. Secondary contraceptive mechanisms are impaired sperm penetration resulting from thickening of cervical mucus and reduced sperm motility, as well as endometrial thinning and atrophy.

Efficacy

Perfect and typical use of DSG and DRSP pills are associated with contraceptive failure rates within the first year of 0.7% and 9.0%, respectively. The NET and LNG pills are less efficient as they do not rely on

Table 12.4 Progestogen-only pills available in Europe

Progestogen	Daily dosage	Advised use	Window for missed pills
Norethisterone (NET)	0.35 mg	Every day without interruption	3 hours
Levonorgestrel (LNG)	0.030 mg	Every day without interruption	3 hours
Desogestrel (DSG)	0.075 mg	Every day without interruption	12 hours
Drospirenone (DRSP)	4 mg	24 days with 4 days interruption	24 hours

ovulation inhibition. Increased metabolism as a result of interactions with liver enzyme-inducing drugs such as many anticonvulsant medicaments (except for lamotrigine), rifampicin and St John's wort (*Hypericum perforatum*) can reduce the contraceptive efficacy of POPs. Available evidence does not indicate a decreased efficacy of POPs in obese women. Due to possible decreased efficacy, the use of POPs in patients after malabsorptive bariatric procedures is not recommended for 12–24 months.

Benefits and Risks

Progestogen-only pills have a very low impact on plasma lipids, carbohydrate metabolism and haemostasis. They reduce complaints of dysmenorrhea and are not associated with an increased risk of VTE or ATE. The DSG pill has a positive effect on the course of migraine with and without aura in the majority of women [14]. Use of the DSG pill by breastfeeding women within 21 days postpartum is generally advantageous above the theoretical or proven risks [5]. Data on the DRSP pill are not available yet, but the amount of DRSP 4 mg in breast milk is negligible as it is only 0.11% of the daily use of 4 mg. During prolonged immobilization POPs are preferably stopped.

Adverse Events and Side Effects

Unpredictable bleeding occurs in around 40% of POP users, including frequent and infrequent bleeding and spotting, or prolonged bleeding. Bleeding problems usually decrease with longer duration of use. Women should be appropriately informed about these changes, which are the main reason for early discontinuation. No evidence is available that changing the type of POP will improve bleeding patterns in women with unscheduled bleeding, although it may help some women. As the DRSP pill is administered with a pill-free period and the other POPs without, comparison of unscheduled bleeding profiles between types of POPs is difficult. Amenorrhoea occurs in up to 20% of POP users.

Other adverse events include ovarian cysts, headache, acne, breast discomfort, nausea, depression and vaginitis. No evidence supports a causal association between POP use and weight change.

In case of emergency contraception with LNG, it is advised to continue the DSG pill and use back-up contraception for 5 days. The DSG pill reduces the ability of ulipristal acetate (UPA) to delay ovulation but the interaction between DRSP and UPA has not been studied yet. In case UPA is needed, current DSG pill users are advised to take a pill break for 5 days and restart on day 6, using back-up contraception from the day of UPA intake for 12 days [15].

Progestogen-Only Implant

Formulation and Release Rate

The only progestogen-only implant available across Europe is a single rod made of evatane, 40 mm in length and 2 mm in diameter [16]. It contains 68 mg etonogestrel (the active 3-keto metabolite of desogestrel) and provides contraception for 3 years. The initial release rate of 60–70 µg/day at week 5 or 6 falls gradually to around 25–30 µg/day at the end of 3 years.

No additional contraceptive precautions are needed if the implant is inserted on days 1–5 of the menstrual cycle, following a first-trimester abortion or ultimately on the day after stopping any other hormonal contraceptive method. Otherwise additional contraceptive measures are recommended for the first 7 days.

Etonogestrel levels during the third year of use are lower in overweight women, although a negative influence on contraceptive efficacy has not been demonstrated yet [17]. Early replacement after 2 years is therefore disputable in obese women. No additional contraceptive precautions are needed after immediate exchange.

Insertion and Removal

To avoid neurovascular damage, the rod is inserted under local anaesthesia just under the skin on the inner side of the non-dominant upper arm about 8–10 cm above the medical epicondyle, 3–5 cm posterior of the sulcal line between brachialis/biceps anteriorly and triceps posteriorly. A preloaded inserter facilitates insertion. Correct insertion of the implant should be confirmed by palpation.

Although the rod is easy to insert, removal can be troublesome, particularly if the implant is inserted subcutaneously rather than subdermally. In the most recent version, 15 mg barium sulphate is added to the implant core, making it detectable by x-ray. Usually a small, longitudinal skin incision at the distal end of the implant is sufficient to grab and extract it when pushing on the proximal end. An experienced surgeon should be consulted when the implant is located too deep or cannot be felt.

Efficacy

The implant is highly effective with an identical extremely low perfect and typical use failure rate of 0.05 within the first year of use. Ovulations were not observed in the first 2 years of use of the implant and only rarely in the third year. Recent data indicate that the implant might provide protection for 2 years more as serum etonogestrel median levels remain above the ovulation threshold of 90 pg/ml for women of all BMI classes [18], but longer use is off-label.

Benefits and Risks

Benefits and risks of the implant are comparable with those of POPs. It has a very low impact on plasma lipids, carbohydrate metabolism and haemostasis, and reduces complaints of dysmenorrhea in women with endometriosis. The implant is not associated with an increased risk of VTE or ATE. It is a possible contraceptive option for smoking women older than 35 years of age and for women with medical conditions such as hypertension (≥ 160/≥ 100 mmHg), multiple risk factors for arterial cardiovascular disease, diabetes, thrombophilia and history of VTE or PE.

Drugs or herbal products that induce certain liver enzymes may decrease the etonogestrel concentration and diminish the effectiveness or increase breakthrough bleeding. Carbamazepine use significantly reduces serum etonogestrel concentrations in women using an etonogestrel contraceptive implant, with the majority of participants having etonogestrel concentrations below the threshold for ovulatory suppression.

Adverse Events

Etonogestrel implant use is associated with an unpredictable bleeding pattern, which includes amenorrhoea (22.2%) and infrequent (33.6%), frequent (6.7%) and/or prolonged bleeding (17.7%) [19]. The bleeding pattern experienced during months 5 and 6 after implantation generally indicates the future bleeding pattern and predicts the subsequent bleeding in the first 2 years of use. Discontinuation rates during the first year of use due to bleeding irregularities vary in studies from 10.4% to 33% of women, mainly because of prolonged flow and frequent irregular bleeding. Amenorrhoea varies in studies from 19% to 25% of users.

Effective pre-insertion counselling on the possible changes in bleeding patterns may improve continuation rates. Available therapies that might stop unscheduled bleeding after at least 6 months of implant use are shown in Table 12.3 [7]. If no acceptable bleeding pattern can be achieved, remove the implant and change the contraceptive method. The most commonly reported drug-related adverse event is headache (15.3%) followed by weight gain (11.8%), acne (11.4%), breast tenderness (10.2%), mood variations (5.7%) and abdominal pain (5.2%) [20].

Progestogen-Only Injectable

Formulations

Two depot preparations available in Europe contain medroxyprogesterone acetate (MPA): 1 ml (150 mg) administered intramuscularly every 12 weeks and 0.65 ml (104 mg) administered subcutaneously every 13 weeks. Both doses reduce ovarian activity stronger than the POPs and protect immediately from pregnancy if started on days 1–7 of the cycle [21].

Benefits and Risks

Health benefits of DMPA are reduction of heavy menstrual bleeding, protection against iron-deficiency anaemia, reduction in dysmenorrhea, positive impact on endometriosis and inhibition of growth of uterine fibroids. Depot medroxyprogesterone acetate is also associated with a reduced risk of endometrial cancer and a reduction of sickle cell crises in women with sickle cell anaemia.

Depot medroxyprogesterone acetate is associated with a small increase in insulin levels, but overall not with significant changes in carbohydrate metabolism or coagulation factors. It should not be used in breastfeeding women within 6 weeks postpartum or in women with thrombophilia or a history of VTE or PE. The current guidelines do not impose a restriction on the use of DMPA after bariatric surgery.

Adverse Events

Due to bleeding irregularities and adverse events, DMPA discontinuation rates are comparable with those of other POC methods. Some 47–60% of women become amenorrhoeic after 1 year of use, but a few will have persistent heavy and prolonged bleeding (6%) or irregular bleeding (15%) [22]. Clinical experience suggests to shorten the interval between injections in these women. Relevant adverse events are weight gain, headache, nausea, acne, depression or mood changes, decreased libido and injection site reactions (in subcutaneous use) [21].

A major concern is the negative effect on bone mineral density (BMD). Due to the high doses of progestogen, suppressing ovarian activity and causing lower oestrogen levels in comparison with other POC, BMD decreases over 2 or 3 years in new starters. This bone loss is at least to a certain degree reversible after discontinuation of DMPA. Although the risk of osteoporosis is increased, there is limited evidence from studies that long-term DMPA exposure might be associated with increased fracture risk. It is not recommended for adolescents as it exerts a negative impact on the development of peak bone mass [23]. As return to fertility is delayed after discontinuation, DMPA is unsuitable for women who wish to have children in the near future.

Recent evidence could not demonstrate increased HIV acquisition among DMPA users, but the risk of HSV-2 infection might be increased. It is suggested that DMPA self-administration might improve contraceptive access, continuation and autonomy [24].

Hormonal Intra-uterine Systems

Formulations

In Europe, three hormonal IUSs are currently available, all of which release levonorgestrel (LNG) into the uterine cavity. The characteristics of the different types are shown in Table 12.5 [25–29]. In the 16 and 12 versions, a silver ring is located close to the horizontal arms to aid in detection by sonography.

Mode of Action

Although systemic progestin exposure is 10–30 times lower than with other POCs, intra-uterine concentrations of LNG-IUS 20 are 1,000 times higher than those associated with subdermal implants and around 200–800 times higher than after daily POPs [25]. The LNG-IUSs mainly act at the endometrial level. The LNG alters the endometrial receptivity and suppresses endometrial proliferation, resulting in marked endometrial atrophy with inhibition of implantation. In addition, the foreign body induces a local inflammatory reaction inhibiting sperm survival. The LNG also leads to thickening of cervical mucus, blocking transport of spermatozoa, thus preventing fertilization of the ovum. The effect of LNG on ovarian activity is minimal and dose-related. Most women continue to ovulate and, despite the decreasing LNG plasma levels over time, the frequency of ovulations increases (Table 12.5) [26].

Insertion and Efficacy

It is advisable to screen for sexually transmitted infections prior to insertion. If this extra visit is inconvenient, antibiotic prophylaxis is not needed in asymptomatic women. The woman can be contacted and treated promptly in the event of a positive result. A routine follow-up visit can be advised after the first menses following insertion or 3–6 weeks later. However, it is not essential and it may be more important to advise women as to signs and symptoms of infection, perforation and expulsion, returning if they have any problems relating to their intra-uterine method.

As shown in Table 12.5, the contraceptive effectiveness of the IUSs is very high and starts immediately if inserted during days 1–7 of the menstrual cycle or following a first-trimester abortion. After delivery it can be inserted within 48 hours in non-breastfeeding women or after 4 weeks if the size of the uterus has returned to normal. Recent data indicate that the LNG-IUS 20 might provide protection for 2 years longer, but longer use is off-label [18]. The risk of ectopic pregnancy is lower in all three types of LNG-IUS than in women without contraception. Return of fertility is rapid after discontinuation of use.

Table 12.5 Characteristics of the three types of LNG-IUS [25–29]

	LNG-IUS 20	LNG-IUS 16	LNG-IUS 12
Dimensions			
T-frame	32 x 32 mm	30 x 28 mm	30 x 28 mm
Insertion tube diameter	4.4 mm	3.8 mm	3.8 mm
LNG content reservoir	52 mg	19.5 mg	13.5 mg
Approved contraceptive period	5 years	5 years	3 years
Daily release rate			
Initially	20 µg	16 µg	12 µg
After 3–5 years	10.7 µg	7.6 µg	5.5 µg
Ovulation rates			
Year 1	76.5%	88.5%	97%
Year 3	91%	100%	100%
Contraceptive effectiveness			
Cumulative 3–5 years Pearl Index (all pregnancies/100 woman-years)	0.2	0.29	0.2–0.3
Ectopic pregnancy rate for the first year of use (ectopic pregnancies/100 woman-years)	0.02	0.18	0.23
Adverse events			
Amenorrhoea at fourth trimester of use	23.6%	18.9%	12.7%
Expulsion rate (complete and partial) over 3–5 years	1.6–6.3%	2–3.6%	0.4–4.6%
Ovarian cyst formation	22%	9%	6%
Three-year adverse events			
Breast pain/discomfort	7–22%	11–18%	6–19%
Acne	28%	22%	26%
Headache	17%	13%	12%
Altered mood	10%	10%	14%
Increased weight	8%	11%	11%
Pelvic pain	9.8%	8.6%	8.7%

Non-contraceptive Benefits

Endometrial atrophy generally results in marked reduction of the amount and duration of uterine bleeding. The LNG-IUS 20 has been approved to treat menorrhagia and is more effective than any other medication. The LNG-IUS 20 also reduces dysmenorrhea and chronic pelvic pain associated with endometriosis and decreases the postoperative recurrence of endometriosis. It also protects against iron-deficiency anaemia and inhibits growth of uterine fibroids. The LNG-IUS 20 is licenced for endometrial protection during oestrogen replacement.

Adverse Events

The three LNG-IUS types are typically associated with transient irregular bleedings during the first few months of use, but this usually settles over time. Frequent, prolonged and irregular bleeding episodes tend to decrease. Infrequent bleeding rates increase over time in users of all three types of LNG-IUS, but significantly more with the LNG-IUS 20 than with the lower-dose LNG-IUS products [27]. By the end of the first year, most women have very light, short, unpredictable and infrequent bleeding episodes which follow a regular menstrual pattern in only 20% of them.

In all three types of LNG-IUS the proportion of women with amenorrhea increases gradually [28]. In addition, transient irregular bleeding does not reoccur in women who opt for a subsequent LNG-IUS 20 after 5 years of use provided that the old LNG-IUS is replaced immediately. Of these women, 60% are amenorrhoeic. Expulsion rates (complete and partial) are comparable between the three LNG-IUS versions. The number of complete expulsions is approximately equal to the number of partial expulsions. About half of all expulsions occur during the first 6 months. The development of unruptured oestrogen-producing follicles may lead to breast tension and breakthrough bleeding. These mostly harmless cysts are more frequent in LNG-IUS 20 users.

The percentages of 3-year adverse events of the three types of LNG-IUS are comparable and include breast pain or discomfort, acne, headache, altered mood, increased weight and pelvic pain [29]. The LNG-IUS improves complaints of dysmenorrhoea, has no adverse effects on bone health and does not increase the risk of adverse cardiovascular events or uterine cancers. However, the LNG-IUS 20 is associated with a minimal but significantly increased risk of breast cancer in premenopausal users [9]. An increased risk for older peri- and postmenopausal women was not found.

The overall 1-year discontinuation rate varies greatly between studies from 7.3% to 27%. Most common reasons for requesting early removal are pain or cramping (2–13%), irregular or frequent bleeding (2–26%) and the aforementioned hormonal side effects (1–5%). Adolescents and nulliparous women tend to have higher removal rates for pain. This might change with the now available smaller devices which are easier and less painful to insert [29]. The LNG-IUS is not suitable for emergency contraception.

References

1. Trussell J. Contraceptive failure in the United States. *Contraception*. 2011;**83**:397–404.

2. Palacios S, Colli E, Regidor PA. Multicenter, phase III trials on the contraceptive efficacy, tolerability and safety of a new drospirenone-only pill. *Acta Obstet Gynecol Scand*. 2019;**98**:1549–57.

3. Philips SJ, Tepper NK, Kapp N et al. Progestogen-only contraceptive use among breastfeeding women: A systematic review. *Contraception*. 2016;**94**:226–52.

4. Tepper NK, Whiteman MK, Marchbanks PA, James AH, Curtis KM. Progestin-only contraception and thromboembolism: A systematic review. *Contraception*. 2016;**94**:678–800.

5. World Health Organization. *Medical eligibility criteria for contraceptive use*. 5th edition. Geneva: World Health Organization, 2015. bit.ly/3RiJdHy.

6. Zigler RE, McNicholas C. Unscheduled vaginal bleeding with progestin-only contraceptive use. *Am J Obstet Gynecol*. 2017;**5**:443–50.

7. Abdel-Aleem H, d'Arcangues C, Vogelsong KM, Gaffield ML, Gülmezoglu AM. Treatment of vaginal bleeding irregularities induced by progestin only contraceptives. *Cochrane Database Syst Rev*. 2013; CD003449.

8. Lopez LM, Ramesh S, Chen M et al. Progestin-only contraceptives: Effects on weight. *Cochrane Database Syst Rev*. 2016;CD008815.

9. Mørch LS, Skovlund CW, Hannaford PC et al. Contemporary hormonal contraception and the risk of breast cancer. *N Engl J Med*. 2017;**377**:2228–39.

10. Skovlund CW, Mørch LS, Kessing LV, Lidegaard Ø. Association of hormonal contraceptives with depression. *JAMA Psychiatry*. 2016;**73**:1154–62.

11. Benagiano G, Primiero FM. Seventy-five microgram desogestrel minipill, a new perspective in estrogen-free contraception. *Ann N Y Acad Sci*. 2003;**997**:163–73.

12. Archer DF, Ahrendt H-J, Drouin D. Drospirenone-only oral contraceptive: Results from a multicenter noncomparative trial of efficacy, safety and tolerability. *Contraception*. 2015;**92**:439–44.

13. Duijkers IJ, Heger-Mahn D, Drouin D, Skouby S. A randomised study comparing the effect on ovarian activity of a progestogen-only pill (POP) containing desogestrel and a new POP containing drospirenone in a 24/4 regimen. *Eur J Contracept Reprod Health Care*. 2015;**20**:419–27.

14. Sacco S, Merki-Feld GS, Aegidius KL et al. Effect of exogenous estrogens and progestogens on the course of migraine during reproductive age: A consensus statement by the European Headache Federation (EHF) and the European Society of Contraception and Reproductive health (ESCRH). *Journal of Headache and Pain*. 2018;**19**:76–96.

15. Brache V, Cochon L, Duijkers IJM et al. A prospective, randomized, pharmacodynamic study of quick-starting a desogestrel progestin-only pill following ulipristal acetate for emergency contraception. *Hum Reprod*. 2015;**13**:2785–93.

16. Palomba S, Falbo A, Di Cello A, Materazzo C, Zullo F. Nexplanon: The new implant for long-term contraception. A comprehensive descriptive review. *Gynecol Endocrinol*. 2012;**9**:710–21.

17. Lazorwitz A, Aquilante CL, Sheeder J, Guiahi M, Teal S. Relationship between patient characteristics and serum etonogestrel concentrations in contraceptive implant users. *Contraception*. 2019;**100**:37–41.

18. McNicholas C, Swor E, Wan L, Peipert JF. Prolonged use of the etonogestrel implant and levonorgestrel intrauterine device: 2 years beyond FDA-approved duration. *Am J Obstet Gynecol*. 2017;**6**:586.e1–586.e6.

19. Mansour D, Korver T, Marintcheva-Petrova M, Fraser IS. The effects of Implanon on menstrual bleeding patterns. *Eur J Contracept Reprod Health Care*. 2008;**13**(Suppl 1):13–28.

20. Blumenthal PD, Gemzell-Danielsson K, Marintcheva-Petrova M. Tolerability and clinical safety of Implanon. *Eur J Contracept Reprod Health Care*. 2008;**13**(Suppl 1):29–36.

21. Kaunitz AM, Darney PD, Ross D, Wolter KD, Speroff L. Subcutaneous DMPA vs. intramuscular DMPA: A 2-year randomized study of contraceptive efficacy and bone mineral density. *Contraception*. 2009;**80**:7–17.

22. Said S, Omar K, Koetsawang S et al. A multicentered phase III comparative clinical trial of depot-medroxyprogesterone acetate given three-monthly at doses of 100 mg or 150 mg. II: The comparison of bleeding patterns. *Contraception*. 1987;**35**:591–607.

23. Lange HLH, Manos BE, Gothard MD, Rogers LK, Bonny AE. Bone mineral density and weight changes in adolescents randomized to 3 doses of depot medroxyprogesterone acetate. *J Pediatr Adolesc Gynecol*. 2017;**30**:169–75.

24. Kohn JE, Simons HR, Badia LD et al. Increased 1-year continuation of DMPA among women randomized to self-administration: Results from a randomized controlled trial at Planned Parenthood. *Contraception*. 2018;**97**:198–204.

25. Reinecke I, Hofmann B, Mesic E, Drenth HJ, Garmann D. An integrated population pharmacokinetic analysis to characterize levonorgestrel pharmacokinetics after different administration routes. *J Clin Pharmacol*. 2018;**58**:1639–54.

26. Apter D, Gemzell-Danielsson K, Hauck B, Rosen K, Zurth C. Pharmacokinetics of two low-dose levonorgestrel-releasing intrauterine systems and effects on ovulation rate and cervical function: Pooled analyses of phase II and III studies. *Fertil Steril*. 2014;**101**:1656–62.e1–4.

27. Goldthwaite LM, Creinin MD. Comparing bleeding patterns for the levonorgestrel 52 mg, 19.5 mg, and 13.5 mg intrauterine systems. *Contraception*. 2019;**100**:128–31.

28. Sergison JE, Maldonado LY, Gao X, Hubacher D. Levonorgestrel intrauterine system associated amenorrhea: A systematic review and metaanalysis. *Am J Obstet Gynecol*. 2019;**220**:440–8.e8.

29 Gemzell-Danielsson K, Schellschmidt I, Apter D. A randomized, phase II study describing the efficacy, bleeding profile, and safety of two low-dose levonorgestrel-releasing intrauterine contraceptive systems and Mirena. *Fertil Steril*. 2012;**97**:616–22.e1–3.

Nonhormonal Contraception

Kristina Gemzell-Danielsson, Juan Acuna and Helena Kopp Kallner

General Concepts

For the past decade there has been an increased interest in nonhormonal contraceptive methods. In the United States the trend is an increase of 1.1–2.2% users with almost 1.4 million women in 2014 and an estimated 2.5 million women in 2020 in this category [1]. Nonhormonal, traditional or natural methods of contraception include fertility awareness–based methods (FABM), barrier, rhythm (periodic abstinence), withdrawal and lactational amenorrhea, abstinence, breastfeeding, douching or traditional folk methods. Sterilization and copper intrauterine devices (Cu-IUDs) are also nonhormonal but are not discussed further in this chapter. Here we cover methods that are not hormone-based and that are included in the barrier/spermicide or natural/traditional categories (Figure 13.1). It is important to mention that there is an abundance of adequate resources on the Internet for counseling. A limited but carefully chosen list is provided at the end of the chapter (Appendix 1).

Fertility Awareness–Based Methods (or Fertility-Awareness Methods)

General Concepts

Fertility awareness–based methods (FABM), sometimes controversially called natural contraception methods [2–4], for family planning include a series of techniques that rely on the identification, recording, analysis and interpretation of symptoms associated with ovulation in order to estimate fertile days during which intercourse should not happen (intermittent abstinence) or protection for conception (such as barrier methods) should be used [5]. Specific counseling and education are needed for these methods to be effective.

The potential for failure, given the high user-dependent practice, is high and the range of effectiveness is wide, reported to be from 27% for typical use to 1% for perfect use [4, 6]. This gap is reported as smaller for a newer and controversial subset of these methods (discussed further later in this chapter) – digital fertility awareness–based methods (d-FABM), specifically the "contraceptive or cycle-monitoring apps" [7–10]. Use of multiple contraceptive methods is frequent in nonhormonal contraception users (16.5%), at least in the United States [7]. Much of the theoretical foundation relies on the biological events of the menstrual cycle. Thus, a short explanation of such events is part of the revision of FABM.

Biological Background

The quintessential foundation of all FABM is counseling regarding the events of the menstrual cycle and the estimation of fertile (and sub-fertile) days. These topics are frequently confused or ignored by most patients and not enough health providers explain the failure rates these methods have, thus the need to review here what we consider the minimum knowledge base required. The menstrual cycle has three distinct phases: the follicular phase, the ovulation phase and the luteal phase. Estimated survival of the gametes is 5 days for the sperm and 24 hours for the ovum. The most important predictor for fertile days in a given cycle is the estimation of the more regular and stable luteal phase based on the duration of the previous cycles. For most women with regular cycles (26–32 days), the prediction of fertile days is easy and fairly accurate. In women with irregular cycles, this estimation fails frequently or will yield a very large number of days labeled as fertile when indeed they most likely are at no risk of pregnancy.

Ovulation occurs, in most cases of regular 28-day cycles, at around day 14. The oocyte is susceptible to fertilization by a sperm during this time only. Based on gamete survival, we consider that a woman under usual conditions is fertile a maximum of 6 days per

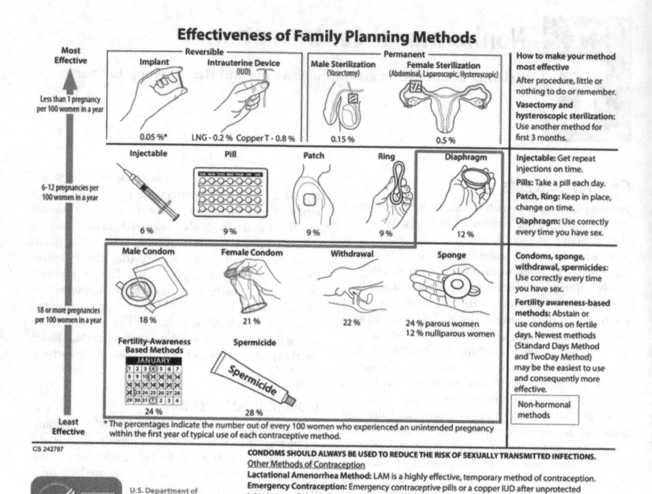

Figure 13.1 Effectiveness of contraception methods with emphasis (red box) on nonhormonal methods of contraception. CDC, 2020

cycle. Although this survival is a probabilistic estimate (most sperm would be dead after 36 hours and only 1% will survive more than 5 days), it is very widely accepted for the estimation of the fertile window.

The luteal phase is accompanied by an increase in progesterone by the corpus luteum after ovulation. The temperature regulatory centers in the central nervous system (CNS) are sensitive to progesterone. The basal body temperature (BBT) increases by about half a degree centigrade (0.6 ± 0.2 C°) after ovulation and this change may be distinctly detected by a thermometer sensitive enough to measure tenths of a degree. Measuring BBT is a delicate process as true basal conditions are needed such as immediately after waking up but before any substantial movement or activity happens. A daily record should be entered into charts (available on the Internet).

The corpus luteum produces both estradiol and progesterone after ovulation that is maintained during luteal phase. The duration of the luteal phase is usually less variable than the follicular phase. Menstruation occurs after the decline in estradiol and progesterone. The follicular phase varies in length depending on the variable process of the recruitment and selection of the dominant follicle. The estimation of the possible length of the follicular phase is thus difficult (Figure 13.2).

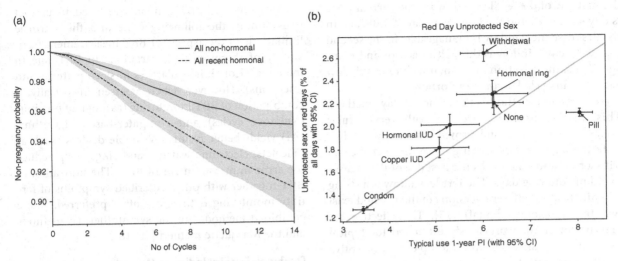

Figure 13.2 Changes and stages in the menstrual cycle

During the follicular phase, pre-ovulatory events produce detectable signs and symptoms that can predict ovulation. During the menstrual cycle, the cervical secretion (cervical mucus) changes, as does the cervix consistency and position. Of those changes, the change in consistency and production of secretions is the easiest to monitor by far. Specific training is needed and only highly committed women will be able to successfully use this for contraception. If they commit, the Pearl Index can reach 1 [3, 11]. Monitoring of cervical secretions has the highest success rate if an almost perfect vaginal condition exists. No inflammatory or infectious processes should be present.

During approximately the first half of the follicular phase (in regular cycles, or before estrogen levels have started to increase), the cervical mucus is scant ("dry days") and thick due to a trabecular microstructure. After estradiol starts rising, the mucus adopts a linear structure, is abundant ("wet days"), becomes translucid and elongates (such as egg white). Maximum clarity and elongation are achieved around the estrogen peak (ovulation day/maximum day of fertility). Accompanying changes in sodium chloride content cause the phenomenon called "ferning." Using a low-power microscope, women (and health practitioners) may determine the possibility of ovulation.

Fertility awareness–based methods, albeit feasible to use in irregular cycles, are mostly recommended for those women with cycles between 26 and 32 days of duration when ovulation is fairly predictable [12]. The use of the natural signs of ovulation in the determination of fertile days is carried out by several contraceptive methods. This next section briefly describes the characteristics of the most popular and well known. The principles of these methods are:

- The identification of the fertile and the non-fertile days as accurately as possible.
- During fertile days, use of periodic abstinence or another form of contraception is needed if intercourse should happen.
- For the labeled non-fertile days, unprotected coitus is possible and safe.

Calendar-based methods: These methods rely on the cumulative information previous cycles provide with respect to fertile days in the current cycle being predicted [2, 13, 14]. In essence, the longer the time of the observations used to calculate the current cycle probabilities the better, and the more stable the cycles the better. The method works better in woman with 26–32-day cycles. There are two common methods: the calendar method and the standard days method.

The calendar method takes the shortest and longest cycles reported and subtracts 18 days from the shortest and 11 days from the longest cycles, respectively. These two numbers provide the first and last fertile days of the current cycle, respectively. For example, for cycles of 26–32 days for a year, the fertile window would be between day 8 (26−18 = 8) and day 21 (32−11 = 21). For cycles between 22 and 40 days, the first day of the fertile window for the current cycle is day 4 (22–18) and the last day is day 29 (40–11). In the first case the window is manageable. In the second case a 25-day window is difficult to accept and manage. Thus, the selection of women with relatively low variation in cycle length is important.

The second method is the standard days method. This method preselects women with very regular cycles of 26–32 days and provides a 12-day window of fertile days. It uses a string of beads (cycle beads) with a red bead that marks the first day of the menses to aid in counting days. The fertile window is a string of white beads. Different versions of the method exist (wristband, analog, digital) [15]. The effectiveness may be lower than previously estimated for typical use where counseling for multiple contraceptive methods use may be appropriate.

Cervical Secretions Monitoring Methods

John and Evelin Billings described the use of cervical mucus for monitoring fertility in the mid-1950s. The Billings method relies on daily observation of the vaginal secretion to identify the characteristics related to hormonal changes. No hormonal preparations may be used concomitantly with any cervical secretion monitoring method (CSMM) as they modify the cervical mucus characteristics.

The CSMMs rely on the appearance (thick, cloudy, clear, transparent), feeling (dry, damp, wet) and stretchiness/elongation (not present, intermediate, maximum/peak) characteristics of the mucus evaluation [3]. Women evaluate these characteristics as well as make other notations for each evaluated cycle. Some model charts are widely available for this purpose in the open web.

The 2-day method of CSMM simplifies the assessment of the appearance of secretions/cervical mucus from absence to presence, over two consecutive days, to define a change. Any day and consecutive days when secretions (as opposed to "dry" days of increasing elongating nature) are present, compared with absence the previous day, are considered fertile days.

Basal Body Temperature

As explained before, changes in the BBT with an increase of around half a degree Celsius from the follicular to the luteal phase are associated with ovulation. However, BBT measurements alone are less than ideal to predict ovulation and to be used as contraceptive method in a given cycle, due to at least

two reasons: the BBT can only be used to predict ovulation in the following cycle and the intrinsic limitations in the aspects of BBT measurement (sensitivity of thermometers, variations in BBT due to intake of alcohol, irregularities in sleep patterns and infections). However, when assessed historically, a combination of BBT monitoring (as a sign of previous ovulatory cycles) and computer-based algorithms (AI) yields better results. Wearable devices (such as bracelets, electronic watches and rings) help reduce the error in measurement of BBT. The utilization of BBT together with other described symptoms of fertility monitoring is therefore often preferred. These combined methods are the symptothermal methods and the Marquette method [16–18].

Combined Fertility Indicator Methods

A combination of the symptoms and signs of fertility done simultaneously and well increases the effectiveness of the method. These methods may also add monitoring of estradiol degradation products in urine (ovulation detection technologies). These FABMs are more effective, reporting 2–4% perfect use pregnancy rate by Pearl Index. Nevertheless, effectiveness for typical use range from close to 30% for symptothermal to 7% for symptoms and urinary hormones monitoring (such as in the Marquette method) pointing to a highly user-dependent variability. Knowledge about these methods is not widespread among general practitioners or even gynecologists, making them even more difficult to implement and use. Extensive counseling is needed and a period of trial and error may be required before a couple (or more concretely the woman) is ready for their use.

Digitally Assisted Fertility Awareness–Based Methods

The essential success of any FABM relies on a correct identification of fertile days *and* successful avoidance of pregnancy during the fertile window by a second method in case of intercourse. The consistent and accurate calculation of the fertile window, a process limited by the potential for human error, is improved in d-FABMs by providing storage of accurate and more complete data and calculations based on algorithms that are more sophisticated than those done by hand. The d-FABMs, represented by computer programs (less frequent) or phone apps (very common today), especially in younger generations, provide easy access to accurate calculations without, many times, the participation of health providers.

The d-FABMs provide a method of including statistical probabilities for deviation from the cycle mean length and a probabilistic approach may be used to define fertile days more accurately using historical data and their variations over time. Algorithms further modify these probabilities through integrated "self-learning" as more information is fed into the app. Some devices/tests (such as Natural Cycles, Persona and Clearblue Easy monitor)[19] have room to input or even to measure hormones, such as luteinizing hormone (LH) and estrone-3-gloconoride (EG), in urine [12, 20] for additional use in their algorithms. Available reports show failure rates of 1–8% for perfect to typical use [10].

After a fertile window is identified, the principle is the same as for other FABMs: use of intermittent abstinence or, if intercourse is going to happen, the use of a secondary form of contraception (most commonly barrier methods). Based on available data, the use of d-FABMs for contraception (they may be used for fertility purposes as well) is growing among women seeking more effective, natural, nonhormonal contraception. Evidence (of low-to-intermediate scientific rigor and quality) supports that these apps, probably by facilitating more complete cycle data recording and by facilitating more complex and accurate calculations, are more effective than other barrier methods or nondigital FABMS [10].

The d-FABMs' most important contribution is probably overcoming user-dependent issues (such as knowledge of physiology, ability to perform calculations, recollection and timing of such measurements) and yet identifying the fertile window through an automated and user-friendly interface. Prediction of ovulation is not the purpose of these apps, but rather prediction of days when intercourse may happen safely without addition methods of contraception. And reminding automatically of fertile days when other contraceptive methods should be used.

Today more than 1,000 apps and many websites are available [21–24]. The purpose behind the use of these apps by women is mixed. In a recent mixed methods study, most users wanted to "monitor the cycle," with other motivations being to conceive, monitor fertility treatments and contraception [24].

Almost all of these apps are promoted as cycle-monitoring devices or as fertility apps (to seek fertile days to support conception). To our knowledge, only one has been certified by the Food and Drug Administration (FDA) as a contraceptive app: Natural Cycles (NC) (Figure 13.3). Surveillance data from NC suggest that women of mid-reproductive age

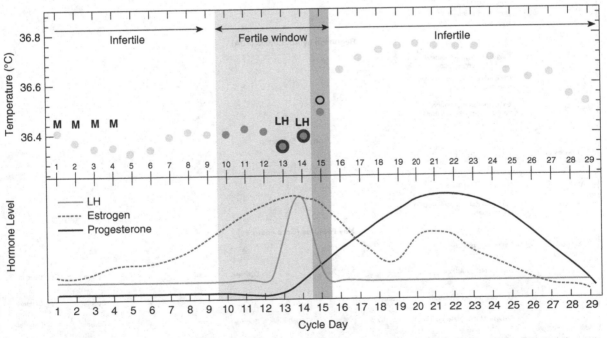

Figure 13.3 Effectiveness of the use of d-FABM (NC) given previous use of hormonal vs. nonhormonal contraception and by specific method of previous use

and regular lifestyle prefer this d-FABM, which often involves BBT data imputed into the app [25, 26]. Data show that most unplanned pregnancies occurring during use of d-FABMs occur during days marked as fertile – that is, couples have unprotected intercourse when they should have used additional protection according to the instructions.

The effectiveness of the d-FABMs may also be linked to the ability to use other contraceptive methods. If women using the app have previously used the methods that are most commonly used to prevent pregnancy during the fertile days (e.g., barrier), the effectiveness of the d-FABMs is increased as shown in the following figures from NC data [26]. Furthermore, the specific method of previous contraceptive use further define these differences. Women who previously used barrier methods, which are more user dependent and require a learning phase, perform better than women who used more user-independent methods such as intrauterine devices

(IUDs). Table 13.1 provides a summary of the most frequently available d-FABMs, with information obtained from available app sites and publications.

Barrier Methods

Male Condoms

Male condoms provide a physical barrier to spermatozoa and are the most common barrier method due to popularity and frequency of use. Increased popularity is linked, especially after the 1980s with the appearance of HIV, to the prevention of sexually transmitted infections (STIs) [27]. The use of "rubber" for the production of male condoms is the probable origin to the name "rubbers" for male condoms. Latex is currently the most common material by far. High emphasis is placed on quality testing as mandated by the FDA and the European Medicines Agency (EMA) since the mid-1970s. Improvement

Table 13.1 Summary of the most frequently available digital fertility awareness–based methods

Category	Sub-category	Natural Cycles	Dot	Clue	Glow	Eve	Ava	Flo	Apple
App (algorithm) optimized for intended use for									
	Period tracking	☑	☑	☑	☑	☑	☑	☑	☑
	Pregnancy planning	☑	☑	☑	☑	x	☑	☑	x
	Birth control	☑	x	x	x	x	x	x	x
Regulated by Authorities (FDA)									
	Cleared by FDA as medical device for contraception	☑	x	x	x	x	x	x	x
	CE-marked in EU as a medical device for contraception	☑	x	x	x	x	x	x	x
	Effectiveness in contraception based on published clinical studies	☑	☑	x	x	x	x	x	x
Body of Evidence									
Peer-reviewed publications		☑	☑	x	x	x	☑	x	x
	Number of publications	7	1	0	0	0	3	x	x
	Published data on contraceptive effectiveness	☑	☑	x	x	x	x	x	x
Key Features (Core Features)									
Period tracking Fertility tracking	Period logging	☑	☑	☑	☑	☑	☑	☑	☑
	BBT (detect ovulation)	☑	x	x	Optional	x	x	Optional	Optional
	LH Tests (detect ovulation)	Supportive	x	x	x	x	x	Optional	Optional
	Cervical Mucus (detect ovulation)	x	x	Optional	Optional	x	x	Optional	Optional
Additional Features Get to Know your body	Educates user on body and cycle	☑	☑	☑	☑	☑	STI	☑	☑
Follow a pregnancy	Track development of pregnancy	☑	x	x	☑	x	☑	☑	x

of feeling and temperature transmission improve user satisfaction, one main barrier for condom use [2, 28]. Polyisoprene condoms are an alternative to latex condoms for people with allergies. Improved flexibility and heat conduction in these have improved feeling during coitus. They can also be used with any type of commonly available lubricants as opposed to latex condoms, which should be used with water-based or silicone-based lubricants only. One downside is that they are more expensive than latex condoms.

Condoms come in many sizes, shapes and forms. They may have an end reservoir and may be textured and in original colors and designs. Condoms with spermicides are as effective as those without it. The effectiveness of the condom is mostly determined by its correct use [29]. The most common error is that condom use is the intended method of contraception but for various reasons the condom is never put on. Guidelines are easily available on the topic, especially for young potential users [2, 30]. (CDC Condom effectiveness www.cdc.gov/condomeffectiveness/index .html)

The most common problems with condom use include the following:

- Late application in 17.0–51.1% of cases (6 studies).
- Incorrect use (including incorrect application or removal, opening the package with a sharp object and any other issue with use) in 2% (completely unrolling condom before putting it on) to above 80% (not inspecting condom before use) of cases.
- Breakage in 0.8–40.7% of cases across 15 studies.
- Condom-associated erection problems during application and intercourse in 5.3–28.1% and 6.0–20.2%, respectively, of cases across 6 studies.

Vaginal Barrier Methods

All of these methods are women's methods. They are female-initiated and considered female-empowering. They have the same mechanism of action (sperm blockage to the upper female genital track) and they also provide good (female condom) to intermediate (others) protection against STIs [31, 32]. Although the dental dam is not a contraceptive method, it is included in this section to recognize its role in the prevention of STIs during oral sex.

The main difference is that the cervical cap covers the cervix and the diaphragm covers the cervix and part of the vagina, while the female condom, with the outer edge located at the pelvic floor, covers the cervix

and vagina completely. The female condom, designed in the 1980s, is a good barrier method. However, it is very rarely used. Several models exist, with the FC2 being the most common. The FC2 is a nitrile synthetic latex condom. Other models include the VA wow condom (latex), the women's condom (polyurethane) and the cupid condom (latex), available outside the United States. All models have an outer ring (larger than the inner ring) – the pouch condom – and an inner ring or doughnut-shaped structure that fits in the vagina near the cervix. One great advantage for women, contrasting with the male condom, is that it may be placed on site hours before intercourse [33].

Diaphragms, Contoured Diaphragms and Cervical Caps

All these methods should be placed deep into the vaginal canal and can be placed hours before intercourse. They should be used with spermicidal compounds. Most are reusable and provide limited protection against STIs [2, 34]. Their use is much less common than the use of male condoms. Fitted diaphragms are made from different materials (latex, silicone) and available in 5 mm increments from 60 mm to 90 mm with a population normal distribution of sizes (the most commonly used is 75 mm). They are not widely or easily available today and must often be ordered directly from the manufacturer, sometimes with a prescription.

The single-sized newest contoured diaphragm, the Caya Diaphragm, has replaced many of the fitted diaphragms. The PI for the Caya is around 14% for typical use. It fits a wider range of women without a consultation and may be demonstrated for adequate insertion technique and positioning to any woman during a regular consultation. Due to its shape, removal is easier than for similar devices.

The cervical cup is a similar, albeit smaller silicone-based device designed to fit snuggly onto the cervix. The natural vacuum action provided by the snug fitting over the cervix keeps the cap in place. The use of spermicide to achieve an acceptable level of effectiveness is also recommended. The most common cervical cap available (and the only one available in many countries such as the United States) is the FemCap. Difficult removal and discomfort during coitus are commonly reported. However, it may be left longer in the vagina (but not more than 36 hours). Cervical caps are available in three sizes: nulliparous, multiparous (no vaginal births) and multiparous (vaginal births).

Fitting is also recommended. Comparative studies show that it is more difficult to use and therefore is less effective than the vaginal diaphragm [35].

Spermicides

Spermicides have the lowest reported effectiveness among all methods if used alone. It works by being toxic to sperm or by inhibiting motility of sperm. Nonoxynol-9 (N-9) is the only widely available and widely used spermicide in the global market [36]. Other spermicides (phenylmercury acetate, octoxynol-9, benzalkonium chloride, mephengol, C31 G, propranolol) and lactic acid compounds do not provide proven increased effectiveness. The mechanism of action is that of cytotoxicity for the sperm, for most of these, except for lactic acid derivatives.

Spermicides are recommended as an adjuvant method to be used with condoms, vaginal barrier methods or during early use of oral contraceptives or IUDs, and are not recommended as the only method. Despite their low effectiveness, spermicides are relatively popular and used, alone or in combination with other barrier methods, by around 15% or more of women in the United States who use contraception. Due to the possibility of vaginal irritation, spermicides are often associated with an increased risk for HIV and other STIs. Discontinuation and adverse secondary effects (mainly local irritation and discomfort) are common.

The sponge is a device perceived by patients and inexperienced healthcare providers as offering a barrier plus a spermicidal effect. However, the sponge's effectiveness is comparable to other spermicides, among the lowest of contraceptives. Allergic reactions are more common with the sponge than with other barrier methods.

Lactational Amenorrhea

Due to the suppression of the hypothalamic-hypophysis-ovarian axis by prolactin, amenorrhea is common during breastfeeding. Prolactin remains high as long as lactation is maintained exclusively, making pregnancy unlikely. If lactation episodes are skipped (e.g., by the use of formula or sleep), the probability of ovulation, and so of pregnancy, increases. As per the Bellagio Consensus, exclusive lactation maintained during 6 months leads to a very low risk of pregnancy. Ovulation is likely to occur after this period and pregnancy may then occur without awareness of it. Success of lactational amenorrhea as contraception, especially in developing countries, is highly related to women's education and social support and nonuse of formula [37].

Copper Intrauterine Device

Copper intrauterine devices are highly effective reversible nonhormonal contraceptive methods with similar perfect-and typical-use Pearl Index numbers. The efficacy is user independent and is not affected by any drug interaction. The copper surface of the IUD determines efficacy and an IUD with a copper surface of at least 300 mm^2 with proven efficacy in clinical trials should be recommended. The most effective Cu-IUDs are recommended for 5–10 (12) years of use. The mechanism of action is mainly by preventing fertilization. Copper ions reduce sperm motility and have a toxic effect on both sperm and eggs while ovulation remains unaffected. If fertilization still occurs, endometrial receptivity is impaired and implantation prevented [38].

Intrauterine devices are a preferred choice for women of all ages with high user compliance and satisfaction [39]. A Cu-IUD inserted after the age of 40 can be kept until menopause. Previous IUD rejection, IUD pregnancy including ectopic pregnancy, or genital infection (including pelvic inflammatory disease (PID)) are not contraindications for IUD insertion [40]. Copper IUDs are associated with a reduced risk of cervical and endometrial cancer [41].

Placement

Counseling should include information on the size of the IUD and expected effects on bleeding and pain. Copper IUDs do not affect bleeding pattern but increase the volume by an average of 55%. They may also increase dysmenorrhea [42]. In case of irregular bleeding pathology or pregnancy should be excluded. Non-steroidal anti-inflammatory drugs (NSAIDs) are proven to alleviate pain and reduce bleeding. Fibrinolysis inhibitors (tranexamic acid) can also be used to reduce bleeding. When a menstrual cup is used, care should be taken that threads are not caught between the vaginal wall and the cup and the vacuum should be released before the menstrual cup is removed to reduce the risk of removing the IUD.

An IUD can be inserted at any time during the menstrual cycle if ongoing pregnancy can be ruled out [43]. It is important to avoid delaying insertion. For women who have not given birth, interval insertion appears to be less painful. Abstinence or other contraceptives should be recommended 1 week prior to insertion. A Cu-IUD is inserted immediately at surgical abortion and after completion of medical abortion (within 1 week of mifepristone). Postpartum it is inserted 6–8 weeks or immediately after expulsion of the placenta [44].

Pain

For most women insertion is not or only mildly painful. A paracervical block (PCB) can be used to reduce pain in connection with or after insertion. "Verbocaine" – that is, a safe environment with experienced personnel and good information – and post-insertion NSAIDs provide the best conditions for reducing pain in connection with inserting IUDs. There is no evidence of efficacy of misoprostol for the purpose of pain relief, but misoprostol may facilitate insertion (or removal) [45, 46].

In case of bacterial vaginosis, treatment can be given at the time of or prior to insertion. Screening for STIs should be performed if indicated. There is no evidence that vaginal washing before IUD insertion reduce the risk of infection, so this can be avoided. There is also a lack of studies on the use of non-sterilized instruments and any increase in the risk of infection, but it is recommended that the forceps and sound should be sterile [47, 48].

The threads on the IUD are cut after insertion to a length of approximately 2–3 cm beyond the outer cervical os. If they are cut too short, this increases the risk of them bothering the partner during sexual intercourse. In breastfeeding women who have a smaller uterus than normal, the threads should be cut longer as otherwise they risk ending up out of reach when the uterus regains its normal size. In rare cases, a woman may experience a vasovagal reaction and drop in blood pressure during IUD insertion.

Complications

- Perforation at insertion is rare (< 1/1,000) but increases with malformation/anatomic variations and breastfeeding when the uterus is atrophic.
- Expulsion occurs in 3–7% of users with a slightly higher risk among parous versus nulliparous women.
- The Cu-IUD has among the lowest absolute risk of ectopic pregnancy. However, in case of a pregnancy, the risk that it is ectopic is increased.
- Within 3 weeks of placement there is a slight increased risk for PID. Thereafter Cu-IUD use is not associated with any increased risk for PID [49].

- After removal fertility returns immediately and previous use of Cu-IUD among nulliparous women is not associated with tubal infertility [50].

If an IUD user becomes pregnant, a gynecological and ultrasound examination must be performed as soon as possible to assess the location and gestational age. If possible, the IUD should always be removed as soon as the intrauterine pregnancy is discovered, regardless of whether it is being terminated or continued, as the risk of complications is significant if the IUD is left in place [51]. Current PID in a woman who has an IUD is treated with the device in place [52]. However, removal should be considered if the infection does not respond to the given treatment, although it is then important to recommend another method of contraception. Placement of a Cu-IUD within 120 hours of an unprotected sexual intercourse is the most effective method for emergency contraception.

Appendix 1

Internet-Based Resources as of October 30, 2020

These are specialty sites that contain information on statistics, epidemiology, resources and other websites and services on natural contraception as well as other methods for contraception. This is not intended to be a comprehensive list but more a list of trusted institutions for further expansion into more internet-based searches for contraception resources.

1. Contraception page, Centers for Disease Control and Prevention, National Center for Chronic Disease Prevention and Health Promotion, Division of Reproductive Health www.cdc.gov/reproductivehealth/contraception/index.htm
2. National Institutes of Health, Eunice Kennedy Shriver National Institute of Child Health and Human Development, Contraception Resources www.nichd.nih.gov/health/topics/contraception/more_information/resources
3. European Contraception Atlas www.contraceptioninfo.eu
4. World Health Organization www.who.int/reproductivehealth/topics/family_planning/en
5. Guttmacher Institute www.guttmacher.org
6. Medicine Net www.medicinenet.com/natural_methods_of_birth_control/article.htm

7. New Zealand Family Planning
www.familyplanning.org.nz/advice/contraception/contraception-methods

8. EngenderHealth
www.engenderhealth.org/our-work/family-planning/index

9. Everyday Health
www.everydayhealth.com/birth-control/resource-center

10. Family Planning Association – UK
www.fpa.org.uk/professionals/resources/leaflet-and-booklet-downloads

11. Department of Health and Human Services (HHS)
www.hhs.gov/opa/pregnancy-prevention/birth-control-methods/lam/index.html

12. National Institute for Health and Care Excellence (NICE)
www.nice.org.uk/guidance/health-and-social-care-delivery/contraception

References

1. Kavanaugh ML, Jerman J. Contraceptive method use in the United States: Trends and characteristics between 2008, 2012 and 2014. *Contraception*. 2018;97:14–21. https://doi.org/10.1016/j.contraception.2017.10.003.

2. Hassoun D. [Natural family planning methods and barrier: CNGOF contraception guidelines]. *Gynecol Obstet Fertil Senol*. 2018;46:873–82. https://doi.org/10.1016/j.gofs.2018.10.002.

3. Han L, Taub R, Jensen JT. Cervical mucus and contraception: What we know and what we don't. *Contraception*. 2017;96:310–21. https://doi.org/10.1016/j.contraception.2017.07.168.

4. Sung S, Abramovitz A. *Natural family planning*. Bethesda, MD: StatPearls, 2020.

5. Klaus H. Natural family planning: A review. *Obstet Gynecol Surv*. 1982;37:128–50. https://doi.org/10.1097/00006254-198202000-00026.

6. Bradley SEK, Polis CB, Bankole A, Croft T. Global contraceptive failure rates: Who is most at risk? *Stud Fam Plann*. 2019;50:3–24. https://doi.org/10.1111/sifp.12085.

7. Polis CB, Jones RK. Multiple contraceptive method use and prevalence of fertility awareness based method use in the United States, 2013–2015. *Contraception*. 2018;98:188–92. https://doi.org/10.1016/j.contraception.2018.04.013.

8. Duane M, Contreras A, Jensen ET, White A. The performance of fertility awareness–based method apps marketed to avoid pregnancy. *J Am Board Fam Med*. 2016;29:508–11. https://doi.org/10.3122/jabfm.2016.04.160022.

9. Grimes DA, Gallo MF, Grigorieva V et al. Fertility awareness-based methods for contraception: Systematic review of randomized controlled trials. *Contraception*. 2005;72:85–90. https://doi.org/10.1016/j.contraception.2005.03.010.

10. Peragallo Urrutia R, Polis CB, Jensen ET et al. Effectiveness of fertility awareness–based methods for pregnancy prevention: A systematic review. *Obstet Gynecol*. 2018;132:591–604. https://doi.org/10.1097/AOG.0000000000002784.

11. Daunter B, Counsilman C. Cervical mucus: Its structure and possible biological functions. *Eur J Obstet Gynecol Reprod Biol*. 1980;10:141–61. https://doi.org/10.1016/0028-2243(80)90056-8.

12. Su H-W, Yi Y-C, Wei T-Y et al. Detection of ovulation: A review of currently available methods. *Bioeng Transl Med*. 2017;2:238–46. https://doi.org/10.1002/btm2.10058.

13. Johnson S, Marriott L, Zinaman M. Can apps and calendar methods predict ovulation with accuracy? *Curr Med Res Opin*. 2018;34:1587–94. https://doi.org/10.1080/03007995.2018.1475348.

14. Nilsson A, Ahlborg T, Bernhardsson S. Use of non-medical contraceptive methods: A survey of women in western Sweden. *Eur J Contracept Reprod Health Care*. 2018;23:400–6. https://doi.org/10.1080/13625187.2018.1541079.

15. Marston CA, Church K. Does the evidence support global promotion of the calendar-based Standard Days Method® of contraception? *Contraception*. 2016;93:492–7. https://doi.org/10.1016/j.contraception.2016.01.006.

16. Pyper C. Natural family planning: Low failure rate with symptothermal method. *BMJ*. 1993;307:1359–60. https://doi.org/10.1136/bmj.307.6915.1359-c.

17. Soler F, Barranco-Castillo E. The symptothermal (double check) method: An efficient natural method of family planning. *Eur J Contracept Reprod Health Care*. 2010;15:379–80, author reply at 381. https://doi.org/10.3109/13625187.2010.505990.

18. Geerling JH. Natural family planning. *Am Fam Physician*. 1995;52:1749–56, 1759.

19. Bouchard TP, Genuis SJ. Personal fertility monitors for contraception. *Can Med Assoc J*. 2011;183:73–6. https://doi.org/10.1503/cmaj.090195.

20. Bonnar J, Flynn A, Freundl G et al. Personal hormone monitoring for contraception. *Br J Fam Plann*. 1999;24:128–34.

21. Moglia ML, Nguyen HV, Chyjek K et al. Evaluation of smartphone menstrual cycle tracking applications using an adapted APPLICATIONS scoring system. *Obstet Gynecol*. 2016;127:1153–60. https://doi.org/10.1097/AOG.0000000000001444.

22. Freis A, Freundl-Schütt T, Wallwiener LM et al. Plausibility of menstrual cycle apps claiming to support conception. *Front Public Health*. 2018;6: 98–102. https://doi.org/10.3389/fpubh.2018.00098.

23. Zwingerman R, Chaikof M, Jones C. A critical appraisal of fertility and menstrual tracking apps for the iPhone. *J Obstet Gynaecol Can*. 2019. https://doi.org/10.1016/j.jogc.2019.09.023.

24. Gambier-Ross K, McLernon DJ, Morgan HM. A mixed methods exploratory study of women's relationships with and uses of fertility tracking apps. *Digit Health*. 2018;4:2055207618785077. https://doi.org/10.1177/2055207618785077.

25. Berglund Scherwitzl E, Lindén Hirschberg A, Scherwitzl R. Identification and prediction of the fertile window using NaturalCycles. *Eur J Contracept Reprod Health Care*. 2015;20:403–8. https://doi.org/10.3109/13625187.2014.988210.

26. Berglund Scherwitzl E, Lundberg O, Kopp Kallner H et al. Perfect-use and typical-use Pearl Index of a contraceptive mobile app. *Contraception*. 2017;96:420–5. https://doi.org/10.1016/j.contraception.2017.08.014.

27. Evans WD, Ulasevich A, Hatheway M, Deperthes B. Systematic review of peer-reviewed literature on global condom promotion programs. *Int J Environ Res Public Health*. 2020. https://doi.org/10.3390/ijerph17072262.

28. Gossman W, Shaeffer AD, McNabb DM. *Condoms*. StatPearls, 2020.

29. Sanders SA, Yarber WL, Kaufman EL et al. Condom use errors and problems: A global view. *Sex Health*. 2012;9:81–95. https://doi.org/10.1071/SH11095.

30. Raidoo S, Kaneshiro B. Contraception counseling for adolescents. *Curr Opin Obstet Gynecol*. 2017;29:310–15. https://doi.org/10.1097/GCO.0000000000000390.

31. Beksinska M, Wong R, Smit J. Male and female condoms: Their key role in pregnancy and STI/HIV prevention. *Best Pract Res Clin Obstet Gynaecol*. 2020;66:55–67. https://doi.org/10.1016/j.bpobgyn.2019.12.001.

32. Maksut JL, Eaton LA. Female condoms = missed opportunities: Lessons learned from promotion-centered interventions. *Women's Health Issues*. 2015;25:366–76. https://doi.org/10.1016/j.whi.2015.03.015.

33. Bounds W. Female condoms. *Eur J Contracept Reprod Health Care*. 1997;2:113–16. https://doi.org/10.3109/13625189709167464.

34. Edouard L. The renaissance of barrier methods. *J Fam Plann Reprod Health Care*. 2012;38:131–3. https://doi.org/10.1136/jfprhc-2012-100314.

35. Mauck C, Callahan M, Weiner DH, Dominik R. A comparative study of the safety and efficacy of FemCap, a new vaginal barrier contraceptive, and the Ortho All-Flex diaphragm: The FemCap Investigators' Group. *Contraception*. 1999;60:71–80. https://doi.org/10.1016/s0010-7824(99)00068-2.

36. Lech MM. Spermicides 2002: An overview. *Eur J Contracept Reprod Health Care*. 2002;7:173–7.

37. Dev R, Kohler P, Feder M et al. A systematic review and meta-analysis of postpartum contraceptive use among women in low- and middle-income countries. *Reprod Health*. 2019;16:154. https://doi.org/10.1186/s12978-019-0824-4.

38. Tredway DR, Umezaki CU, Mishell DR Jr, Settlage DS. Effect of intrauterine devices on sperm transport in the human being: Preliminary report. *Am J Obstet Gynecol*. 1975;123(7):734–5.

39. Winner B, Peipert JF, Zhao Q et al. Effectiveness of long-acting reversible contraception. *N Engl J Med*. 2012;366(21):1998–2007.

40. World Health Organization. *Medical eligibility criteria for contraceptive use*. 5th edition. Geneva: World Health Organization, 2015. www.who.int/publications/i/item/9789241549158.

41. Castellsagué X, Thompson WD, Dubrow R. Intra-uterine contraception and the risk of endometrial cancer. *Int J Cancer*. 1993;54(6):911–16.

42. Milsom I, Andersson K Jonasson K, Lindstedt G, Rybo G. Contraception: The influence of the Gyne-T 380S IUD on menstrual blood loss and iron status. *Contraception*. 1995;52(3):175–9.

43. Whiteman MK, Tyler CP, Folger SG, Gaffield ME, Curtis KM. When can a woman have an intrauterine device inserted? A systematic review. *Contraception*. 2013;87(5):666–73.

44. Lopez LM, Bernholc A, Hubacher D, Stuart G, Van Vliet HA. Immediate postpartum insertion of intrauterine device for contraception. *Cochrane Database Syst Rev*. 2015;(6):CD003036.

45. Gemzell-Danielsson K, Jensen JT, Monteiro I et al. Interventions for the prevention of pain associated with the placement of intrauterine contraceptives: An updated review. *Acta Obstet Gynecol Scand*. 2019;98(12):1500–13.

46. Sääv I, Aronsson A, Marions L, Stephansson O, Gemzell-Danielsson K. Cervical priming with sublingual misoprostol prior to insertion of an intrauterine device in nulliparous women: A randomized controlled trial. *Hum Reprod*. 2007;22(10):2647–52.

47. Mishell DR Jr, Bell JH, Good RG, Moyer DL. The intrauterine device: A bacteriologic study of the endometrial cavity. *Am J Obstet Gynecol*. 1966;96

(1):119–26. https://doi.org/10.1016/s0002-9378(16)
34650-6.

48. FSRH Guidance. Intrauterine contraception. 2015.
     bit.ly/3kVvj1Y.

49. Farley TM, Rosenberg MJ, Rowe PJ, Chen JH, Meirik
     O. Intrauterine devices and pelvic inflammatory
     disease: An international perspective. *Lancet*.
     1992;**339**(8796):785–8.

50. Hubacher D, Lara-Ricalde R, Taylor DJ, Guerra-
     Infante F, Guzmán-Rodríguez R. Use of copper
     intrauterine devices and the risk of tubal infertility
     among nulligravid women. *N Engl J Med*. 2001;**345**
     (8):561–7.

51. Brahmi D, Steenland MW, Renner RM, Gaffield ME,
     Curtis KM. Pregnancy outcomes with an IUD in situ:
     A systematic review. *Contraception*. 2012;**85**(2):
     131–9.

52. Tepper NK, Steenland MW, Gaffield ME,
     Marchbanks PA, Curtis KM. Retention of
     intrauterine devices in women who acquire pelvic
     inflammatory disease: A systematic review.
     Contraception. 2013;**87**(5):655–60.

Permanent Methods of Contraception in Women

Omar Thanoon, Chu Chin Lim, and Tahir A. Mahmood

Efficacy

The US Collaborative Review of Sterilization investigated the efficacy of various tubal sterilization techniques in 1996. These procedures included clip sterilization, unipolar coagulation, bipolar coagulation, and postpartum partial salpingectomy. Cumulative 10-year probability of pregnancy was determined to be about 18.5 per 1,000 female sterilization procedures [2]. The failure rate range was 7.5–36.5 per 1,000. This included tubal sterilization methods such as postpartum partial salpingectomy, laparoscopic unipolar coagulation, Falope rings, interval partial salpingectomy, bipolar coagulation, and spring clips. Table 14.1 shows the failure rate for the different sterilization techniques after 1 year.

Causes of Failure of Sterilization in Women Include

- Undetected luteal pregnancy.
- Occlusion of the incorrect structure (most commonly, the round ligament).
- Incomplete or inadequate occlusion, slippage of a mechanical device.
- Development of a tubo-peritoneal fistula.
- Spontaneous re-anastomosis or recanalization of the cut ends. [3]

Table 14.1 Failure rates for different methods of sterilization

METHOD	FAILURE RATE 1 YEAR/ 1,000 PROCEDURES
BIPOLAR	2.3
MONOPOLAR	0.7
RINGS	3.9
CLIPS	18.2
POSTPARTUM PARTIAL SALPINGECTOMY	0.6
ALL METHODS	5.5

Timing

- **Postpartum**: Mostly done at the time of caesarean section. Most experts recommend an interval of 4–6 weeks following a vaginal delivery.
- **Postabortion**: Female sterilization can be done following an abortion; however, it is associated with higher levels of regret.
- **At any time not related to pregnancy**: At any time of the menstrual cycle providing that the woman is not at risk of having conceived prior to the procedure.

Contraindications

- Medical comorbidities and significant contraindication to anesthesia.
- Obesity (especially patients with morbid obesity) can also limit laparoscopic approaches by preventing adequate ventilation.
- Patients with extensive history of abdominal surgery should be counseled on the possibility that their fallopian tubes may not be accessible at the time of abdominal or laparoscopic surgery.
- Allergy to the device used in the sterilization procedure.

Approaches

Female sterilization can be performed through different approaches to gain access to the fallopian tubes. These include laparoscopy, laparotomy, and hysteroscopy approaches (Table 14.2).

Female Sterilization through Laparotomy

Tubal ligation through an open abdominal incision can be carried out during elective caesarean section or other elective abdominal surgery. Mini-laparotomy (2–5 cm length suprapubic transverse incision) is an alternative for interval sterilization when equipment

Table 14.2 Different approaches for sterilization

Laparotomy	Laparoscopy	Hysteroscopy
Inspect abdominal and pelvic organs	Inspect abdominal and pelvic organs	Inspect uterine cavity
Larger abdominal incision	Small incision	No incision
Effective immediately	Effective immediately	Needs to confirm effective after 3 months
General or regional anesthetic	General anesthetic	Local anesthetic
Needs operative theater setting	Needs operative theater setting	Can be done in outpatient setting

for laparoscopic or transcervical hysteroscopic tubal occlusion is unavailable or too expensive [4].

Madlener (1919) introduced tubal occlusion through an abdominal incision based on double clamping of each tube and suturing the two clamp grooves to tie the in-between segment. The most widely used technique of abdominal sterilization is the Pomeroy technique introduced in 1929. It involves grasping the tubal isthmic part with an atraumatic clamp, ligation of the loop with absorbable suture, and excision. Both tubal ends separate after resorption of the suture and in-between fibrotic tissue is formed [5]. A modification of the Pomeroy technique introduced by Pritchard adds an extra step where the avascular section of the mesosalpinx is sutured with absorbable material, avoiding blood vessels. The thread is tied around the proximal and distal part of the loop of the tube; subsequently the loop is excised.

The use of occlusive mechanical devices can also be introduced through an open sterilization. The most commonly used is the Filshie clip at the time of caesarean sections; however, several studies have demonstrated that, compared with partial salpingectomy, the clips are significantly less effective [6]. Postpartum partial salpingectomy is the most effective method of sterilization, with a 10-year cumulative failure rate of 7.5 failures per 1,000 procedures [7].

Laparoscopic Sterilization

Laparoscopic sterilization has been performed for more than 30 years. This is the most common method to gain access to the fallopian tubes; it has low complication rates and quicker recovery. For that reason laparoscopy is usually preferred for interval sterilization over laparotomy and mini-laparotomy. Laparoscopic sterilization is usually performed under general anesthesia with carbon dioxide used to provide abdominal distension. It requires a two-puncture technique, but refinement of the instruments has led to procedures being carried out through a single, sub-umbilical puncture.

After abdominal insufflation, tubal occlusion can be achieved in different ways. Unipolar electrocoagulation was first used in the laparoscopic approach. It requires electrocoagulation of the tubal isthmus followed by tubal transaction and re-coagulation of cut edges. It causes destruction of at least 3 cm of the tube. The use of monopolar diathermy can lead to surgical complications such as thermal injury to visceral organs such as bladder and bowel. The safest alternative to unipolar diathermic electro-surgery is bipolar diathermy [5]. It is different from unipolar diathermy as the current passes selectively through the tissue grasped between the jaws of the forceps, leading to a diathermy effect of the tissues between the jaws of the forceps or grasper used, reducing the complication rate [4].

The 10-year cumulative failure rate for monopolar electrocoagulation is 7.5 failures per 1,000 procedures [7]. The 10-year cumulative failure rate for bipolar electrocoagulation is 24.8 failures per 1,000 procedures [7]. Sterilization failures occur with bipolar electrocoagulation when there is incomplete coagulation of the fallopian tubes. Methods to decrease the high rates of failure rates with bipolar sterilization include use of more than 25 W of current in cutting mode, use of an inline current meter to ensure the appropriate energy is delivered, and coagulation of three or more sites of the fallopian tube [8].

In 1973, another occlusion method was introduced – the Yoon Ring (barium sulfate-impregnated silicone rubber). Later, devices with a similar mechanism of action were introduced for laparoscopic tubal sterilization (Hulka Clemens clip and Filshie clip). Filshie clips (Cooper Surgical) are silicone-lined titanium clips placed across the fallopian tubes to cause occlusion. The clip is placed approximately 3 cm from the cornua and both sides of the tube are visualized to ensure the entire tube is crushed and occluded by the clip. The

Hulka clip (Richard Wolf Medical) is a hinged spring clip placed across the isthmic portion of the tube. The Hulka clip has a high failure rate (36.5 failures per 1,000 procedures) compared to the Filshie clip (9.7 per 1,000 procedures), making it a less popular choice of tubal occlusion [7].

Another method of sterilization, where sterilization can be performed through an open or laparoscopic approach, is total bilateral salpingectomy. The findings of premalignant cells in the epithelium of the fallopian tube has led to theories of a tubal origin of ovarian cancer and the hypothesis that salpingectomy may decrease ovarian cancer risk. Bilateral total salpingectomy is now being considered as a method of sterilization that could potentially decrease ovarian cancer risk. Theoretically, bilateral salpingectomy is 100% effective. Salpingectomy is the preferred method for women who have become pregnant after a tubal ligation.

Hysteroscopic Sterilization

Hysteroscopic sterilization has been researched for more than 150 years [9]. In the 1970s, Quinones had the largest experience in electrocoagulation. He performed around 1,284 hysteroscopic tubal sterilizations using electrosurgical energy. The overall bilateral tubal occlusion rate was 80% [10]; it had a high failure rate (up to 35%) and serious complications including perforation of the uterus and thermal bowel injury. Since hysteroscopy became widely available for use in an outpatient setting, many hysteroscopic sterilization methods started gaining popularity.

The two most widely used hysteroscopic sterilization devices are Essure hysteroscopic sterilization (Bayer) and Adiana hysteroscopic sterilization (Hologic). The Essure hysteroscopic sterilization device was approved by the Food and Drug Administration (FDA) in 2002. It involves inserting a nickel-steel alloy implant in the fallopian tubes, causing tubal occlusion by inducing fibrosis [11].

According to Miño et al., Essure insertion should be performed in the early proliferative menstrual phase (days 7–14 of the cycle) because the tubal ostium is better visualized [11]. Insertion of the Essure implant can be performed in an outpatient setting even though the most frequently used anesthetic technique is a paracervical block with or without oral or intravenous sedation [11]. Recovery takes generally less than 24 hours.

Various studies have reported initial placement success at a rate of 84–98%. The results of a prospective Phase III clinical trial funded by Conceptus Inc. were reported in July 2003. This study demonstrated that bilateral placement of the Essure device was achieved in 464 (90%) of the 518 women participating in their study.

Appropriate follow-up is necessary to determine the efficacy of this product. Patients must understand the importance of confirming tubal blockage and proper device placement with a subsequent imaging study. Without this objective evidence of tubal occlusion and/or device placement, they cannot rely on the Essure for contraception [12]. Until this confirmatory test, another reliable form of contraception must be used. The type of imaging study used for the Essure confirmation test varies according to location. The hysterosalpingogram (HSG) is the method utilized in the United States, but other countries rely on plain x-ray or transvaginal ultrasound to document placement. The manufacturer of Essure reports effectiveness rates of 99%.

Complications following Essure were high and difficult to treat, and these included device breakage, uterine perforation, distal placement of the device, allergic reactions, and chronic pain. For that reason, the Essure hysteroscopic sterilization devise was withdrawn from the European market in 2017 and from the US market in 2018.

The FDA approved the Adiana hysteroscopic sterilization system in 2009. It involves delivering less than 3 W of bipolar radiofrequency energy within the fallopian tubes lumen, creating a superficial lesion. After the radiofrequency energy is delivered, a silicone matrix is placed into the tubal lumen in the region where the lesion was formed. The endothelial damage provided by the radiofrequency energy encourages a tissue ingrowth response consisting primarily of fibroblasts infiltrating the porous structure of the silicone matrix [13]. Similarly to the Essure system, the FDA requires tubal occlusion confirmation by HSG three months after the Adiana procedure [14]. In early studies, the Adiana system had an efficacy rate of 99% [15]. However, in 2012, the Adiana system was withdrawn from the market due to high failure rates and high legal costs. Other hysteroscopic sterilization techniques include Ovabloc (insertion of a silicone plug in the tube) and YAG laser, but these have very limited use.

Complications

Female sterilization is a well-tolerated form of permanent contraception with no major side effects compared to hormonal contraception [16, 17].

Immediate Complications

- Anesthetic complications.
- Infection: Infections of the wound, bladder, bowel, or pelvic organs occur in less than 1% of sterilizations and are more common with open procedures (laparotomy/mini-laparotomy) compared to laparoscopy.
- Hemorrhage: Hemorrhage is rare, occurring in 30–90 per 100,000 procedures. This can be due to major vessel injury (inferior epigastric, aorta, and iliac) during laparoscopic entry and occasionally following meso-salpingeal vessel injury during the occlusion procedure.
- Visceral injury: Bowel, bladder, blood vessel.
  - Injuries can occur from sharp trauma (i.e., from a Veress needle, trocar, scalpel).
  - Blunt trauma (e.g., from dissecting adhesions).
  - Electrical-thermal trauma.
  - Inadvertent application of the occlusion device to the incorrect structure.
  - Bowel and bladder injuries are more common in the presence of pelvic and abdominal adhesions. If recognized at the time of occurrence, injuries to the bladder and bowel are relatively easy to manage and will not result in long-term adverse sequelae. The high mortality rate (2.5%) results from the fact that most injuries to bowel and bladder are not recognized until delayed peritonitis occurs 5–10 days postoperatively.
  - Injuries to the uterus, most often caused by uterine manipulators.

Long-Term Complications

- Ectopic pregnancy
  - Because of its efficacy in preventing pregnancy, female sterilization has an overall protective effect on the risk for ectopic pregnancy.
  - When pregnancy does occur in a woman who has been sterilized, the chance that the pregnancy is ectopic is 16–76% versus 0.5% in women who have not been sterilized.

- The highest percentage of ectopic pregnancy occurs when sterilization was performed using electro-diathermy.
- Regret
  - Approximately 1–3% of women will seek reversal at a later date, especially when the procedure was done when the woman was younger than 30 years of age.
  - The vast majority of women do not regret sterilization.
  - Measuring regret is a challenge because it is difficult to determine what actually indicates significant regret. Studies have reported regret rates of 0.9–26%.
  - An attempt to seek reversal is considered an indication of significant regret.
  - The factors most commonly associated with regret are young age at sterilization and unpredictable life events such as the death of a child or a new spouse.
  - Data are conflicting regarding whether women are more likely to experience regret if sterilization is performed after a vaginal delivery or caesarean section.
- Port-site hernia
  - This is a rare complication associated with laparoscopic sterilization when the bowel can herniate through the site of an umbilical or lower abdominal puncture.
  - This complication is more likely when the puncture site is more than 8 mm.
  - Preventive techniques include fascial closure for ports larger than 7 mm, using the smallest punctures possible, and removing trocars slowly under direct visualization after air is released to prevent entrapment of omentum or bowel.

Reversal of Sterilization

Although sterilization is a form of permanent contraception, some women who experience regret will want to have their tubal patency restored through re-anastomosing the fallopian tubes via laparotomy, laparoscopy, or robotic surgery. Women who have had hysteroscopic sterilization cannot have their sterilization reversed. Women who have their sterilization through a laparotomy or laparoscopy can choose to try reversing the sterilization procedure.

In a recent systematic review of reversal of sterilization, the pooled pregnancy rate after sterilization reversal was 42–69%. The reported ectopic pregnancy rate was 4–8%. The only prognostic factor affecting the chance of conception was female age. The surgical approach (laparotomy, laparoscopy, or robotic) had no impact on the outcome [18]. Factors affecting the success of reversal include the woman's age, the skill of the surgeon, and the length of the remaining undamaged tube.

Clips, which destroy less than 1 cm of tube, are generally the most reversible procedure compared with Pomeroy ligation, which destroys 2–3 cm of tube. Electrical methods are usually the least reversible, with unipolar sterilization more difficult to reverse than bipolar. Ectopic pregnancy should always be ruled out in any woman who is pregnant after a reversal.

Non-contraception Effects of Sterilization

Ovarian cancer: A number of studies have demonstrated a protective effect of sterilization on ovarian cancer [19, 20].

Sexually transmitted diseases: Sterilization does not protect against sexually transmitted diseases. Sterilization has, however, been shown to reduce the spread of organisms from the lower genital tract to the peritoneal cavity and thus protect against pelvic inflammatory disease.

References

1. Daniels K, Daugherty J, Jones J. Current contraceptive status among women aged 15–44: United States, 2011–2013. *NCHS Data Brief*. 2014;**173**:1–8.

2. March CM. Female tubal sterilization. In Shoupe D (ed.), *The handbook of contraception*. 3rd edition. Cham: Humana, 2020, pp. 193–238.

3. Hulka JF. Methods of female sterilization. In Nichols DH, Clarke-Pearson DL (eds.), *Gynecologic and obstetric surgery*. St. Louis, MO: Mosby, 2000, pp. 626–40.

4. Beerthuizen R. State-of-the-art of non-hormonal methods of contraception: V. Female sterilisation. *Eur J Contracept Reprod Health Care*. 2010;**15**:124–35.

5. Steele SJ. The potential for improved abdominal procedures and approaches for tubal occlusion. *Int J Gynaecol Obstet*. 1995;**51**:S17–S22.

6. Rodriguez M, Seuc A, Sokal D. Comparative efficacy of postpartum sterilization with the titanium clip versus partial salpingectomy: A randomized controlled trial. *BJOG*. 2013;**120**(1):108–12.

7. Peterson HB, Xia Z, Hughes JM et al. The risk of pregnancy after tubal sterilization: Findings from the U.S. Collaborative Review of Sterilization. *Am J Obstet Gynecol*. 1996;**174**:1161–8.

8. Peterson HB, Xia Z, Wilcox LS et al. Pregnancy after tubal sterilization with bipolar electrocoagulation: U.S. Collaborative Review of Sterilization Working Group. *Obstet Gynecol*. 1999;**94**:163–7.

9. Abbott J. Transcervical sterilization. *Best Pract Res Clin Obstet Gynaecol*. 2005;**19**:743–56.

10. Quiñones R, Alvarado A, Ley E. Hysteroscopic sterilization. *Int J Gynaecol Obstet*. 1976;**14**:27–34.

11. Miño M, Arjona JE, Cordón J et al. Success rate and patient satisfaction with the Essure sterilisation in an outpatient setting: A prospective study of 857 women. *BJOG*. 2007;**114**:763–6.

12. Walter R, Ghobadi C, Haymen E, Xu S. Hysteroscopic sterilization with Essure. *Obstetrics & Gynecology*. 2017;**129**(1):10–19.

13. Vancaillie TG, Harrington DC, Anderson JM. Mechanism of action of the Adiana device: A histologic perspective. *Contraception*. 2011;**84**:299–301.

14. Herbst SJ, Evantash EG. Clinical performance characteristics of the Adiana system for permanent contraception: The first year of commercial use. *Rev Obstet Gynecol*. 2010;**3**:156–62.

15. Johns DA. Advances in hysteroscopic sterilization: Report on 600 patients enrolled in the Adiana EASE pivotal trial. *J Minim Invasive Gynecol*. 2005;**12**:39–40.

16. Westburg J, Scott F, Creinin F. Safety outcomes of female sterilization by salpingectomy and tubal occlusion. *Contraception*. 2017;**95**:505–8.

17. Peterson HB, DeStefano F, Rubin GL et al. Deaths attributable to tubal sterilization in the United States, 1977 to 1981. *Am J Obstet Gynecol*. 1983; **146**:131–6.

18. Van Seeters JAH, Chua SJ, Mol BWJ, Koks CAM. Tubal anastomosis after previous sterilization: A systematic review. *Human Reproduction Update*. 2017;1–13.

19. Whittemore AS, Wu ML, Paffenbarger RS et al. Personal and environmental characteristics related to epithelial ovarian cancer-exposures to talcum powder, tobacco, alcohol and coffee. *Am J Epidemiol*. 1988;**128**:1228.

20. Cibula D, Widschwendter M, Majek O et al. Tubal ligation and the risk of ovarian cancer: Review and meta-analysis. *Hum Reprod Update*. 2011;**17**:55–67.

Emergency Contraception

Sharon T. Cameron

Introduction

Emergency contraception (EC) is defined as any drug or device used after sexual intercourse to prevent pregnancy. The recommended options for oral EC are ulipristal acetate (UPA), a progesterone receptor modulator (30 mg), and the progestogen levonorgestrel (LNG) (1.5 mg or 3 mg dose depending on weight). Ulipristal acetate is licenced to be used within 120 hours of sexual intercourse and LNG within 72 hours. Mifepristone, a progesterone receptor modulator, is also used as an oral EC, but it is only available for this purpose in China, Vietnam, Russia, Armenia, Moldova and Ukraine. Although the copper intrauterine device is the most effective form of EC, oral EC remains the more commonly used approach [2].

Availability and Barriers to Access

The World Health Organization (WHO) lists EC as an essential medicine [3]. In spite of this, availability of EC varies widely across the world. Although 147 countries currently have at least one brand of oral EC registered, access to EC is often restricted due to myths or misconceptions about its use [1]. Currently EC can be obtained in all countries in Europe, with the exception of Hungary and Poland, from a pharmacy without a prescription [1]. This is safe and improves access to EC for women. Better access to EC increases timely use of EC but is not associated with any increase in sexually transmitted infections or unintended pregnancies [4].

Effectiveness of Emergency Contraception

There are no randomised placebo-controlled trials of EC, as this would be considered unethical given that oral EC can delay or inhibit ovulation and so on that basis must be better than no method. The efficacy of EC is therefore calculated from clinical trials that compare the number of observed pregnancies after EC to the numbers of *expected* pregnancies that would occur in the absence of EC (based on likelihood of conception at the time of the menstrual cycle when sex occurred) [5].

In the meta-analysis of two clinical trials (more than 3,400 women) comparing UPA and LNG, UPA was shown to be more effective than LNG, almost halving the risk of pregnancy for women treated within 120 hours of unprotected sex (1% UPA versus 2% LNG pregnancy rates, respectively) [6]. The expected pregnancy rates (if no EC was used) in these trials were calculated at around 5% [6]. One might therefore conclude that oral EC prevents around one half to two thirds of pregnancies that would otherwise have occurred.

Mechanism of Action

Both UPA and LNG work by delaying or inhibiting ovulation until sperm are no longer viable (presumed lifespan of sperm in the female reproductive tract is 5 days) [7]. The superior effectiveness of UPA is attributed to the ability of UPA to delay ovulation even after the onset of the (ovulatory trigger) luteinising hormone (LH) surge, whereas LNG can no longer delay ovulation once the LH surge has commenced [7]. There is good evidence that LNG and UPA do not prevent implantation and are not abortifacient. Studies using in vitro models of blastocyst implantation have shown that nether LNG nor UPA can prevent implantation in vitro [8, 9]. Clinical data have also been consistent with no increased rate of miscarriage or ectopic or congenital abnormality in babies after exposure to LNG or UPA used for EC [10–12].

Safety and Side Effects

There are no absolute contraindications to oral EC. The WHO medical eligibility criteria for contraceptive use advises that the advantages of using UPA or

LNG for EC outweighs any real or potential risks (MEC1) [13]. Repeat administration of oral EC in the same menstrual cycle is also considered safe.

Both LNG and UPA are well tolerated and associated with a similar side effect profile (nausea, headache). Both may be associated with the next period arriving a few days earlier or later [6]. Emergency contraception is not required before 21 days postpartum. Women who take LNG whilst breastfeeding can continue to breastfeed [13]. There are no data on effects of UPA on breastfeeding nor on infant outcomes. Since UPA is lipophilic it could be expected to be secreted to breast milk. However, levels are likely extremely low and unlikely have any adverse effects on either breastfeeding or the baby/infant. Nevertheless, based upon the manufacturer's summary of product characteristics, guidelines currently advise that women should discard breast milk for 7 days after UPA [14].

Factors Associated with Failure of Emergency Contraception

A Cochrane review reported that women who had further episodes of sex in the same cycle but after EC had a fourfold increase in the risk of pregnancy [15]. It is therefore clearly important that an ongoing method of effective contraception is commenced following EC. For women using LNG, a hormonal method of contraception can be started immediately, but women are currently advised to wait at least 5 days after UPA before starting a hormonal method as there is some evidence that starting a progestogen-containing contraception before this may affect the ability of UPA, a progesterone receptor modulator, to delay ovulation (Table 15.1) [14].

In clinical trials, women with obesity had a higher risk of pregnancy after EC compared to those with a normal body mass index (BMI), especially if they received LNG rather than UPA (Tables 15.2 and 15.3)

Table 15.1 Risk factors for failure of oral emergency contraception (adapted from [16])

	Odds Ratio [95% CI]
Cycle day at intercourse *	4.4 [2.3–8.2]
Further unprotected sex in same cycle after EC	4.6 [2.2–9.0]
Body mass index Obese vs. normal	3.6 [1.96–6.53]

* Higher risk in sex that occurred close to mid-cycle

Table 15.2 Risk of pregnancy in women with body mass index in obese range vs. normal range and treatment with levonorgestrel (LNG) or ulipristal acetate (UPA) from [16]. *P = 0.0002

Body Mass Index	LNG OR (95% CI)	UPA OR (95% CI)
Obese vs. normal	4.41 (2.05–9.44) *	2.62 (0.89–7.00)

Table 15.3 Strategies to prevent unintended pregnancies after emergency contraception

- Increase use of copper intrauterine device
- Abstain from further sex in same cycle
- Commence preferred effective method of contraception
- Use bridging contraception until the preferred contraceptive method can be accessed
- Develop a more effective method of oral EC

[16]. Pharmacokinetic studies support this finding and have demonstrated that the EC dose of LNG takes a longer time to reach steady state levels in women with obesity, but this is improved by doubling the dose of LNG [17]. In contrast, the dose of UPA does not need to be adjusted for obesity [18]. Clinical guidelines from the United Kingdom now advise that women with a BMI higher than 26 Kg/m2 who choose oral EC rather should have UPA as first-line contraception but, if not, a double dose of LNG may be provided (i.e. 3 mg) [14].

Starting Effective Contraception after Emergency Contraception

Given the higher risk of pregnancy if further unprotected sex occurs after EC, it is important that women start an effective method of ongoing contraception as soon as possible. Increasingly women are choosing to access EC from a pharmacy and then there can be a delay in getting an appointment at a clinic for ongoing contraception. A robust randomised controlled trial, the 'Bridge-It Study', showed that community pharmacy provision of a 3-month supply of progestogen-only pill as an interim or 'bridging' method of contraception along with EC resulted in around a 20% increase in the subsequent use of effective contraception, compared to provision of EC alone [18]. If provision of a bridging supply of an oral contraceptive along with EC became standard practice in pharmacies, this could prevent more unintended pregnancies for women after using EC.

Copper Intrauterine Device for Emergency Contraception

The copper intrauterine device (Cu-IUD) induces a local inflammatory reaction in the endometrium that is thought to prevent implantation if fertilization has occurred [20]. The Cu-IUD is by far the most effective method of EC. In a systematic review of use of the Cu-IUD for EC of more than 40 studies with more than 7,000 women, the observed pregnancy rate after Cu-IUD was just 1 in 1,000 [20]. The Cu-IUD can also be used over a wider time frame than oral EC; it can be inserted up to 5 days after the earliest estimated date of ovulation [14]. It also can be retained as a method of highly effective, long-acting reversible contraception. Its use is limited, however, by acceptability to women, the need for an invasive procedure and the availability of a skilled provider.

Future, More Effective Oral Emergency Contraception

Although EC prevents pregnancy for individuals, there is no good evidence that it reduces abortion rates at population level [4]. This may be because EC is not always used when required, even when it is available [21]. In addition, existing oral methods of EC are of limited use and effective only if ovulation has not yet occurred. Also, oral EC does not prevent pregnancy from subsequent episodes of unprotected sex after EC. A more effective oral EC is therefore desirable.

Prostaglandins play a critical role in follicle rupture and the cyclo-oxygenase-2 inhibitor meloxicam inhibits prostaglandin synthesis. A study comparing the effect of LNG plus meloxicam versus LNG and placebo on follicle rupture when administered to healthy female volunteers in the pre-ovulatory phase of the cycle demonstrated that ovulation was inhibited at 5 days in 39% of participants receiving LNG and meloxicam versus 16% of those receiving LNG and placebo [22]. Large robust trials are therefore required to determine if this combination might increase the efficacy of LNG for EC.

Mifepristone has the potential to be developed as an oral method that might prevent implantation through effects on the endometrium [23]. Mifepristone in combination with misoprostol has also been used successfully in clinical studies in China as a 'missed menses pill' – that is, to disrupt implantation in a very early abortion amongst women seeking to avoid pregnancy who presented with a menstrual delay of one week or more [24]. In a survey of more than 450 women in the United Kingdom seeking sexual and reproductive healthcare, 83% stated that they would be prepared to use a pill that works by preventing implantation and 75% to use a pill that might disrupt implantation. This shows that there may be widespread acceptability amongst women towards post-fertilization mechanisms of action [25].

Conclusions

Emergency contraception provides a chance to prevent an unintended pregnancy. Given that the Cu-IUD is the most effective method of EC, increased use of this method should be an effective strategy to prevent more unintended pregnancies. However, if a Cu-IUD is not acceptable to a woman or is unavailable, then UPA should be used as it is more effective than LNG. It is also important that an ongoing method of contraception is established. If the woman's chosen method cannot be provided, then a supply of a bridging method of contraception should be offered along with oral EC. In addition, researchers need to develop a more effective oral EC (Table 15.3).

References

1. International Consortium for Emergency Contraception. In depth country information. www.cecinfo.org/country-by-country-information/in-depth.

2. Cleland K, Zhu H, Goldstuck N, Cheng L, Trussell J. The efficacy of intrauterine devices for emergency contraception: A systematic review of 35 years of experience. *Hum Reprod*. 2012;27(7): 1994–2000.

3. WHO Model list of essential medicines April 2015. www.who.int/medicines/publications/essentialmedicines/en.s.

4. Polis CB, Schaffer K, Blanchard K et al. Advance provision of emergency contraception for pregnancy prevention (full review). *Cochrane Database Syst Rev*. 2007;2:CD005497.

5. Trussell J, Ellertson C, von Hertzen H et al. Estimating the effectiveness of emergency contraceptive pills. *Contraception*. 2003;67(4):259–65.

6. Glasier A, Cameron ST, Fine PM et al. Ulipristal acetate versus levonorgestrel for emergency contraception: A randomised non-inferiority trial and meta-analysis. *Lancet*. 2010;375:555–62.

7. Brache V, Cochon L, Deniaud M, Croxatto HB. Ulipristal acetate prevents ovulation more effectively than levonorgestrel: Analysis of pooled data from three randomized trials of emergency contraception regimens. *Contraception*. 2013;**88**(5):611–18.

8. Lalitkumar PG, Lalitkumar S, Meng CX et al. Mifepristone, but not levonorgestrel, inhibits human blastocyst attachment to an in vitro endometrial three-dimensional cell culture model. *Hum Reprod*. 2007;**22**(11):3031–7.

9. Berger C, Boggavarapu NR, Menezes J, Lalitkumar PG, Gemzell-Danielsson K. Effects of ulipristal acetate on human embryo attachment and endometrial cell gene expression in an in vitro co-culture system. *Hum Reprod*. 2015;**30**(4):800–11.

10. Zhang L, Ye W, Yu W et al. Physical and mental development of children after levonorgestrel emergency contraception exposure: A follow-up prospective cohort study. *Biol Reprod*. 2014;**91**(1):27.

11. Cleland K, Raymond E, Trussell J et al. Ectopic pregnancy and emergency contraceptive pills: A systematic review. *Obstet Gynecol*. 2010;**115**:1263–6. https://doi.org/10.1097/AOG.0b013e3181dd22ef.

12. Levy DP, Jager M, Kapp N, Abitbol JL. Ulipristal acetate for emergency contraception: Postmarketing experience after use by more than 1 million women. *Contraception*. 2014;**89**(5):431–3.

13. World Health Organization. *Medical eligibility criteria for contraceptive use*. 5th edition. Geneva: World Health Organization, 2015. www.who.int/publications/i/item/9789241549158.

14. Faculty of Sexual & Reproductive Healthcare. Emergency contraception (March 2017, amended December 2017). bit.ly/3Y2277Q.

15. Shen J, Che Y, Showell E, Chen K, Cheng L. Interventions for emergency contraception. *Cochrane Database Syst Rev*. 2019;**1**(1):CD001324. https://doi.org/10.1002/14651858.CD001324.pub6. PMID: 30661244; PMCID: PMC7055045.

16. Glasier A, Cameron ST, Blithe D et al. Can we identify women at risk of pregnancy despite using emergency contraception? Data from randomized trials of ulipristal acetate and levonorgestrel. *Contraception*. 2011;**84**(4):363–7.

17. Edelman AB, Cherala G, Blue SW, Erikson DW, Jensen JT. Impact of obesity on the pharmacokinetics of levonorgestrel-based emergency contraception: Single and double dosing. *Contraception*. 2016;**94**(1):52–7.

18. Praditpan P, Hamouie A, Basaraba CN et al. Pharmacokinetics of levonorgestrel and ulipristal acetate emergency contraception in women with normal and obese body mass index. *Contraception*. 2017;**95**(5): 464–9. Published Online First: 23 January 2017. https://doi.org/10.1016/j.contraception.2017.01.004. Epub 2017 Jan 23.

19. Cameron ST, Glasier A, McDaid L et al. Use of effective contraception following provision of the progestogen-only pill for women presenting to community pharmacies for emergency contraception (Bridge-It): A pragmatic cluster-randomised crossover trial. *Lancet*. 2020;**396** (10262):1585–94. https://doi.org/10.1016/S0140-6736(20)31785-2. PMID: 33189179; PMCID: PMC7661838.

20. Stanford JB, Mikolajczyk RT. Mechanisms of action of intrauterine devices: Update and estimation of postfertilization effects. *Am J Obstet Gynecol*. 2002;**187**:1699–1708.

21. Moreau C, Bouyer J, Goulard H, Bajos N. The remaining barriers to the use of emergency contraception: Perception of pregnancy risk by women undergoing induced abortions. *Contraception*. 2005;**71**:202–7.

22. Massai MR, Forcelledo ML, Brache V et al. Does meloxicam increase the incidence of anovulation induced by single administration of levonorgestrel in emergency contraception? A pilot study. *Hum Reprod*. 2007;**22**:434–9.

23. Cameron ST, Critchley HOD, Buckley CH, Kelly RW, Baird DT. Effect of two antiprogestins (mifepristone and onapristone) on endometrial factors of potential importance for implantation. *Fertility and Sterility*. 1997;**67**:1046–53.

24. Willetts SJ, MacDougall M, Cameron ST. A survey regarding acceptability of oral emergency contraception according to the posited mechanism of action. *Contraception*. 2017;**96**(2):81–8. https://doi.org/10.1016/j.contraception.2017.03.012. Epub 2017 Apr 3. PMID: 28385554.

25. Xiao B, von Hertzen H, Zhao H, Piaggio G. Menstrual induction with mifepristone and misoprostol. *Contraception*. 2003;**68**(6):489–94.

Management of Issues Associated with Female Contraceptives
Bleeding

Katarina Sedlecky and Johannes Bitzer

Introduction

Unscheduled bleeding is common during hormonal contraception (HC) use. It increases the likelihood of poor adherence and premature discontinuation of the contraceptive method. In users of combined hormonal contraception (CHC) bleeding disturbances are more frequent in the first months, occurring in up to one third of women in the first cycle and decreasing afterwards to about 5% at the sixth month [1].

The frequency of irregular bleeding depends on the dose of both oestrogen and progestin, the type of progestin and the route of hormone administration. Irregular bleeding is more frequent in the users of ≤ 20 mcg ethynil-oestradiol (EE) than with combined oral contraceptives (COC) with ≥ 30 mcg of EE [2]. Combined oral contraceptives containing more natural oestrogens are characterized by similar bleeding patterns to those seen with EE [3]. Cycle control was similar or better in the users of triphasic COC compared to monophasic COC [4]. Furthermore, COC preparations containing third-generation progestins were associated with less irregular bleeding compared to COCs with levonorgestrel (LNG) [5]. With respect to the route of hormone administration, in the majority of studies spotting and breakthrough bleeding were not as common in the users of combined vaginal ring (CVR) as in the users of various COCs. Differences in cycle control between COC and the combined transdermal patch (CTP) were less evident [6].

With progestin-only contraceptive (POC) methods unpredictable bleeding patterns are more common than with CHC use with no tendency to settle over time. Cycle control in POC users depends on the type and dose of progestin, the route of hormone administration, the length of use and the mechanism by which the contraceptive effect is achieved. The proportion of women with unscheduled bleeding is lower in the users of progestin-only pills (POPs) with drospirenone compared to desogestrel POPs [7]. Due to the persistence of

nuisance bleeding, 25% of POP users will discontinue the method by the end of the first year [8]. Among discontinuers of other POCs, bleeding changes were the reason given by 25.6% of depot medroxyprogesterone acetate (DMPA) users, 45.5% of progestin implant users and 19.1% of levonorgestrel-releasing intrauterine system (LNG-IUS) users [9]. Women who have been informed about the possibility of bleeding disorders before using HC better tolerate unscheduled bleeding. It is important to discuss this issue in advance, during contraceptive counselling, particularly in POC users [10].

Pathophysiology of Unscheduled Uterine Bleeding

The bleeding occurring during a normal cycle (menstruation) is provoked by the withdrawal of the natural progesterone in a cycle in which ovulation did not lead to pregnancy. Menstruation is thus called withdrawal bleeding. This type of bleeding is also produced by the withdrawal of the synthetic progestins in hormonal contraceptives leading to regular cycles. Irregular cycles and bleeding are not induced by this withdrawal mechanism but occur under hormone treatment and are therefore called breakthrough bleeding.

The underlying mechanism of this bleeding is complex. During CHC use endometrium is continuously exposed to oestrogen and progestin. The effect of progestin on the endometrium dominates, preventing oestrogen from stimulating endometrial proliferation. The endometrium becomes thin, atrophic and decidedly changed [8]. Alterations in endometrial morphology in women who use POC are similar but more pronounced. Vascular changes are considerable, with an increase of microvascular density and enhanced fragility of superficial venules [11].

It was hypothesized that the use of hormonal contraception may disrupt the balance in the growth of various components of the endometrium. An association between endometrial instability leading to degradation and changes in the production and activity of certain matrix metalloproteinases (MMPs) has been demonstrated [12]. Of particular interest for endometrial integrity are MMP-2 and MMP-9. These enzymes degrade the extracellular matrix and major components of the sub-endothelial basement membrane, which increases vessel fragility [13]. In the endometrium of COC users increased activity of both MMP-2 and MMP-9 were found. With continuation of COC use in an extended regimen MMP-2 and MMP-9 activity decreases. It has been observed that exogenous progestins in the form of DMPA, LNG-IUS and LNG implants initially increased endometrial MMP-9 activity, as well as MMP-2 activity in the areas of endometrial focal degradation. With continuation of exposure to POC, both MMP-2 and MMP-9 activity decreased [13].

Management of Unscheduled Bleeding

Unscheduled bleeding during the first 3 months of HC use is common. However, in users of COCs and POPs, it is necessary to check whether the method is used regularly and correctly. Inconsistent use of oral contraception increases the risk of withdrawal bleeding by 60–70% [8]. Examination includes the exclusion of disorders that may reduce the absorption of hormones from the digestive system (severe vomiting or diarrhoea) and chronic diseases/conditions accompanied by malabsorption.

The HC user should be asked if she smokes as smoking has an anti-oestrogenic effect. She should also be asked if she uses liver enzyme–inducing drugs, such as antiepileptic drugs, some antiretrovirals (efavirenz, nevirapine or protease inhibitors boosted with ritonavir), ryfamycin or rifabutin, St John's wort (*Hypericum perforatum*), as well as some other medications (e.g. bosentan, modafinil, aprepitant, isotretinoin) [8, 14]. If no organic cause of bleeding (e.g. inflammation, pregnancy, genital neoplasm) or reduced contraceptive efficacy has been identified, reassurance is usually sufficient. However, when irregular bleeding occurs after a period of good cycle control, the organic cause should be ruled out first, in addition to all of these. Baseline examination includes screening for chlamydial infection and gonorrhoea, assessment of cervical cancer screening status, exclusion of both pelvic inflammatory disease and uterine/ovarian pathology, especially intrauterine and ectopic pregnancy (Table 16.1).

Table 16.1 Management of hormonal contraceptive user with unscheduled bleeding

First three cycles of hormonal contraceptive use

- Adherence to the recommended regimen of use
- Severe vomiting or diarrhoea, chronic diseases/conditions accompanied by malabsorption
- Smoking
- Use of liver enzyme–inducing drugs:
  - antiepileptic drugs
  - some antiretrovirals (efavirenz, nevirapine, protease inhibitors boosted with ritonavir)
  - ryfamycin or rifabutin
  - herbal products – St John's wort (*Hypericum perforatum*)
  - other drugs (e.g. bosentan, modafinil, aprepitant, isotretinoin)

Onset of bleeding after a period of good cycle control

- All of the above
- Screening for chlamydial infection and gonorrhoea
- Assessment of cervical cancer screening status
- Examination for pelvic inflammatory disease
- Exclusion of uterine/ovarian pathology, primarily intrauterine and ectopic pregnancy

Treatment Options

The treatment of unscheduled bleeding in HC users is largely based on clinical experience and, to a lesser extent, on research results. During the first 3 months of use, explanation of the nature of bleeding and reassurance are usually sufficient. If bleeding persists after the first 3 months and an organic cause is excluded, additional therapeutic options should be considered.

Combined Hormonal Contraception

Several treatment options have been proposed for unscheduled bleeding during CHC use (Table 16.2). According to available evidence, COCs containing third-generation progestins may be associated with less unscheduled bleeding than COC with second-generation progestins. This is explained by different oestrogenic, progestogenic and androgenic properties of different progestins. Generally, characteristics of progestin have a much greater impact on cycle control than the dose and type of oestrogen [5]. However, the oestrogen component matters, and thus in women with persistent unscheduled bleeding a favourable therapeutic effect may be achieved by increasing the dose of EE or switching to COC with more natural oestrogens [2, 14].

Table 16.2 Treatment options for unscheduled bleeding in combined hormonal contraceptive users

What is changing	How to change
Progestin component of COC	Switching to COC containing third-generation progestin
Oestrogen component of COC	Increasing the dose of EE or switching to COC with more natural oestrogens (oestradiol-valerate, 17β-oestradiol)
Combined oral contraceptive	Combined vaginal ring
COC in standard regimen	COC in extended or continuous regimen
COC in continuous regimen	Introducing 4-day hormone free period
COC in continuous regimen	Prophylactic use of 40 mg/daily doxycycline

Legend: COC – combined oral contraception

When considering increasing the dose of EE, one should take into account the fact that it also increases the risk of serious adverse events, primarily venous thromboembolism [1]. Also a change in the route of hormone administration is one of the options, as cycle control is better in 15 mcg EE/120 mcg etonogestrel CVR users than in COC or CTP users [6]. It seems that cycle control could be better if EE in CVR were replaced by more natural 17β-oestradiol (E2) [15]. A new 17.4 mg EE/103 mg segesterone acetate CVR that is reusable for 13 cycles also seems to have a good cycle control [16].

Use of CHC in extended or continuous regimen reduces the number of bleeding days. In the case of unscheduled bleeding lasting 3 or more days during extended or continuous CHC use, it is recommended to start a 4-day hormone-free period, which will allow the endometrium to shed completely [14].

Doxycycline has been shown to reduce the likelihood of irregular bleeding in hormonal contraceptive users. This effect is due to inhibition of MMP activity achieved by much lower doses (e.g. 20–40 mg/day) of doxycycline than required for the antimicrobial effect (100–200 mg/day). However, doxycycline treatment should be started prophylactically before unscheduled bleeding begins because, once bleeding is established, endometrial stability cannot be achieved with even higher doses of the antibiotic [17]. The use of sub-antimicrobial doses of doxycycline in the prevention of

irregular bleeding has been most studied in women who have been on an extended or continuous CHC regimen.

Progestin-Only Contraception

The therapeutic options used so far in the treatment of unscheduled bleeding during the use of progestin-only contraceptives are presented in Table 16.3.

Non-steroidal Anti-inflammatory Medications

The primary mechanism of action of non-steroidal anti-inflammatory drugs (NSAIDs) is inhibition of cyclooxygenase, which is a prostaglandin synthase. As elevated levels of prostaglandins (PGE2 and PGF2) in the endometrium were found in some women with irregular bleeding, it is reasonable to believe that a short course of NSAIDs may have a favourable effect [11].

It was demonstrated that mefenamic acid reduces the number of bleeding days in DMPA users in the short-term, and in both etonogestrel (ENG) and LNG implant users in short- and long-term, while it was not effective in LNG-IUS users [11]. In LNG-IUS users preventive treatment with naproxen reduced a number of bleeding/spotting days by 10%, but this effect persisted for only 4 weeks [18].

The results of these studies indicate that short-term use of NSAIDs may have a beneficial effect on irregular bleeding in some women. These results can likely be applied to all types of POCs. However, use of NSAIDs may be contraindicated in women with history of gastrointestinal bleeding or renal insufficiency.

Oestrogen

As bleeding in users of POC may be associated with a very pronounced atrophy and decidualization of the endometrium, oestrogen administration can have a beneficial effect by stimulating endometrial proliferation and regeneration. Oestrogen can be used alone or in the form of a COC. Both treatment options have proven successful [11]. A less favourable effect was observed with the use of transdermal oestrogen [18]. This type of treatment should not be used in women with contraindications to oestrogen.

Doxycycline

Doxycycline inhibits MMPs, which are determinants of endometrial stability, and has antibacterial properties that can treat endometritis. The potential of this antibiotic to improve the cycle control in the users of progestin-based long-acting reversible contraceptives

Table 16.3 Treatment options for unscheduled bleeding in progestin-only contraceptive users

Medical treatment	DMPA	LNG implant	ENG implant	LNG-IUS
NSAIDs				
mefenamic acid (500 mg 2–3 times/day x 5 days)	effective	effective	effective	not effective
naproxen (500 mg 2 times/day x 5 days)	no data	no data	no data	effective
Oestrogen				
conjugated oestrogen (1.25 mg/day) or oestradiol (2 mg/day) x 7–14 days	effective	effective	no data	no data
combined oral contraceptives (1–3 cycles)	no data	effective	effective	no data
doxycycline (100 mg 2 times/day x 5 days)	effective	no data	effective	no data
tranexamic acid (250–500 mg 2–4 times/day x 5 days, or until a day after bleeding cessation)	effective	effective	no data	not effective
mifepristone (50–100 mg/day x 1 or 2 days, or prophylactically 50 mg once in 14 days)	effective	effective	effective	not effective
tamoxifen (10 mg 2 times/day x 7 days)	no data	no data	effective	no data
ulipristal acetate (15 mg/day x 7 days)	no data	no data	effective	no data

Legend: DMPA – depot-medroxyprogesterone acetate; LNG implant – levonorgestrel implant; ENG implant – etonogestrel implant; LNG-IUS – levonorgestrel-intrauterine system; NSAIDs – non-steroidal anti-inflammatory drugs

(LARC) has been investigated in several studies. The available data indicate that short-term use of doxycycline in antibacterial doses is not more effective than placebo in reducing the number of bleeding days in DMPA users, but it significantly improved cycle control in ENG implant users [9, 19].

However, the impact of doxycycline treatment on long-term bleeding patterns in progestin-based LARC users has not been established [11]. Additionally, this antibiotic may cause side-effects like gastrointestinal symptoms and repeated use increases the risk of developing antibiotic resistance.

Tranexamic Acid

Tranexamic acid (TXA) is an anti-fibrinolytic drug with a potential of reducing heavy menstrual bleeding. Short-term treatment with TXA demonstrated positive effect on unscheduled bleeding in DMPA users in the acute phase and up to 4 weeks, while in ENG implant users it was effective during its use only [11]. No positive effect was found in the users of LNG-IUS [20].

Mifepristone

Mifepristone is a progesterone receptor antagonist that may up-regulate oestrogen receptors in endometrium, thus reducing the likelihood of irregular bleeding. When used prophylactically, mifepristone has been found to decrease the number of bleeding days in the users of DMPA and the ENG implant, but not LNG-IUS users [11, 21]. There is a concern that mifepristone may induce ovulation and compromise the contraceptive efficacy of progestin-based LARC [19]. Further disadvantage of mifepristone is its use as an abortifacient, which is not usually available in pharmacies.

Tamoxifen

Tamoxifen is a selective oestrogen receptor modulator that exerts a beneficial effect in LNG and ENG implant users by reducing the number of bleeding and spotting days. This favourable bleeding profile is maintained within 1 month following treatment, without compromising ovulation suppression [22, 23]. However, further studies are needed before giving a general recommendation for the use of tamoxifen in progestin-based LARC users.

Ulipristal Acetate

A randomized placebo-controlled trial found that treatment of ENG implant users with UPA reduced the number of bleeding days in the short term, without compromising contraceptive efficacy [24].

References

1. Bitzer J, Simon JA. Current issues and available options in combined hormonal contraception. *Contraception*. 2011;**84**(4):342–56.

2. Sabatini R, Cagiano R. Comparison profiles of cycle control, side effects and sexual satisfaction of three hormonal contraceptives. *Contraception*. 2006;**74**(3):220–3.

3. Yu Q, Huang Z, Ren M et al. Contraceptive efficacy and safety of estradiol valerate/dienogest in a healthy female population: A multicenter, open-label, uncontrolled Phase III study. *Int J Womens Health*. 2018;**10**:257–66.

4. Van Vliet HA, Grimes DA, Lopez LM, Schulz KF, Helmerhorst FM. Triphasic versus monophasic oral contraceptives for contraception. *Cochrane Database Syst Rev*. 2011;**11**:CD003553.

5. Lawrie TA, Helmerhorst FM, Maitra NK et al. Types of progestogens in combined oral contraception: Effectiveness and side-effects. *Cochrane Database Syst Rev*. 2011;**5**:CD004861.

6. Lopez LM, Grimes DA, Gallo MF, Stockton LL, Schulz KF. Skin patch and vaginal ring versus combined oral contraceptives for contraception. *Cochrane Database Syst Rev*. 2013;**4**:CD003552.

7. Palacios S, Colli E, Regidor PA. A multicenter, double-blind, randomized trial on the bleeding profile of a drospirenone-only pill 4 mg over nine cycles in comparison with desogestrel 0.075 mg. *Arch Gynecol Obstet*. 2019;**300**(6):1805–12.

8. ESHRE Capri Workshop Group. Ovarian and endometrial function during hormonal contraception. *Hum Reprod*. 2001;**16**(7):1527–35.

9. Diedrich JT, Zhao Q, Madden T, Secura GM, Peipert JF. Three-year continuation of reversible contraception. *Am J Obstet Gynecol*. 2015;**213**(5):662. e1–8.

10. Fruzzetti F, Paoletti AM, Fidecicchi T et al. Contraception with estradiol valerate and dienogest: Adherence to the method. *Open Access J Contracept*. 2019;**10**:1–6.

11. Zigler RE, McNicholas C. Unscheduled vaginal bleeding with progestin-only contraceptive use. *Am J Obstet Gynecol*. 2017;**216**(5):443–50.

12. Vincent AJ, Zhang J, Ostör A et al. Decreased tissue inhibitor of metalloproteinase in the endometrium of women using depot medroxyprogesterone acetate: A role for altered endometrial matrix metalloproteinase/tissue inhibitor of metalloproteinase balance in the pathogenesis of abnormal uterine bleeding? *Hum Reprod*. 2002;**17**(5):1189–98.

13. Hickey M, Crewe J, Mahoney LA et al. Mechanisms of irregular bleeding with hormone therapy: The role of matrix metalloproteinases and their tissue inhibitors. *J Clin Endocrinol Metab*. 2006;**91**(8):3189–98.

14. Foran T. The management of irregular bleeding in women using contraception. *Aust Fam Physician*. 2017;**46**(10):717–20.

15. Duijkers I, Klipping C, Heger-Mahn D et al. Phase II dose-finding study on ovulation inhibition and cycle control associated with the use of contraceptive vaginal rings containing 17β-estradiol and the progestagens etonogestrel or nomegestrol acetate compared to NuvaRing. *Eur J Contracept Reprod Health Care*. 2018;**23**(4):245–54.

16. Virro JJ, Besinque K, Carney CE et al. Long-lasting, patient-controlled, procedure-free contraception: A review of Annovera with a pharmacist perspective. *Pharmacy (Basel)*. 2020;**8**(3):156–61.

17. Kaneshiro B, Edelman A, Carlson NE et al. A randomized controlled trial of subantimicrobial-dose doxycycline to prevent unscheduled bleeding with continuous oral contraceptive pill use. *Contraception*. 2012;**85**(4):351–8.

18. Madden T, Proehl S, Allsworth JE, Secura GM, Peipert JF. Naproxen or estradiol for bleeding and spotting with the levonorgestrel intrauterine system: A randomized controlled trial. *Am J Obstet Gynecol*. 2012;**206**(2):129.e1–8.

19. Weisberg E, Hickey M, Palmer D et al. A pilot study to assess the effect of three short-term treatments on frequent and/or prolonged bleeding compared to placebo in women using Implanon. *Hum Reprod*. 2006;**21**(1):295–302.

20. Sørdal T, Inki P, Draeby J, O'Flynn M, Schmelter T. Management of initial bleeding or spotting after levonorgestrel-releasing intrauterine system placement: A randomized controlled trial. *Obstet Gynecol*. 2013;**121**(5):934–41.

21. Papaikonomou K, Kopp Kallner H, Söderdahl F, Gemzell-Danielsson K. Mifepristone treatment prior to insertion of a levonorgestrel releasing intrauterine system for improved bleeding control: A randomized controlled trial. *Hum Reprod*. 2018;**33**(11):2002–9.

22. Cohen MA, Simmons KB, Edelman AB, Jensen JT. Tamoxifen for the prevention of unscheduled bleeding in new users of the levonorgestrel 52-mg intrauterine system: A randomized controlled trial. *Contraception*. 2019;**100**(5):391–6.

23. Simmons KB, Edelman AB, Fu R, Jensen JT. Tamoxifen for the treatment of breakthrough bleeding with the etonogestrel implant: A randomized controlled trial. *Contraception*. 2017;**95**(2):198–204.

24. Zigler RE, Madden T, Ashby C, Wan L, McNicholas C. Ulipristal acetate for unscheduled bleeding in etonogestrel implant users: A randomized controlled trial. *Obstet Gynecol*. 2018;**132**(4):888–94.

17 Management of Issues Associated with Female Contraceptives
Mood

Johannes Bitzer

Definition

Mood as a category can be subdivided into different states of mind. Bad mood includes an aggressive component such as being angry, frustrated, dissatisfied. Changing mood indicates instability and includes irritability. Depressed mood indicates sadness, lack of motivation, negative outlook and pessimism.

Mood Status and Changes: A Multifactorial Process

Pre-existing Vulnerability to Psychiatric Disorders

In women with negative mood and affect change related to oral contraceptive (OC) use, potential mediators of the relationship between OCs and mood or affect have been identified:

- A history of depression, psychiatric symptoms, dysmenorrhoea and premenstrual mood symptoms prior to OC use.
- A history of pregnancy-related mood symptoms.
- A family history of OC-related mood complaints, being in the postpartum period and age.

Psycho-endocrine Mechanisms

Researchers have published a huge body of literature about the impact of steroid hormones on the brain and the most important neurotransmitter pathways related to affective state. Oestrogen interacts with synapsis formation and serotonin activation and has been found to have a psychotropic mood-elevating effect. This has been mainly shown in studies of women with perimenopausal depression. A possible pathway of this action is via the serotonin system.

Research shows that high levels of serotonin in the brain are linked to elevated mood and feeling happy, whereas low levels of serotonin are linked to the symptoms of depression, including feeling sad, upset and generally low in mood. The idea that serotonin levels are related to depression is further supported by the fact that people who are experiencing a 'comedown' after drinking alcohol or taking drugs report feeling sad and depressed. This is because alcohol and drugs such as ecstasy/MDMA cause levels of serotonin to peak and then reduce very quickly. This sudden reduction in serotonin levels has a negative impact on mood during the drug comedown stage. Premenstrual dysphoric disorder (PMDD) studies have shown that women suffering from PMDD have low serotonin levels in platelets.

Progesterone interacts with gamma-aminobutyric acid (GABA) and with the serotonin system by itself, but mainly by neuroactive metabolites, especially allopregnanolone and pregnanolone. These neurosteroids potentiate the inhibitory actions of GABA, having an antianxiety and partial antidepressive effect. The impact is complicated, however, and depends not only on the presence or level of hormones but also on the hormone receptors in the brain.

Animal studies suggest that pregnanolone increases anxiety after a period of low allopregnanolone concentration. This effect is potentially mediated by the amygdala and related to the negative mood symptoms in humans that are observed during increased allopregnanolone levels. Thus metabolites of progesterone may have adverse mood effects, depending on the concentrations and receptor environment.

The vulnerability of women to endogenous steroid hormones has been very well studied in research aimed at trying to understand the hormonal mechanisms involved in premenstrual syndrome (PMS) and premenstrual dysphoric disorder (PMDD). These studies show that in vulnerable women the use of progestogens may increase the symptoms of depressed mood. There seems to be a difference between progestogens: antiandrogenic or neutral progestogens show a more favourable action compared with androgenic progestogens.

The final action in the individual patient is, however, complicated by the fact that the oestrogen component has a mood-elevating effect while at the same time reducing circulating levels of free testosterone, which may have a mood-lowering effect. It is known from studies of the progestogen drospirenone that this combined oral contraceptive (COC) can treat the psychiatric affective disorder PMDD as effectively as the gold standard treatment with selective serotonin reuptake inhibitors [6].

Other studies have shown the complexity and sometimes the contradictory actions of synthetic steroids on the brain: Oinonen and Mazmanian [7] found that, compared with non-users, oral contraceptive (OC) users experience less variability in affect across the entire menstrual cycle and less negative affect during menstruation (i.e. during withdrawal bleeding).

Furthermore, a lower ratio of progestogen to oestrogen is associated with more negative mood changes in women with a history of premenstrual mood symptoms; a higher progestogen-to-oestrogen ratio is associated with increased negative mood effects in women without such a history; monophasic OCs have a greater stabilising effect on mood compared to triphasic OCs. In an important study, Rapkin et al. showed that in healthy women without underlying mood or anxiety disorder the use of a low-dose OC did not result in adverse psychological symptoms despite a significant reduction in neuroactive steroids, indicating that individual vulnerability to steroid action in the brain – as we know from PMS and PMDD – is a precondition for adverse effects and that in healthy women fluctuations of neurosteroids are well tolerated [8].

Psychosocial Factors

Distress, defined as a state of imbalance between the stressors and the coping capacity of the individual, leads to feelings of being overwhelmed, frustrated, having no more energy and so forth. There is a correlation between these feelings and the endocrine stress response, especially the cortisol secretion pattern. If this state of distress persists the system faces a brain and psycho-endocrine dysfunctional response. Sadness cannot be resolved by good feeling and thus becomes depression. Frustration and lack of energy cannot be counteracted or compensated for by feelings of control and become helplessness and loss of motivation.

Epidemiological Studies

Hormonal contraceptives have been reported to have various effects on mood.

- Improvement of mood in women with PMDD.
- Irritability and depressed mood in women.
- No impact on mood.

Keyes et al. indicated a protective effect of hormonal contraception with respect to affective disorders [2]. A Swedish observational study published in the *European Journal of Contraception & Reproductive Health Care* found a positive association between the use of progestogen-only contraception and antidepressants, particularly among teenagers [3, 4]. Regarding combined hormonal contraception, teenage users were more likely, but older women were less likely, to be prescribed antidepressants compared with non-users.

Another study, not mentioned in the Skovlund et al. article [1], may contribute to understanding of the complexity [5]. This study included women under the age of 40 years suffering from major depression: 223 used combined hormonal contraceptives, 58 used progestogen-only preparations and 948 did not use hormonal contraceptives. The women who used combined hormonal contraceptives were significantly less depressed than the women who did not. Users also showed higher physical fitness and less comorbidity with compulsive disorders. The various factors contributing to the affective state of the OC user are summarized in Figure 17.1.

Counselling

Before starting hormonal contraceptives a thorough history, not only about physical symptoms and diseases, but also about mental health status and mental health history, is important and may frequently be forgotten.

- History of depressed mood during adolescence or postpartum.
- Cycle-related mood changes, PMS, PMDD.
- Present psychological well-being.
- Major stressors.

Information about the Possible Impact of Hormonal Contraceptives on Mood

- The majority of women experience no change.
- Some women experience improvement.
- Some women experience negative mood changes.

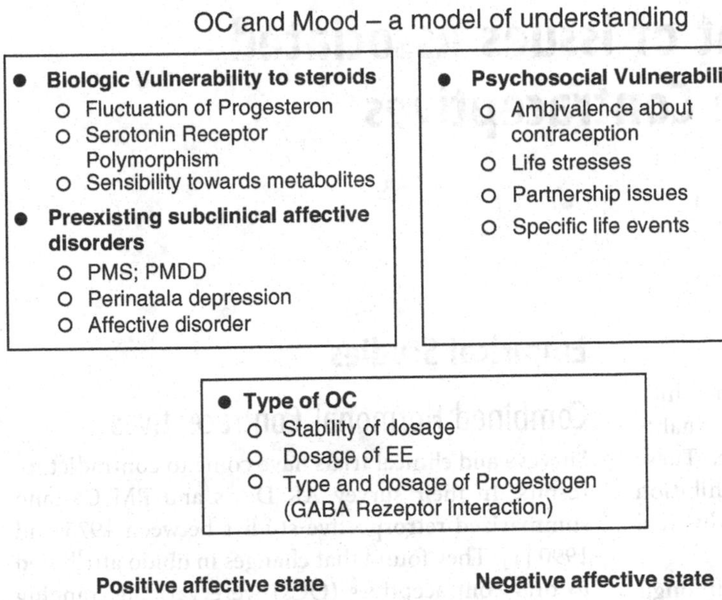

OC and Mood – a model of understanding

- ● **Biologic Vulnerability to steroids**
  - ○ Fluctuation of Progesteron
  - ○ Serotonin Receptor Polymorphism
  - ○ Sensibility towards metabolites
- ● **Preexisting subclinical affective disorders**
  - ○ PMS; PMDD
  - ○ Perinatala depression
  - ○ Affective disorder

- ● **Psychosocial Vulnerability**
  - ○ Ambivalence about contraception
  - ○ Life stresses
  - ○ Partnership issues
  - ○ Specific life events

- ● **Type of OC**
  - ○ Stability of dosage
  - ○ Dosage of EE
  - ○ Type and dosage of Progestogen (GABA Rezeptor Interaction)

Positive affective state   Negative affective state

Figure 17.1 Oral contraceptives and mood. The determinants of outcome

Follow-Up

- During use, ask proactively about side effects, including sexual function and affective symptoms, and explore factors contributing to any complaints that may be due to the contraceptive being used or to other causes.
- Carry out a biopsychosocial assessment of the woman, including her mental condition and environmental distress.
- Provide a choice of contraceptive method.
  - ○ Hormonal contraceptives.
  - ○ Increase oestrogen component (estradiol-valerate to estradiol).
  - ○ Change progestogen (androgenic to anti-androgenic).
  - ○ Change to non-hormonal contraception.

References

1. Skovlund CW, Mørch LS, Kessing LV, Lidegaard Ø. Association of hormonal contraception with depression. *JAMA Psychiatry*. 2016:73:1154–62.

2. Keyes KM, Cheslack-Postava K, Westhoff C et al. Association of hormonal contraceptive use with reduced levels of depressive symptoms: A national study of sexually active women in the United States. *Am J Epidemiol*. 2013;178:1378–88.

3. Wien AB, Foldemo A, Josefsson A, Lindberg M. Use of hormonal contraceptives in relation to antidepressant therapy: A nationwide population-based study. *Eur J Contracept Reprod Health Care*. 2010;15:41–7.

4. Lindberg M, Foldemo A, Josefsson A, Wiréhn AB. Differences in prescription rates and odds ratios of antidepressant drugs in relation to individual hormonal contraceptives: A nationwide population-based study with age-specific analyses. *Eur J Contracept Reprod Health Care*. 2012;17: 106–18.

5. Young EA, Kornstein SG, Harvey AT et al. Influences of hormone-based contraception on depressive symptoms in premenopausal women with major depression. *Psychoneuroendocrinology*. 2007;32: 843–53.

6. Pearlstein TB, Bachmann GA, Zacur HA, Yonkers KA. Treatment of premenstrual dysphoric disorder with a new drospirenone-containing oral contraceptive formulation. *Contraception*. 2005;72:414–21.

7 Oinonen KA, Mazmanian D. To what extent do oral contraceptives influence mood and affect? *J Affect Disord*. 2002;70:229–40.

8. Rapkin AJ, Morgan M, Sogliano C et al. Decreased neuroactive steroids induced by combined oral contraceptive pills are not associated with mood changes. *Fertil Steril*. 2006;85:1371–8.

Management of Issues Associated with Female Contraceptives
Sexuality

Johannes Bitzer

Basics

There are several levels or dimensions on which contraceptive methods can interact with the sexuality of the woman (or man) and of the couple. These interactions can result in enhancement or inhibition of the sexual response depending on the individual characteristics of the user.

a) Separating reproduction from sexuality, although being the rationale for contraception and having a liberating effect, can also be experienced on an emotional level as a deprivation of a profound potency and a feeling of sense of the sexual encounter.

b) Contraceptive methods can interfere with the physiology and neurobiology of the human sexual response. This is mainly mediated by hormonal changes which may go unnoticed or may facilitate or inhibit the sexual response cycle [1–3].

   a. Sexual arousal (and libido) is mediated by neurotransmitter action. Noradrenalin, dopamin, melanocortin and oxytocin are considered to enhance the sexual response while prolactin, opioids and especially serotonin are viewed as inhibiting the response.

   b. Sex steroids have a direct impact on these neurotransmitters, partially pro-sexual and partially inhibiting, depending on the receptors especially in the serotonin pathway.

c) Contraceptive methods can have both a negative and a positive impact on general physical and mental well-being.

d) Contraceptive methods can directly impact the relationship and the sexual encounter.

e) Contraceptive methods can have a social image which may influence sexual well-being (e.g., anxiety regarding risks may have a negative effect on sexual arousal).

Empirical Studies

Combined Hormonal Contraceptives

Surveys and clinical trials have come to contradictory results. In their survey AR Davis and PM Castano summarized retrospective studies between 1975 and 1990 [1]. They found that changes in libido attributed to oral contraceptives (OCs) were variable, ranging from large increases to modest decreases. 'It was found that most women did not report large negative effects on libido but changes did occur during OC use in some women' [4].

Some randomized placebo-controlled studies found controversial results. In a Scottish study 50% of Scottish women taking a combined oral contraceptive (COC) reported reduced sexual interest. In the same study this was not the case in women from the Philippines [5]. Other studies reported similar increases and decreases in desire with a majority of women not reporting any changes in sexual function [6–11]. Sanders reported that, among 107 women receiving two types of COCs, 36% reported a lower frequency of intercourse and 80% of these women discontinued or switched OC, whilst 39% of participants had a reduction in sexual thoughts, of whom 89% discontinued or switched OC [12].

In this context it is important to mention a placebo study in which 147 women received an OC placebo during 424 months of observation. Aznar-Ramos et al. found that, following administration of the placebo OC, decreased sexual desire was the most commonly reported effect with 29.5% of women presenting. Interestingly, only 33.2% of women remained asymptomatic during observation [13].

In a comparative study of changes in sexual desire in women using either OCs or a non-hormonal intrauterine device (IUD) found that the majority of women reported no change in sexual desire while the proportion of women reporting a reduction in desire was comparable between the two groups (OC 10.4%, IUD 12.1%) [14].

Taking these results together, it seems that the independent effect of COCs is very difficult to determine and that for the majority of women the use of OCs is not associated with a deterioration of their sexual function. However, a subgroup of women may be vulnerable to the impact of synthetic steroid hormones on the female sexual response. Furthermore it seems even more difficult to differentiate between different dosages and types of oestrogens and progestogens [15].

Progestogen-Only Contraceptives

None of the women taking the progestogen-only pill in the aforementioned study comparing Scottish women and women from the Philippines reported any adverse effects on sexuality [5]. This is consistent with the available data from other studies, which suggest that progesterone-only contraceptives have little effect on sexual desire [15]. There may, however, be indirect negative effects due to bleeding irregularities and impact on mood.

Contraceptive Methods and Sexual Side Effects

Combined Hormonal Contraceptives

Combined hormonal contraceptives can interact with the sexual physiology on several levels:

a) They reduce the fluctuation of ovarian hormones through the cycle and block ovulation. This reduction of fluctuation may be experienced as positive, especially in women with pre-existing premenstrual syndrome (PMS). It may also be experienced as reducing energy and desire.

b) Sex hormone-binding globulin (SHBG) is increased by the ethinyl-estradiol component of CHCs, and this leads to a diminution of testosterone levels. Testosterone interacts with receptors in the brain located in the midbrain and hypothalamic centres and is linked to sexual desire. Lowering free testosterone may reduce sexual desire in some women.
Reduction of testosterone may, on the other hand, lead to improvement of the skin and thus contribute to a better body image with a positive effect on sexual activity.

c) They partly replace the natural hormones and change in that way the sum of estrogenic and progestogenic actions.

d) The integrity of the vaginal mucosa is maintained by oestrogen. Lack of oestrogen leads to atrophic changes. Progestogen-dominant hormonal contraceptives may contribute to these changes.

It is important to realize that most women do not become aware of these changes as physical or mental symptoms. This is probably due to the fact that the female body is used to hormonal fluctuations and changes in concentrations (menstrual cycle, pregnancy, etc.).

Impact on General Well-Being

Combined hormonal contraceptives can have positive or negative effects on general well-being which indirectly can influence sexual well-being. Possible positive effects are:

- Reduction of heavy menstrual bleeding and dysmenorrhea.
- Reduction of PMS/PMDD, especially when used in a long-cycle manner.
- Improvement of hyperandrogenic skin and hair disorders (acne, hirsutism) with a positive impact on body image.

Possible negative effects are:

- Irregular bleeding, subjective weight gain, irritability, mood instability, skin symptoms.

Impact on the Relationship

Combined hormonal contraceptives (CHC) can help partners enjoy sexuality without fear of pregnancy and the consequences of unintended pregnancies on the relationship. The responsibility for practising contraception can, however, be viewed by one partner, especially the woman, as unjust. The user may feel forced into taking hormones which may change the individual's view on the tolerability of the method and on the sexual encounter.

The Role of Social Image

As mentioned before CHCs can be perceived as welcome tools of female emancipation on one hand or tools of manipulation by Big Pharma. Depending on the media presence and availability of information, including pictures and stories, the threats and dangers of taking the pill may be dominant on one hand while,

127

on the other, the beneficial effects do not get great attention (only bad news is good news).

Progestogen-Only Contraceptives

Progestogen contraceptives include progestogen-only pills, LNG IUDs and implants and Depo progestogen injections.

Separating Sexuality and Reproduction

The impact on the level of separation sexuality/reproduction is basically the same as described earlier in this chapter. When it comes to long-acting methods like LNG IUDs and implants, the fact that the method needs a medical professional for insertion and removal may increase feelings of loss of control, which may have a negative impact on the inner perception of the method and the emotional reaction to it (foreign body which is not under control like ingesting a pill).

Physiology of the Sexual Response

Progestogen-only contraceptives inhibit ovulation effectively. The main differences in comparison to CHCs are the following:

a) There is no increase in SHGB and thus no reduction of free testosterone: It has been shown in observational studies that progestogen only users do not observe a loss of interest or desire as seen in users of CHCs.

b) There is a reduction of oestrogen supply with different degrees with respect to different methods. This is dependent on the dose of the progestogen applied. The highest exposure is in depot progestogen injections users. The most negative impact could be reduction in the thickness of the vaginal wall and a reduction of blood flow during arousal.

Impact on General Well-Being

Possible positive effects

Progestogens can improve well-being by reducing dysmenorrhea and heavy menstrual bleeding. In some women they may reduce pre-existing PMS.

Possible negative effects

Irregular bleeding, unwanted amenorrhea, acne, weight gain (Depo-Provera).

The impact on relationship can be the same as with CHCs.

The Role of Social Image

This depends very much on whether progestogen-only contraceptives are perceived as hormones like in the pill (bad news) or as how dose preparations without thrombotic risks (good news). Another aspect of the social image is concerning news about depression, mainly in adolescents.

Copper Intrauterine Devices

Copper IUDs are very effective contraceptive methods with a good safety profile. There is no impact on the physiology of the sexual response. An indirect negative impact would be in women who have heavy menstrual bleeding or pain during or between menstruations. The psychological impact of a very effective method outside the control of the woman may also have an indirect negative effect on the inner representation of the method which could theoretically be experienced as less pleasurable sexuality. There are, however, no studies proving such an association.

Local Barrier Methods

When properly used the condom protects against unwanted pregnancies and many sexually transmitted infections. It is therefore a very important preventive instrument in sexual and reproductive healthcare. This aspect can be very motivating regarding the use of the condom, which can be then be experienced as the expression of a shared responsibility among partners, which then can improve the sexual experience.

On the other hand, the use of the condom demands the interruption of the sexual interaction in the moment of arousal of the male or of both partners. This interruption can lead to a problem in maintaining the state of arousal or being able to increase arousal. Men can experience condom use as a reduction in pleasurable feelings coming from penetration and movement of the penis in the vagina. The female partner may have an unpleasant feeling or sometimes a little pain during intercourse, which may reduce lubrication, thus increasing the problem. Finally, there may be a negative impact on the enjoyment of the sexual encounter due to insecurity and fears regarding the possible failure in preventing a pregnancy

Fertility Awareness–Based Methods

Fertility-awareness methods have no impact on the physiology or anatomy or the sexual response, nor do they have negative side effects which may impact sexuality besides the insecurity and fears regarding a possible failure in preventing a pregnancy. They may have a positive effect on the sexual experience through the fact that women using fertility awareness–based methods are usually very interested in knowing more about their body and its responses. They feel empowered and developing security and a positive feeling towards their body may facilitate a sexual response which is welcome and enjoyable.

Counselling

Based on the these described possible positive and negative effects of contraceptive methods on sexual function, it is evident that sexual counselling must be tailored to the individual patient. It is helpful to structure the counselling process into different steps

Initial Visit

Taking a sexual history is an important part of the initial contraceptive counselling session.

- Are you satisfied with your sexual life?
- Are there any issues like low desire, arousal or orgasmic problems?
- Does it hurt during sex?

When patients chooses HC, they address in advance the possible impact of methods on sexuality and encourage reporting.

Example: 'The purpose of contraception is to help you enjoy sexuality without any fear of an unintended pregnancy. For the large majority of women the use of contraceptives has therefore a positive effect on their sexual life. Nonetheless some women may feel changes in their desire or their arousal or other aspects of their sexual life and then it is important to talk about it and to see what we can do.'

Follow-Up Visit with a Patient Using Hormonal Contraceptives

Example: The user complains about negative changes in her sexual life and/or sexual function. Take the complaint seriously.

- ○ Find a common language to talk about sex.
- ○ Clarify the diagnosis.

    Is the complaint due to a lack of desire, arousal difficulty, anorgasmia or sexual pain? Is it a combination of complaints? What came first?

- ○ If not assessed before, ask about pre-existing sexual function and take a sexual history.

- ○ Briefly assess other factors having a possible impact on sexual function:
    - ▪ Changes at work.
    - ▪ Changes in the relationship.
    - ▪ Stresses.
    - ▪ Ask patients whether they think these other factors have an impact.
- ○ If psychosocial factors have no or minimal impact, assess whether method-typical changes could contribute to the problem (look for possible negative effects on physiology and anatomy).
    - ▪ The dosage and type of oestrogen (higher oestrogen dosage may lead to reduced free testosterone; low oestrogen may induce vaginal atrophy; androgenic progestogens may contribute to free testosterone levels but cause androgenic side effects; anti-androgenic progestogens improve skin condition but may lead to suppression of androgenic action on the brain, etc.).
- ○ Come to a shared decision.
    - ▪ Change composition and type of hormonal contraception.
    - ▪ Reduce oestrogen component.
    - ▪ Change progestogen.
        I. Not enough oestrogen action: difficulty in arousal, vaginal dryness.
        II. Too much oestrogen action: reduction of free testosterone with subsequent low desire.
        III. Not enough testosterone action: low desire.
        IV. Too much testosterone action: skin and hair problems.
    - ▪ Change contraceptive method.
    - ▪ If psychosocial factors have a larger impact, invite the patient for sexual counselling.

References

1. Pfaus JG. Pathways of sexual desire. *J Sex Med.* 2009;6:1506–33.

2. Brotto LA, Bitzer J, Laan E, Leiblum S, Luria M. Women's sexual desire and arousal disorders. *J Sex Med.* 2010;7:586–614.

3. Dei M, Verni A, Bigozzi L, Bruni V. Sex steroids and libido. *Eur J Contracept Reprod Health Care.* 1997;**2** (4):253–8.

4. Davis A, Castano P. Oral contraceptives and libido in women. *Annu Rev Sex Res*. 2004;**15**:297–320.

5. Graham CA, Ramos R, Bancroft J, Maglaya C, Farley TM. The effects of steroidal contraceptives on the well-being and sexuality of women: A double-blind, placebo-controlled, two-centre study of combined and progestogen-only methods. *Contraception*. 1995;**52**:363–9.

6. Cullberg J, Gelli MG, Jonsson CO. Mental and sexual adjustment before and after six months' use of an oral contraceptive. *Acta Psychiatrica Scandinavica*. 1969;**45**: 259–76.

7. Graham C, Sherwin B. The relationship between mood and sexuality in women using an oral contraceptive as a treatment for premenstrual symptoms. *Psychoneuroendocrinology*. 1993;**18**(4):273–81.

8. Plewig G, Cunliffe W, Binder N, Höschen K. Efficacy of an oral contraceptive containing ethinyl estradiol 0.03 mg and chlormadinone acetate 2 mg (EE/CMA; Belara®) in moderate acne resolution: A randomised, double-blind, placebo-controlled phase III trial. *Contraception*. 2008:123–30.

9. Erkkola R, Hirvonen E, Luikku J et al. Ovulation inhibitors containing cyproterone acetate or desogestrel in the treatment of hyperandrogenic symptoms. *Acta Obstetricia et Gynecologica Scandinavica*. 1990;**69**:61–5.

10. Endrikat J, Hite R, Bannemerschult R, Gerlinger C, Schmidt W. Multicenter, comparative study of cycle control, efficacy and tolerability of two low-dose oral contraceptives containing 20 microg ethinylestradiol/ 100 microg levonorgestrel and 20 microg ethinylestradiol/500 microg norethisterone. *Contraception*. 2001;**64**(1):3–10.

11. Worret I, Arp W, Zahradnik H, Andreas J, Binder N. Acne resolution rates: Results of a single-blind, randomized, controlled, parallel phase III trial with EE/CMA (Belara) and EE/LNG (Microgynon). *Dermatology*. 2001;**203**(1):38–44.

12. Sanders S, Graham C, Bass J, Bancroft J. A prospective study of the effects of oral contraceptives on sexuality and well-being and their relationship to discontinuation. *Contraception*. 2001;**64**(1):51–8.

13. Aznar-Ramos R, Ginger-Velazquez J, Lara-Ricalde R, Martinez-Manautou J. Incidence of side effects with contraceptive placebo. *Am J Obstet Gynecol*. 1969;**105** (7):1144–9.

14. Martin-Loeches M, Orti R, Monfort M, Ortega E, Rius J. A comparative analysis of the modification of sexual desire of users of oral hormonal contraceptives and intrauterine contraceptive devices. *Eur J Contracept Reprod Health Care*. 2003;**8**(3):129–34.

15. Schaffir J. Hormonal contraception and sexual desire: A critical review. *J Sex Marital Ther*. 2006;**32**(4):305–14.

Chapter 19

Management of Issues Associated with Female Contraceptives
Drug–Drug Interactions

Katarina Sedlecky, Gabriele S. Merki-Feld and Frans J. M. E. Roumen

Introduction

Assessing the safety and efficacy of hormonal contraception involves examining possible interactions between contraceptives and concomitant medications or herbal supplements. The effects of hormonal contraception may be altered by changes in the resorption, metabolism, secretion or activity of sex hormones. Hormonal contraception, on the other hand, can affect the metabolism or therapeutic effect of drugs.

Resorption of Steroid Contraceptive Hormones

Drugs that increase gastric pH, like proton pump inhibitors, antacids and H2-receptor antagonists, might reduce the effectiveness of ulipristal acetate (UPA) emergency contraception due to its low solubility at neutral conditions and consequently reduced gastrointestinal resorption [1]. Also, regular use of laxatives or medications whose common side effects are vomiting or diarrhoea may reduce the resorption of ethinyl-oestradiol (EE) and progestins from the small intestine. Overdosing of activated charcoal can prevent absorption of oral contraceptive pills. Changes in the release and systemic absorption of sex hormones have also been observed in EE/nestorone contraceptive vaginal ring users treated with miconazole. Systemic exposure to EE and nestorone was highest in women treated with a single dose of miconazole suppository, slightly lower in those treated with multiple doses of vaginal suppositories and unchanged in women who received multiple-dose cream compared to the cycle without miconazole treatment [2].

Metabolism of Steroid Contraceptive Hormones

Most interactions between hormonal contraception and drugs are achieved by induction or inhibition of enzymes involved in their metabolism. After oral ingestion, oral bioavailability of EE is 20–65%, while for progestins it is higher and variable for different products. Metabolism of EE involves hydroxylation (app. 30%) via cytochrome P450 iso-enzymes CYP3A4 (app. 66%), CYP2C9 (app. 25%) and, to a lesser extent, CYP2C8, CYP2C19 and CYP3A5. First-pass biotransformation of EE also occurs through conjugation via sulphation (up to 38% in the gut) and glucuronidation (app. 20%) via UDP-glucuronosyltransferase (UGT) 1A1. For progestins the extent of first-pass metabolism depends on the type of progestin (high for norethisterone, desogestrel and norgestimate, none for levonorgestrel). Although it is not fully understood, metabolism of progestins also includes CYP-mediated hydroxylation (mainly CYP3A4), as well as conjugation reactions, but with no active forms of these compounds entering enterohepatic recirculation [3, 4].

For drug–drug interactions (DDIs) it is important that hormonal contraceptives may change the activity of enzymes involved in the metabolism of some drugs. Combined oral contraceptives (COCs) are moderate inhibitors of CYP1A2 and weak inhibitors of CYP3A4, CYP2C19 and CYP2D6 enzymes. On contrary, EE may induce UGT enzymes and affect the metabolism of drugs that use that metabolic route. It was not found that progestins have any impact on the activity of CYP450 enzymes. For a complete overview of DDIs it is necessary to take into account whether hormonal contraception is used continuously or in a cyclic regime [3, 4].

Interactions between Drugs and Hormonal Contraception

Clinically relevant is considered the change for a certain pharmacokinetic parameter outside the interval 80–125%, within 90% confidence interval (CI). Changes within this range can be statistically significant but are clinically irrelevant [4]. Enzyme-inducing drugs, like some antiepileptics, antibiotics, antiretrovirals and herbal remedies, may decrease the effectiveness of hormonal contraceptives. As strong and moderate enzyme inducers are considered those drugs that lower the area under the curve (AUC) for the substrate, or other co-administered drug by more than 80% and between 50 and 80%, respectively. The degree of AUC reduction for the substrate in weak inducers is 20–50%. On the contrary, enzyme-inhibiting drugs may increase the risk of side effects and serious adverse events (SAE) due to higher blood levels of EE and/or progestin. Drugs that increase AUC of another co-administered drug by more than five fold, or between two and five fold, are estimated to be strong and moderate enzyme inhibitors, respectively [5]. The following is an overview of DDIs between hormonal contraception and most important

groups of drugs, except those used in the treatment of HIV disease, which are presented in Chapter 24.

Antiepileptic Drugs

Many antiepileptic drugs (AEDs) have the potential to affect metabolism of hormonal contraception (Table 19.1). Hormonal contraceptives may also have an effect on the pharmacokinetics (PK) of AEDs.

Some AEDs, like carbamazepine, phenobarbital, primidone and phenytoin, are inducers of CYP450 enzymes and have the potential to lower EE and progestin levels, increasing the risk of unplanned pregnancy [6]. Oxcarbazepin is a weaker inducer of liver enzymes than the previous ones but has a similar effect on the metabolism of hormonal contraception. Some less-potent enzyme inducers, like topiramate, significantly affect the PK of EE at doses higher than

Table 19.1 Interactions between hormonal contraceptives and antiepileptic drugs

Antiepileptic drug (AED)	Changes in serum concentration of AED	Changes in serum concentration of ethinyl-oestradiol	Changes in serum concentration of progestin
Strong enzyme inducers			
Carbamazepine	no data	decrease	decrease
Felbamate	no data	decrease	decrease
Eslicarbazepine	no data	decrease	decrease
Oxcarbazepin	no data	decrease	decrease
Primidone	no data	decrease	decrease
Phenobarbitone	no data	decrease	decrease
Phenytoin	no data	decrease	decrease
Topiramate	no data	decrease*	none
Perampanel	no data	none	decrease*
Weak enzyme inducers			
Lamotrigine	decrease	none	decrease
No enzyme inducers			
Valproate	decrease	none	none
Gabapentin	no data	none	none
Lacosamide	none	none	none
Levitiracetam	none	none	none
Zonisamide	none	none	none
Retigabine/ezogabine	none	none	none
Pregabalin	no data	no data	no data
Vigabatrin	none	none	none

* dose-dependent effect

200 mg. Similarly, perampanel dose-dependently enhances progestin metabolism and may decrease the efficacy of progestin-only pills (POPs) at daily doses higher than 12 mg.

Valproate, gabapentin, levetiracetam, and lacosamide have no effect on the metabolism of COCs. Lamotrigine induces the metabolism of some progestins, like levonorgestrel (LNG), and may reduce contraceptive efficacy of some low-dose COCs and POPs. The impact of lamotrigine on the efficacy of progestin-only emergency contraception has not been evaluated [3, 6].

Conversely, metabolism and serum concentrations of some AEDs may be affected by EE. Serum concentration of valproate is moderately reduced probably by accelerating glucuronidation. In the same way, serum concentration of lamotrigine is reduced by more than 50%, resulting in therapeutic failure. The effect of COCs on the metabolism of lamotrigine is achieved quickly, but it also disappears within a few days. Therefore, in the hormone-free period serum concentration of lamotrigine becomes twice as high, carrying the risk of drug intoxication. Thus, women who are on lamotrigine monotherapy are not advised to take combined hormonal contraception (CHC), but they can safely use some of the progestin-only contraceptive methods. However, women who are on combination therapy with lamotrigine and valproate can use CHC because valproate counteracts the effect of CHC on the metabolism of lamotrigine [3].

The impact of hormonal contraception on the metabolism of AEDs has been studied for a small number of medications. Eslicarbazepine and licarbazine are metabolised by UGT enzymes and therefore may be affected by EE. Available data suggest that hormonal contraception does not affect the metabolism of levitiracetam, zonisamide, lacosamide and retigabine/ezogabine [3, 6].

Based on patient reports, frequency of epileptic seizures is significantly different, dominantly increased, in hormonal contraception users compared to non-hormonal contraception users. These changes were most often recorded among women who were on valproate monotherapy (29.4%), and least often in patients who received antiepileptics that do not induce cytochrome P450 enzymes (11.6%) [7].

Psychotropic Drugs

The number of people with mental illness is on the rise. Women are at higher risk of developing depression and/or anxiety disorders. About 40–50% of affected persons are receiving prescription pharmacotherapy. Some of these psychotropic drugs may affect metabolism of hormonal contraceptives (Table 19.2). No psychotropic drug has been shown to induce liver enzymes and decrease EE and progestin serum concentrations. Some of these drugs are inhibitors of the CYP450 enzymes, like fluoxetine (inhibitor of CYP2C19 enzyme), but the only one that inhibits both CYP3A4 and CYP2C9 is fluvoxamine [5].

Selective serotonin reuptake inhibitors (SSRIs). No clinically significant DDIs were found between fluoxetine or citalopram and CHC in terms of the rates of unintended pregnancy and treatment response to psychotropic drugs. Concomitant use of vortioxetine and COC resulted in clinically insignificant decrease of EE by 6.1% and increase of LNG by 7.1% [8].

Tricyclic antidepressants (TCAs). No differences in the treatment response and side effects, as well as mean plasma concentrations of clomipramine were found with respect to the use of COCs. Small-scale PK studies found an increase in both AUC of imipramine by 104.4% and mean serum concentrations of amitriptyline by 89.7% in COC users, compared to women not using hormonal contraception. This observation that the use of COCs can significantly increase the concentration of some TCAs raises the concern that many TCAs have narrow therapeutic windows [8].

Bupropion. Bupropion is commonly used in the treatment of mental disorders and nicotine addiction. In COC users a modest decrease in AUC of both bupropion (19%), and its active metabolite hydroxybupropion (31%) were registered. Hence, a weaker therapeutic effect of bupropion in COC users may be expected [5, 8].

Atypical antipsychotics. No DDIs between COC and ziprasidone were perceived. In patients treated with olanzapine CHC use decreased by 33% concentration of the metabolite N-desmethyl olanzapine, but similar changes were not observed in users of progestin-only contraception.

Lurasidone did not demonstrated any impact on PK of COC. On the other hand, COC use demonstrated a considerable effect on PK of clozapine, inducing approximately twofold increase in plasma drug concentrations [9]. No data exist for DDIs between COC and duloxetine or mirtazapine [5, 8].

Table 19.2 Interactions between hormonal contraceptives and psychotropic drugs

Psychotropic drug	Changes in serum concentration of psychotropic drug	Changes in serum concentration of oestrogen/progestin
Selective serotonin reuptake inhibitors (SSRIs)		
fluoxetine, citalopram	none	none
vortioxetine	none	decrease of EE and increase of progestin
fluvoxamine	none	increase of EE and progestin
Tricyclic antidepressants (TCAs)		
clomipramine	none	none
imipramine	app. twofold increase	none
amitriptyline	app. twofold increase	none
Atypical antidepressant		
bupropion	modest decrease	none
Atypical antipsychotics		
ziprasidone	none	none
olanzapine	modest decrease with CHC; no changes with POC	none
lurasidone	none	none
clozapine	app. two-fold increase	none
duloxetine	no data	no data
mirtazapine	no data	no data
Oral benzodiazepines		
oxazepam	decrease	no data
lorazepam	decrease	no data
temazepam	decrease	no data
triazolam	none	no data
alprazolam	increase	no data
chlordiazepoxide	no data	breakthrough bleeding
meprobamate	no data	breakthrough bleeding

* app. – approximately

Oral benzodiazepines. Metabolism of some, but not all, benzodiazepines includes CYP450 enzymes. In COC users no significant differences in volume distribution of oxazepam were detected, although the clearance increased by 157%. In COC users treated with either lorazepam or temazepam a higher elimination rate was recorded with lower AUC of temazepam compared to women not taking hormonal contraception. It was not found that COC use affects any PK parameter of triazolam, but it decreased elimination rate of alprazolam, resulting in higher AUC. Furthermore, COC users treated with alprazolam, lorazepam and triazolam were found to have a higher degree of psychomotor dysfunction that did not correlate with PK changes. Differences in sedation and memory were not found for any of these benzodiazepines concerning the use of COC.

An impact of benzodiazepines on the clinical outcomes of COC use was evaluated by recording the incidence of breakthrough bleeding. Treatment with diazepam, chlordiazepoxide, nitrazepam or meprobamate resulted in one third (36.1%) of COC users experiencing breakthrough bleeding, with the vast majority of those taking chlordiazepoxide and meprobamate [8, 10].

Opioids and Psychostimulants

The data on DDIs between opioids and hormonal contraception are scarce. Theoretically, DDIs might be expected having in mind the fact that both groups of drugs are metabolized by CYP450 and UGT enzymes [5, 10]. Since the majority of opioid substances do not induce or inhibit CYP450 enzymes, there should be no concern for the effectiveness of hormonal contraceptives (Table 19.3). On the other hand, as EE acts as inhibitor of some CYP450 enzymes, it is possible to theoretically assume an increase in serum concentrations of some opioids, like hydrocodone, meperidine, oxycodone and tramadol, which carries the risk of overdose. The EE is also an inducer of UGT enzymes and could increase clearance and decrease serum concentrations of some opioids (codeine, hydromorphone, morphine and oxymorphone) which are substrates for these enzymes [10].

Cannabinoids are extensively metabolized by cytochrome P450 enzymes and have a potential to either induce or inhibit some of liver enzymes, with a predominant effect on inhibiting many CYP450 enzymes [11]. However, there are currently no data on the clinically significant DDIs between these opioids and hormonal contraception. It should also be borne in mind that women who use opioids are more likely to use hormonal contraception irregularly, so they are at higher risk of unplanned pregnancy.

Modafinil is used in the treatment of narcolepsy, but it is also widely used for certain professions in which a state of wakefulness should be maintained. Students often use it during exams. In vitro studies imply that modafinil acts as an inducer of CYP1A2, CYP3A4 and CYP2B6 enzymes, and as inhibitor of CYP2C9 and CYP2C19 enzymes [12]. Treatment with modafinil of COC users resulted in a moderate decrease in AUC and Cmax of EE, while the half-life of EE was not affected [13].

Antibiotics

Rifamycin antibiotics are used to treat tuberculosis. As strong inducers of CYP3A and CYP2C19 and moderate inducers of CYP2C8 and CYP2C9, these antibiotics may enhance the metabolism of EE and progestin, thus increasing the risk of unplanned pregnancy [5]. Administration of rifamycin to COC users resulted in a decrease in AUC for progestin by 30–83% and for EE by 42–66%. Concurrent use of COC and rifabutin decreased AUC for progestin by 13–46% and for EE by 35%. There is no evidence that hormonal contraception affects exposure or a therapeutic response to rifamycin antibiotics [14].

In hormonal contraception users treated with non-rifamycin antibiotics no significant increase in unplanned pregnancy rate was found (Table 19.4). Concurrent use of antibiotic and hormonal contraception was not identified as a risk factor for unintended

Table 19.3 Interactions between hormonal contraceptives and opioids/psychostimulants

Drug type	Changes in serum concentration of drug	Changes in serum concentration of oestrogen/progestin
Opioids		
hydrocodone	increase	none
meperidine	increase	none
oxycodone	increase	none
tramadol	increase	none
codeine	decrease	none
hydromorphone	decrease	none
morphine	decrease	none
oxymorphone	decrease	none
cannabis	no data	no data
Psychostimulants		
modafinil	none	decrease

135

Table 19.4 Interactions between hormonal contraceptives and antibiotics

Antibiotic	Changes in serum concentration of antibiotic	Changes in serum concentration of oestrogen/progestin
Rifamycin		
rifamycin, rifabutin	none	decrease of EE and progestin
Non-rifamycin antibiotics		
Penicillins and cephalosporins		
ampicillin	insignificant decrease	none
cephaloridine	insignificant decrease	none
Tetracyclines		
tetracycline	none	none for EE, increase of progestin
doxycycline	none	none
oxtetracycline	no data	no breakthrough bleeding
Fluoroquinolones		
ciprofloxacin, temafloxacin, ofloxacin	none	none
Trovafloxacin, moxifloxacin	decrease	none
Macrolides		
erythromycin	no data	increase
dirithromycin	no data	decrease of EE
azithromycin	increase	no data
clarithromycin	no data	none
roxithromycin	no data	none
Other		
metronidazole	no data	none
sulfamethoxasole/trimethoprim	no data	breakthrough bleeding
nitrofurantoin	no data	none
dapsone	no data	increase of EE, no changes for progestin
griseofulvin	none	decrease of EE, no changes for progestin

pregnancy and the incidence of antibiotic use was not different between women with COC failure pregnancies and non-gravid women [15].

In COC users treated with ampicillin a slight increase (10%) in cycle disturbances without changes in EE and progestin plasma values was found. The use of COCs induced a slight decrease in mean plasma concentrations of ampicillin 1 hour after dosing without changes later on. In users of combined vaginal ring no changes in both EE and etonogestrel plasma concentrations were observed with concurrent use of amoxicillin or doxycycline compared with the antibiotic-free cycle [16].

Concomitant use of tetracycline and COC did not affect contraceptive efficacy and EE metabolism, while plasma norethindrone concentrations increased.

Doxycycline did not alter EE or norethindrone levels. Treatment of COC users with oxtetracycline was not associated with bleeding disturbances [15]. Treatment of COC users with fluoroquinolones (ciprofloxacin, temafloxacin or ofloxacin) has no impact on cycle control or EE and levonorgestrel plasma levels. On the contrary, COC use resulted in a decrease of trovafloxacin and moxifloxacin plasma concentrations [15].

Macrolides (roxithromycin, clarithromycin or dirithromycin) do not reduce the effectiveness of COCs. Still, dirithromycin induced significant decrease in mean EE AUC. Conversely, treatment with erythromycin of postmenopausal women taking oestradiol-valerate and dienogest resulted in a significant increase of both steroid hormones. On the other hand, COC use increases AUC of azithromycin [15].

Treatment with metronidazole or nitrofurantoin has no impact on the efficacy of COC while very few (10%) COC users treated with sulfamethoxasole/trimethoprim report breakthrough bleeding. Concurrent use of COC and dapsone for leprosy results in significant increase of EE AUC [15]. In relation to the effects of antibiotic therapy, no differences in the outcomes of isoniazid-based antibiotic regimens between COC users and non-users were found. Erythromycin treatment did not affect the efficacy of UPA. An increase in systemic exposure to UPA in the presence of erythromycin was well tolerated, and no SAE were recorded [15].

Other Drugs

Isotretinoin is used to treat acne in adolescents and young women. Since isotretinoin is a known teratogen, effective contraceptive protection is extremely important. A PK study suggested that isotretinoin decreased AUC of EE by 9% and Cmax of norethindrone by 11% [17]. Therefore, women treated with isotretinoin are advised to use COCs with a higher dose of hormones, shorten intervals between depot-medroxyprogesterone acetate injections, or to switch to intrauterine contraception (Table 19.5).

An antiemetic drug aprepitant was found to decrease AUC of both EE (43%) and norethindrone (8%). Therefore, COC users treated with aprepitant need to take additional contraceptive precautions [18]. Bosentan is moderate inducer of CYP3A and moderately decreases AUC for both EE and progestin [19]. On the contrary, antifungals (fluconazole, ketoconazole, voriconazole posakonazole) are inhibitors of several CYP450 enzymes, including CYP3A4, CYP2C9 and CYP2C19 [5]. The increase in systemic exposures of both EE and several progestins (e.g. norethindrone,

drospirenone) with voriconazole, ketoconazole and fluconazole was demonstrated [20]. Similar changes were perceived in EE/etonogestrel vaginal ring users treated with antifungals [21]. Therefore, it is better to prescribe progestin-only contraception or combined hormonal products with low doses of EE in women on long-term antifungal treatment [22].

Griseofulvin is used orally for dermatophytosis. In COC users griseofulvin may increase the metabolism of EE, resulting in breakthrough bleeding and unplanned pregnancy [23]. The effectiveness of progestin-only contraception is not affected by concurrent use of griseofulvin.

Herbal Remedies

St. John's wort (SJW), containing *Hypericum perforatum*, is used as treatment for depression. As a strong inducer of CYP3A this product may increase a risk of contraceptive failure in a dose-dependent manner [24]. The risk of contraceptive failure is greatest in women who use very low COCs and POPs.

Direct Effect on the Efficacy of Hormonal Contraception

Ulipristal acetate is the most effective hormonal emergency contraceptive (EC). The question has arisen whether hormonal contraception can reduce the effectiveness of UPA if use is started immediately after EC. It has been observed that initiation of COC use 2 days after the UPA significantly reduced the effectiveness of UPA to prevent ovulation in the next 5 days [25]. Therefore, hormonal contraception can be initiated after 5 days of taking UPA with additional contraceptive precautions for the next 7 days. Another study demonstrated that

Table 19.5 Interactions between hormonal contraceptives and other drugs

Drug	Changes in serum concentration of drug	Changes in serum concentration of oestrogen/progestin
isotretinoin	none	decrease in both EE and progestin
aprepitant	none	decrease in both EE and progestin
bosentan	decrease	decrease in both EE and progestin
Antifungals		
fluconazole, ketoconazole, voriconazole, posakonazole	increase of voriconazole	increase in both EE and progestin
Herbal products		
St John's wort (SJW): *Hypericum perforatum*	none	decrease in both EE and progestin

UPA has no influence on the ability of COC to suppress ovulation when initiated the next day after EC was used [26].

References

1. Pohl O, Osterloh I, Lecomte V, Gotteland JP. Changes in gastric pH and in pharmacokinetics of ulipristal acetate: A drug–drug interaction study using the proton pump inhibitor esomeprazole. *Int J Clin Pharmacol Ther*. 2013;**51**(1): 26–33.

2. Simmons KB, Kumar N, Plagianos M et al. Effects of concurrent vaginal miconazole treatment on the absorption and exposure of Nestorone® (segesterone acetate) and ethinyl estradiol delivered from a contraceptive vaginal ring: A randomized, crossover drug–drug interaction study. *Contraception*. 2018;**97** (3):270–6.

3. Reimers A, Brodtkorb E, Sabers A. Interactions between hormonal contraception and antiepileptic drugs: Clinical and mechanistic considerations. *Seizure*. 2015;**28**:66–70.

4. Lee CR. Drug interactions and hormonal contraception. *Trends in Urology Gynaecology & Sexual Health*. 2009:23–6.

5. US Food and Drug Administration. Drug development and drug interactions: Table of substrates, inhibitors and inducers. http://bit.ly/3JpjGL7.

6. Reddy DS. Clinical pharmacokinetic interactions between antiepileptic drugs and hormonal contraceptives. *Expert Rev Clin Pharmacol*. 2010;**3** (2):183–92.

7. Herzog AG, Mandle HB, Cahill KE, Fowler KM, Hauser WA. Differential impact of contraceptive methods on seizures varies by antiepileptic drug category: Findings of the Epilepsy Birth Control Registry. *Epilepsy Behav*. 2016;**60**:112–17.

8. Berry-Bibee EN, Kim MJ, Simmons KB et al. Drug interactions between hormonal contraceptives and psychotropic drugs: A systematic review. *Contraception*. 2016;**94**(6):650–67.

9. Schoretsanitis G, Kane JM, de Leon J. Adding oral contraceptives to clozapine may require halving the clozapine dose: A new case and a literature review. *J Clin Psychopharmacol*. 2020;**40**(3):308–10.

10. Ti A, Stone RH, Whiteman M, Curtis KM. Safety and effectiveness of hormonal contraception for women who use opioids: A systematic review. *Contraception*. 2019;**100**(6):480–3.

11. Qian Y, Gurley BJ, Markowitz JS. The potential for pharmacokinetic interactions between cannabis products and conventional medications. *J Clin Psychopharmacol*. 2019;**39**(5):462–71.

12. Robertson P, DeCory HH, Madan A, Parkinson A. In vitro inhibition and induction of human hepatic cytochrome P450 enzymes by modafinil. *Drug Metab Dispos*. 2000;**28**(6):664–71.

13. Robertson P, Jr, Hellriegel ET, Arora S, Nelson M. Effect of modafinil on the pharmacokinetics of ethinyl estradiol and triazolam in healthy volunteers. *Clin Pharmacol Ther*. 2002;**71**(1):46–56.

14. Simmons KB, Haddad LB, Nanda K, Curtis KM. Drug interactions between rifamycin antibiotics and hormonal contraception: A systematic review. *BJOG*. 2018;**125**(7):804–11.

15. Simmons KB, Haddad LB, Nanda K, Curtis KM. Drug interactions between non-rifamycin antibiotics and hormonal contraception: A systematic review. *Am J Obstet Gynecol*. 2018;**218**(1):88–97.e14.

16. Dogterom P, van den Heuvel MW, Thomsen T. Absence of pharmacokinetic interactions of the combined contraceptive vaginal ring NuvaRing with oral amoxicillin or doxycycline in two randomised trials. *Clin Pharmacokinet*. 2005;**44** (4):429–38.

17. Hendrix CW, Jackson KA, Whitmore E et al. The effect of isotretinoin on the pharmacokinetics and pharmacodynamics of ethinyl estradiol and norethindrone. *Clin Pharmacol Ther*. 2004;**75** (5):464–75.

18. Bailard N, Rebello E. Aprepitant and fosaprepitant decrease the effectiveness of hormonal contraceptives. *Br J Clin Pharmacol*. 2018;**84**(3):602–3.

19. Van Giersbergen PL, Halabi A, Dingemanse J. Pharmacokinetic interaction between bosentan and the oral contraceptives norethisterone and ethinyl estradiol. *Int J Clin Pharmacol Ther*. 2006;**44**(3):113–18.

20. Zhang N, Shon J, Kim MJ et al. Role of CYP3A in oral contraceptives clearance. *Clin Transl Sci*. 2018;**11** (3):251–60.

21. Verhoeven CH, van den Heuvel MW, Mulders TM, Dieben TO. The contraceptive vaginal ring, NuvaRing, and antimycotic co-medication. *Contraception*. 2004;**69**(2):129–32.

22. Ezuruike U, Humphries H, Dickins M et al. Risk-benefit assessment of ethinylestradiol using a physiologically based pharmacokinetic modeling approach. *Clin Pharmacol Ther*. 2018;**104**(6): 1229–39.

23. Catalano PM, Blank H. Griseofulvin–oral contraceptive interaction. *Arch Dermatol*. 1985;**121** (11):1381–7.

24. Berry-Bibee EN, Kim MJ, Tepper NK, Riley HE, Curtis KM. Co-administration of St. John's wort and hormonal contraceptives: A systematic review. *Contraception.* 2016;94(6): 668–77.

25. Edelman AB, Jensen JT, McCrimmon S et al. Combined oral contraceptive interference with the ability of ulipristal acetate to delay ovulation: A prospective cohort study. *Contraception.* 2018;98(6):463–6.

26. Cameron ST, Berger C, Michie L, Klipping C, Gemzell-Danielsson K. The effects on ovarian activity of ulipristal acetate when 'quickstarting' a combined oral contraceptive pill: A prospective, randomized, double-blind parallel-arm, placebo-controlled study. *Hum Reprod.* 2015;30(7):1566–72.

Chapter 20

Contraception in Women with Cancer

Anne Gompel

Introduction

Cancer, although more frequent after menopause, can reach younger and fertile patients or occur during childhood. Contraception in women during the treatment of or after cancer is an important subject and too often neglected. Studies show that counseling on contraception in women with cancer is often missing [1]. Some treatment can alter the ovarian reserve even in children but in adult women it can be only transitory and it is not easy to evaluate accurately the potential fertility after the treatment of a cancer. Follicular and AMH counts are not so well contributive, and thus preventing pregnancy has to be systematic if it is not wished or allowed. During the treatment of any cancer in premenopausal women, providing an efficient contraception without interfering with the treatment of the cancer and without adverse effects is mandatory. A recent study highlighted the fact that many women think they are not anymore fertile after the treatment of cancer and, as a consequence, they neglect to use an efficient contraception [2]. In all cases, however, the combined estro-progestin contraception (CC) is contraindicated during the acute phase of treatment because of the increasing risk of venous thrombosis (VTE) associated with cancer, surgery, and chemotherapy [3].

There is increasing possibilities to spare fertility during the treatment of cancer, including gynecological cancers. During the consultation for fertility preservation or in combination with it, contraceptive options can be discussed with the patient [4]. Contraception will help program a pregnancy when allowed by the clinical evolution. It is thus important to know the potential impact of various contraception on the cancer and include its management in the general counseling.

During both long-term and short-term treatment of cancer, the choice can be different according to the clinical context of the patient and the risk of recurrence. The cardiovascular risk of the patient can be worsened by some of the oncologic treatments [5]. Anthracyclines, cyclophosphamide, 5-Fluorouracil, trastuzumab, taxanes, platinum, and tyrosine kinase inhibitors can be associated with cardiac side effects (heart failure, ischemia, or arrhythmia), mostly in the short term, and it is reversible in most instances but not for anthracyclines [5].

Radiotherapy of the left breast and mediastinum can increase the risk of heart failure, myocardial infarction, and lung cancer (in smokers) in the long term [6]. One of the frequent problem occurring during chemotherapy is aplasia leading to abnormal gynecological bleeding and severe anemia. The choice of the contraceptive can help control these occurrences.

Breast Cancer

Breast cancer is the most common cancer in many Western countries. About 20% of the women with breast cancer in Europe and North America are premenopausal whereas this proportion is higher in Africa and Asia [7]. It is the paradigm of hormone-dependent cancer. A majority of BC is estradiol receptor positive (ER+) but the most aggressive ones are those which express an amplification of HER2 (HER2 +) and the triple negative (TN) (devoid of HER2 amplification, ER, and progesterone receptor (PR)).

Breast cancer treatments in the more aggressive cases consist of surgery, radiotherapy and chemotherapy ± hormonotherapy (if ER+). The first chemotherapy indicated in young women includes anthracyclines and taxanes but can also include cyclophosphamide; these treatments may be associated with amenorrhea and ovarian failure (OF) according to the dose administered and the age of the women [8].

Tamoxifen, prescribed as adjuvant therapy in ER+ patients, in addition to chemotherapy, may increase the duration of amenorrhea even in the absence of complete OF. Tamoxifen is administered, usually for

5 years, in premenopausal women. The GnRH agonist may be associated with tamoxifen or aromatase inhibitors in the most severe patients for 5 years, as well as an extension of hormonotherapy up to 10 years in the most aggressive forms [8]. Of course, during the GnRH agonist therapy, no contraception is necessary. The GnRH agonist also may help preserve fertility and can be used with this purpose in women in whom ovarian oocyte and embryo cryopreservation are not feasible [4, 9].

In the youngest population, fertility may persist and because amenorrhea does not necessarily mean complete OF it is mandatory to provide effective contraception. Several studies analyzed the occurrence of amenorrhea during chemotherapy ± tamoxifen and the probability for recovering ovarian function and were reviewed in reference [10]. It is not clear what proportion of women will become postmenopausal with current therapeutic sequences. Nevertheless, because amenorrhea does not coincide systematically with definitive OF, contraception is needed in these women. The average duration of hormone therapy before allowing a pregnancy is in most cases 5 years. In some cases, because of the age of the patient and low ovarian reserve, pregnancy may be permitted before 5 years have elapsed. Ideally, the woman should wait a minimum of 2 years after BC treatment. A meta-analysis however, suggested that a delay of 10 months was sufficient and that pregnancy did not impact survival [11].

The World Health Organization (WHO) contraindicate all hormone contraception in women with BC [12]. Copper IUD is the contraception recommended during the treatment of the cancer. After 5 years, the WHO stated, "an hormonal contraception has to be as possible avoided but if there is no other solution then discuss any hormonal contraception." The risk of infection during chemotherapy for BC is relatively low and does not contraindicate use of the copper IUD. Intolerance and bleeding can occur during the treatment of cancer using copper IUD.

In case of bleeding, antifibrinolytic agents may be used but scarcely because of the risk of VTE. Tamoxifen can induce or promote the growth of polyps and myoma and (rarely) hyperplasia. Several trials have evaluated the efficacy of a high-dose levonorgestrel IUD (LNG-IUD) on the prevention of the benign uterine diseases in women with BC and tamoxifen. The results were analyzed in a Cochrane review [13].

There was a decrease in the number of polyps in the group using the LNG-IUD: OR 0.22 (0.13 to 0.39, 4 studies, n = 417) [13]. Less hyperplasia was observed based on six cases. Interestingly, there was no difference in BC recurrence in LNG-IUD users (14.3%) compared to the control group (9.1%), based on 77 patients in two randomized trials. Deaths were not different (5.8% vs. 5.7%) based on three trials and 277 patients [13].

Bleeding was more frequent during the first year than in the control group. Newer systems containing lower dosages of LNG compared with the original dosage are now available. No data are available on their use and the risk of BC recurrence. However, when bleeding occurs spontaneously or with a copper IUD, it is usually admitted by various groups of experts that a high-dose LNG-IUD can be used in women with BC [4, 10]. There is no contraindication to use an hormonal emergency contraception in women with BC, but copper IUD is the first line if possible [4].

If the woman agrees to a good compliance to condoms or diaphragms or equivalent, then she can be proposed taking into account the fertility, some anatomical situations, and the age of the woman. Female or male sterilization may also be discussed in couples who do not wish to have another pregnancy. Medroxyprogesterone acetate (MPA) and megestrol acetate are used in high doses in metastatic BC patients and in those patients are contraceptive.

In women with hereditary BC carriers of a BRCA mutation, a hormonal contraception can be used up to the age of prophylactic oophorectomy because of its beneficial effect on the ovarian cancer (OC) risk, and despite a possible increase in the risk of BC. Using a long term CC at a young age could be associated with a higher risk of BC [14]. As a consequence, some authors advise the use of CC for ovarian protection after the age of 25 years and up to the age of oophorectomy (30/35 years) [14]. Alternatively, a copper IUD or barrier methods can be used. Emergency contraception is not contraindicated.

Endometrial Cancer

Endometrial cancer is the sixth most common cancer in women [15]. It has two principal differentiations. Type I is highly estrogen dependent, endometrioid, well differentiated, and of good prognosis. Type II is more aggressive and less hormone dependent (constituted of the types serous and clear cells). Endometrial cancer is essentially occurring in postmenopausal women but can occur in premenopausal women in the context of hyperestrogenism, obesity, polycystic ovary syndrome or hereditary EC with mismatch repair abnormalities (Lynch syndrome). In the context of a Lynch syndrome, hysterectomy (and ovariectomy) are performed after the age of 40 years or more according to the type of genetic abnormality [16]. Before this age, because of its efficacy on the risk of EC and OC, a CC can be used or alternatively a progestin.

In atypical hyperplasia and well differentiated endometrial cancer grade 1 stage 1a, occurring in premenopausal women, an LNG-IUD can be used as a treatment, if efficient, in women wishing to spare their fertility up to the will of pregnancy or alternatively a strong antigonadotropic progestin [17, 18]. When the will of pregnancy is reached, or in case of inefficacy, a hysterectomy will be performed. In the other grade and stage, unfortunately the treatment consists in hysterectomy.

Cervical Cancer

Cervical cancer is the highest or second-highest among cancers in women in developing countries, whereas in Western countries, including Europe, cervical cancer does not even rate within the top five leading cancers in women [19]. Forty-six percent of cases of cervical cancer are diagnosed in women younger than 45 years of age. Cervical cancer can display two histology. The squamous type is not hormone dependent and there is no contraindication to any hormonal contraception if the surgery was conservative.

The WHO authorizes the use of CC or progestins. They contraindicate to insert a IUD in women awaiting treatment but authorize to keep them if they were in place before [20]. They promote the use of condoms with a more efficient contraception. If the conservative, fertility-sparing treatment was trachelectomy, there is some concern on the efficacy of POP because of its lasting effect on cervical mucus in those patients. Concerning CIN, they wrote "Evidence: Among women with persistent human papillomavirus (HPV) infection, long-term DMPA use (≥ 5 years) may increase the risk of carcinoma in situ and invasive carcinoma" [12].

Adenocarcinoma of the cervix, representing about 10% of cervical cancers, is usually treated by hysterectomy. It is considered hormone-dependent, contraindicating estrogen-containing treatment. Emergency contraception is not contraindicated.

Ovarian Cancer

Most OCs are treated by an extensive surgery removing the ovaries and uterus. In some cases, however a conservative surgery can be performed. This is the case for borderline tumors and germinal tumors [21]. For granulosa cell tumors, contraception-containing estrogens are contraindicated but not progestins [21]. A high-dose progestin contraception is preferable. Emergency contraception is not contraindicated.

Gastrointestinal Cancers

Colorectal cancer (CRC) is the second most common cancer in Europe. Gastrointestinal cancers occur predominantly in postmenopausal women. About 5% of CRCs occur in mutation carriers and in young patients. Hereditary GI cancers can occur in the context of hereditary non-polyposis CRC (Lynch syndrome, caused by germline mutations in the MisMatch Repair system), familial adenomatous polyposis and attenuated familial adenomatous polyposis, both caused by a germline mutation in the adenomatous polyposis coli gene), polyposis associated with the MUTYH gene), Peutz-Jeghers syndrome (mutation of the STK 11 gene), juvenile polyposis syndrome (mutations in the SMAD4 or BMPR1A gene), Cowden syndrome (multiple hamarthomas, mutations in the PTEN gene), serrated (hyperplastic) polyposis syndrome, hereditary pancreatic cancer, and hereditary gastric cancer [22]. In Lynch syndrome, EC and OC can be part of the spectrum, as well as small bowel, gastric and urothelial cancers.

In women with a POLE/POLD1 mutation (associated with a high risk of CRC), endometrial cancer (of good prognosis) and possibly brain tumors can occur. In Peutz-Jeghers syndrome, CRC, breast, pancreatic, gynecological (uterus, cervix, ovaries), small bowel, lung, and gastroesophageal cancers can be observed.

Juvenile polyposis is associated with a high risk of colon cancer and an increased risk for gastric, duodenal, and pancreatic cancers. Cowden syndrome is caused by mutations in the PTEN gene. Its spectrum is large with colon, stomach, small bowel, thyroid, breast, uterine, kidney, and skin (melanoma) cancers. The standard chemotherapy used for CRC is called FOLFOX. The effects of FOLFOX on the ovarian reserve is less important that those with other chemotherapies [23].

Concerning contraception, in women with a treated CRC and in hereditary CRC, if there is no risk of BC associated, CC is not contraindicated nor any contraception. Colon cnacer is associated with a decrease in the risk of CRC in women. In Lynch syndrome, CC or progestin contraception could help decrease the risk of endometrial and ovarian cancer up to the age of prophylactic hysterectomy [24]. Emergency contraception is always allowed.

Hepatocellular Carcinoma

The incidence of this cancer is low in Europe, but it is the fifth most common cancer worldwide. It is even more rare in premenopausal women. If the liver function is correct or in the absence of a transplantation, there is no evidence to contraindicate any hormonal contraception. A nonhormonal contraceptive should be the first line if the liver function is altered. In case of transplantation, CC is not recommended as well as the copper IUD because of immunosuppressant agents

Skin Cancer

Skin cancer is the most common form of cancer, globally accounting for at least 40% of cases. There are three main types of skin cancer: basal-cell skin cancer, squamous-cell skin cancer, and melanoma. The first two types are not influenced by the hormones and all types of contraception can be allowed.

Melanoma has one of the higher survival rates among cancers, with about 90% of people surviving more than 5 years. It is the most common cancer for people 20–29 years of age. Survivors have a nine-fold increase of developing a secondary melanoma, most of within the first 2 years. Thus contraception has to be taken into account in those women. No data are available on hormonal contraception in women after a treatment for melanoma. In newer and larger studies no association could be found between use of hormonal contraceptives and melanoma risk. Based on these publications, any type of contraception can be used after skin cancer. In aggressive melanoma, however, it could be wise not to use estrogens since melanoma contain ER. The WHO does not address this disease in its "Medical Eligibility Criteria for Contraceptive Use" [25].

Hematological Malignancies

They can originate from the lymphoid lineage that includes white blood cells such as T lymphocytes and B lymphocytes. These include acute lymphoblastic leukemia, chronic lymphocytic leukemia, lymphomas, and multiple myeloma. Among lymphomas, they can belong to the Hodgkin type (HL), and the non-Hodgkin (NHL) type. Hodgkin lymphoma accounts for less than 1% of all new cancer cases in the United Kingdom [26]. It shows a bimodal age distribution, with the first peak in incidence rates in young adults and the second peak in older females [26]. Non-Hodgkin lymphoma accounts for 4% of all new cancer cases in the United Kingdom and is much frequent after menopause and with aging [27]. They can also originate from the myeloid lineage (precursor cells to red blood cells, platelets, and white blood cells). They include acute myelogenous leukemia, chronic myelogenous leukemia, myelodysplastic syndromes, and the myeloproliferative neoplasms (essential thrombocythemia, polycythemia vera, and myelofibrosis). In females, leukemia is the twelfth most common cancer in the United Kingdom (2% of all new female cancer cases) [28]. Its incidence increases with age.

Most of the malignant diseases are treated by chemotherapy. The influence on the ovarian function depends on the nature of the chemotherapy. Alkylating agents are the most associated with OF. Taxanes, anthracyclines, and platine are mildly associated with OF. Allogeneic hematopoietic stem cell transplants are associated with a relatively high risk of OF. The GnRH agonist therapy during chemotherapy could help preserve fertility with a limited efficacy [9].

During treatment amenorrhea or bleeding can occur and an efficient contraception with a low risk of breakthrough bleeding is recommended. A GnRH agonist or progestin (MPA) can be used [29, 30]. However, the risk of VTE is major especially in myeloproliferative disease and as MPA can be associated with a weak risk of VTE, it should be avoided in this context. Copper IUD is contraindicated because of the risk of bleeding and infection. The LNG-IUD also is associated with the risk of bleeding and is probably not suitable during the chemotherapy associated with aplasia.

In cancer survivors, hormonal contraception is not expected to influence their course or rate of recurrence in most of types of lymphoma. Only follicular lymphoma seems to be mildly favored by the use of COC [31]. Since there are no data on recurrence, it seems prudent not to use CC in survivors of follicular lymphoma [23, 31]. Emergency contraception is always allowed.

Others

Thyroid and pancreatic cancers are not aggravated by hormonal contraception. Pancreatic cancer, however, is associated with a very high risk of VTE, which contraindicate CC during treatment. Lung cancer in smokers might be impacted by exogenous hormones, including CC [32]. It occurs at a younger age in women smokers than men. This could thus contraindicate CC in premenopausal women with a history of lung cancer [33]. Smoking being a condition that also contraindicate CC, this probably is more theoretical than a real question.

Conclusions: During the treatment of cancers, when the risk of VTE is increased, CC is contraindicated. Breast cancer and some types of ovarian tumors contraindicate the use of progestin contraception. Copper IUD is neutral on the cancer but the risk of bleeding and infection limit its use in conditions with aplasia, thrombocytopenia, and aggressive chemotherapy. A GnRH agonist can be a transitory solution in these contexts but expose users to the risk of poor tolerance. In survivors of cancer, the choice is larger and has to be adapted to the risk of recurrence and hormone-dependency of the cancer (Table 20.1).

Table 20.1 Contraindications to contraceptive methods according to the cancer

1) During the treatment of cancer:
   a. CC is contraindicated
      i. If Risk of VTE during the treatment of cancer
      ii. In BC patient
      iii. In endometrial cancer patient
      iv. In granulosa cell tumors
      v. In myeloproliferative disease
   b. Low-dose progestin contraceptives are contraindicated
      i. In BC patient
      ii. In women at risk of bleeding (chemotherapy with aplasia/thrombopenia)
   c. Copper IUD is contraindicated
      i. In conditions with risk of bleeding and infection
2) In cancer survivors
   a. CC is contraindicated
      i. In BC patient
      ii. In endometrial cancer patient
      iii. In granulosa cell tumors
      iv. In myeloproliferative disease
   b. Low dose Progestin contraceptives are contraindicated
      i. In BC patient

References

1. Dominick SA, McLean MR, Whitcomb BW et al. Contraceptive practices among female cancer survivors of reproductive age. *Obstet Gynecol.* 2015;**126**(3):498–507.
2. Hadnott TN, Stark SS, Medica A et al. Perceived infertility and contraceptive use in the female, reproductive-age cancer survivor. *Fertil Steril.* 2019;**111**(4):763–71.
3. Plu-Bureau G, Maitrot-Mantelet L, Hugon-Rodin J, Canonico M. Hormonal contraceptives and venous thromboembolism: An epidemiological update. *Best Pract Res Clin Endocrinol Metab.* 2013;**27**(1):25–34.
4. Chelmow D, Pearlman MD, Young A et al. Executive summary of the Early-Onset BC Evidence Review Conference. *Obstet Gynecol.* 2020;**135**(6):1457–78.
5. Thavendiranathan P, Nolan MT. An emerging epidemic: Cancer and heart failure. *Clin Sci (Lond).* 2017;**131**(2):113–21.
6. Taylor C, Correa C, Duane FK et al. Estimating the risks of BC radiotherapy: Evidence from modern radiation doses to the lungs and heart and from previous randomized trials. *J Clin Oncol.* 2017;**35**(15):1641–9.
7. Heer E, Harper A, Escandor N et al. Global burden and trends in premenopausal and postmenopausal BC: A population-based study. *Lancet Glob Health.* 2020;**8**(8):e1027–37.
8. Parisi F, Razeti MG, Blondeaux E et al. Current state of the art in the adjuvant systemic treatment of premenopausal patients with early BC. *Clin Med Insights Oncol.* 2020;**14**:1179554920931816.
9. Sofiyeva N, Siepmann T, Barlinn K, Seli E, Ata B. Gonadotropin-releasing hormone analogs for gonadal protection during gonadotoxic chemotherapy: A systematic review and meta-analysis. *Reprod Sci.* 2019;**26**(7):939–53.
10. Gompel A, Ramirez I, Bitzer J, European Society of Contraception Expert Group on Hormonal Contraception. Contraception in cancer survivors: An expert review Part I. Breast and gynaecological cancers.*Eur J Contracept Reprod Health Care.* 2019;**24**(3):167–74.
11. Valachis A, Tsali L, Pesce LL et al. Safety of pregnancy after primary breast carcinoma in young women: A meta-analysis to overcome bias of healthy mother effect studies. *Obstet Gynecol Surv.* 2010;**65**(12):786–93.
12. World Health Organization. *Medical eligibility criteria for contraceptive use.* 5th edition. Geneva: World Health Organization, 2015. www.who.int/publications/i/item/9789241549158.

13. Dominick S, Hickey M, Chin J, Su HI. Levonorgestrel intrauterine system for endometrial protection in women with BC on adjuvant tamoxifen. Cochrane Database Syst Rev. 2015;**12**:CD007245.

14. Kotsopoulos J, Lubinski J, Moller P et al. Timing of oral contraceptive use and the risk of BC in BRCA1 mutation carriers. *BC Res Treat*. 2014;**143**(3):579–86.

15. Endometrial cancer statistics [Internet]. World Cancer Research Fund. 2018. https://bit.ly/3HmkBJI.

16. Dominguez-Valentin M, Sampson JR, Seppälä TT et al. Cancer risks by gene, age, and gender in 6350 carriers of pathogenic mismatch repair variants: Findings from the Prospective Lynch Syndrome Database. *Genet Med*. 2020;**22**(1):15–25.

17. Baker J, Obermair A, Gebski V, Janda M. Efficacy of oral or intrauterine device-delivered progestin in patients with complex endometrial hyperplasia with atypia or early endometrial adenocarcinoma: A meta-analysis and systematic review of the literature. *Gynecol Oncol*. 2012;**125**(1):263–70.

18. Koskas M, Azria E, Walker F et al. Progestin treatment of atypical hyperplasia and well-differentiated adenocarcinoma of the endometrium to preserve fertility. *Anticancer Res*. 2012;**32**(3):1037–43.

19. Bray F, Ferlay J, Soerjomataram I et al. Global cancer statistics 2018: GLOBOCAN estimates of incidence and mortality worldwide for 36 cancers in 185 countries. *CA: A Cancer Journal for Clinicians*. 2018;**68**(6):394–424.

20. Summary Chart of U.S. Medical Eligibility Criteria for Contraceptive Use.: 2.

21. Rousset-Jablonski C, Selle F, Adda-Herzog E et al. Fertility preservation, contraception and menopause hormone therapy in women treated for rare ovarian tumours: Guidelines from the French national network dedicated to rare gynaecological cancers. *Eur J Cancer*. 2019;**116**:35–44.

22. Syngal S, Brand RE, Church JM et al. ACG clinical guideline: Genetic testing and management of hereditary gastrointestinal cancer syndromes. *Am J Gastroenterol*. 2015;**110**(2):223–62.

23. Cagnacci A, Ramirez I, Bitzer J, Gompel A. Contraception in cancer survivors: An expert review Part II. Skin, gastrointestinal, haematological and endocrine cancers. *Eur J Contracept Reprod Health Care*. 2019;**24**(4):299–304.

24. Dashti SG, Chau R, Ouakrim DA et al. Female hormonal factors and the risk of endometrial cancer in Lynch syndrome. *JAMA*. 2015;**314** (1):61–71.

25. Medical Eligibility Criteria for Contraceptive Use: A WHO Family Planning Cornerstone. 4th edition. Geneva: World Health Organization, 2010. (WHO Guidelines Approved by the Guidelines Review Committee.) www.ncbi.nlm.nih.gov/books/ NBK138639.

26. Hodgkin lymphoma incidence statistics. Cancer Research UK. 2015. www.cancerresearchuk.org/healt h-professional/cancer-statistics/statistics-by-cancer-type/hodgkin-lymphoma/incidence.

27. Non-Hodgkin lymphoma incidence statistics. Cancer Research UK. 2015. www.cancerresearchuk.org/healt h-professional/cancer-statistics/statistics-by-cancer-type/non-hodgkin-lymphoma/incidence.

28. Leukaemia (all subtypes combined) incidence statistics. Cancer Research UK. 2015. www .cancerresearchuk.org/health-professional/cancer-statistics/statistics-by-cancer-type/leukaemia/ incidence.

29. Meirow D, Rabinovici J, Katz D et al. Prevention of severe menorrhagia in oncology patients with treatment-induced thrombocytopenia by luteinizing hormone-releasing hormone agonist and depo-medroxyprogesterone acetate. *Cancer*. 2006;**107** (7):1634–41.

30. Bates JS, Buie LW, Woodis CB. Management of menorrhagia associated with chemotherapy-induced thrombocytopenia in women with hematologic malignancy. *Pharmacotherapy*. 2011;**31**(11):1092–1110.

31. Kane EV, Roman E, Becker N et al. Menstrual and reproductive factors, and hormonal contraception use: Associations with non-Hodgkin lymphoma in a pooled analysis of InterLymph case-control studies. *Ann Oncol*. 2012;**23**(9):2362–74.

32. Iversen L, Sivasubramaniam S, Lee AJ, Fielding S, Hannaford PC. Lifetime cancer risk and combined oral contraceptives: The Royal College of General Practitioners' Oral Contraception Study. *Am J Obstet Gynecol*. 2017;**216**(6):580.e1–580.e9.

33. Stapelfeld C, Dammann C, Maser E. Sex-specificity in lung cancer risk. *Int J Cancer*. 2020;**146**(9): 2376–82.

Chapter 21

Contraception in Women with Benign Breast Disease and Benign Uterine and Ovarian Conditions

Giovanni Grandi, Maria Chiara Del Savio, and Fabio Facchinetti

Contraception in Women with Benign Breast Disease

Benign breast diseases (BBDs) deserve attention because of their high prevalence, their impact on women's quality of life (QoL) and, only for some histologic types, their cancerous potential. Fibrocystic breast disease (FBD), recently called "fibrocystic changes," is the most frequent BBD, diagnosed in 50% of clinically and 90% of histopathologically examined women [1].

Another common benign breast lesion is fibroadenoma, characterized by a nodule of fibrous tissue with epithelial cells. Fibroadenomas confer a moderate increased risk (~two- to threefold) of developing breast cancer (BC) [2]. Evidence of an association between age of menarche, age of menopause, and hormonal therapy, including oral contraceptives (OC), has been less consistently shown for fibroadenoma.

The relationship between OC use and the risk of BC has been investigated in numerous epidemiological studies. Most studies have considered the relationship between combined oral contraceptives (COCs) use and BC risk [3]. Only smaller studies have been performed about the relation between COCs use and BBD. Most studies have concluded that COCs use offers some protection against BBD, in particular fibroadenoma and fibrocystic disease, with an increased effect with a longer duration of use, and this was recently confirmed also with the use of new COC formulations [4]. However, some studies have shown that the protective effect of COC use is related only with BBD without atypia and that risk of BBD with atypia was not decreased and possibly even increased by COC use [5]. This observation is consistent with the fact that synthetic progestins may act as mitogenic agents on transformed cells but as anti-proliferative agents in normal or non-transformed breast epithelial cells [6].

There is a lack of studies about the long-term effect of hormonal contraceptives on existing BBD. A number of studies conducted in the 1970s and 1980s showed that OC use, especially combined hormonal contraceptives (CHCs), decreased the incidence of BBD (including fibroadenoma), and this protective effect against BBD has been regarded as a noncontraceptive health benefit of OC. However, the reduced risk associated with BBD contradicts the known link between OC and increased BC risk: such opposing effects may be partly explained by the opposite effect induced by OC on transformed and non-transformed cells [5]. However, no associations have been observed between COC use and direct transitions to fibroadenoma or to BC [7].

The United Kingdom Medical Eligibility Criteria for Contraceptive Use (UKMEC) updated in 2019 offer recommendations about methods that could be used safely by individuals with certain health conditions or characteristics to prevent an unintended pregnancy. For each of the personal characteristics or medical conditions considered by the UKMEC, a category 1, 2, 3, or 4 is given (Table 21.1). The United States Centers for Disease Control and Prevention (USCDC) in 2016 and the World Health Organization (WHO) in 2015 provided similar recommendations on this topic.

Focusing on BBD, including FBD and fibroadenoma, WHO, USCDC, and UKMEC guidelines do not report any contraindications, nor for intrauterine devices, also containing levonorgestrel, nor for other hormonal contraceptives (category 1) [8–10].

Contraception in Women with Benign Uterine Disease

There is a wide spectrum of causes of benign uterine disease, classified by the PALM-COEIN classification system adopted by the International Federation of

Table 21.1 Categories for contraceptive use established by International Medical Eligibility Criteria for Contraceptive use [8–10]

UKMEC	Definition
Category 1	A condition for which there is no restriction for the use of the method.
Category 2	A condition where the advantages of using the method generally outweigh the theoretical or proven risks.
Category 3	A condition where the theoretical or proven risks usually outweigh the advantages of using the method. The provision of a method requires expert clinical judgment and/or referral to a specialist contraceptive provider, since use of the method is not usually recommended unless other, more appropriate methods are not available or not acceptable.
Category 4	A condition that represents an unacceptable health risk if the method is used.

Table 21.2 PALM-COEIN FIGO classification of abnormal uterine bleeding

P	Polyps
A	Adenomyosis
L	Leiomyoma
M	Malignant and premalignant
C	Coagulation
O	Ovarian dysfunction
E	Endometrial dysfunction
I	Iatrogenic
N	Not otherwise classified

Gynaecology and Obstetrics (FIGO) in 2010 to describe the causes underling the abnormal uterine bleeding (AUB) during a woman's lifetime. In this system, PALM refers to the structural causes of AUB, while COEIN refers to the nonstructural causes of AUB (Table 21.2). Contraception in benign uterine diseases can be analyzed starting from this classification system, in particular in the presence of a structural condition (PALM).

Polyps

Polyps are epithelial proliferations of the endometrial glands and stromal tissue, with a vascular pedicle. The etiology of endometrial polyps is proposed to be related to estrogenic stimulation [11], which is manifested by induction of polyps after the treatment with tamoxifen for BC that provides an estrogenic stimulus to the endometrium [12]. In menstruating women, they may cause AUB, hypermenorrhea, or infertility.

Wada-Hiraike et al. studied the relation between the OC and the endometrial polyp (both sessile and pedunculated) pathogenesis, trying to confirm its expected effect to decrease the volume of endometrial polyp by suppressing endogenous estrogens [13]. The study demonstrates that sessile polyps can regress at a higher rate than pedunculated polyps under OC treatment. Several mechanisms can be speculated in OC-induced regression of the polyps. Apoptosis

might be a mechanism in light of the finding that exposure to a monophasic OC for 30 days significantly increases endometrial apoptosis, in both epithelial and stromal cells [14]. Another mechanism could be that the establishment of a steady estrogen–progestin milieu induces endometrial quiescence, leading to the regression of endometrial polyps. Anti-inflammatory effects of progesterone might also be involved given that mast cell-associated inflammation is associated with endometrial polyp growth. Chowdary et al. demonstrated the role of levonorgestrel-releasing intrauterine systems (LNG-IUSs) in the treatment of endometrial polyps found at outpatient hysteroscopy [15]. The higher intrauterine progestin concentration provided by the LNG-IUS rather than oral progestins can explain the apparent regression of endometrial polyps. The effects of LNG on the endometrium seem to be mediated by a decrease in the expression of Bcl-2 and Ki-67, and this may prevent polyp formation or cause regression in polyps. Until now, there is no proper guideline for the treatment of endometrial polyps and no specific contraindication for hormonal contraception use in this situation [8–10].

Adenomyosis

The rationale for using COCs in adenomyosis is related to the induced decidualization and subsequent atrophy of the endometrium, reducing pain and bleeding. Patients with dysmenorrhea, dyspareunia, or menorrhagia in fact may benefit from the resulting amenorrhea, which may provide relief of symptoms [16]. In addition, COCs suppress aromatase expression in the ectopic endometrium and in adenomyotic foci.

Despite the common off-label use of COCs for adenomyosis-related symptoms with satisfactory long-term pain control, no well-conducted randomized controlled trials (RCTs) are available supporting the pharmacological treatment of adenomyosis using COCs.

Healthcare personnel have used LNG-IUS 52 mg to successfully treat adenomyosis with the aim to reduce menstrual blood loss and pain via a reduction in thickness of the myometrial junctional zone and total uterine volume [17]. The reduction of menstrual blood loss is attributed to both the direct effect of LNG on adenomyosis foci with decidualization and the increase in apoptosis in endometrial glands and stroma.

In fact, local LNG release caused atrophy and shrinkage of adenomyotic lesions through a downregulation of estrogen receptors, preventing further stimulation by estrogens [18]. The LNG-IUS guarantees reduction in side effects caused by other oral treatment providing, in contrast with low serum levels, locally high concentrations of LNG in the endometrium and adjacent tissues.

The LNG-IUS 52 mg is a cost-effective, reversible, and long-term treatment for women with pelvic pain associated with adenomyosis, especially mild and moderately severe, reducing the need for surgical intervention (reduction of need of hysterectomy in ~70% of the cases).

In women treated with LNG-IUS 52 mg for 3 years there was an overall satisfaction rate of 72%, with continued significant decrease in dysmenorrhea and uterine volume compared to baseline [19]. An RCT on 75 women undergoing either LNG-IUS 52 mg or hysterectomy showed that 6 months post treatment hemoglobin levels were comparable, and QoL increased more with LNG-IUS in comparison to hysterectomy [20].

Another RCT comparing COCs and LNG-IUS 52 mg showed both reduced pain and menstrual loss, but the intrauterine device is more effective in these outcomes [21]. To date, the cut-off value of uterine volume more than 150 mL was significantly associated with failure of LNG-IUS, thus the insertion of an LNG-IUS in a large-volume uterus has a significantly higher failure rate than its insertion into a small-volume uterus [22].

Leiomyoma

Uterine leiomyoma (fibroid or myoma) is a benign tumor of smooth muscle origin that may produce symptoms including menorrhagia, dysmenorrhea, pelvic pressure and pain, and reproductive dysfunction, although most women with uterine fibroids gave no symptoms. Fibroids are most commonly diagnosed during reproductive life, usually in the fourth decade, and they tend to shrink or fibrose after menopause [23].

The beneficial effects of the LNG-IUS 52 mg in treating excessive menstrual bleeding in the subgroup of women with fibroids [24–26] and its superior effectiveness in reducing menstrual blood loss compared to COC are clearly demonstrated [27]. Among women with uterine fibroids using an LNG-IUS, most experienced improvements in serum levels of hemoglobin, hematocrit, and ferritin and in menstrual blood loss [28]. Rates of LNG-IUSs expulsion were higher in women with uterine fibroids (11%) than in women without fibroids (up to 3%); these findings were not statistically significant or significance testing was not conducted [28]. Rates of expulsion found in noncomparative studies ranged from 0% to 20% [28]. The study conducted by Ross et al. provides the first real evidence that the risk of fibroids is reduced by use of OCs – roughly a 17% reduction in risk with each 5 years of OC use [23]. The "unopposed" estrogens seem to be the strongest suspect as an underlying cause of fibroids: the decreased risk associated with the use of COC would be explained most readily by the estrogen-modifying effect of progestins. However, these contraceptives are not a treatment for fibroids, acting more on the endometrium [29]. The specific effects of different treatments used in women with fibroids on fibroid size and endometrial thickness are reported in Figure 21.1.

The WHO and UKMEC guidelines defined the use of LNG-IUSs and copper intrauterine devices (IUDs) in women with fibroid without distortion of the uterine cavity as category 1 while involvement of the cavity was placed in category 3 [8] or 4 [10]; for the US-CDC all types of fibroids are in category 2 [9]. There are no specific limitations regarding other contraceptive methods (category 1). Hormonal contraception, oral patch, or ring do not appear to cause growth of uterine fibroids.

Malignant and Premalignant: Endometrial Hyperplasia

Endometrial hyperplasia commonly results from continuous estrogen stimulation unopposed by adequate levels of progesterone/progestins. Among reproductive-aged women, the most common source of endogenous-unopposed estrogen is likely chronic anovulation, a common feature of conditions

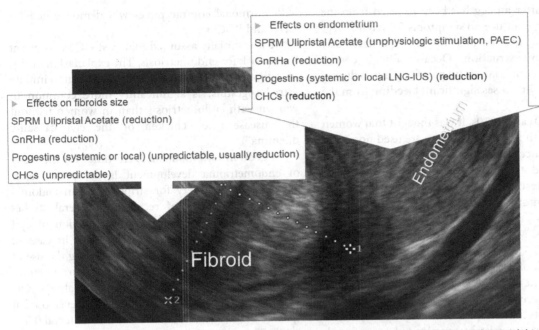

> ▶ Effects on endometrium
>
> SPRM Ulipristal Acetate (unphysiologic stimulation, PAEC)
> GnRHa (reduction)
> Progestins (systemic or local LNG-IUS) (reduction)
> CHCs (reduction)

> ▶ Effects on fibroids size
>
> SPRM Ulipristal Acetate (reduction)
> GnRHa (reduction)
> Progestins (systemic or local) (unpredictable, usually reduction)
> CHCs (unpredictable)

Figure 21.1 Differential effects of common treatments used in women with fibroids on fibroid size and endometrial thickness. CHC: combined hormonal contraceptive; GnRHa: gonadotropin-releasing hormone analogs; LNG-IUS: levonorgestrel-releasing intrauterine systems; PAEC: progesterone receptor modulator–associated endometrial changes; SPRM: selective progesterone receptor modulator

such as polycystic ovary syndrome (PCOS) (see Chapter 3). The likelihood of progression from endometrial hyperplasia to endometrial cancer varies according to its classification (simple/complex, atypical/non-atypical), with atypical hyperplasia being the type most strongly associated with progression to endometrial cancer. Conservative management with progestin therapy has been used in clinical practice for women with non-atypical endometrial hyperplasia (low and medium risk), although consensus regarding optimal progestin agent, dose, and therapy duration has never been established [30]. Whiteman et al. conducted a systematic review on the use of hormonal contraceptives with endometrial hyperplasia: LNG-IUS 52 mg use is safe and may have therapeutic effects [31]. They did not identify any studies regarding the safety of contraceptive methods other than LNG-IUS 52 mg in women with endometrial hyperplasia. Given the established therapeutic effects of oral progestin on endometrial hyperplasia, there generally has been no concern about safety of other hormonal contraceptives [31].

All contraceptive methods are considered safe for women with endometrial hyperplasia [8–10]: most women experienced disease regression during the use of LNG-IUS 52 mg [31].

Contraception in Women with Ovarian Conditions

Benign Ovarian Tumors (Mucinous or Serous Cystadenoma)

Most (~ 90%) ovarian cancers are of epithelial origin and can be further classified into five major histological types, with serous (high- and low-grade) being the most common (~ 75%), followed by mucinous (~ 13%), endometrioid (~ 13%), and clear-cell cancers (~ 6%) [32]. However, the exact relationship between functional ovarian cyst and ovarian cancer development is completely unknown.

A recent meta-analysis concluded that, although widely used for treating functional ovarian cysts, COCs appear to be of no benefit [33]. Watchful waiting for two or three cycles is more appropriate. Should cysts persist, surgical management is often indicated. The vast majority of ovarian cysts are benign and are often described as physiologic or functional.

Follicle cysts can form when ovulation does not occur or when the mature follicle involutes. Rupture of the cyst during ovulation can cause mid-cycle pain, but persistent follicle cysts usually produce no symptoms and regress spontaneously. Corpus luteum cysts, which occur after an egg has been released from the follicle, usually produce no symptoms. When no pregnancy occurs, the corpus luteum spontaneously regresses at menstruation. Occasionally, a corpus luteum cyst becomes large and painful, persists during the next cycle, or causes significant bleeding from the rupture site.

In the 1960s and 1970s, it was thought that women taking OC (with higher doses than are used now) had a lower incidence of functional cysts and that the pills could be used to suppress pituitary hormones as a diagnostic test. It was reasoned that suppressing pituitary hormone production would cause these cysts to regress, and this became a common therapy for many years. More recently, it has been shown that low-dose OC does not substantially decrease a woman's risk of ovarian cysts formation [34].

Placing patients on OCs, in the doses currently used, is no more effective in producing resolution of physiologic cysts than simple observation. Nonoperative management of a persistent ovarian cyst is preferred, particularly in a young woman, because most cysts eventually spontaneously regress. Too often, ultrasound visualization of a small asymptomatic ovarian cyst in a young woman leads to laparoscopy and removal of a normal corpus luteum cyst. Ovarian surgery carries a risk of subsequent adhesions and infertility, so surgical management is rarely indicated unless the cyst is symptomatic or its documented persistence suggests it is an adnexal mass of another etiology. Benign ovarian tumors, mucinous and serous cystadenoma in particular, do not represent at all a contraindication to contraception. The use of IUDs and LNG-IUSs is classified as category 1 by the UKMEC, similarly to OCs, vaginal rings, and patches [8–10].

Ovarian Endometriosis

A recent systematic review [35] shows that hormonal contraceptive use (both CHCs and progestin-only contraceptives [POCs]) results in a statistically significant reduction from baseline in endometriosis-related pain, resulting in QoL improvement from baseline. During CHC treatment, it was found clinically significant reductions in dysmenorrhea in almost all the reviewed studies, often associated with a concomitant reduction in noncyclical pelvic pain and dyspareunia. Similarly, during POC treatment, researchers found a significant reduction in dysmenorrhea, often associated with a decrease in noncyclical pelvic pain and dyspareunia. The concomitant improvement in QoL

with hormonal contraceptives was demonstrated for CHC and POC use.

It was initially assumed that past OC users are at higher risk for endometriosis. The explanation of this paradigm is that dysmenorrhea, as a reason to initiate estro-progestins, is significantly more common in women with endometriosis than in women without the disease (the "chicken or the egg causality dilemma").

A good in vivo model of "zero-time" for the study of endometrioma development is the period after a conservative surgery for stripping of an endometrioma and the risk of recurrence. Several studies have demonstrated the important reduction of cyst recurrence after surgery for cystectomy in case of prolonged ovulation inhibition, like during the use of CHCs. A recent meta-analysis found a recurrent endometrioma one year after surgery in 8% of "always" OC users and in 34% of women who have never used it (pooled odds ratio 0.12; 95% confidence interval 0.05–0.29). This rate of recurrence, also during constant ovulation inhibition, may indicate that ovulation is not the only mechanism involved in endometrioma development. However, the presence of bias such as the presence of residual cyst after an incomplete surgery cannot be excluded [36]. Following conservative surgery, continuous instead of cyclic administration of CHCs, avoiding cyclic menstrual flows, is associated with a greater reduction of endometrioma recurrence and more effective pain management. These findings empirically suggest that the development of endometrioma not only is dependent on ovulation but also is intrinsically connected with menstruation [36]. These findings should be taken into consideration when counseling patients on the most effective therapies capable of avoiding recurrence of clinical disease, pain, and associated infertility.

However, POCs have fewer contraindications than CHCs, due to the absence of thrombotic risk, and they can be prescribed in particular situations – for example, to women with migraine or who are breastfeeding. No data are available regarding the postoperative use of POCs and the risk of disease recurrence. The most-studied POC was surprisingly the LNG-IUS 52 mg. The advantages of LNG-IUS 52 mg for the treatment of endometriosis are that medical treatment may continue for up to 5 years, the device is simple to remove if it is not tolerated, the cumulative costs are low, and the systemic LNG dose is low (no first hepatic passage) in association with a high local intrauterine dose. The disadvantages are possible menstrual irregularities, the risk of spontaneous expulsion (5%), and the fact that ovulation is not constantly inhibited. Indeed, the only RCT that evaluated the rate of endometrioma recurrence during LNG-IUS 52 mg use in comparison with placebo failed to find a protective effect of the LNG-IUS [35].

Polycystic Ovarian Syndrome

Another benign ovarian condition is polycystic ovarian syndrome (PCOS), characterized by chronic anovulation, polycystic ovary morphology, and hyperandrogenism. Related to these clinical situations, CHCs are the first-line management option, specifically for menstrual irregularity, hirsutism, and acne. The complete rationale for their use to treat this syndrome in comparison to other medical therapies is explained in Figure 21.2. Polycystic ovarian syndrome is associated with clinical and metabolic comorbidities that may limit the prescription of CHC in women with PCOS [37]. Common risk factors for cardiovascular diseases, such as systemic arterial hypertension, obesity, dyslipidemia, metabolic syndrome, and type 2 diabetes mellitus, can develop in women with PCOS by the fourth decade of life. Although PCOS by itself is not a contraindication for contraception, some of these comorbidities have to be considered in the contraception decision, especially for CHCs.

Hyperandrogenism is the most prominent diagnostic component of PCOS and the use of CHC can decrease the androgens levels. First, estrogens increase the hepatic synthesis of sex hormone–binding globulin (SHBG), subsequently reducing the free testosterone that can bind to the androgen receptor: this antiandrogenic effect is more prominent with the use of ethinylestradiol (EE) than with the use of natural estrogens such as estradiol [38]. In addition, progestins promote negative feedback on the surge of luteinizing hormone, as a result reducing ovarian androgen production. Some progestins, like norgestimate, can directly antagonize the effects of androgen receptors and also reduce the activity of the 5α reductase enzyme, which converts testosterone to di-hydrotestosterone, a highly potent androgen. The COCs containing cyproterone acetate have been shown to have higher antiandrogenic activity than desogestrel and drospirenone (DRSP) in long-term users (12 months or more), but not in short-term users (up to 6 months) [39].

The Endocrine Society Clinical Practice Guideline, the American Society of Reproductive Medicine, and the European Society of Human Reproduction and Embryology recommend CHCs (including vaginal ring and patch) for first-line treatment of menstrual irregularity, acne, and hirsutism in women with PCOS, but the guidelines do not suggest any specific combination [40, 41]. The European Society of Endocrinology specifically recommends COCs containing cyproterone acetate for more effective management of hyperandrogenism [42].

With regard to management of acne and hirsutism, there is no good evidence for any differential effectiveness of CHCs containing different progestins. Recent studies have focused on the effects of COCs containing DRSP, an antiandrogenic, spironolactone-derivative progestin. A systematic review that included 18 RCTs of EE/DRSP versus standard treatment options concluded that EE/DRSP combinations was very effective in treating the symptoms of PCOS [43]. In the presence of estrogen contraindication, POP, in particular containing DRSP, or drugs with antiandrogenic effects (such as spironolactone,

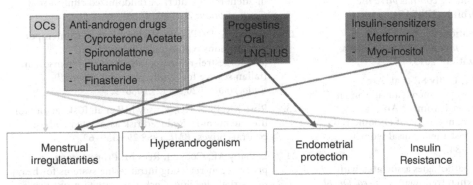

Figure 21.2 Rationale for the use of different medical therapies in woman with polycystic ovarian syndrome. OC: oral contraceptives; LNG-IUS: levonorgestrel-releasing intrauterine systems

cyproterone, flutamide, and finasteride) should be used in combination with other effective contraceptives such as IUDs or LNG-IUSs [44].

References

1. Milosevic ZC, Nadrljanski MM, Milovanovic ZM et al. Breast dynamic contrast enhanced MRI: Fibrocystic changes presenting as a non-mass enhancement mimicking malignancy. *Radiol Oncol.* 2017;**51**(2):130–6.

2. Dupont WD, Page DL, Parl FF et al. Long-term risk of breast cancer in women with fibroadenoma. *N Engl J Med.* 1994;**331**(1):10–15.

3. Collaborative Group on Hormonal Factors in Breast Cancer. Breast cancer and hormonal contraceptives: Collaborative reanalysis of individual data on 53,297 women with breast cancer and 100,239 women without breast cancer from 54 epidemiological studies. *Lancet.* 1996;**347**:1713–22.

4. Vessey M, Yeates D. Oral contraceptives and benign breast disease: An update of findings in a large cohort study. *Contraception.* 2007;**76**:418–24.

5. Rohan TE, Miller AB. A cohort study of oral contraceptive use and risk of benign breast disease. *Int J Cancer.* 1999;**82**:191–6.

6. Cibula D, Gompel A, Mueck AO et al. Hormonal contraception and risk of cancer. *Hum Reprod Update.* 2010;**16**(6):631–50.

7. Li J, Humphreys K, Ho PJ et al. Family history, reproductive, and lifestyle risk factors for fibroadenoma and breast cancer. *JNCI Cancer Spectr.* 2018;**2**(3):pky051.

8. Faculty of Sexual & Reproductive Healthcare. *UK medical eligibility criteria for contraceptive use (UKMEC).* London: Faculty of Sexual & Reproductive Healthcare,2016. www.fsrh.org/standards-and-guidance/documents/ukmec-2016.

9. Centers for Disease Control and Prevention. *US medical eligibility criteria for contraceptive use (USCDC).* 2016. http://bit.ly/3RhFASx.

10. World Health Organization. *Medical eligibility criteria for contraceptive use.* 5th edition. Geneva: World Health Organization, 2015.

11. McGurgan P, Taylor LJ, Duffy SR et al. Are endometrial polyps from pre-menopausal women similar to post-menopausal women? An immunohistochemical comparison of endometrial polyps from pre- and post-menopausal women. *Maturitas.* 2006;**54**:277–84.

12. Cohen I. Endometrial pathologies associated with postmenopausal tamoxifen treatment. *Gynecol Oncol.* 2004;**94**:256–66.

13. Wada-HiraikeE O, Osuga Y, Hiroi H et al. Sessile polyps and pedunculated polyps respond differently to oral contraceptives. *Gynecol Endocrinol.* 2011;**27**(5):351–5.

14. Meresman GF, Auge L, Baranao RI et al. Oral contraceptives suppress cell proliferation and enhance apoptosis of eutopic endometrial tissue from patients with endometriosis. *Fertil Steril.* 2002;**77**:1141–7.

15. Chowdary P, Maher P, Ma T et al. The role of the Mirena intrauterine device in the management of endometrial polyps: A pilot study. *J Minim Invasive Gynecol.* 2019;**26**(7):1297–1302.

16. Vannuccini S, Luisi S, Tosti C et al. Role of medical therapy in the management of uterine adenomyosis. *Fertil Steril.* 2018;**109**(3):398–405.

17. Fedele L, Portuese A, Bianchi S et al. Treatment of adenomyosis-associated menorrhagia with a levonorgestrel-releasing intrauterine device. *Fertil Steril.* 1997;**68**:426–9.

18. Critchley HOD, Wang H, Kelly RW et al. Progestin receptor isoforms and prostaglandin dehydrogenase in the endometrium of women using a levonorgestrel-releasing intrauterine system. *Hum Reprod.* 1998;**13**:1210–17.

19. Sheng J, Zhang WY, Zhang JP et al. The LNG-IUS study on adenomyosis: A 3-year follow-up study on the efficacy and side effects of the use of levonorgestrel intrauterine system for the treatment of dysmenorrhea associated with adenomyosis. *Contraception.* 2009;**79**:189–93.

20. Ozdegirmenci O, Kayikcioglu F, Akgul MA et al. Comparison of levonorgestrel intrauterine system versus hysterectomy on efficacy and quality of life in patients with adenomyosis. *Fertil Steril.* 2011;**95**:497–502.

21. Shaaban OM, Ali MK, Sabra AM et al. Levonorgestrel-releasing intrauterine system versus a low-dose combined oral contraceptive for treatment of adenomyotic uteri: A randomized clinical trial. *Contraception.* 2015;**92**(4):301–7.

22. Grandi G, De Fata R, Varliero F et al. Contemporary prescriptions pattern of different dose levonorgestrel-releasing intrauterine systems in an Italian service for family planning. *Gynecol Endocrinol.* 2020;**36**(12):1086–9.

23. Ross RK, Pike MC, Vessey MP et al. Risk factors for uterine fibroids: Reduced risk associated with oral contraceptives. *BMJ.* 1988;**293**:359–62.

24. Lethaby AE, Cooke I, Rees M. Progesterone or progestogen-releasing intrauterine systems for heavy menstrual bleeding. *Cochrane Database Syst Rev.* 2006:CD002126.

25. Starczewski A, Iwanicki M. Intrauterine therapy with levonorgestrel releasing IUD of women with hypermenorrhea secondary to uterine fibroids. *Ginekol Pol.* 2000;**71**(9):1221–5.

26. Soysal S, Soysal ME. The efficacy of levonorgestrel-releasing intrauterine device in selected cases of myoma-related menorrhagia: A prospective controlled trial. *Gynecol Obstet Invest.* 2005;**59**(1):29–35.

27. Sayed GH, Zakherak MS, El-Nashar SA et al. A randomized clinical trial of levonorgestrel-releasing intrauterine system and a low-dose combined oral contraceptive for fibroid-related menorrhagia. *International Journal of Gynecology and Obstetrics.* 2011;**112**:126–30.

28. Zapata LB, Whiteman MK, Tepper NK et al. Intrauterine device use among women with uterine fibroids: A systematic review. *Contraception.* 2010;**82**:41–55.

29. Marret H, Fritel X, Ouldamer L et al. Therapeutic management of uterine fibroid tumors: Updated French guidelines. *Eur J Obstet Gynecol Reprod Biol.* 2012;**165**:156–64.

30. Sletten ET, Arnes M, Vereide AB et al. Low-dose LNG-IUS as therapy for endometrial hyperplasia: A prospective cohort pilot study. *Anticancer Res.* 2018;**38**(5):2883–9.

31. Whiteman MK, Zapata LB, Tepper NK et al. Use of contraceptive methods among women with endometrial hyperplasia: A systematic review. *Contraception.* 2010;**82**(1):56–63.

32. Coburn SB, Bray F, Sherman ME et al. International patterns and trends in ovarian cancer incidence, overall and by histologic subtype. *Int J Cancer.* 2017;**140**(11):2451–60.

33. Grimes DA, Jones LB, Lopez LM et al. Oral contraceptives for functional ovarian cysts. *Cochrane Database Syst Rev.* 9:CD006134.

34. Holt VL, Daling JR, McKnight B et al. Functional ovarian cysts in relation to the use of monophasic and triphasic oral contraceptives. *Obstet Gynecol.* 1992;**79**:529–33.

35. Grandi G, Barra F, Ferrero S et al. Hormonal contraception in women with endometriosis: A systematic review. *Eur J Contracept Reprod Health Care.* 2019;**24**(1):61–70.

36. Grandi G, Toss A, Cortesi L et al. The association between endometriomas and ovarian cancer: Preventive effect of inhibiting ovulation and menstruation during reproductive life. *Biomed Res Int.* 2015:751571.

37. De Melo AS, Dos Reis RM, Ferriani RA et al. Hormonal contraception in women with polycystic ovary syndrome: Choices, challenges, and noncontraceptive benefits. *Open Access J Contraception.* 2017;**8**:13–23.

38. Charitidou C, Farmakiotis D, Zournatzi V et al. The administration of estrogens, combined with anti-androgens, has beneficial effects on the hormonal features and asymmetric dimethyl-arginine levels, in women with the polycystic ovary syndrome. *Atherosclerosis.* 2008;**196**(2):958–65.

39. Bhattacharya SM, Jha A. Comparative study of the therapeutic effects of oral contraceptive pills containing desogestrel, cyproterone acetate, and drospirenone in patients with polycystic ovary syndrome. *Fertil Steril.* 2012;**98**(4):1053–9.

40. Legro RS, Arslanian SA, Ehrmann DA et al. Diagnosis and treatment of polycystic ovary syndrome: An Endocrine Society clinical practice guideline. *J Clin Endocrinol Metab.* 2013;**98**:4565–92.

41. Fauser BC, Tarlatzis BC, Rebar RW et al. Consensus on women's health aspects of polycystic ovary syndrome (PCOS): The Amsterdam ESHRE/ASRM–Sponsored 3rd PCOS Consensus Workshop Group. *Fertil Steril.* 2012;**97**(1):28–38.

42. Conway G, Dewailly D, Diamanti-Kandarakis E et al. The polycystic ovary syndrome: A position statement from the European Society of Endocrinology. *Eur J Endocrinol.* 2014;**171**(4):P1–29.

43. Li J, Ren J, Sun W. A comparative systematic review of Yasmin (drospirenone pill) versus standard treatment options for symptoms of polycystic ovary syndrome. *Eur J Obstet Gynecol Reprod Biol.* 2017;**210**:13–21.

44. Del Savio MC, De Fata R, Facchinetti F et al. Drospirenone 4 mg-only pill (DOP) in 24+4 regimen: A new option for oral contraception. *Expert Rev Clin Pharmacol.* 2020;**13**(7):685–94.

Contraception in Women with Cardiovascular Conditions

Angelo Cagnacci, Claudia Massarotti, Laura Gabbi, and Anjeza Xholli

Introduction

Cardiovascular conditions include arterial disease, mainly myocardial infarction, ischemic stroke, peripheral artery disease, and venous thromboembolism (VTE). A combination of multiple risk factors or evidence of microvascular diseases can be considered as risky as a cardiovascular event.

Myocardial Infarction, Ischemic Stroke, and Peripheral Artery Diseases

Myocardial infarction, ischemic stroke, and peripheral artery diseases are rather rare in women of reproductive age and, in general, are associated with the presence of cardiovascular risk factors. Risk factors are represented by age $\geq$ 35 years of age, smoking, hypertension, diabetes, diminished apo A/apo B ratio, and valvular heart disease [1, 2].

Arterial events are consequent to sudden occlusion of blood flow in an artery consequent to atherosclerotic plaque rupture, platelet activation, and formation of an obstructing blood clot. Ischemic stroke can also be consequent to blood clot emboli in cerebral vessels [2]. A history of myocardial infarction, ischemic stroke, angina, or peripheral artery occlusions indicates advanced atherosclerosis with a high risk of recurrence of the event. In these conditions, external stimuli, such as estrogen administration, leading to atherosclerotic plaque destabilization and blood clot activation should be avoided. Women with these disturbances can be on chronic low-dose aspirin. Aspirin has no interaction with contraceptives.

Contraception

Combined Hormonal Contraception

Use of combined hormonal contraceptives (CHCs) with high doses of ethinyl estradiol represents per se a risk factor for myocardial infarction and ischemic stroke [3–5]. Doses of ethinyl estradiol $\leq$ 20 mcg do not increase the risk of ischemic stroke and only slightly increase the risk of myocardial infarction [5, 6]. Arterial risk is negligible with the use of CHCs containing non-androgenic progestins, such as cyproterone acetate [7] and drospirenone [7, 8], or CHCs containing estradiol [9]. Yet in women with a history of myocardial infarction or ischemic stroke, guidelines indicate that CHCs of any type, administered as pill, patch, or ring, are highly contraindicated [10].

Progestin-Only Contraceptives

Progestin-only contraceptives (POCs) can be administered to women with myocardial infarction or ischemic stroke [10]. This is true for oral pills or subcutaneous implants. Injection of medroxyprogesterone is not indicated because the glucocorticoid properties of the molecule may increase coagulation activity [11]. Progestins may have an influence on the metabolic pathways, leading to atherosclerotic plaque formation. To this end the stimulus on androgen receptors should be minimized by using progestins with a lower androgenic (desogestrel vs. levonorgestrel) or non-androgenic (chlormadinone, drospirenone) activity [12]. If myocardial infarction or stroke develop during contraception, POCs should be withdrawn [10].

Other Contraceptive Options

There is no contraindication to the use of intrauterine devices (IUD), levonorgestrel intrauterine systems (LNG-IUS), barrier methods, natural methods, or sterilization [10]. Sterilization usually requires a surgical approach with anesthesia. There may be contraindications due to the cardiovascular status of the woman.

Multiple Cardiovascular Risk Factors, Evidence of Microvascular Disease

The combination of two or more cardiovascular risk factors without a history of cardiovascular events can be considered as risky as a history of cardiovascular events [10]. Cardiovascular risk factors to consider are: age older than 40 years, smoking, diabetes, known dyslipidemia, and history of controlled hypertension [1, 2]. In women with two or more of these risk factors contraceptive prescription should follow the indications given for women with history of myocardial infarction or ischemic stroke [10].

Venous Thromboembolism

Venous thromboembolism is consequent to the Virchowood triad of endothelial damage, blood stasis, and increased blood coagulation. Increased blood coagulation is the parameter influenced by contraception and is associated with the estrogenic component of the CHC [12, 13]. Accordingly, VTE is not a contraindication for the use of POC, IUD, LNG-IUS, barrier methods, natural methods or sterilization. Also, during acute VTE on anticoagulant therapy, limited evidence indicates the possibility to use POC [10]. Accordingly, limitations refer only to the use of CHC. When considering the risk of VTE we should investigate personal history of VTE or superficial vein thrombosis and familial history of VTE, known thrombophilia, varicose veins, or single acquired risk factors for VTE [13].

Women with Personal History of Venous Thromboembolism

Women with a personal history of VTE cannot use CHCs even if on anticoagulant therapy [10]. Progestin-only contraceptives can be used except during acute VTE, and it can be used in established VTE on prolonged anticoagulant therapy [10]. In this case LNG-IUS may be useful in order to reduce menstrual bleeding to amenorrhea [14, 15].

Women with Personal History of Superficial Vein Thrombosis

Although it is not considered a main contraindication for CHC use [10, 16], superficial vein thrombosis (SVT) seems to increase the risk of VTE, in particular when associated with other risk factors such as smoking, obesity, surgery, hospitalization, and CHC use [17]. Accordingly, in women with a history of SVT it would be useful to use CHC at lower VTE risk, such as those containing ≤ 30 mcg ethynilestradiol and levonorgestrel, 20 mcg ethynilestradiol and gestodene [18], or estradiol and dienogest [9]. Data on CHCs

containing estradiol and nomegestrol acetate are not yet available.

Women with Inherited Thrombophilia

Medical eligibility criteria indicate that inherited thrombophilia represents an absolute contraindication to CHC [10, 16]. Indeed, not all thrombophilia induce the same VTE risk. Any homozygous inherited thrombophilia or the association of two heterozygous deficits is also an absolute contraindication to CHC use. The single heterozygous mutation of factor V of Leiden or prothrombin gene increases from two to seven times the risk of VTE, but the aggravating effect of CHC is not always evident [19]. Thus, following extensive multidisciplinary counseling and a clear evaluation of the risk/benefit ratio, CHC can be administered if required or necessary [19]. Indication is to use CHC associated with a lower VTE risk such as those containing ≤ 30 mcg cthynilestradiol and levonorgestrel, 20 mcg ethynilestradiol and gestodene [18], or estradiol and dienogest [9, 20].

Women with Familial History of Venous Thromboembolism

Investigation of familial history of VTE is the only requirement to determine the risk of VTE induced by CHCs [21, 22]. Combined hormonal contraceptives cannot be used in women whose first-degree relatives have a history of idiopathic VTE prior to 45 years of age [21]. Analysis of coagulation or of inherited thrombophilia does not change the indication and should not be performed [19, 21]. All other contraceptive methods, including POCs, can be used.

Women with Varicose Veins

Presence of varicose veins is not a risk factor for VTE. All contraceptive options, including CHCs, can be used in women with varicose veins [10, 16].

Women with Isolated Risk Factors for Cardiovascular Disease

The presence of isolated risk factors for cardiovascular disease allows the use of any type of contraception with the exception of CHC, whose prescription could be contraindicated or may need personalization.

155

Age At or Older Than 40 Years

Aging is an aggravating factor of any cardiovascular risk [22, 23]. In the absence of additional cardiovascular risks, women of older age can use any CHC. Yet in premarketing studies only a few CHCs, those containing estradiol or estradiol valerate, were tested up to 50 years of age. In general, CHC combining a lower risk of arterial and venous disease should be used in women of an older age [8, 9, 12]. The CHC with estradiol appears to posses this characteristic [9, 20]. Otherwise, we should consider that VTE risk is lower in women using CHC containing ≤ 30 mcg ethynilestradiol and levonorgestrel, or 20 mcg ethynilestradiol and gestodene [16], but that these CHC may induce a higher risk of arterial disease [12]. Arterial risk is lower with CHCs containing drospirenone [8], that on the other hand seems to be associated with a slightly higher risk of VTE [18]. Accordingly, patient selection is important in order to decide the type of CHC to be used.

Obesity

Obesity is a risk factor for arterial diseases and VTE [22–25]. Guidelines differ about the indication of using CHC in obese women. In the World Health Organization (WHO) medical eligibility criteria obesity of any type does not contraindicate [10], while in the United Kingdom Medical Eligibility Criteria for Contraceptive Use (UKMEK) criteria [16] a body mass index equal to or greater than 35 contraindicates the use of CHC.

When prescribing a CHC the healthcare provider should take into consideration the efficacy that is dependent on the pharmacokinetic of the components, the influence of the contraceptive on body weight, and obviously the cardiovascular risk factors for both arteries and veins [26].

Smoking

Smoking represents a risk factor for arterial events but also, to some extent, for VTE. Smokers can use all types of contraceptives, but a limitation is given for CHCs. In women younger than 35 years of age, CHCs are permitted. In smokers 35 years of age or older CHCs should be avoided [10, 16]. Women who stopped smoking at least 1 year before can use CHCs [10, 16].

Hypertension

Hypertension is a risk factor for arterial events. Measurement of blood pressure is the only exam requested prior to CHC prescription. The estrogenic component of the CHC is responsible for inducing an increase of blood pressure that is type and dose dependent [12]. Hypertension is a contraindication to the use of CHCs, while POCs can be used. There are no data on the use of CHC in women with medically controlled hypertension. For these women CHC use remains prudentially contraindicated. In the case CHC is administered as therapy, its use can be considered. In this case associations proven not to increase blood pressure, such as CHCs containing drospirenone or estradiol, should be used [8, 27, 28].

Diabetes

It is a risk factor for arterial events. Diabetes is not a contraindication to the use of CHCs, but personalization of the treatment is advisable [10, 16].

Dyslipidemia

Dyslipidemia is a risk factor for arterial events and, to some extent, also for VTE. By itself it is not a contraindication to CHC use, but personalization of treatment is necessary [10, 16].

Systemic Lupus Erythematous with Anti-phospholipid Antibodies

Systemic lupus erythematous with anti-phospholipid antibodies represents a risk factor for arterial events and VTE [29]. It represents a contraindication to the use of CHCs and POCs [10, 16]. All other contraceptive options can be used.

Headache

Migrainous headache represents a risk factor for stroke. The risk is increased by CHCs [30, 31]. The condition is a clear contraindication to the use of CHCs only for women older than 35 years of age. If migrainous headache is associated with aura, the contraindication to the use of CHCs extends to all ages and POCs can be used [10].

Valvular Heart Disease

Valvular heart disease is not a contraindication to the use of CHCs. It becomes a contraindication when complicated by endocarditis, atrial fibrillation, or pulmonary hypertension [10]. All other contraceptive options, including POCs, can be used. These women can be in continuous anticoagulant therapy. The

LNG-IUS may be useful to reduce menstrual bleeding up to amenorrhea [14, 15].

Surgery with Immobilization

Surgery with immobilization increases the risk of VTE by four or five times. The risk is magnified up to seven times in overweight women [24]. Venous thromboembolism can occur in the 12 weeks following surgery, and prophylaxis should be continued for this period. It is recommended that CHCs are discontinued for the 4 weeks preceding and the 3 months following major surgery [16].

References

1. Yusuf S, Hawken S, Ounpuu S et al. Effect of potentially modifiable risk factors associated with myocardial infarction in 52 countries (the INTERHEART study): Case-control study. *Lancet.* 2004;**364** (9438):937–52.

2. O'Donnell MJ, Xavier D, Liu L et al. Risk factors for ischaemic and intracerebral haemorrhagic stroke in 22 countries (the INTERSTROKE study): A case-control study. *Lancet.* 2010;**376**(9735):112–23.

3. Hannaford PC, Croft PR, Kay CR. Oral contraception and stroke: Evidence from the Royal College of General Practitioners' Oral Contraception Study. *Stroke.* 1994;**25**:935–42.

4. Poulter NR for the WHO Collaborative Study of Cardiovascular Disease and Steroid Hormone Contraception. Ischaemic stroke and combined oral contraceptives: Results of an international, multicentre, case-control study. *Lancet.* 1996;**348**:498–505.

4. Weill A, Dalichampt M, Raguideau F et al. Low dose oestrogen combined oral contraception and risk of pulmonary embolism, stroke, and myocardial infarction in five million French women: Cohort study. *BMJ.* 2016;**353**:i2002.

5. Roach RE, Helmerhorst FM, Lijfering WM et al. Combined oral contraceptives: The risk of myocardial infarction and ischemic stroke. *Cochrane Database Syst Rev.* 2015;**8**:CD011054.

6. Lidegaard Ø, Kreiner S. Contraceptives and cerebral thrombosis: A five-year national case-control study. *Contraception.* 2002;**65**:197–205.

7. Lidegaard Ø, Løkkegaard E, Jensen A, Skovlund CW, Keiding N. Thrombotic stroke and myocardial infarction with hormonal contraception. *N Engl J Med.* 2012;**366**(24):2257–66.

8. Dinger J, Mohner S, Heinemann K. Cardiovascular risks associated with the use of drospirenone-containing combined oral contraceptives. *Contraception.* 2016;**93**:378–85.

9. Dinger J, Mohner S, Heinemann K. Combined oral contraceptives containing dienogest and estradiol valerate may carry a lower risk of venous and arterial thromboembolism compared to conventional preparations: Results from the extended INAS-SCORE study. *Front Women's Health.* 2020; **5**:1–8.

10. World Health Organization. *Medical eligibility criteria for contraceptive use.* 5th edition. Geneva: World Health Organization, 2015. www.who.int/pub lications/i/item/9789241549158.

11. Ezihe-Ejifor JA, Hutchinson N. Anticlotting mechanisms I: Physiology and pathology. *Contin Educ Anaesth Crit Care Pain.* 2013;**13**:87–92.

12. Cagnacci A. Hormonal contraception: Venous and arterial disease. *EJCRHC.* 2017;**22**:191–9.

13. Rosendaal FR, Van Hylckama Vlieg A, Tanis BC, Helmerhorst FM. Estrogens, progestogens and thrombosis. *J Thromb Haemost.* 2003;**1**:1371–80.

14. Pisoni CN, Cuadrado MJ, Khamashta MA, Hunt BJ. Treatment of menorrhagia associated with oral anticoagulation: Efficacy and safety of the levonorgestrel releasing intrauterine device (Mirena coil). *Lupus.* 2006;**15**:877–80.

15. Kilic S, Yuksel B, Doganay M et al. The effect of levonorgestrel-releasing intrauterine device on menorrhagia in women taking anticoagulant medication after cardiac valve replacement. *Contraception.* 2009;**80**:152–7.

16. Faculty of Sexual & Reproductive Healthcare. UK medical eligibility use. UKMEK 2016 (amended September 2019).

17. Roach RE, Lijfering WM, Van Hylckama Vlieg A et al. The risk of venous thrombosis in individuals with a history of superficial vein thrombosis and acquired venous thrombotic risk factors. *Blood.* 2013;**122**:4264–9.

18. De Bastos M, Stegeman BH, Rosendaal FR et al. Combined oral contraceptives: Venous thrombosis. *Cochrane Database Syst Rev.* 2014;CD010813.

19. Reich LM, Bower M, Key NS. Role of the geneticist in testing and counseling for inherited thrombophilia. *Genet Med.* 2003;**5**:133–43.

20. Fruzzetti F, Cagnacci A. Venous thrombosis and hormonal contraception: What's new with estradiol-based hormonal contraceptives? *Open Access J Contracept.* 2018;**9**:75–9.

21. Prandoni P, Prins MH, Ghirarduzzi A et al. Family history of venous thrombosis or sudden death as a risk factor for venous thromboembolism. *Thromb Haemost.* 2012;**107**:1191–2.

22. Oger E. Incidence of venous thromboembolism: A community-based study in Western France. EPI-GETBP Study Group. Groupe d'Etude de la Thrombose de Bretagne Occidentale. *Thromb Haemost.* 2000;**83**:657–60.

23. Sugiura K, Ojima T, Urano T, Kobayashi T. The incidence and prognosis of thromboembolism associated with oral contraceptives: Age-dependent difference in Japanese population. *J Obstet Gynaecol Res.* 2018;**44**:1766–72.

24. Parkin L, Sweetland S, Balkwill A et al. Body mass index, surgery, and risk of venous thromboembolism in middle-aged women: A cohort study. *Circulation.* 2012;**125**:1897–1904.

25. Horton LG, Simmons KB, Curtis KM. Combined hormonal contraceptive use among obese women and risk for cardiovascular events: A systematic review. *Contraception.* 2016;**94**:590–604.

26. Merki-Feld GS, Skouby S, Serfaty D et al. European society of contraception statement on contraception in obese women. *Eur J Contracept Reprod Health Care.* 2015;**20**:19–28.

27. Cagnacci A, Ferrari S, Napolitano A et al. Combined oral contraceptive containing drospirenone does not modify 24-h ambulatory blood pressure but increases heart rate in healthy young women: Prospective study. *Contraception.* 2013;**88**:413–17.

28. Grandi G, Napolitano A, Cagnacci A. Metabolic impact of combined hormonal contraceptives containing estradiol. *Expert Opin Drug Metab Toxicol.* 2016;**12**:779–87.

29. Sánchez-Guerrero J, Uribe AG, Jiménez-Santana L et al. A trial of contraceptive methods in women with systemic lupus erythematosus. *N Engl J Med.* 2005;**353**:2539–49.

30. Etminan M, Takkouche B, Isorna FC, Samii A. Risk of ischaemic stroke in people with migraine: Systematic review and meta-analysis of observational studies. *BMJ.* 2005;**8**:330(7482):63.Erratum in: BMJ. 2005;330(7487):345.Erratum in: BMJ. 2005;**330** (7491):596.

31. Edlow AG, Bartz D. Hormonal contraceptive options for women with headache: A review of the evidence. *Rev Obstet Gynecol.* 2010;3:55–65.

Chapter 23

Contraception in Women with Metabolic Conditions

Angelo Cagnacci, Anna Biasioli, Claudia Massarotti, Laura Gabbi, Anjeza Xholli

Introduction

Diabetes and known dyslipidemia represent the main metabolic risk factors for cardiovascular disease [1, 2]. No contraceptive method has a clear contraindication in the presence of a single metabolic disease. Yet limitations, particularly to hormonal contraceptive methods, may apply when diseases develop that are associated with such methods of contraception or with additional cardiovascular risk factors [3, 4]. No contraindication applies to natural methods, barrier and interceptive contraception, or sterilization [3, 4]. Presence of a metabolic disease may require personalization of hormonal contraception, in particular combined hormonal contraceptives (CHCs) and systemic progestin-only contraceptives (POCs). In order to understand how hormonal contraception can be used in women with metabolic disease, it is useful to understand how exogenous hormones influence glucose and lipid metabolism.

Glucose Metabolism

Influence of Sex Hormones

Several factors regulate glucose metabolism: rapidity and quantity of insulin released by the pancreas, insulin clearance by the liver, peripheral tissue insulin sensitivity, insulin-independent glucose utilization, gut hormones released during oral ingestion of carbohydrates, and gut microbiota. Modulation of many of these mechanisms by estrogens has been revealed in postmenopausal women, in whom estrogen manipulation is easier [5, 6]. Overall, the data indicate that estrogens, when given in the right quantity, improve glucose metabolism. The opposite occurs when estrogens are absent or are given in excessive quantities [5–7]. How estrogens of CHCs modulate the different aspects of glucose metabolism is not completely clear. Levels of ethinyl-estradiol of 30 or 20 mcg do

not seem to deteriorate glucose metabolism when associated with non-androgenic progestins [8–10]. The same applies to CHC with doses of 15 mcg ethinyl-estradiol and slight androgenic progestins (the vaginal ring) [10], or with CHCs containing estradiol [11–13]. The CHCs containing a high quantity of estrogens and androgenic progestin may deteriorate glucose metabolism [14, 15].

Progestins derive from three different molecules: testosterone and its derivatives, progesterone and its derivatives, and spironolactone. They can be classified in different ways, but in terms of glucose metabolism what is important is the glucocorticoid property and the androgenic/non/antiandrogenic activity of the progestin molecule [16]. Progesterone, gestodene, cyproterone acetate, and medroxyprogesterone acetate are progestins with a glucocorticoid activity. Yet this activity is not exerted at the concentration these progestins reach in blood during contraceptive use. The only exception is medroxyprogesterone acetate depot [16]. Because androgens reduce insulin sensitivity [17], the androgenic potency of a progestins is of paramount importance. Levonorgestrel and gestodene have an androgenic potency higher than desogestrel. Norgestimate is partially transformed into levonorgestrel (25%). Nomegestrol acetate, chlormadinone acetate, dienogest, and spironolactone are non-androgenic progestins [16]. Norethisterone can be considered androgenic, but it is partially converted into ethynylestradiol and it does not seem to markedly deteriorate insulin metabolism [8, 15].

Contraception in Women with Insulin-Dependent Type 1 Diabetes

In women with type 1 insulin-dependent diabetes contraception is necessary for the appropriate timing of reproductive events [18]. Indeed, women with diabetes use contraception more than others [19].

In diabetic women with evidence of microangiopathy, such as nephropathy/retinopathy/neuropathy, presence of other cardiovascular risk factors or suffering from diabetes for more than 20 years, CHCs are contraindicated because of the high risk of inducing cardiovascular events. In women with only diabetes, without evidence of microangiopathy or suffering from diabetes for less than 20 years, CHCs can be administered [3, 4]. In general, any CHC can be used, the slight alteration of glucose metabolism being easily compensated for by minimal modification of insulin administration. Yet CHCs containing less than 30 mcg ethynylestradiol or estradiol in conjunction with non-androgenic progestin may have a lower negative impact on glucose metabolism [13, 16, 20]. Limited evidence indicates that the clinical evolution toward microalbunuria is less evident in women using CHC containing less androgenic (desogestrel) than more androgenic (levonorgesterel) progestins [21]. Presence of comorbidities favoring venous thromboembolism (VTE) should be considered because VTE is increased in diabetic women. Use of CHCs with estradiol is associated with a low impact on glucose metabolism [11–13] and VTE risk [22].

A POC contains either androgenic (levonorgestrel, desogestrel, or etonorgestrel) or non-androgenic compounds (drospirenone). A POC with androgenic progestins negatively influences glucose metabolism [23–27], but a POC administered as implants, in particular etonorgestrel, proved safe [28]. It is tempting to speculate that POCs with drospirenone can be more safely used in diabetic women [16]. Progestins with glucocorticoid activity may deteriorate glucose metabolism and increase the risk of VTE [16]. Accordingly, medroxyprogesterone acetate depot should be avoided. Medroxyprogesterone acetate depot is contraindicated in women with diabetes for more than 20 years, in women with additional risk factors for cardiovascular disease, or in women with evidence of microangiopathy [3, 4].

Contraception in Women with Insulin-Dependent Type 2 Diabetes

Women with insulin-dependent type 2 diabetes may be on therapy with insulin-sensitizing medicine. In this case maintaining appropriate insulin sensitivity is probably more important than in women with insulin-dependent diabetes. The purpose is to reduce the excessive stimulus on pancreatic beta-cells in order to avoid their exhaustion. In terms of contraceptive use the same considerations expressed for insulin-dependent type 1 diabetes are valid [3, 4]. Personalization of therapy is important.

Contraception in Women with Polycystic Ovarian Syndrome

Classification of polycystic ovarian syndrome (PCOS) has been highly debated in the literature, with several PCOS phenotypes characterized. Modification of glucose metabolism, and in particular insulin resistance, is not included among the diagnostic criteria of PCOS, but is considered one of the main pathogenetic mechanisms of the syndrome [29]. A high percentage of women with PCOS develop clinical manifestations of the metabolic syndrome, whose pathogenesis impinges upon insulin resistance [30]. Among the phenotypic manifestations of PCOS, oligomenorrhea, unbalanced hyperestrogenism, ovarian hyperandrogenism, and peripheral manifestation of hyperandrogenism can be ameliorated by CHCs [31, 32]. Hyperandrogenism induces insulin resistance and its suppression improves insulin sensitivity [17, 33–35]. Because of the already critical glucose metabolism, the use of CHCs that induce a lower stimulus [15, 36, 37] or do not stimulate androgen receptors [10–13, 20, 38–40] may be preferred. In addition, the possibility to stimulate sex hormone–binding globulin (SHBG) by the estrogenic component, and thus reduce free available testosterone, make CHC with more potent estrogens (ethynylestradiol vs. estradiol or estetrol) more indicated [16]. Some evidence shows that in hyperandrogenic PCOS the use of CHC with ethinylestradiol and potent antiandrogenic progestins ameliorates insulin sensitivity [41].

Personalization of contraception should also take into consideration the presence of other risk factors for cardiovascular disease, in particular the presence of obesity, which may increase the risk of VTE. It has to be considered that women with PCOS are young and the risk of VTE in young women is minimal if not negligible [42]. The possibility of doubling the VTE risk by obesity should be referred to as a minimal baseline. When VTE is considered a risk, CHCs containing estradiol or estetrol and antiandrogenic progestins can be a useful option [43, 44].

A POC does not increase the risk of VTE but is made mainly by androgenic progestins such as levonorgestrel, desogestrel, and its active form, etonorgestrel. These progestins may induce insulin resistance and stimulate androgen receptors to some extent. A POC with non-androgenic or antiandrogenic (drospirenone) progestins could be more indicated.

Contraception in Women at Risk of Type 2 Insulin-Independent Diabetes

Women with a familial history of type 2 diabetes or who developed diabetes during pregnancy may be at higher risk. In these women there is no contraindication to any contraceptive option. Yet it is preferable to use CHCs or POCs that do not increase insulin resistance. A CHC with non-androgenic progestins [11–13, 20, 38–40, 44], a vaginal ring [10], or a POC with drospirenone should be preferred.

Lipid Metabolism

Influence of Sex Hormones

A major cardiovascular risk factor is represented by low-HDL cholesterol or apoprotein A, and high-LDL cholesterol or apoprotein B. A better relation to the cardiovascular risk is given by the apoA/apoB ratio and to a lesser extent by the HDL/LDL cholesterol ratio [1, 2]. Elevated triglycerides can also be considered a cardiovascular risk factor, but only when associated with other lipoprotein abnormalities, in particular low HDL-cholesterol levels [45].

Exogenous estrogens stimulate liver synthesis of apoprotein A and consequently HDL cholesterol, and of free fatty acids, to form triglycerides of very-low-density lipoprotein (VLDL) [46]. In the presence of elevated HDL cholesterol, VLDL is rapidly metabolized and not converted into LDL cholesterol [46]. Accordingly, the resulting effect exerted by exogenous estrogen on lipoprotein balance appears to be protective against cardiovascular diseases [45, 46]. The effect is dependent on the estrogen molecule administered (ethynylestradiol stronger than estradiol) and is linearly related to the dose of the estrogen administered, while is not dependent on the route of administration, at least in the case of ethynylestradiol administration [47].

Progestins with androgenic properties exert effects opposite to those of estrogens by reducing the synthesis of apoprotein A and HDL cholesterol and of free fatty acids and VLDL. The effect is greater for progestins with higher androgenic potency. Progestins with non-androgenic properties do not affect lipoprotein synthesis by the liver [16].

When a CHC is administered the final result is dependent on the balance between the estrogen stimulus on the liver and its antagonization by the progestin molecule. Antagonism can be absent in the case of non-androgenic progestins [13, 20] or very pronounced, up to reversal of the favorable effect of estrogens, when potent androgenic progestins are administered in high doses [48–50]. The CHCs containing estradiol [11–13] or estetrol [44] and non-androgenic progestins are almost neutral on lipid metabolism. In case of POCs the effect is the results of the androgenic potency and of the administered dose of that progestin. Androgenicity decreases from levonorgestrel to desogestrel or ketogestrel, up to non-androgenic progestins such as medroxyprogesterone acetate, chlormadinone acetate, or drospirenone [16, 51–53].

Contraception in Women with Known Dyslipidemia

Alteration in circulating lipoproteins does not represent a contraindication to any type of contraceptive method, including sterilization [3, 4]. Even hormonal contraceptives can be used [3, 4]. Women with lipid abnormalities are at higher risk of arterial cardiovascular events and VTE. Poor-quality observational studies indicate that the rate of these events may be slightly increased by use of unselected CHCs [54]. No effect of increased rates of pancreatitis or worsening of the lipid abnormality was found [54]. Personalization may be necessary for both CHCs and POCs.

A CHC with an equilibrium toward estrogenicity [13, 20] should be preferred over a CHC with an equilibrium toward androgenicity [48–50]. Very high VLDL/triglycerides may require a low estrogenic stimulus, which can be achieved by reducing the dose of ethynylestradiol or by using a CHC with estradiol [11–13] or eventually estetrol [44], rather than by using a CHC with potent androgenic progestins. It is important to note that the effects on lipoprotein are reduced with the vaginal ring [10] and CHCs containing estradiol or estetrol. The latter can be used safely without significantly modifying any parameter of lipid metabolism [11–13, 44].

A POC with lower androgenic potency, as those containing oral drospirenone, but to a lesser extent desogestrel, or ketogestrel implants, is probably more indicated than oral or implanted levonorgesterel [16]. Use of LNG-IUS is safe because the low levels of levonorgestrel in blood seems unable to influence lipid metabolism [55, 56].

References

1. Yusuf S, Hawken S, Ounpuu S et al. Effect of potentially modifiable risk factors associated with myocardial infarction in 52 countries (the INTERHEART study): Case-control study. *Lancet.* 2004;**364**(9438):937–52.

2. O'Donnell MJ, Xavier D, Liu L et al. Risk factors for ischaemic and intracerebral haemorrhagic stroke in 22 countries (the INTERSTROKE study): A case-control study. *Lancet.* 2010;**376**(9735):112–23.

3. World Health Organization. *Medical eligibility criteria for contraceptive use.* 5th edition. Geneva: World Health Organization, 2015.

4. Faculty of Sexual and Reproductive Healthcare. UK medical eligibility use. UKMEK 2016 (amended September 2019).

5. Cagnacci A, Tuveri F, Cirillo R et al. The effect of transdermal 17-beta-estradiol on glucose metabolism of postmenopausal women is evident during the oral but not the intravenous glucose administration. *Maturitas.* 1997;**28**:163–7.

6. Lindheim SR, Presser SC, Ditkoff EC et al. A possible bimodal effect of estrogen on insulin sensitivity in postmenopausal women and the attenuating effect of added progestin. *Fertil Steril.* 1993;**60**:664–7.

7. De Pirro R, Fusco A, Bertoli A, Greco AV, Lauro R. Insulin receptors during the menstrual cycle in normal women. *J Clin Endocrinol Metab.* 1978;**47**:1387–9.

8. Kojima T, Lindheim SR, Duffy DM et al. Insulin sensitivity is decreased in normal women by doses of ethinyl estradiol used in oral contraceptives. *Am J Obstet Gynecol.* 1993;**169**:1540–54.

9. Sitruk-Ware R, Nath A. Characteristics and metabolic effects of estrogen and progestins contained in oral contraceptive pills. *Best Pract Res Clin Endocrinol Metab.* 2013;**27**:13–24.

10. Cagnacci A, Ferrari S, Tirelli A, Zanin R, Volpe A. Route of administration of contraceptives containing desogestrel/etonorgestrel and insulin sensitivity: A prospective randomized study. *Contraception.* 2009;**80**:34–9.

11. Junge W, Mellinger U, Parke S, Serrani M. Metabolic and haemostatic effects of estradiol valerate/dienogest, a novel oral contraceptive: A randomized, open-label, single-centre study. *Clin Drug Investig.* 2011;**31**:573–84.

12. Ågren UM, Anttila M, Mäenpää-Liukko K et al. Effects of a monophasic combined oral contraceptive containing nomegestrol acetate and 17β-oestradiol compared with one containing levonorgestrel and ethinylestradiol on haemostasis, lipids and carbohydrate metabolism. *Eur J Contracept Reprod Health Care.* 2011;**16**:444–57.

13. Grandi G, Piacenti I, Volpe A, Cagnacci A. Modification of body composition and metabolism during oral contraceptives containing non-androgenic progestins in association with estradiol or ethinyl estradiol. *Gynecol Endocrinol.* 2014;**30**:676–80.

14. Waine HFE. Metabolic effects of Enovid in rheumatoid patients. *Arthritis Rheum.* 1963;**6**:796.

15. Godsland I, Walton C, Felton C, Proudler A. Insulin resistance, secretion and metabolism in users of oral contraceptives. *J Clin Endocrinol Metab.* 1991;**74**:64–70.

16. Cagnacci A. Hormonal contraception: Venous and arterial disease. *EJCRHC.* 2017;**22**:191–9.

17. Corbould A. Chronic testosterone treatment induces selective insulin resistance in subcutaneous adipocytes of women. *J Endocrinol.* 2007;**192**:585–94.

18. National Institute for Health and Clinical Excellence. Management of diabetes from preconception to the postnatal period: Summary of NICE guidance. *BMJ.* 2008;**336**:714–17.

19. Napoli A, Colatrella A, Botta R et al. Contraception in diabetic women: An Italian study. *Diabetes Res Clin Pract.* 2005;**67**:267–72.

20. Cagnacci A, Ferrari S, Tirelli A, Zanin R, Volpe A. Insulin sensitivity and lipid metabolism with oral contraceptives containing chlormadinone acetate or desogestrel: a randomized trial. *Contraception.* 2009;**79**:111–16.

21. Monster TB, Janssen WM, De Jong PE, De Jong–Van den Berg LT. Prevention of renal and vascular end stage disease study group: Oral contraceptive use and hormone replacement therapy are associated with microalbuminuria. *Arch Intern Med.* 2001;**161**:2000–5.

22. Dinger J, Mohner S, Heinemann K. Combined oral contraceptives containing dienogest and estradiol valerate may carry a lower risk of venous and arterial thromboembolism compared to conventional preparations: Results from the extended INAS-SCORE study. *Front Women's Health.* 2020;**5**:1–8.

23. Kivelä A, Ruuskanen M, Agren U, Dieben T. The effects of two progestogen-only pills containing either desogestrel (75 microgram/day) or levonorgestrel (30 microgram/day) on carbohydrate metabolism and adrenal and thyroid function. *Eur J Contracept Reprod Health Care.* 2001;**6**:71–677.

24. Benagiano G, Primiero FM. Seventy-five microgram desogestrel mini pill, a new perspective in estrogen-free contraception. *Ann N Y Acad Sci.* 2003;**997**:163–73.

25. Grandi G, Cagnacci A, Volpe A. Pharmacokinetic evaluation of desogestrel as a female contraceptive. *Expert Opin Drug Metab Toxicol.* 2013;**10**:1–10.

26. Biswas A, Viegas OA, Coeling Bennink HJ, Korver T, Ratnam SS. Implanon® contraceptive implants: Effects on carbohydrate metabolism. *Contraception.* 2001;**63**:137–41.

27. Cagnacci A, Tirelli A, Cannoletta M, Pirillo D, Volpe A. Effect on insulin sensitivity of Implanon vs. GnRH agonist in women with endometriosis. *Contraception.* 2005;**72**:443–6.

28. Vicente L, Mendonça D, Dingle M, Duarte R, Boavida JM. Etonogestrel implant in women with diabetes mellitus. *Eur J Contracept Reprod Health Care.* 2008;**13**:387–95.

29. Rosenfield RL, Ehrmann DA. The pathogenesis of polycystic ovary syndrome (PCOS): The hypothesis of PCOS as functional ovarian hyperandrogenism revisited. *Endocr Rev.* 2016;**37**:467–520.

30. Randeva HS, Tan BK, Weickert MO et al. Cardiometabolic aspects of the polycystic ovary syndrome. *Endocr Rev.* 2012;**33**:812–41.

31. Dokras A. Noncontraceptive use of oral combined hormonal contraceptives in polycystic ovary syndrome: Risks versus benefits. *Fertil Steril.* 2016;**106**:1572–9.

32. De Medeiros SF. Risks, benefits size and clinical implications of combined oral contraceptive use in women with polycystic ovary syndrome. *Reprod Biol Endocrinol.* 2017;**15**:93.

33. Cagnacci A, Paoletti AM, Arangino S, Melis GB, Volpe A. Effect of ovarian suppression on glucose metabolism of young lean women with and without ovarian hyperandrogenism. *Hum Reprod.* 1999;**14**:893–7.

34. Dahlgren E, Landin K, Krotkiewski M, Holm G, Janson PO. Effects of two antiandrogen treatments on hirsutism and insulin sensitivity in women with polycystic ovary syndrome. *Hum Reprod.* 1998;**13**:2706–11.

35. Moghetti P. Insulin resistance and polycystic ovary syndrome. *Curr Pharm Des.* 2016;**22**:5526–34.

36. Van der Mooren MJ, Klipping C, Van Aken B et al. A comparative study of the effects of gestodene 60 microg/ethinylestradiol 15 microg and desogestrel 150 microg/ethinylestradiol 20 microg on hemostatic balance, blood lipid levels and carbohydrate metabolism. *Eur J Contracept Reprod Health Care.* 1999;**4**(Suppl 2):27–35.

37. Lüdicke F, Gaspard UJ, Demeyer F, Scheen A, Lefebvre P. Randomized controlled study of the influence of two low estrogen dose oral contraceptives containing gestodene or desogestrel on carbohydrate metabolism. *Contraception.* 2002;**66**:411–15.

38. De Medeiros SF. Risks, benefits size and clinical implications of combined oral contraceptive use in women with polycystic ovary syndrome. *Reprod Biol Endocrinol.* 2017;**15**:93.

39. Amiri M, Ramezani Tehrani F, Nahidi F et al. Effects of oral contraceptives on metabolic profile in women with polycystic ovary syndrome: A meta-analysis comparing products containing cyproterone acetate with third generation progestins. *Metabolism.* 2017;**73**:22–35.

40. De Leo V, Fruzzetti F, Musacchio MC et al. Effect of a new oral contraceptive with estradiol valerate/dienogest on carbohydrate metabolism. *Contraception.* 2013;**88**:364–8.

41. Cagnacci A, Paoletti AM, Renzi A et al. Glucose metabolism and insulin resistance in women with polycystic ovary syndrome during therapy with oral contraceptives containing cyproterone acetate or desogestrel. *J Clin Endocrinol Metab.* 2003;**88**:3621–5.

42. Oger E. Incidence of venous thromboembolism: A community-based study in Western France. EPI-GETBP Study Group. Groupe d'Etude de la Thrombose de Bretagne Occidentale. *Thromb Haemost.* 2000;**83**:657–60.

43. Fruzzetti F, Cagnacci A. Venous thrombosis and hormonal contraception: What's new with estradiol-based hormonal contraceptives? *Open Access J Contracept.* 2018;**9**:75–9.

44. Klipping C, Duijkers I, Mawet M et al. Endocrine and metabolic effects of an oral contraceptive containing estetrol and drospirenone. *Contraception.* 2021;**103**:213–21.

45. Salazar MR, Carbajal HA, Espeche WG et al. Identifying cardiovascular disease risk and outcome: Use of the plasma triglyceride/high-density lipoprotein cholesterol concentration ratio versus metabolic syndrome criteria. *J Intern Med.* 2013;**273**:595–601.

46. Knopp RH, Zhu X, Bonet B. Effects of estrogens on lipoprotein metabolism and cardiovascular disease in women. *Atherosclerosis.* 1994;**110**(Suppl):S83–S91.

47. Sitruk-Ware R, Plu-Bureau G, Menard J et al. Effects of oral and transvaginal ethinyl estradiol on hemostatic factors and hepatic proteins in a randomized, crossover study. *J Clin Endocrinol Metab.* 2007;**92**:2074–9.

48. La Rosa JC. The varying effects of progestins on lipid levels and cardiovascular disease. *Am J Obstet Gynecol.* 1988;**158**:1821–9.

49. Upton V. Lipids, cardiovascular disease, and oral contraceptives: A practical perspective. *Fertil Steril.* 1990;**53**:1–12.

50. Godsland IF, Crook D, Simpson R et al. The effects of different formulations of oral contraceptive agents on lipid and carbohydrate metabolism. *N Engl J Med.* 1990;**323**:1375–81.

51. Barkfeldt J, Virkkunen A, Dieben T. The effects of two progestogen-only pills containing either desogestrel (75 μg/day) or levonorgestrel (30 μg/day) on lipid metabolism. *Contraception.* 2001;**64**:295–9.

52. Suherman SK, Affandi B KT. The effects of Implanon on lipid metabolism in comparison with Norplant. *Contraception.* 1999;**60**:281–7.

53. Mascarenhas L, Van Beek A, Bennink HC NJ. Twenty-four month comparison of apolipoproteins A-1, A-II and B in contraceptive implant users (Norplant and Implanon) in Birmingham, United Kingdom. *Contraception.* 1998;**58**:215–19.

54. Dragoman M, Curtis KM, Gaffield ME. Combined hormonal contraceptive use among women with known dyslipidemias: A systematic review of critical safety outcomes. *Contraception.* 2016;**94**:280–7.

55. Ng YW, Liang S, Singh K. Effects of Mirena (levonorgestrel-releasing intrauterine system) and Ortho Gynae T380 intrauterine copper device on lipid metabolism: A randomized comparative study. *Contraception.* 2009;**79**:24–8.

56. Zueff LFN, Melo AS de, Vieira CS, Martins WP, Ferriani RA. Cardiovascular risk markers among obese women using the levonorgestrel-releasing intrauterine system: A randomised controlled trial. *Obes Res Clin Pract.* 2017;**11**:687–93.

Chapter 24

Contraceptive Choices for Women with HIV Infection

Katarina Sedlecky, Gabriele S. Merki-Feld and Frans J. M. E. Roumen

Introduction

Women account for more than half of the individuals infected with human immunodeficiency virus (HIV), and at particularly high risk are those aged 15–24 years [1]. In the era of combined antiretroviral treatment (ART), HIV has become a chronic manageable condition, and many more affected women can nowadays re-evaluate their reproductive choices, including childbearing and prevention of pregnancy [2].

Use of efficient contraception is very important for women living with HIV in order to reduce health risks related to unintended pregnancies, especially perinatal HIV transmission and poor perinatal outcomes. Women with HIV have the right to decide whether they want motherhood. Therefore contraceptive counselling should include the issue of return to fertility and impact of a method on future generative capacity [3]. Regular condom use as a component of a dual protection should be highlighted because sexually transmitted infections (STIs) facilitate the transmission of HIV, which in turn worsens the course and consequences of STIs.

Contraception and HIV can interact in several ways. These include influence of contraception on progression of HIV infection/disease, HIV transmission and acquisition, risks of contraceptive use related to HIV infection/disease and drug interactions between hormonal contraceptives and ART [4].

Influence of Contraception on the Progression of HIV Infection/Disease

Contraception and HIV could theoretically interact, on one hand, by reduction of the effect of ART through drug–drug interactions (DDIs) between ARTs and concurrently used hormonal contraceptives (HCs) or through further suppression of the immune system by combined hormonal contraceptives (CHCs).

In a few studies significantly lower concentrations of ART (e.g. efavirenz, ritonavir, nelfinavir, atazanavir) were found in users of combined oral contraceptives (COCs), combined transdermal patch, progestin-injectables and, to a lesser extent, in users of combined vaginal rings [5, 6]. However, these reductions in ART exposure are of no clinical relevance. The pharmacokinetics (PK) of many antiretrovirals (e.g. lamivudine/stavudine, zidovudine, emtricitabine, tenofovir, nevirapine, elvitegravir/cobicistat) are not changed in COC users. Depot-medroxyprogesterone acetate (DMPA) use did not change the PK of lopinavir/ritonavir, efavirenz or nevirapine, and a levonorgestrel (LNG) implant did not influence the serum concentrations of efavirenz or nevirapine [5, 7]. In conclusion there is at present no evidence for a reduction in the efficacy of ART by HC.

For the second hypothetical mechanism the majority of studies did not find significant changes in CD4+ cell count and plasma HIV-RNA levels in CHC users [8]. In the study that compared markers of HIV disease progression between women randomized to DMPA, copper intrauterine device (IUD) or LNG implant, markers were more favourable in the groups of women on HC methods than in copper IUD users [9]. This confirmed the results of previous investigations that HC does not increase the risk for the progression of HIV disease [10]. No changes in HIV disease progression were found in the users of copper-bearing IUDs and levonorgestrel-releasing intrauterine systems (IUSs) [11]. Further, among women living with HIV who were randomized to a copper IUD or an LNG-IUS, no significant differences in genital and plasma HIV viral loads were found at 6 months, while expulsion and discontinuation rates were lower in LNG-IUS than in copper-IUD users [12]. There is no evidence that contraceptive methods have a significant impact on the progression of HIV infection/disease.

Influence of Contraception on HIV Transmission and Acquisition

Concerns about the impact of different methods of contraception on HIV transmission and acquisition have become less important after the World Health Organization (WHO) recommended ART for all persons living with HIV. Namely, ART contributes the most to reducing the risk of HIV transmission in serodiscordant couples. The risk of HIV transmission in women not on ART has been the subject of extensive research. A study with serodiscordant couples in Uganda demonstrated that not using ART or condoms elevated only moderately the risk for HIV transmission and acquisition (1.4) in DMPA users [13].

Another prospective trial (n = 3,790 serodiscordant couples) indicated that HC use was associated with a twofold increased risk of HIV-1 acquisition by women and HIV-1 transmission from women to men. The majority of women in that study used injectables. Compared to women who were not using HC, in women who used injectables, mostly DMPA, HIV-1 RNA was more commonly detected in cervical mucus, and genital HIV-1 RNA concentrations were higher [14]. On the contrary, in the multicentre, recently conducted study in Africa that included 7,829 HIV-negative women randomly assigned to use DMPA, a copper IUD or a levonorgestrel implant for 18 months, differences in HIV acquisition between investigated groups were insignificant [15]. Therefore, in order to reduce the risk of HIV transmission or acquisition regular condom use should be strongly recommended, particularly in women who use DMPA.

Infection with herpes simplex virus type 2 (HSV-2) can also facilitate HIV transmission and acquisition in injectable contraceptive users. The WHO therefore also recommends concomitant use of condoms and other HIV-preventive measures in women who use progestin-only injectables [16]. No relationship between the use of other HC methods and both HIV transmission and genital viral shedding was observed in studies [17].

The risk for HIV transmission in the users of copper IUDs and LNG-IUSs was assessed using HIV-1 genital shedding as a marker, and no changes were found. The risk for HIV acquisition was investigated in copper-IUD users, and no significant differences in HIV incidence were observed compared to women who underwent tubal ligation or were not using any contraception, as well as to the users of DMPA or levonorgestrel implants [17, 18].

Health Risks of Contraceptive Use Related to HIV Infection/Disease

Contraceptive efficacy of hormonal methods might be reduced in women with HIV due to DDIs between oestrogen/progestin and drugs these women use for HIV infection and HIV-related diseases (e.g. rifamycins or antiepileptics) [19]. Still, despite a possible decreased contraceptive efficacy, the rate of unintended pregnancy remains lower in women using HC compared to women not using contraception, indicating that careful consideration is needed before withholding a certain method from women with HIV [17].

The efficacy of LNG-IUS is not reduced, even when the systemic exposure to levonorgestrel is lower due to DDIs, because the contraceptive effect of this device is mainly achieved by the local action on the uterus. So far, there are no data on whether the non-contraceptive benefits of LNG-IUS, primarily the improvement of menorrhagia and the resulting anaemia, are diminished due to DDIs [17].

A particular problem in women living with HIV is the increased risk for venous thromboembolism (VTE). Factors related to HIV disease, antiretroviral treatment, comorbidities, infections and lifestyle characteristics (smoking and alcohol consumption) contributes to an increased risk for VTE [20]. This fact should be taken into account when women living with HIV need COC with higher doses of ethinyloestradiol (EE). HIV infection increases the risk of cardiovascular diseases, possibly due to chronic inflammation, ART, and high rates of typical risk factors in persons who live with HIV [21].

HIV-positive copper-IUD/LNG-IUS users are at increased risk of pelvic inflammatory disease (PID) due to their immunocompromised status. Still, rates of symptomatic PID with IUD are low [12]. As asymptomatic STIs increases the risk of PID in IUD users, screening for at least chlamydia and gonorrhoea is necessary before inserting a copper IUD/LNG-IUS. However, in the systematic review the rates of STIs and PID after IUD insertion were low, without differences in the incidence of inflammatory complications among women with different degrees of HIV disease severity [11, 12]. Hence, laboratory STI screening can be replaced in resource-poor areas with syndromic screening and treatment of all STIs that present within the certain syndrome. According to the WHO medical eligibility criteria (MEC) for contraceptive use, there are differences in the safety of copper-IUD/LNG-IUS use among women with varying severity of HIV disease. In women with HIV who are stable on ART, the use of IUD/IUS outweighs potential risks (MEC category 2). However, risks outweigh benefits of starting a copper IUD/LNG-IUS in women with severe or advanced HIV clinical disease (MEC category 3), and therefore in such cases, if IUD use continues, close monitoring for inflammatory complications is strongly recommended [16].

Interactions of Hormonal Contraception and Antiretroviral Drugs

Lifelong ART is recommended for all persons who live with HIV, regardless of the stage of HIV infection and CD4 cell count. There are several classes of antiretroviral drugs: nucleotide reverse transcriptase inhibitors (NRTIs) and non-nucleotide reverse transcriptase inhibitors (NNRTIs) prevent reverse transcription of viral RNA into DNA; protease inhibitors (PIs) inhibit maturation of HIV by blocking an HIV enzyme protease; fusion and entry inhibitors prevent HIV from entering the CD4 cell; integrase strand transfer inhibitors (INSTIs) prevent replication of HIV by blocking integration of viral DNA into the DNA of the host CD4 cell.

As the first-line ART for adults, the WHO recommends a combination of two NRTIs with either an NNRTI or an INSTI. The preferred option consists of tenofovir disoproxil fumarate (TDF), lamivudine and efavirenz. Instead of efavirenz, ART regimens may also contain other NNRTI (e.g. nevirapine), PIs (e.g. lopinavir, atazanavir, darunavir, all boosted with ritonavir) or INSTI (e.g. dolutegravir, elvitegravir, raltegravir). Fusion inhibitors (enfuvirtide), gp120 attachment inhibitors (fostemsavir), CCR5 inhibitors (maraviroc) and post-attachment inhibitors or monoclonal antibody (ibalizumab) are used in salvage therapy for HIV-infected people who do not respond favourably to common treatment regimens [2].

Some antiretrovirals have an effect on liver enzymes involved in the metabolism of oestrogen and progestin from hormonal contraception. By acting as inducers, inhibitors or substrates of cytochrome P450 (CYP450) enzymes, these drugs may alter the PK of hormones and their serum concentrations (Table 24.1). The assessment of DDIs is further complicated by the fact that ART regimens consist of at least three different drugs which can also interact with each other.

Table 24.1 The most important drug–drug interactions between antiretroviral drugs and hormonal contraceptives

Antiretroviral drug	Significant effect on oestrogen/progestin	Contraceptive efficacy
Nucleotide reverse transcriptase inhibitors		
tenofovir disoproxil fumarate, emtricitabine, lamivudine, zidovudine	none	unchanged
Non-nucleotide reverse transcriptase inhibitors		
efavirenz	lowers progestin	decreased for both combined and progestin-only methods
nevirapine	lowers EE	possibly decreased
etravirine, rilpivirine	none	unchanged
Protease inhibitors boosted with		
ritonavir	lowers EE	maintained in ≥ 30 μg EE COC
cobicistat	increases DRSP, unchanged LNG	DRSP use not recommended
Entry inhibitor		
maraviroc	none	unchanged
Integrase strand transfer inhibitors		
elvitegravir/cobicistat	lowers EE; increases progestin	≥ 30 μg EE COC recommended
raltegravir, dolutegravir, cabotegravir	None	unchanged

Nucleotide Reverse Transcriptase Inhibitors

As the backbone of most ART regimens, NRTIs are renally eliminated and have no effect on CYP450 enzymes. Therefore NRTIs do not have any impact on the effectiveness and safety of HC [17].

Non-nucleotide Reverse Transcriptase Inhibitors

Most NNRTIs act as both inducers and inhibitors of various CYP enzymes, but with the exception of efavirenz, they do not significantly affect the efficacy of HC [5]. A slight decrease in EE exposure and significant decrease in progestin exposure was found in women who used both COC and efavirenz. Similar decrease in levonorgestrel exposure occurred in volunteers treated with efavirenz who received progestin-only emergency contraception [5]. On the other hand, in COC users on nevirapine-based ART, EE concentrations were 58% lower and etonogestrel concentrations 22% lower. In HIV-positive women using progestin implants, the pregnancy incidence was three times higher for efavirenz-based ART in relation to nevirapine-based ART (3.3 vs. 1.1 per 100 woman-years). Differences between efavirenz and nevirapine-based ART were smaller during DMPA use (5.4 vs. 4.5 per 100 woman-years). The newer NNRTIs etravirine and rilpivirine do not significantly alter EE and progestin levels when used concurrently with COC [22].

Protease Inhibitors

In order to enhance the PK of PIs, either ritonavir or cobicistat is used as a booster. The changes in PK of HCs were noticed in women who used PIs boosted with ritonavir. Co-administration of atazanavir, darunavir and lopinavir, all boosted with ritonavir, with HC, resulted in reduced EE exposure, but with variable effect on progestin exposure. Darunavir/ritonavir and lopinavir/ritonavir did not significantly decrease norethindrone/etonogestrel exposure, while norgestimate exposure was significantly (50–85%) increased when used with atazanavir/ritonavir. Contraceptive efficacy of progestin-only methods is unchanged in women treated with PIs [5, 16].

Much less is known about the interactions of HC and PIs boosted with cobicistat. An increase in drospirenone exposure with decreased or unchanged levels of EE was found in both darunavir/cobicistat and atazanavir/cobicistat regimens, compared to HC use without ART. Avoiding the use of HC with drospirenone in women receiving atazanavir/cobicistat and monitoring for drospirenone-associated hyperkalaemia in those treated with darunavir/cobicistat are recommended [22]. However, atazanavir/cobicistat did not demonstrate a significant impact on PK of EE/levonorgestrel COC [23].

Entry Inhibitor

Maraviroc has no significant clinical impact on the metabolism of combined or progestin-only contraceptive methods [4, 7].

Integrase Strand Transfer Inhibitors

Raltegravir led to insignificant increase in progestin exposure in COC users, whereas dolutegravir did not change EE or progestin levels. On the contrary, elvitegravir boosted with cobicistat induce considerable changes with the reduction of EE exposure by 25% and increase in norethindrone exposure by 126%. There are no data regarding elvitegravir boosted with ritonavir; women taking these drugs should be advised, therefore, to use non-HC methods [17]. No significant DDIs were detected between cabotegavir and COCs [24].

Pre-exposure Prophylaxis

Antiretroviral therapy is recommended for HIV-negative persons who are at increased risk of HIV infection. Currently the only drug approved for use is Truvada®. It is a combination of tenofovir disoproxil fumarate and emtricitabine, both NRTIs. Truvada® can be safely used with HC, as no significant DDIs exist between these two groups of drugs [7, 16].

Post-exposure Prophylaxis

Antiretovirals should be initiated within 72 hours after a persons has been accidentally exposed to HIV. A combination of two NRTIs (tenofovir combined with either lamivudine or emtricitabine) and ritonavir-boosted lopinavir is the WHO-recommended regimen for adults. There are no significant DDIs between these antiretroviral drugs and HC [7].

References

1. UN Women. Facts and figures: HIV and AIDS. 2018. https://bit.ly/3wGpmsu.

2. World Health Organization. *Consolidated guidelines on the use of antiretroviral drugs for treating and*

preventing HIV infection: Recommendations for a public health approach. 2nd edition. Geneva: World Health Organization, 2016. www.who.int/hiv/pub/arv/arv-2016/en.

3. Amin A. Addressing gender inequalities to improve the sexual and reproductive health and wellbeing of women living with HIV. *J Int AIDS Soc.* 2015;**18** (Suppl 5):20302.

4. Sharma M, Walmsley SL. Contraceptive options for HIV-positive women: Making evidence-based, patient-centred decisions. *HIV Med.* 2015;**16**(6): 329–36.

5. Scarsi KK, Darin KM, Chappell CA, Nitz SM, Lamorde M. Drug–drug interactions, effectiveness, and safety of hormonal contraceptives in women living with HIV. *Drug Saf.* 2016;**39**(11):1053–72.

6. Scarsi KK, Cramer YS, Rosenkranz SL et al. Antiretroviral therapy and vaginally administered contraceptive hormones: A three-arm, pharmacokinetic study. *Lancet HIV.* 2019;**6**(9):e601–e612.

7. Nanda K, Stuart GS, Robinson J et al. Drug interactions between hormonal contraceptives and antiretrovirals. *AIDS.* 2017;**31**(7):917–52.

8. Hel Z, Stringer E, Mestecky J. Sex steroid hormones, hormonal contraception, and the immunobiology of human immunodeficiency virus-1 infection. *Endocr Rev.* 2010;**31**(1):79–97.

9. Morrison CS, Hofmeyr GJ, Thomas KK et al. Effects of depot medroxyprogesterone acetate, copper intrauterine devices, and levonorgestrel implants on early HIV disease progression. *AIDS Res Hum Retroviruses.* 2020;**36**(8):632–40.

10. Curtis KM, Hannaford PC, Rodriguez MI et al. Hormonal contraception and HIV acquisition among women: An updated systematic review. *BMJ Sex Reprod Health.* 2020;**46**(1):8–16.

11. Tepper NK, Curtis KM, Nanda K, Jamieson DJ. Safety of intrauterine devices among women with HIV: A systematic review. *Contraception.* 2016;**94**(6):713–24.

12. Todd CS, Jones HE, Langwenya N et al. Safety and continued use of the levonorgestrel intrauterine system as compared with the copper intrauterine device among women living with HIV in South Africa: A randomized controlled trial. *PLoS Med.* 2020;**17**(5):e1003110.

13. Lutalo T, Musoke R, Kong X et al. Effects of hormonal contraceptive use on HIV acquisition and transmission among HIV-discordant couples. *AIDS.* 2013;**27**(Suppl 1):S27–34.

14. Heffron R, Donnell D, Rees H et al. Use of hormonal contraceptives and risk of HIV-1 transmission: A prospective cohort study. *Lancet Infect Dis.* 2012;**12** (1):19–26.

15. Evidence for Contraceptive Options and HIV Outcomes (ECHO) Trial Consortium. HIV incidence among women using intramuscular depot medroxyprogesterone acetate, a copper intrauterine device, or a levonorgestrel implant for contraception: A randomised, multicentre, open-label trial. *Lancet.* 2019;**394**(10195):303–13.

16. World Health Organization. *Medical eligibility criteria for contraceptive use.* 5th edition. Geneva: World Health Organization, 2015.

17. Patel RC, Bukusi EA, Baeten JM. Current and future contraceptive options for women living with HIV. *Expert Opin Pharmacother.* 2018;**19**(1):1–12.

18. Hannaford PC, Ti A, Chipato T, Curtis KM. Copper intrauterine device use and HIV acquisition in women: A systematic review. *BMJ Sex Reprod Health.* 2020;**46**(1):17–25.

19. Majeed SR, West S, Ling KH, Das M, Kearney BP. Confirmation of the drug–drug interaction potential between cobicistat-boosted antiretroviral regimens and hormonal contraceptives. *Antivir Ther.* 2019;**24** (8):557–66.

20. Agrati C, Mazzotta V, Pinnetti C, Biava G, Bibas M. Venous thromboembolism in people living with HIV infection (PWH). *Transl Res.* 2020;S1931–5244 (**20**):30174–2.

21. Hsue PY, Waters DD. HIV infection and coronary heart disease: Mechanisms and management. *Nat Rev Cardiol.* 2019;**16**(12):745–59.

22. Patel RC, Onono M, Gandhi M et al. A retrospective cohort analysis comparing pregnancy rates among HIV-positive women using contraceptives and efavirenz or nevirapine-based antiretroviral therapy in Kenya. *Lancet HIV.* 2015;**2**(11):e474–e482.

23. Elliot ER, Bisdomini E, Penchala SD et al. Pharmacokinetics (PK) of ethinylestradiol/ levonorgestrel co-administered with atazanavir/ cobicistat. *HIV Res Clin Pract.* 2019;**23**:1–10.

24. Trezza C, Ford SL, Gould E et al. Lack of effect of oral cabotegravir on the pharmacokinetics of a levonorgestrel/ethinyl oestradiol-containing oral contraceptive in healthy adult women. *Br J Clin Pharmacol.* 2017;**83**(7):1499–1505.

Contraception in Women with Neurological Conditions

Gabriele S. Merki-Feld, Frans J. M. E. Roumen and Katarina Sedlecky

Multiple Sclerosis

Introduction

Multiple sclerosis (MS) is an inflammatory disease characterised by demyelination and axonal degeneration in the central nervous system with a probable autoimmune aetiology [1]. In advanced stages of the disease persons may develop muscle stiffness and paralyses of the leg. Female hormones seem to play a role and could impact the course of the disease. Multiple sclerosis does not significantly impair fertility, although there is emerging evidence on decreased ovarian reserve. Pregnancy is associated with lower rates of MS relapse, while postpartum rates increase again [2].

Women with MS should plan their pregnancy carefully. Many patients use disease-modifying drugs which might be teratogenic and are not approved for use during pregnancy. For most of those a washout period before conception is recommended. Washout periods of 2–4 months are, for example, recommended for fingolimod, teriflunomide, alemtuzumab, natalizumab and daclizumab [3]. Provision of efficient contraception for MS patients is required during most of their reproductive life, if they are sexually active.

Contraception in Multiple Sclerosis

Present evidence suggests that short-term or long-term use of combined hormonal contraceptives (CHCs) is associated neither with an increased risk to develop MS nor an increased risk for worsening its clinical course [1, 3]. Although most guidelines may classify nearly all contraceptive options as category 1, this does not mean that all methods are the best choice for an individual woman. Stage of the disease, medication and private and social circumstances are very relevant. Some MS patients might face difficulties with swallowing pills, while others may experience problems with insertion of the vaginal ring or a barrier method like the diaphragm. If management of menstrual hygiene is difficult, a contraceptive method with few or no bleeding days might be the first choice. Multiple sclerosis patients with immobility are at higher risk for venous thromboembolism (VTE) (Table 25.1) [4].

Combined Hormonal Contraceptives

A pill, patch or vaginal ring can be used as long as there is no prolonged immobility, and if the woman does not use medications which accelerate the metabolism of CHCs.

Progestin-Only Methods

Progestin-only pills (POP) and implants can be used without restriction. Also progestin-only contraceptives (POCs) can interact with medications. When using depo-medroxyprogesterone acetate (DMPA), take care for potentially reduced bone density related to corticoid use and immobility, and balance risks and benefits.

Copper Intrauterine Device and Levonorgestrel-Releasing Intrauterine System

There are no restrictions for use of a copper intrauterine device (Cu-IUD) or levonorgestrel-releasing intrauterine system (LR-IUS). Insertion can be more difficult and inconvenient in nulliparous women and those with restricted mobility.

Barrier Methods

All barrier methods have the disadvantage of low efficacy.

Female and Male Sterilization

Permanent methods of female and male sterilization can be very convenient and a relief for women with a chronic condition if no more children are planned.

Epilepsy

Epilepsy is a common brain condition characterised by a lasting predisposition to generate spontaneous epileptic seizures. Classification is made by seizure

Table 25.1 Multiple sclerosis: Aspects for contraceptive counselling and during regular check-ups in women with multiple sclerosis

Situation	Associated risk	Aspects for contraception
Impaired mobility	Increased VTE risk	Strict contraindication for CHC! Possible are progestogen-only methods, IUDs and operative procedures as efficient methods
	Increased risk for osteopenia	DMPA: no first-choice method
Long-term corticoid use	Increased risk for osteopenia	DMPA: no first-choice method
Uses of teratogenic medications		Use a highly efficient method
Problems to swallow		Use a non-oral method
Desire to become pregnant soon		Check if there is need for a washout period of medication; refer to obstetrician for counselling
Use of concomitant medications, which interact with hormones (modafinil, anticonvulsants, others)	Pregnancy	Consider DMPA or Cu-IUD
Annual control		Check new medications and risk factors for VTE
No wish for more children in the future		Consider male or female sterilization, long-term methods

type, epilepsy type and syndrome. Causes range from strong genetic predisposition to structural, metabolic, immune, infectious and unknown causes [5]. Long-term use of seizure medication is associated with a reduction in bone density [6]. In women of child-bearing age the risk of teratogenicity of the medication needs to be balanced against available alternatives. Especially valproate should be avoided in women without efficient contraception [7]. Many antiseizure medications reduce the efficacy of hormonal contraceptives, while on the other hand CHCs increase lamotrigine levels [8].

Catamenial Epilepsy

One third of women with epilepsy have catamenial epilepsy, defined as seizures occurring at certain times of the menstrual cycle. Even though oestrogen is a proconvulsant, CHCs have not been associated with an increase in seizures. There is no clear evidence if continuously used contraceptive hormones like CHCs in the long cycle or DMPA have a positive impact.

Contraception

There are no data that any types of hormonal or intrauterine contraception have a negative impact on the course of epilepsy. Drug–drug interactions of

hormonal contraception and antiepileptic drugs are frequent and, as mentioned, several antiepileptic medications are teratogenic, especially valproate [7]. This has to be addressed and discussed with the patient during counselling. Efficient contraceptive options for women using antiepileptic drugs interacting with hormone metabolism are copper or hormone-releasing IUDs, DMPA in higher dosages or permanent methods. It might also be worthwhile to discuss with the patient's neurologist whether the anticonvulsants can be switched to a substance that does not induce liver enzymes (Table 25.2). Further information can be found in the World Health Organization (WHO) practice recommendations on contraceptive use [9].

Combined Hormonal Contraceptives and Progestin-Only Contraceptives

Both CHCs and POCs are safe and efficient in women with epilepsy, if no anticonvulsants which increase metabolism of these compounds are used. If the latter are used, a CHC can be combined with a barrier method or another contraceptive method can be recommended. Use of a high-dose CHC (≥ 50 µg EE) is not recommended as the risk for cardiovascular events is too high. Shortening the interval between injections increases the efficacy of DMPA in women using a drug, which is a stronger inducer of liver enzymes.

Table 25.2 Frequently used antiepileptic drugs interacting with combined hormonal contraceptives or progestin-only contraceptives

Liver enzyme inducers
Carbamazepine
Felbamate
Oxcarbazepine
Phenobarbital
Phenytoin
Primidone
Rufinamide
Topiramate

Table 25.3 Diagnostic criteria for migraine adapted from the International Headache Society

Migraine	Aura
Attacks last 4–72 h	Visual symptoms: scotoma, zigzag lines, flashes
Unilateral location	Sensory symptoms: numbness, tingling, muscle weakness
Pulsating quality	Speech/language symptoms: difficulty to talk
Moderate to severe intensity	Duration >5 min
Aggravation by physical activity	Accompanied or followed by headache
Nausea, photophobia, phonophobia	

Copper Intrauterine Devices and Levonorgestrel-Releasing Intrauterine Systems

Both Cu-IUDs and LR-IUSs are safe and efficient in woman with epilepsy.

Barrier Methods

Barrier methods might not be the first-choice contraceptives as many antiseizure drugs are teratogenic. They could, however, be used for protection against sexually transmitted infections or to increase efficacy of hormonal methods.

Male and Female Sterilization

Permanent methods of sterilization can be very convenient for couples if no more children are planned.

Migraine

After puberty the prevalence of migraine is around 18%, and it is two to three times higher in women than in men [10]. Hormonal factors, especially hormone fluctuations and oestrogen withdrawal at the end of the menstrual cycle or before the hormone-free interval of CHCs, play a pivotal role. For the gynaecologist it is relevant to differentiate between migraine with aura (MA) and migraine without aura (MO), as MA is associated with a high risk for ischemic stroke, whereas MO is associated with a lower risk (Table 25.1) [11, 12]. For this reason CHCs are not recommend for MA patients [13]. The International Headache Society has defined diagnostic criteria for both forms of migraine (Table 25.3). Depression and endometriosis are comorbidities of migraine, which might impact the gynaecologist's recommendation for contraceptive choices.

Risk for Ischemic Stroke

The risk for ischemic stroke is higher in migraineurs with aura and higher in younger women. It increases multiplicative with additional risk factors (Table 25.4).

Contraception in Women with Migraine

Combined Hormonal Contraceptives

Combined hormonal contraceptives can initiate migraine, worsen existing migraine and cause auras in patients who suffered from MO before CHC use. Further, they increase significantly the risk for ischemic stroke, which is of concern as stroke occurs especially in young migraineurs [11]. Migraine with aura is therefore an absolute contraindication for CHC, while for MO risks and benefits have to be balanced. If migraine worsens or changes to MA, the CHC should be stopped immediately. Other factors like increased age and smoking multiply the stroke risk in migraineurs. This recommendation is based on consensus and new evidence and differs from the WHO recommendations [9].

Progestin-Only Contraceptives

Progestin-only contraceptives, which inhibit ovulation and are used continuously, might theoretically have a positive impact on hormonal migraines as the fluctuations in hormone plasma levels are small. For the desogestrel 75 µg pill it has been shown that this pill not only does not worsen migraine, but also reduces significantly frequency and intensity of migraine

Table 25.4 Migraine and risk for ischemic stroke in combined hormonal contraception users

	OR for ischemic stroke
All migraine	2.3–3.7
Migraine without aura	2.3–3.8
Migraine with aura	3.8–8.6
Migraine and COCs	13.9–16.9
Migraine, smoking and COCs	34.4

attacks and thus causes a major improvement in quality of life [14–16]. It is therefore a first-choice option for women with MA and MO. The improvement occurs over time. It has not been studied whether the injection (DMPA) or the implant or the drospirenone-only pill have such an impact. Progestin-only contraceptives do not increase the risk for ischemic stroke.

Levonorgestrel-Releasing Intrauterine Systems

Clinical experience with the LNG-IUS shows that women with migraine experience more attacks since insertion; others, however, experience fewer attacks, especially those who suffer exclusively from menstrual-related migraines. Both aspects have to be addressed during counselling and follow-up visits. A worsening can also happen stepwise over several months.

Copper Intrauterine Device, Barrier Methods, Male and Female Sterilization

There is no restriction for the use of the Cu-IUD, barrier methods, or sterilization in migraineurs.

References

1. Alonso A, Clark CJ. Oral contraceptives and the risk of multiple sclerosis: A review of the epidemiologic evidence. *J Neurol Sci.* 2009;**286**(1–2):73–5.

2. Confavreux C, Hutchinson M, Hours MM et al. Rate of pregnancy-related relapse in multiple sclerosis. Pregnancy in Multiple Sclerosis Group. *N Engl J Med.* 1998;**339**(5):285–91.

3. Houtchens MK, Zapata LB, Curtis KM, Whiteman MK. Contraception for women with multiple sclerosis: Guidance for healthcare providers. *Mult Scler.* 2017;**23**(6):757–64.

4. Peeters PJ, Bazelier MT, Uitdehaag BM et al. The risk of venous thromboembolism in patients with multiple sclerosis: The Clinical Practice Research Datalink. *J Thromb Haemost.* 2014;**12** (4):444–51.

5. Thijs RD, Surges R, O'Brien TJ, Sander JW. Epilepsy in adults. *Lancet.* 2019;**393**(10172):689–701.

6. Beerhorst K, Van der Kruijs SJ, Verschuure P et al. Bone disease during chronic antiepileptic drug therapy: General versus specific risk factors. *J Neurol Sci.* 2013;**331**(1–2):19–25.

7. Harris L, Lowes O, Angus-Leppan H. Treatment decisions in women of childbearing age on valproate. *Acta Neurol Scand.* 2020;**141**(4):287–93.

8. Rauchenzauner M, Deichmann S, Pittschieler S et al. Bidirectional interaction between oral contraception and lamotrigine in women with epilepsy: Role of progestins. *Seizure.* 2020;**74**:89–92.

9. World Health Organization. *Selected practice recommendations for contraceptive use.* Geneva: World Health Organization, 2016.

10. Vetvik KG, Macgregor EA, Lundqvist C, Russell MB. Prevalence of menstrual migraine: A population-based study. *Cephalalgia.* 2014;**34** (4):280–8.

11. Tzourio C, Kittner SJ, Bousser MG, Alperovitch A. Migraine and stroke in young women. *Cephalalgia.* 2000;**20**(3):190–9.

12. Bousser MG, Welch KM. Relation between migraine and stroke. *Lancet Neurol.* 2005;**4**(9):533–42.

13. Sacco S, Merki-Feld GS, Bitzer J et al. Hormonal contraceptives and risk of ischemic stroke in women with migraine: A consensus statement. *J Headache Pain.* 2017;**18**(1):108.

14. Morotti M, Remorgida V, Buccelli E et al. Comparing treatments for endometriosis-related pain symptoms in patients with migraine without aura. *J Comp Eff Res.* 2012;**1**(4):347–57.

15. Merki-Feld GS, Imthurn B, Langner R et al. Headache frequency and intensity in female migraineurs using desogestrel-only contraception: A retrospective pilot diary study. *Cephalalgia.* 2013;**33**(5):340–6.

16. Merki-Feld GS, Imthurn B, Gantenbein AR, Sandor P. Effect of desogestrel 75 microg on headache frequency and intensity in women with migraine: A prospective controlled trial. *Eur J Contracept Reprod Health Care.* 2019;**24**(3): 175–81.

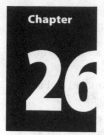

Contraception in Women with Psychiatric Conditions

Gabriele S. Merki-Feld, Frans J. M. E. Roumen and Katarina Sedlecky

Major Depression

This chapter discusses major depression (MD) as defined in the *Diagnostic and Statistical Manual of Mental Disorders, Fifth Edition* (DSM-5) criteria [1]. Mood changes and irritability in the context of hormonal contraception (HC) are discussed in Chapter 17. The most relevant symptoms of MD patients are demonstrated in Table 26.1. Patients with MD are no more capable to function in their daily life.

Prevalence of depression in women of reproductive age is around 14% and the prevalence of postpartum depression is slightly higher (15%) [2]. People with depression can be reluctant to seek help, even though effective treatments are available.

Does Hormonal Contraception Initiate Depression in Healthy Women?

Most studies demonstrate that depression and anxiety scores do not change with the use of combined hormonal contraceptives (CHCs) [3, 4]. There is, however, some evidence that, very rarely, CHC might initiate depression. In a Danish cohort study two more cases of depression were found in 10,000 woman-years compared with a group of nonusers, indicating only a minimal impact of hormones [5]. Similar small numbers were found for users of progestin-only contraceptives (POCs) with desogestrel and low-dose levonorgestrel-releasing intrauterine systems (LNG-IUSs). Adolescents seemed to be more frequently affected [5, 6]. Symptoms occur typically within few months after initiation of the hormones [5]. No data indicate that the injection of depo-medroxyprogesterone acetate (DMPA) or other POCs triggers depression in healthy women [3, 7–10]. However, the evidence for this statement is limited. Barrier methods, copper intrauterine devices (Cu-IUDs) and permanent methods do not initiate depression.

Table 26.1 Symptoms of major depression

- Depressed mood nearly daily, no pleasure in activities
- Fatigue or loss of energy nearly every day, sleeping problems
- Diminished ability to concentrate, slowing down of thoughts
- Feelings of worthlessness or inappropriate guilt

Contraception in Women with Major and Postpartum Depression

The preponderance of the limited evidence does not support an association between CHC or POC use and worsening of depression [3]. While symptoms of depression varied during the natural cycle, they did not change during the hormone-free interval in CHC users [11]. No differences in the course of disease or the frequencies of rehospitalization were observed among CHC users, LNG-IUS users, DMPA users and women with sterilization or using a Cu-IUD in patients with bipolar disorder [12]. Data on the effect of DMPA on postpartum depression are inconsistent. One trial found more women with MD in the DMPA group than in the Cu-IUD group, but this was not confirmed in another trial [3, 13]. Other contraceptive options might therefore be preferred.

Clinical Aspects

Although most studies do not find an association, clinical experience shows that severe depressive moods can arise in a small group of potentially predisposed women, and this effect does not seem to be associated with the progestin dose, as LNG-IUS users can be affected as well. Depressive women are ashamed and have little energy. They might not mention their symptoms. It is the responsibility of the counsellor to actively explore mood changes in the follow-up visit. Fortunately, we know from clinical experience that the negative impact of HC resolves within days after discontinuation [7].

Schizophrenia

Schizophrenia is a mental health disorder with high genetic heritability and a lifetime prevalence of nearly 1% [14, 15]. Medical comorbidities like increased risk for cardiovascular disease (CVD) as consequence of long-term use of antipsychotics and smoking, contribute to the high global burden [15]. Cognitive deficiencies, absence of emotional support and cumulative effects of antipsychotic medications impede the counselling of these patients (Table 26.2). Not only insufficient awareness that these women need contraception, but also the limited capability of some patients to use their contraceptive correctly contribute to the high rate of unwanted pregnancies (24–47%) [16].

Table 26.2 Reproductive health issues in women with schizophrenia

Circumstance	Consequence
Less stable partnerships/ casual sexual encounters	High number of sexual partners High risk of sexually transmitted infections Intercourse without protection
No use of contraceptives or incapability to use the contraceptive method correctly	Very high unplanned pregnancy rates (24–47%)
Cognitive deficiencies, insufficient emotional support	Risk for sexual exploitation
Adverse events of antipsychotic or concomitant antiepileptic medications affecting gynaecologic issues	Hyperprolactinemia Weight increase Metabolic symptoms Sexual dysfunction
Amenorrhea	Frequently associated with drug-induced hyperprolactinemia. Exclude pregnancy if necessary!
Inability to use a method reliably	Patients might not show up for scheduled follow-up visits related to contraception. Daily use of a pill might be difficult.
Interaction between antipsychotic medication and hormonal contraceptive (HC)	This includes increase of plasma levels of the antipsychotic drug by HC (e.g. clozapine) and accelerated metabolism of HC induced from the antipsychotic.

Contraception

Hormonal factors seem to be involved in the course of the disease by, for example, worsening psychotic symptoms in the peri-menstrual phase of the cycle or postpartum. There is, however, no evidence for a negative impact of CHCs or POCs on the course of disease. Table 26.3 summarises points which might be helpful to support a woman in her decision for an efficient contraceptive method.

Combined Hormonal Contraceptives

Use of CHCs is possible if the client is capable of adhering to the instructions for correct use. Exclude cardiovascular risk, especially smoking and obesity.

Progestin-Only Methods and Copper Intrauterine Devices

All POC methods or a Cu-IUD can be used. A progestin-only pill (POP) or etonogestrel-releasing implant might be too low-dosed if there are drug–drug interactions (DDIs). Implant users have to remember

Table 26.3 Points which should be addressed when discussing risks and benefits of contraceptive methods with a client

Exclude gynaecologic condition and take other conditions into account	Hyperprolactinemia with the concomitant irregularities of the menstrual cycle is frequent, also obesity-related metabolic syndrome
Medication and interactions	Potentially discuss with psychiatrist if you are worried the hormone you prescribe interacts with the antipsychotic drug and vice versa
Reliability	This might vary depending on the state of disease. In general less-reliable women should use a long-acting reversible contraceptive (LARC)
Barrier method	Important to protect from sexually transmitted infections
LARC	Explain advantage of user independency
Preference of the woman	It is important that the woman can accept the method she uses and accepts the changes in bleeding pattern associated with most POCs or LARCs

that, after 3 years, the implant needs to be exchanged. Therefore, LARCs are generally the better options for patients with low adherence. The DMPA can be injected in shorter intervals to increase efficacy if there are distinct DDIs. Many women might find long-term amenorrhea convenient. Intrauterine devices are LARCS that do not interact with medications and can be used mostly beyond the licensed duration of use. The continuation rate was higher than that with the injection in women with bipolar disorders [12].

Barrier Methods

Barrier methods should always be recommended in unstable relationships as prevention against sexually transmitted infections.

Female/Male Sterilization

Sterilization might be a good choice for some women or couples if use of other contraceptives is a burden. The decision and its consequences must be well understood by the patient.

Amenorrhea or Oligomenorrhea

Longer use of antipsychotics is often associated with hyperprolactinemia and weight increase. Consequences can be cycle irregularities, amenorrhea, and obesity with metabolic syndrome. If circumstances are not clear, exclude pregnancy in amenorrhoeic patients.

Eating Disorders

Eating disorders (EDs) are classified in the DSM-5 criteria and include anorexia nervosa, bulimia nervosa, binge-eating disorder and other subtypes. Anorexia nervosa (AN) and bulimia nervosa (BN) are the most prevalent types (1–3%) [1]. The long duration of the conditions has severe implications for long-term health. These include loss of bone mineral density (BMD) or lack of achieving peak bone mass (PBM) during adolescence, functional hypothalamic hypogonadism with oestrogen deficiency, loss of brain volume and psychological symptoms like anxiety, depression and obsessive-compulsive disorder [17].

Contraception in Anorexia Nervosa

Women with AN have a twofold higher risk of an unplanned pregnancy [17]. Physicians focusing on weight gain, eating behaviour and restoration of menses might underestimate this risk. On the other hand, anorectic women, based on their fear to gain weight, can be reluctant to use hormones and might be less compliant. Anorectic patients should have the option to discuss their fears during counselling. The risk–benefit balance for a contraceptive method has to include the physical condition and body-mass index (BMI), the duration of disease, the potential effect on bone density and the motivation of the patient. Women with EDs might also practise vomiting after attacks of binge eating. Some women might appreciate menstruation, while others do not. The CHCs do not only provide efficient contraception, but also treat the oestrogen deficiency and contribute to maintenance of bone density. If vomiting is a problem, the patch or the vaginal ring can be used. Women have to be aware that, in spite of regular bleeding, there is need for further weight gain, as CHC withdrawal bleedings are artificial. In a subset of women CHCs exert a positive impact on the course of disease [17]. As anorectic patients have oestrogen deficiency, POCs are not a first choice. Injectables like DMPA will have a further negative impact on BMD. No data on BMD are available for the implant and POPs when used in anorectic patients. The LNG-IUS might not reduce BMD, but suppression of menstruation can influence the course of disease. Copper intrauterine devices do not substitute for oestrogen in women with functional hypothalamic hypogonadism, but will not exert a negative impact on BMD. For unreliable women, risks and benefits of LARCs have to be balanced.

Contraception in Bulimia Nervosa

If low body weight and irregular cycles or amenorrhea indicate oestrogen deficiency, the contraceptive patch or the vaginal ring are of special advantage. Intrauterine devices and the implant can also be used.

References

1. DSM 5 criteria. www.psychiatry.org/psychiatrists/practice/dsm.

2. WHO: Prevalence of mental disorders. https://bit.ly/3wPpx4F.

3. Pagano HP, Zapata LB, Berry-Bibee EN et al. Safety of hormonal contraception and intrauterine devices among women with depressive and bipolar disorders: A systematic review. *Contraception.* 2016;94(6):641–9.

4. Robakis T, Williams KE, Nutkiewicz L, Rasgon NL. Hormonal contraceptives and mood: Review of the

literature and implications for future research. *Curr Psychiatry Rep.* 2019;**21**(7):57.

5. Skovlund CW, Morch LS, Kessing LV, Lidegaard O. Association of hormonal contraception with depression. *JAMA Psychiatry.* 2016;**73**(11):1154–62.

6. De Wit AE, Booij SH, Giltay EJ et al. Association of use of oral contraceptives with depressive symptoms among adolescents and young women. *JAMA Psychiatry.* 2019.

7. Merki-Feld GS, Apter D, Bartfai G et al. ESC expert statement on the effects on mood of the natural cycle and progestin-only contraceptives. *Eur J Contracept Reprod Health Care.* 2017;**22**(4):247–9.

8. Civic D, Scholes D, Ichikawa L et al. Depressive symptoms in users and non-users of depot medroxyprogesterone acetate. *Contraception.* 2000;**61**(6):385–90.

9. Westhoff C, Wieland D, Tiezzi L. Depression in users of depo-medroxyprogesterone acetate. *Contraception.* 1995;**51**(6):351–4.

10. Worly BL, Gur TL, Schaffir J. The relationship between progestin hormonal contraception and depression: A systematic review. *Contraception.* 2018;**97**(6):478–89.

11. Rasgon N, Bauer M, Glenn T et al. Menstrual cycle related mood changes in women with bipolar disorder. *Bipolar Disord.* 2003;**5**(1):48–52.

12. Berenson AB, Asem H, Tan A, Wilkinson GS. Continuation rates and complications of intrauterine contraception in women diagnosed with bipolar disorder. *Obstet Gynecol.* 2011;**118**(6):1331–6.

13. Tsai R, Schaffir J. Effect of depot medroxyprogesterone acetate on postpartum depression. *Contraception.* 2010;**82**(2):174–7.

14. Charlson FJ, Ferrari AJ, Santomauro DF et al. Global epidemiology and burden of schizophrenia: Findings from the Global Burden of Disease Study 2016. *Schizophr Bull.* 2018;**44** (6):1195–1203.

15. Disease GBD, Injury I, Prevalence C: Global, regional, and national incidence, prevalence, and years lived with disability for 328 diseases and injuries for 195 countries, 1990–2016: A systematic analysis for the Global Burden of Disease Study 2016. *Lancet.* 2017;**390**(10100):1211–59.

16. Gonzalez-Rodriguez A, Guardia A, Alvarez Pedrero A et al. Women with schizophrenia over the life span: Health promotion, treatment and outcomes. *Int J Environ Res Public Health.* 2020;**17**(15):n.p.

17. Merki-Feld GS, Bitzer J. Contraception in adolescents with anorexia nervosa: Is there evidence for a negative impact of combined hormonal contraceptives on bone mineral density and the course of the disease? *Eur J Contracept Reprod Health Care.* 2020;**25**(3):213–20.

Chapter 27

Contraception in Disabled Women

Johannes Bitzer

Introduction

The United Nations (UN) Convention on the Rights of Persons with Disabilities (2006) Article 1 identifies persons with disabilities (PwD) as 'those who have long-term physical, mental, intellectual, or sensory impairments which, in interaction with various barriers, may hinder their full and effective participation in society on an equal basis with others' [1].

Article 6 of the UN Convention underlines that women and girls with disabilities are subject to multiple types of discrimination, and, in this regard, the states shall take measures to ensure their full and equal human rights and fundamental freedoms. Articles 23 and 25 of state that PwD are entitled to decide freely and responsibly on the number and spacing of their children, to access age-appropriate information and reproductive and family planning education, to retain fertility to enable them to exercise these rights on equal basis with others, and to receive quality healthcare services equal to others, including sexual and reproductive healthcare.

Definitions and Concepts of Disabilities

The UN Convention defines PwD as individuals who have long-term physical, mental, intellectual or sensory impairments which, in interaction with various barriers, may hinder their full and effective participation in society on an equal basis with others [1]. Another definition comes from the Centers for Disease Control (CDC) [2]. Disability is any condition of the body or mind (impairment) that makes it more difficult for the person with the condition to do certain activities (activity limitation) and interact with the world around them (participation restrictions).

Regarding the different manifestations and the factors contributing to disability the International Classification of Functioning, Disability and Health (ICF) takes a biopsychosocial perspective and defines disability as the result of health condition and contextual factors enumerating the body, activity, participation and environment [3, 4].

- Body functions are physiological functions of body systems (including psychological functions).
- Body structures are anatomical parts of the body such as organs, limbs and their components.
- Impairments are problems in body function or structure such as a significant deviation or loss.
- Activity is the execution of a task or action by an individual.
- Participation is involvement in a life situation.
- Activity limitations are difficulties an individual may have in executing activities.
- Participation restrictions are problems an individual may experience in involvement in life situations.
- Environmental factors make up the physical, social and attitudinal environment in which people live.

Based on this biopsychosocial model the ICF has two parts, each with two components to define the individual experience of a disabled person.

Part 1. Functioning and Disability

a) These include body functions and structures thus evaluating physical and mental health impairments

b) These include activities and participation thus evaluating the degree of restrictions and limitations of activity and participation in social life

Part 2. Contextual Factors

c) Environmental factors refer to the degree of existing support or difficulties from the family and the society

d) Personal factors refer to stress and resources regarding the coping with the disability. [4]

For clinical purposes disabilities are divided into five groups: [5]

1. Physical, which is expressed in difficulties of movement (for example, cerebral palsy, hemiplegia, paraplegia etc.)
2. Sensory, which is caused by hearing and visual impairments (for example, severe deterioration of eyesight, deafness etc.)
3. Intellectual, which is related to mental retardation (for example, Down syndrome, autistic spectrum, cerebral palsy etc.)
4. Psychical, related to mental health difficulties (for example, schizophrenia, bipolar disorders, severe depression disorders, post-traumatic stress disorders etc.)
5. Multiple disorders: intellectual and sensor, sensor and physical, psychic and intellectual and so forth.

Contraceptive Needs of Individuals with Disabilities and Good Contraceptive Counselling and Care

Women and men with disabilities, like individuals without disabilities, need contraception to allow them to live their sexuality free from fear of an unwanted pregnancy. Good contraceptive counselling and care for women and men with disabilities should follow specific standards of communication and interaction on one side and a joint search for methods which fit best the needs and the biopsychosocial profile of the user.

Standards of Communication to Establish a Helpful Patient–Healthcare Provider Relationship

Healthcare providers (HCPs) should respect all patients, regardless of disability status. Disability is still stigmatized in our society, which becomes one of the reasons for low referral to healthcare services by persons with disabilities. This is especially common when it comes to sensitive issues like sexual and reproductive health [6]. The healthcare professional should observe interpersonal skills in order to support people with disabilities and provide any services needed. Feedback, of course, largely depends on verbal and non-verbal communication – for example,

provision of hearing aids and translation for people with hearing impairments, or using short sentences and easy-to-understand words with people with intellectual disabilities, or providing information using visual material.

The provision of information should follow the principles of eliciting what the individual already knows and which questions they want to ask. Giving information in small units and summarizing what is very important can help the patient to understand. In each conversation the HCP will need to find the language and the words which correspond to the way the patient talks, thus trying to find a common language. Sign language translators should be present for persons with disabilities in need of such services. At the end of each consultation, the doctors should ask questions to determine whether the patient understood the information provided [7].

Selection of the Method Based on Needs, Individual Health Conditions and Psychosocial Environment

To find the best method for the individual the HCP needs to follow a structured approach [8, 9].

Understand the Needs and Concerns of the Person

What about the wish for a child? What does the patient know? What are her desires and fears? The answers to these questions will vary largely in women with different disabilities and may be difficult with patients with mental and intellectual disabilities. It may then be important that the HCP puts herself or himself as far as possible into the position of the patient (directive counselling).

Take a Medical History to Look for Comorbidities and General Risk Factors

Other comorbidities described in the World Health Organization's (WHO) Medical Eligibility Criteria (MEC) or the United Kingdom's MEC Faculty include pregnancy, postpartum depression, cardiovascular diseases, cancer and neurological psychiatric morbidity.

Examination

Gynaecological examination may be undertaken (only if necessary for symptoms or if an intrauterine device (IUD) is considered). Specific positions can help to make the examination less bothersome:

- Knee-chest position: A woman lies down on her side with bended knees. This position could be used for women who cannot spread legs apart and feel more protected or balanced in this position.
- Diamond position: a woman lies on her back with feet joined together and knees apart. This position can be used for PwD women who cannot place legs on a gynaecological chair.
- M-position: A woman lies on her back with bended knees. This is more useful for women who need to fully lean on the table.
- V-position: A woman lies on her back with legs spread apart and knees straight like a V shape. This position is for women who have trouble manipulating their legs.
- OB position: Use of handles to support knees is often most comfortable for women with disabilities.

(Shared) Choice of the Method

Depending on the specific disability the HCP will look (together with the patient if possible) into the different methods of contraception and their advantages and disadvantages, as well as possible contraindications based on the disability and other medical conditions [7–11]. See also Table 27.1.

Non-hormonal Methods

There are two major groups of non-hormonal methods of contraception – IUDs and barrier methods.

Intrauterine contraception provides excellent long-term, reversible contraception and can be a good choice for many women with disabilities. Two main types of IUD contraceptives are currently used. The most frequently employed and most effective is the copper-T IUD, a non-hormonal contraceptive that can remain in place for 10 years. There are no major health risks but the rare side effects include cramping and heavy menses, which are the most important disadvantage (see also Chapter 13).

The IUD containing levonorgestrel (LNG) provides a long-lasting and high effectiveness. This form of contraception has the benefit of decreased menstrual flow to amenorrhea after the first few months of use. It may be an ideal method of contraception as well as provide menstrual regulation for women with menstrual flow management problems The IUD may be used by women at risk for thromboembolism or who

Table 27.1 Selection of contraception method for women with disabilities

Methods	Advantages	Other factors to consider
Hormonal contraception 1. Combined oral contraception 2. Vaginal ring 3. Plaster	- Highly effective method - Regulated menstrual cycle - Reduces menstrual bleeding - Does not require gynaecological examination	- Increased risk of venal thromboembolism and thrombophlebitis in case of physical disorders, resulting from estrogenic component - Less contraceptive effect for women with mental disorders that take barbiturates against convulsions, seizures and epilepsy
1. Progestogen-only pills 2. Injective progesterone contraception 3. Implant	- Injections and Implant - Highly effective methods - Does not require gynaecological examination - No increased risk for deep venous thromboembolism and thrombophlebitis - Injection is performed once every 12 weeks by the doctor - Implant effective for 3–5 years - Long-term use of progestogen-only methods frequently results in amenorrhea - Depo Provera can reduce menstruation related seizures in patients with epilepsy	- Progestogen-only pills need to be taken at exactly the same time - Progestogen injections and implants may initially cause irregular bleeding, which may complicate hygienic care. - After some months of use progestogen-only pills can lead to amenorrhea, especially in Depo Provera users, which can facilitate hygiene

have other barriers to oestrogen-containing contraception, and for those who have difficulty in remembering or administering short-acting contraception.

However, there are instances in which IUD contraception should be considered with caution. Women with a high spinal cord injury may develop autonomic dysreflexia (ADR) as a result of the stimulation caused by the insertion of the IUD. If the patient is at risk for ADR, an anaesthesiologist should be consulted for the insertion. Positioning for IUD insertion may be difficult for some women with contractures or spasms or for those who cannot cooperate with a pelvic exam. In some instances difficult insertions may require anaesthesia.

Barrier methods are of limited value in most disabled patients due to problems with mobility and emotional and practical difficulties to apply these methods in the context of intercourse (see Chapter 13). The condom is, however, an important part of the contraceptive methods disabled patients should be informed about as a means of protection against sexually transmitted infections (STIs) and for use in the context of forgetting a short-acting method like a combined hormonal contraceptive (CHC) or a progestogen-only pill.

Hormonal Methods

With consistent use CHCs have a high effectiveness and there is no need for gynaecological examination, no need for an intervention and no necessity to learn the application of the method (as with barrier methods) but the method is under the control of the woman. Hormonal methods of contraception have several important advantages related to menstruation, especially when used in a continuous regimen.

An important point to consider is the thromboembolic risk, which is increased in patients with reduced mobility or immobility. Another problem is the dependence of the method on regular use (forgetting the pill) and possible interactions with pharmacological treatments.

The main advantage of progestogen-only contraception methods (pill, injection, implant) is that they do not increase the risk of thromboembolism, which is important for patients with immobility or other risk factors. The progestogen-only pill has similar advantages to CHCs (no gynaecological examination, no need for intervention, under the control of the user). Like CHCs progestogen-only pills are user dependent, which may reduce their effectiveness. The major

disadvantage is the possible irregularity of bleeding, which may be irritating to the users and cause problems with hygiene.

Depomedroxyprogesterone acetate (DMPA) injections are largely user independent, but need three monthly injections. Their advantage lies in the reduction of menstrual problems by inducing amenorrhea. In patients with reduced mobility and activity this method may increase or aggravate pre-existing obesity.

The progestogen implant is independent of the user, does not need a gynaecological examination or intervention like IUD contraception and thus presents several advantages. The main disadvantage is the unpredictability of the developing bleeding pattern during use.

Emergency Contraception

Emergency contraception (EC) in the form of LNG or ulipristal tablets is an important option for almost all disabled patients independent of the individual form of disability (see Chapter 15) [12]. The most effective type of EC is the insertion of a copper IUD, which is suitable solution for many disabled patients, excluding those with high spinal injury as mentioned earlier in this chapter.

Permanent Contraception

Permanent contraception (tubal sterilization) with the consequence of infertility for the patient has advantages inherent to the method (highly effective, a one-time intervention under anaesthesia, no long-term health risks etc.). It needs, however, the full and informed consent of the patient. In cases where, due to intellectual or other mental disabilities, this cannot be ensured and the wish for permanent contraception comes from parents or other caregivers, the preference would be for long-lasting reversible contraceptives.

Information and Education about the Chosen Method

The patient should receive information about the effectiveness of different types of contraception and should be informed of the advantages and shortcomings of each. The information about side effects is important to prevent fear and discontinuation if these effects occur. At the same time the HCP can assure patients that these side effects are part of the adaptation to a method and disappear frequently after some time of use. Patients also need to be informed about side effects which indicate a health problem and which should be reported immediately (chest pain, breathlessness, abdominal pain etc.). Encourage women to call or visit if any changes occur which are unexpected or cause concern.

Patients should be provided with clear, practical instructions on how to use specific methods. Patients with intellectual disabilities should be provided with information on the use of alternative methods. Patients should know what to do in case of missing combined oral contraception – for example, use of additional contraception (condom) to prevent undesired pregnancy. Patients with intellectual and/or mental disabilities may need assistance or a reminder on how and when to take pills.

Healthcare providers should offer patients information on STIs and associated risks, including HIV and AIDS, and the use of condoms for protection together with another method for contraception (double protection). Patients should be informed about the possibility of tests regarding different types of STIs.

Follow-up Visits

Many women with disabilities using a contraceptive method need a good follow-up strategy to help them live with their method. Very often it is important to reassure them about the proper use, listen to them about their experience and concerns and encourage them to ask questions. The management of side effects is the same as for non-disabled users.

There may be other reasons for people with disabilities to come back to clinics – for example, to receive further contraception supplies or follow-up medical services – which may be somewhat difficult for people with disabilities due to lack of adapted transportation or other reasons. In this case alternative monitoring methods are selected. Doctors may need to remind patients with intellectual disabilities over the phone on using other means of communication.

Summary

Disability can manifest in different ways, including long-term physical, mental, intellectual or sensory impairments which have to be taken into account in the context of contraceptive counselling and care regarding specific needs, on one hand, with respect to patient-centred communication and, on the other, regarding the choice of the method based on advantages and disadvantages in relation to the individual disability. This selection should be whenever possible made together with the patient based on information and education. In cases of mental disability it is important that the HCP tries to find a solution in the best interest of the patient.

References

1. https://bit.ly/3X3z0jJ.

2. www.cdc.gov/ncbddd/disabilityandhealth/disability.html.

3. http://bit.ly/3YqSCPF.

4. Bickenbach JE, Chatterji S, Badley EM, Üstün TB. Models of disablement, universalism and the ICIDH. *Social Science and Medicine*. 1999;**48**:1173–87.

5. www.cdc.gov/ncbddd/disabilityandhealth/disability.html.

6. https://bit.ly/3RAIUZa.

7. Kripke C. Supported health care decision-making for people with intellectual and cognitive disabilities. *Family Practice*. 2016;**33**(5):445–6.

8. World Health Organization. *Medical eligibility criteria for contraceptive use*. 5th edition, 2015.

9. World Health Organization, Johns Hopkins Bloomberg School of Public Health Center for Communication Programs. *Family planning: A global handbook for providers*. Geneva: World Health Organization, 2018.

10. Wu JP, McKee KS, McKee MM et al. Use of reversible contraceptive methods among US women with physical or sensory disabilities. *Perspect Sex Reprod Health*. 2017;**49**(3):141–7.

11. Dickson J, Thwaites A, Bacon L. Contraception for adolescents with disabilities: Taking control of periods, cycles and conditions. *BMJ Sex Reprod Health*. 2018;**44**(1):7–13. First published as 10.1136/jfprhc-2017–101746 on 8 November 2017. http://jfprhc.bmj.com.

12. International Consortium for Emergency Contraception and International Federation of Gynecology and Obstetrics. *Emergency contraceptive pills (medical and service delivery guidelines)*. 3rd edition. N.p.: International Federation of Gynecology and Obstetrics, 2012.

Contraception in Women with Immunosuppressive Diseases

Charles Savona-Ventura, Alison Fava, and Judith-Marie Mifsud

Introduction

An immunosuppressive state can result from either a primary congenital condition reflecting an abnormality of the immune system or a secondary acquired condition resulting from medical conditions – for example, HIV – associated with a depression of the immune system. It can also be the result of incidental or purposeful effects of medications. Purposeful immunosuppressive therapy is commonly used to prevent the rejection of transplanted organs and tissues, but it may also be used to treat autoimmune disorders such as rheumatoid arthritis, systemic lupus erythematosus (SLE), multiple sclerosis, and inflammatory bowel disease (IBD). It may also be used in the treatment of other non-autoimmune inflammatory diseases such as bronchial asthma and ankylosing spondylitis.

Many oncological agents are associated with immunosuppression. The pathogenesis of the immunesuppressive state can be the result of a malfunction of one or more immune system components, notably deficiencies of the humoral immune system, of T-cell function, or complement deficiency; alternatively, it may be a result of asplenism or neutropenia. The immunocompromised individual is primarily at an increased risk of developing opportunistic infections. There may also be decreased cancer immunosurveillance [1].

Women in a primary or secondary immunosuppressive state may be at increased risk during pregnancy since pregnancy is generally believed to promote a degree of immune tolerance to prevent an immune response against the fetus. The mechanism behind immune tolerance during pregnancy is not, however, the promotion of an immunosuppressed state, but rather the creation of a controlled inflammatory environment leading to a delicate immune balance preventing a graft-versus-host by the fetus while modulating without suppression the mother's immunity [2]. Purposeful pharmacological induction of immunosuppression often relies on medications that may be teratogenic to the developing fetus. The need for adequate contraceptive advice is therefore often an essential component in the management of immunocompromised women. The choice of the right effective contraceptive method may be made difficult owing to physiological changes associated with the immunosuppressive-inducing condition or with the pharmacological agents inducing the immunosuppression.

Pharmacological Considerations

The main physiological effect of the immunosuppressive state is immunodeficiency, resulting in increased susceptibility to infections. This alone can influence the choice of contraceptives available to the women, since some methods of contraceptives, for example, a copper intrauterine device (Cu-IUD) or a levonorgestrel intrauterine system (LNG-IUS) – have been assumed to place the individual at a higher risk of pelvic inflammatory disease (PID). Based on this grade 3 criterion – that is, "theoretical or proved risks generally outweigh the advantages," the use of the Cu-IUD and the LNG-IUS was generally not recommended in HIV-positive women. However, controlled trials have suggested that HIV-positive immunosuppressed women showed no significant difference in PID rates between women using a Cu-IUD and depot progesterone for contraception, and recent guidelines recommend the use of these methods (Table 28.1) [3].

Progesterone has been shown to have immunomodulatory effects through a mechanism of inhibitory modulation of T-cell receptor signal transduction, suppressing cellular cytotoxicity, and inducing tolerant antigen-presenting cells [4]. Progestational agents can therefore be considered as promoting immunosuppression. Studies have shown a decrease in T-cell responsivity during intramuscular depot medroxyprogesterone acetate (DMPA) use. The observed immune suppression response to DMPA was, however, transient. The progestogen norethisterone enanthate does not exhibit any decrease in T-cell responsivity [5]. The use of

Table 28.1 Contraceptive choice in patients with a medical history of immunosuppression

	Cu-IUD		LNG-IUS		IMP	DMPA	POP	COC
Failure rate [after 15]	0.8%		0.2%		0.05%	6.0%	6.0–9.0%	9.0%
High-risk HIV	1		1		1	1	1	1
HIV infected:								
i) CD4 ≥ 200 cells/mm^3	2		2		1	1	1	1
ii) CD ≤ 200 cells/mm^3	Init. 3	Cont. 2	Init. 3	Cont. 2	1	1	1	1
IBD	1		1		1	1	2	2
SLE with no phospholipid antibodies	1		2		2	2	2	2
SLE with positive antiphospholipid antibodies	1		2		2	2	2	4
Rheumatic arthritis	1		2		2	2	2	2

1 = Use method in any circumstances; 2 = Generally use the method (advantages outweigh disadvantages]; 3 = Use of method not usually recommended unless other more appropriate methods are not available or not acceptable; 4 = Use of method pose unacceptable risk. Init. = initiation; Cont. = continuation

progestogen-containing contraceptives is not contraindicated in HIV-positive individuals [6].

The original medical condition may on its own accord affect physiological functions. This may also influence contraceptive method choice. Immunosuppressive medication is the mainstay option in the management of autoimmune disorders and non-autoimmune inflammatory disorders. Autoimmune disorders cause dysregulation of the immune system, generally involving multiple organ systems and causing chronic disease-related damage, with particular significance for the development of renal disease and an increased predisposition to thrombosis – a definite consideration when using hormonal contraception in individuals with conditions increasing the risk of thrombosis. Studies have suggested an increased risk of thrombosis in SLE women with positive antiphospholipid antibodies when using combined hormonal contraceptives. No such associations appear to be present with progesterone-only based contraceptives [7]. Hormonal contraceptives may also influence the susceptibility to autoimmune diseases increasing the risks from the condition [8].

Other autoimmune processes can affect endocrine systems such as thyroid or pancreatic β-cell dysfunction, which can separately affect overall reproductive function. Chronic inflammatory bowel disease, with its attendant chronic diarrhea and malabsorption,

Table 28.2 Medical eligibility criteria categories for contraceptive use [6]

Category 1	A condition for which there is no restriction for the use of the contraceptive method
Category 2	A condition for which the advantages of using the method generally outweigh the theoretical or proven risks
Category 3	A condition for which the theoretical or proven risks usually outweigh the advantages of using the method
Category 4	A condition that represents an unacceptable health risk if the contraceptive method is used

could interfere with the absorption of any oral contraceptive. It is therefore essential to categorize the individual's risk of using the different forms of contraception according to the different medical conditions and/or medications being used (Table 28.2).

The pharmacological treatment administered to manage immunosuppressive disease may itself affect the pharmacokinetics of hormonal contraceptives, potentially reducing bioavailability and hence effectiveness. Immunosuppressive drugs can directly interfere with intestinal absorption of other medications [9], while immunosuppressant medications that may induce vomiting (e.g., cisplatin, cyclophosphamide, doxorubicin) or cause diarrhea (e.g., 5-fluorouracil, irinotecan, capecitabine) will also affect the bioavailability of hormonal contraceptives.

Other medications may act as estrogen-related enzyme-inducers, or inhibitors, to respectively decrease or increase the bioavailability of estrogen and progesterone. The antiretroviral ritonavir is known to induce glucuronidation, thereby reducing the bioavailability of estrogen and progestogens [10]. In contrast, the anti-rejection medication tacrolimus is known to be enzyme-inhibiting, thus increasing the bioavailability of the hormones [11]. Reversely, hormonal contraceptive drugs may alter the bioavailability of immunosuppressant medication, necessitating an assessment of regular serum concentrations of the medication. Ethinyl estradiol and progestogens are known to contribute to an increase in serum concentration of tacrolimus and ciclosporin concentrations. Ulipristal acetate may increase the serum concentrations of the drugs everolimus and sirolimus [12].

Effect of Hormonal Contraceptives on the Evolution of Immunosuppressive Disease

The sex steroids in hormonal contraceptives have been associated with immune system modulation by a yet unspecified mechanism, potentially affecting the development and progression of autoimmune diseases and generally increasing the risks of developing the condition [13]. Estrogen–progestogen combinations have been linked with an increased risk of developing autoimmune conditions such as SLE, ulcerative colitis and Crohn's disease, interstitial cystitis, and multiple sclerosis. Long-term use correlates with an increased need for surgery in IBD [8, 14]. While data regarding the association of hormonal contraception and the risk of developing SLE are not consistent, high-quality cohort studies show a positive correlation between hormonal contraception use (both current and past) and development of SLE.

Data regarding the risk of multiple sclerosis with hormonal contraceptive use are also not consistent, but a meta-analysis of six studies concluded the risk may be increased with hormonal contraceptive use. Evidence regarding hormonal contraception use and rheumatoid arthritis risk is conflicting. In contrast, combined oral contraceptives appear to lower the incidence of hyperthyroidism [8]. Progestogen-only hormonal contraceptives have been associated with progesterone-linked skin disorders such as dermatitis,

eczema, urticaria, alopecia, acne, and pruritus, and to progesterone-linked arthropathies [8]. Clinicians should therefore carefully evaluate contraceptive options and closely monitor the progression of any established autoimmune disease when women opt to use hormonal contraception.

Conclusion

It is clearly evident that contraception for women with immunosuppressive disease or on immunosuppressive therapy is associated with potential risks and must be used judiciously, balancing potential immunosuppression-related side effects and the efficacy of the chosen contraceptive method and its potential effects on the medical condition (Table 28.3).

Table 28.3 Practice guidelines [after 12]

History of immunosuppressant therapy use
When advising on contraception, a thorough history is important

Women taking immunosuppressant therapy should be informed about possible drug interactions when considering starting hormonal contraception.
Women using hormonal contraception should discuss it with a healthcare professional before starting a new immunosuppressant drug.

KEY CONSIDERATIONS
Women on immunosuppressant drugs that cause severe drug-induced vomiting or diarrhea should be cautious when using oral hormonal contraception and concomitant consistent use of condoms is advised.
Women on enzyme-inducing immunosuppressant therapy are not advised to use oral hormonal contraception or a progesterone-only implant.
Women on immunosuppressant therapy can be reassured that the contraceptive efficacy of the Cu-IUD, LNG-IUS, and injectable DMPA are not affected by any immunosuppressant drug therapy interactions.
Women on enzyme-inducing immunosuppressant drugs who require hormonal contraception can be advised on concomitant consistent use of condoms.
Women on enzyme-inducing immunosuppressant drugs who need emergency contraception should be offered a Cu-IUD. If this is not suitable, a double dose of levonorgestrel emergency contraception may be used.
Women who are taking immunosuppressant therapy with known teratogenic potential (e.g., methotrexate) should be advised to use a contraception method that is highly effective, including Cu-IUD, LNG-IUS, and a progesterone-only implant, both during use and for a recommended time frame after stopping. Women using CHC, POP, and DMPA require additional methods of contraception (e.g., condoms) when prescribed teratogenic medications, in view of the failure rate associated with these contraceptives (CHC and POP 9%; DMPA 6%). The failure rates of other forms of contraception are unacceptably high to be considered effective in these circumstances (fertility-awareness-based methods 24%; spermicides 28%; barrier methods 12–24%). Male or female sterilization is also an effective contraceptive option.

References

1. Heise ER. Diseases associated with immunosuppression. *Environ Health Perspect.* 1982;**43**:9–19. https://doi.org/10.1289/ehp.82439.

2. Mor G, Cardenas I. The immune system in pregnancy: a unique complexity. *Am J Reprod Immunol.* 2010;**63** (6):425–33. https://doi.org/10.1111/j.1600-0897 .2010.00836.x.

3. Hofmeyr GJ, Singata M, Lawrie TA. Copper containing intra-uterine devices versus depot progestogens for contraception. *Cochrane Database of Systematic Reviews* 2010;**6**:CD007043. https://doi.org/10.1002/14 651858.CD007043.pub2.

4. Shah NM, Lai PF, Imami N, Johnson MR. Progesterone-related immune modulation of pregnancy and labor. *Front. Endocrinol.* 2019;**10**:1–19. https://doi.org/10.3389/fendo.2019.00198.

5. Matubu A, Hillier SL, Meyn LA et al. Depot medroxyprogesterone acetate and norethisterone enanthate differentially impact T-cell responses and expression of immunosuppressive markers. *Am J Reprod Immunol.* 2020;**83**:e13210. https://doi.org/10.1111/aji .13210.

6. World Health Organization. *Medical eligibility criteria for contraceptive use.* 5th edition. Geneva: World Health Organization, 2015.

7. Culwell KR, Curtis KM. Contraception for women with systemic lupus erythematosus. *Journal of Family Planning and Reproductive Health Care* 2013;**39**:9–11. https://doi.org/10.1136/jfprhc-2012-100437.

8. Williams WV. Hormonal contraception and the development of autoimmunity: A review of the literature. *Linacre Q.* 2017;**84**(3):275–95. https://doi .org/10.1080/00243639.2017.1360065.

9. Aggarwal V, Williams MD, Beath SV. Gastrointestinal problems in the immunosuppressed patient. *Archives of Disease in Childhood* 1998;**78**:5–8.

10. Tseng A, Hills-Nieminen C. Drug interactions between antiretrovirals and hormonal contraceptives. *Expert Opin Drug Metab Toxicol.* 2013;**9**(5):559–72.

11. Migali G, Tintillier M. Interaction between estradiol and tacrolimus in kidney-transplanted menopausal women. *NDT Plus.* 2008;**1**(4):277–8. https://doi.org/ 10.1093/ndtplus/sfn035.

12. Faculty of Sexual and Reproductive Healthcare. *Clinical guidance: Drug interactions with hormonal contraception.* London: Faculty of Sexual and Reproductive Healthcare, 2017.

13. Mann DR, Ansari AA, Akinbami MA et al. Neonatal treatment with luteinizing hormone-releasing hormone analogs alters peripheral lymphocyte subsets and cellular and humorally mediated immune responses in juvenile and adult male monkeys. *J Clin Endocrinol Metab.* 1994;**78**(2):292–8.

14. Khalili H, Granath F, Smedby KE et al. Association between long-term oral contraceptive use and risk of Crohn's disease complications in a nationwide study. *Gastroenterology* 2016;**150**(7):1561–7.e1.

15. Gavin L, Moskosky S, Carter M et al. Providing quality family planning services: Recommendations of CDC and the U.S. Office of Population Affairs. Morbidity and mortality weekly report. *Recommendations and Reports* 2014;**63**(4):1–54.

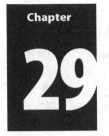

Contraception in Women with Lupus Autoimmune Diseases

Parivakkam S. Arunakumari and Charlotte Gatenby

Introduction

Access to safe and effective contraception is a basic human right for all women, including those with lupus autoimmune diseases (LADs) [1]. Lupus auto-immune diseases predominantly affect young to middle-aged women, a patient population more likely to require contraception [2]. They include systemic lupus erythematosus (SLE) and/or anti-phospholipid syndrome (APS).

Definitions

Systemic lupus erythematosus is a complex systemic autoimmune disease with a probable female-to-male ratio of 10:1 [3]. Anti-phospholipid syndrome is diagnosed based on the persistent presence of anti-phospholipid antibodies (aPLs) and vascular thrombosis and/or pregnancy complications. Three clinically relevant and well-characterized aPLs (antibodies associated with thrombosis) are lupus anticoagulant (LA), anticardiolipin antibodies (ACA, IgG and IgM) and β2 glycoprotein I antibodies (aβ2GPI, IgG and IgM) [4].

Anti-phospholipid syndrome can occur in otherwise healthy people without underlying systemic autoimmune disease (primary APS) or with other systemic autoimmune diseases, particularly SLE. In this population aPLs are common, with 30–40% of SLE patients testing positive for aPL [4, 5].

Pathophysiology

Systemic lupus erythematosus can affect any organ in the body due to autoantibody production, complement activation and immune complex deposition [2]. Women with SLE are at increased risk of ischemic heart disease, stroke and venous thromboembolism (VTE) [3]. Testing positive for aPL is not in itself a disease state and, in the absence of manifestations of APS, stratification of risk with specialist advice, if necessary, is recommended. In particular, persistence of aPL positivity, a high titre of aPL, LA positivity, triple positivity for LA, aCL, aβ2GP1 and IgG aPL have a greater risk of future events [6].

Significance of Contraception

Contraception should be an essential discussion point in all consultations for women with LAD as:

1. The majority of women with LAD have normal fertility.
2. Pregnancy poses additional risks due to:

   a. obstetric complications;
   b. fetal complications;
   c. worsening of disease activity; or
   d. adverse effects of medication on both mother and baby [3].

Medical Eligibility Criteria

The United Kingdom Medical Eligibility Criteria (UK MEC) provide guidance on the use of contraceptive methods through optimizing choice within acceptable margins of safety (see Tables 29.1–29.3) [6].

Table 29.1 Medical Eligibility Criteria

UKMEC/ WHOMEC/ USMEC	Definition
1	No restriction for use of the method.
2	Advantages of the method outweigh the theoretical or proven risks.
3	Theoretical or proven risks usually outweigh the advantages. Provision requires specialist expert opinion as use not usually recommended.
4	Use of this method represents an unacceptable health risk.

Table 29.2 Contraceptive methods and associated Medical Eligibility Criteria scores with systemic lupus erythematosus [6, 11, 12]

Method	Method of action	UKMEC		WHOMEC	USMEC	Failure rates	
		aPL −	aPL +	SLE	SLE	Typical use	Perfect use
POP	Thickens cervical mucus	2	2	3	3	9%	0.3%
IMP	Inhibits ovulation and thickens cervical mucus	2	2	3	3	0.05%	0.05%
DMPA	Prevents follicular maturation and thus ovulation. Also thickens cervical mucus	2	2	3	3	6%	0.2%
CHC	Inhibits follicular development preventing ovulation	2	4	4	4	9%	0.3%
LNG-IUS	Thinning of endometrial lining and thickening of cervical mucus	2	2	3	3	0.2%	0.2%
Cu-IUD	Toxic to sperm and ova. Prevents implantation due to local endometrial inflammation.	1	1	1	1	0.8%	0.8%

Table 29.3 Medical Eligibility Criteria for emergency contraception methods [6,11,12,13]

Method	Method of action	UKMEC	WHOMEC	USMEC	Estimated pregnancy rates
UPA	Progesterone receptor modulator licenced for use up to120 hours after UPSI. Delays ovulation for up to 5 days.	No specific mention	Reduced dose from regular usage therefore safe for use	No specific mention	1–2%
LNG	Inhibits ovulation by delaying follicular rupture resulting in luteal dysfunction. Licenced for use for 72 hours after UPSI.	No specific mention	Reduced dose from regular usage therefore safe for use	No specific mention	0.6–2.6%
Cu-IUD	Toxic effect on sperm and ova. Local endometrial inflammation, prevents implantation. Can be used for up to 120 hours after UPSI or within 5 days of expected ovulation.	1	1	No specific mention	<0.1%

Contraceptive Methods and Lupus Autoimmune Disease

Fertility Awareness Methods

Involves one of more of the following:

- basal body temperature charting;
- cervical mucus monitoring;
- monitoring changes in cervix; and
- calculating fertile days.

Fertility awareness methods of contraception may be appropriate for the highly motivated couple but cannot be recommended on their own due to the serious consequences of unintended pregnancy in women with SLE.

Barrier Methods

Male and female condoms are safe with no restrictions for use for women with LAD. Their additional use is recommended when potential drug interactions (corticosteroids, immunosuppressant and teratogenic medications) pose concerns [7].

Intrauterine Methods

Intrauterine methods of contraception are highly effective with licenced use from 3 to 10 years.

Copper-Bearing Intrauterine Devices

Copper-bearing intrauterine devices (Cu-IUDs) require no restrictions for use in women with LAD with or without aPL positivity. This can increase heavy menstrual bleeding (HMB), potentially resulting in anaemia. Hence, where thrombocytopenia is a feature of the disease or the woman is on anticoagulants, the risks outweigh the benefits for initiation [3, 6].

Levonorgestrel-Releasing Intrauterine Systems

The advantages of levonorgestrel-releasing intrauterine systems (LNG-IUS) outweigh the risks of low-dose exposure to progestogen. They may be positively indicated for women with LAD who also experience HMB as they can reduce menstrual blood loss by up to 96% following the first year of use [6, 8].

Progesterone-Only Contraception

Given the thrombotic concerns with oestrogen, progesterone-only contraception (POC) methods are more popular in women with LAD.

Progesterone-Only Pill

Typical preparations and doses of the progesterone-only pill (POP) per day include:

Norethisterone – 350micrograms

Levonorgestrel – 30micrograms

Desogestrel – 75micrograms

Advantages of this method generally outweigh the benefits. Individualization is necessary in patients with high risk factors for thrombosis. Irregular bleeding patterns can occur in between 20 and 50% patients on this method, resulting in high discontinuation rates [9].

Depo Medroxyprogesterone Acetate

Depo medroxyprogesterone acetate (DMPA) is available in intra-muscular and subcutaneous injections provided at 13 weekly intervals in the United Kingdom (12 weekly outside the United Kingdom). Women with SLE are at increased risk of osteopenia due to both the disease and/or steroid use. These patients should be assessed for additional risk factors for osteopenia prior to prescribing DMPA [6, 7].

Implant

An implant is an attractive option as it is licenced for 3 years with no adverse effect on bone mineral density and increased efficacy as it is non-user dependent. However, as the implant requires an invasive procedure for insertion, haematoma may occur in women with low platelets [10].

Combined Hormonal Contraception

This guidance applies to combined oral contraception (COC), vaginal rings and transdermal patches. There is no association between combined hormonal contraception (CHC) and disease flares in patients with LAD [6]. Combined hormonal contraception is, however, known to increase VTE risk in healthy women of reproductive age. Arterial and venous thromboembolism are major causes of death for women with SLE and this risk is increased by aPL positivity. As such, use of CHC in patients positive for aPL represents an unacceptable health risk [6].

However, for women with SLE without aPL positivity, provided there are no other contraindications to use, the benefits of CHC outweigh the risks. Further, patients may also reap the non-contraceptive benefits of CHC, including reduction in dysmenorrhoea, HMB and acne [3, 6].

i. COC: Consider prescribing second-generation pills containing a lower dose of oestrogen, thus reducing VTE risk [6].
ii. Patches: An average of 33.9 micrograms of ethinylestradiol and 203 micrograms of norelgestromin can be released per day [6]. The same considerations apply as for the COC.
iii. Vaginal rings: Vaginal rings release ethinylestradiol 15 micrograms and etonorgestrel 120 micrograms daily. They require insertion only once every 3

weeks and provide the lowest oestrogen dose; therefore, they offer an attractive alternative [6].

There are no special considerations for sterilization in women with LAD.

Emergency Contraception

Women with LAD are no more or no less at risk of requiring emergency contraception (EC) than the general population. All methods of EC can be used [13].

The Summary of Product Characteristics (SPC) for ulipristal acetate (UPA-EC) advises against its use in women with severe asthma controlled by oral glucocorticoids due to its anti-glucocorticoid effect. It is unknown whether the same consideration applies to women on corticosteroids for SLE [13].

The SPC for Levonelle® (LNG-EC) states its use is not recommended in patients with severe hepatic dysfunction. However, pregnancy poses a significant risk in women with severe hepatic impairment and expert opinion suggests that use of a single dose of LNG 1.5 mg is therefore acceptable [13].

According to the Yuzpe Method, 100 μg of ethinyl estradiol and levonorgestrel 0.5 mg given within 72 hours of intercourse and repeated 12 hours later inhibits ovulation. This is not used in the United Kingdom as studies demonstrate that it is less effective than LNG-EC. However, where used, as its use is short term, it is considered safe [14].

Contraceptive Considerations for Women Using Teratogenic Medications for Disease Control

Practical Tips for Contraception Consultations for Women with Lupus Autoimmune Disease

- Take a detailed history of all organ systems.
- Determine aPL status.
- Assess thrombotic risk.
- Ascertain use of teratogenic medications (Table 29.4).
- Discuss options on an individual basis.
- Refer to MEC for guidance.
- Promote long-acting reversible contraceptives.

Conclusion

Available evidence indicates that many women with LAD can be good candidates for most methods of contraception, including hormonal contraception.

References

1. World Health Organization. *WHO model list of essential medications 21st list 2019*. Geneva: World Health Organization, 2019, pp. 46–7.

2. Parks C, de Souza Espindola Santos A, Barbhaiya M, Costenbader K. Understanding the role of environmental factors in the development of systemic lupus erythematosus. *Best Practice & Research Clinical Rheumatology*. 2017;**31**(3):306–20.

3. Culwell K, Curtis K. Contraception for women with systemic lupus erythematosus. *BMJ Sexual and Reproductive Health*. 2013;**39**(1):9–11. https://srh.bmj.com/content/39/1/9.

4. *Recurrent pregnancy loss*. 2nd edition. Strombek-Bever: European Society of Human Reproduction and Embryology, 2017. http://bit.ly/3RuaUxs.

5. Unlu O, Zuily S, Erkan D. The clinical significance of antiphospholipid antibodies in systemic lupus erythematosus. *European Journal of Rheumatology*. 2016;**3**(2):75–84. https://bit.ly/40pvQts.

6. United Kingdom Medical Eligibility Criteria (UK MEC). 2016. http://ukmec.pagelizard.com/2016.

7. Tesher M, Whitaker A, Gilliam M, Wagner-Weiner L, Onel K. Contraception for adolescents with lupus. *Pediatric Rheumatology*. 2010;**8**(1):10.

8. National Institute for Health and Care Excellence. Heavy menstrual bleeding: Assessment and management. 2018. https://bit.ly/3JEZ3KP.

9. *Progesterone only pill*. 2nd edition. Edinburgh: Clinical Effectiveness Unit, 2015. https://bit.ly/3Y8mVuT.

10. *Progesterone only implants*. 1st edition. Edinburgh: Clinical Effectiveness Unit, 2014. http://bit.ly/3l2xNf7.

11. World Health Organization. *Medical Eligibility Criteria for contraceptive use*. Geneva: World Health Organization, 2015. https://bit.ly/40wrqRt.

12. Centers for Disease Control. US Medical Eligibility Criteria (US MEC) for contraceptive use. 2016 | CDC. Cdc.gov. 2020. http://bit.ly/3RhFASx.

Table 29.4 Teratogenic drugs commonly used in management of lupus [15, 16]

Medication	Method of action	Contraceptive advice
Cyclophosphamide	Alkylating agent. Cytotoxic, could result in congenital or fetal malformations [15, 16]	Commence contraception prior to first dose and continue for 3 months after finishing treatment [16]
Mycophenolate mofetil	Antiproliferative immunosuppressant – suppresses cell-mediated immune responses and antibody formation [16]	Women should use contraception throughout treatment course and for 6 weeks. Female partners of males using this drug should continue contraception for 3 months after their partner has discontinued medication. [15, 16]
Methotrexate	Prevents RNA and DNA synthesis – teratogenic [15, 16]	Contraception required during and for 6 months after treatment for females and males [15, 16]
Glucocorticoids	Immunosuppressant – modulates gene transcription to reduce inflammation [16]	Caution advised, avoid unplanned conception [16]
Hydroxy Chloroquine	Alters stability of cell membranes and signalling pathways [16]	Minimal fetal or maternal risk: hence often continued in pregnancy [16]
Azathioprine	Inhibits DNA and RNA synthesis [16]	Post exposure reports of low birth weight and premature delivery. Effective contraception required during treatment. [16]
Rituximab	Lysis of B lymphocytes [16].	Recommend contraception during and for 12 months post treatment [15, 16]
Leflunomide	Pyramidine synthesis inhibitor – teratogenic in animal studies [15, 16]	Females: Advise contraception for duration of treatment and for at least 2 years after treatment course. Males advised to avoid conception for 3 months after treatment. [15]

13. Faculty of Sexual and Reproductive Healthcare. FSRH clinical guideline: Emergency contraception (March 2017, amended December 2017). 2017. http://bit.ly/3Y26ZKN.

14. World Health Organization. Emergency contraception factsheet. 2018. http://bit.ly/3DFpUTh.

15. Bermas B, Smith NA. UpToDate. 2020. http://bit.ly/3DEDmqI.

16. National Institute for Health and Care Excellence. Cytotoxic drugs | Treatment summary | BNF content published by NICE. 2020. http://bit.ly/3YlspC7.

Chapter 30

Contraception in Women with Chronic Kidney Disease

Jean-Jacques Ries and Johannes Bitzer

Introduction

Chronic kidney disease (CKD), also known as chronic renal disease, is a condition characterized by a gradual loss of kidney function over time. It is a common condition often associated with getting older, but it can affect anyone [1]. The causes are manifold, including kidney diseases, diabetic nephropathy and diabetes, hypertension, immunopathologies like systemic lupus erythematosus (SLE) with and without anti-phospholipid antibodies and kidney transplantation (uncomplicated, complicated).

The gradual loss of function is described in different stages characterized by clinical and functional signs [2].

Stage 1   (G1): A normal estimated glomerular filtration rate (eGFR) above 90 ml/min, but other tests have detected signs of kidney damage. Mild kidney damage with normal function.

Stage 2   (G2): A slightly reduced eGFR of 60–89 ml/min, with other signs of mild kidney damage.

Stage 3a   (G3a): An eGFR of 45–59 ml/min. Slightly reduced function with mild kidney disease.

Stage 3b   (G3b): An eGFR of 30–44 ml/min. Functional reduction with mild and moderate kidney damage.

Stage 4   Severe CKD (glomerular filtration rate (GFR) = 15–29 mL/min): Severe kidney damage close to renal failure.

Stage 5   End-Stage CKD (GFR <15 mL/min): Most severe kidney damage

(www.kidneyfund.org/all-about-kidneys/stages-kidney-disease).

Contraceptive Needs

Adequate counselling about contraception is very important at all stages of the disease and should consider the effect of contraceptive on the disease, but also the effect the disease has on the choice of contraceptive method [3]. A badly timed pregnancy can result in disease progression and exposure of an unborn child to teratogenic medications (e.g. mycophenolate mofetil, angiotensin blockers, cyclophosphamide). Pregnancy in CKD is associated with a higher risk of complications: preeclampsia, fetal growth restriction and preterm delivery increase with the severity of CKD and proteinuria [4]. Pregnancy also can exacerbate comorbidities such as anaemia, vitamin D deficiency and hypertension. Around 33–50% of all pregnancies among renal transplant recipients are unplanned [4].

Chronic kidney disease and dialysis affect hypothalamic-pituitary-gonadal axis function and can lead to menstrual abnormalities, sexual dysfunction, functional menopause and loss of fertility, but a pregnancy incidence of 1–7% has been reported [5–7]. Successful kidney transplantation restores fertility and these patients should be protected by an effective method of contraception [3, 7]. It is advised to avoid a pregnancy for up to 24 months after transplantation [8–10].

Contraceptive Methods

Combined Hormonal Contraceptives

Combined hormonal contraceptives are available in different dosages and galenic forms and are very effective (Pearl Index < 1 if correctly used), but the cardiovascular and thrombotic risk is increased. The World Health Organization (WHO) Medical Eligibility Criteria classification of contraceptives takes into account some nephropathies (cats. 1–2: CHC can be given; cats. 3–4: CHC should be avoided) [11].

- Diabetic nephropathy (category 3 or 4 depending on severity).
- Diabetes without vascular disease, normotensive, well controlled and in remission (category 2).

- SLE (category 2), if anti-phospholipid antibodies are present (category 4).
- Kidney transplantation (category 2 if uncomplicated, up to category 4 in case of organ failure or acute/chronic rejection).
- Hypertension, even moderate and well controlled (category 3).

Some side effects and risks of CHC are particularly important in CKD patients, including thromboembolic and cardiovascular events, induction or worsening of albuminuria. The use of a transdermal patch is associated with higher circulating hormone levels and thus adverse effects. Alternatives should always be sought in advanced and progressive CKD, immunologic diseases and complicated kidney transplantation; proteinuria and hypertension increase the risk of adverse effects [3].

Progestin-Only Contraceptives

The main advantage of progestin-only contraceptives is their lower impact on coagulation and blood pressure, which can be relevant for many women with CKD. The WHO has given no absolute contraindication for progestin-only contraceptive use in CKD patients [3]:

- Hypertension (category 1–2).
- SLE (category 2; if anti-phospholipid antibodies are present, category 3).
- Kidney transplantation (category 2), independent of hypertension, proteinuria or functional reduction.
- Diabetic nephropathy (pills, implants: category 2; injectables: category 3).
- There can be an interaction with calcineurin inhibitors.

Progestin-only contraceptives are not contraindicated in dialysis patients. In case of treatment with heparin during dialysis, patients can have some vaginal spotting. Progestin-only contraceptives can be used in patients with intense bleeding to reduce the intensity of the bleeding. Furthermore they can be used in the postpartum and lactation period. (see also the levonorgestrel-releasing intrauterine device (LNG IUD) later in this chapter).

Intrauterine Devices

Copper IUDs and LNG IUDs are both very effective and, once placed, they can stay for the whole duration of their activity and be removed quickly if necessary – that is, if a pregnancy is planned or if a complication occurs.

Intrauterine devices can be used at any stage of kidney disease. A main advantage, especially regarding CKD patients, is the avoidance of drug interactions There is a concern about infections and failure of IUDs in immunosuppressed patients. The uterine milieu is predominantly populated by macrophages, whereas immunosuppression used in the management of immunological renal disease and following transplantation acts predominantly via lymphocyte inhibition, suggesting that different pathways are involved [3]. As there is in general an increased risk of pelvic infection during the first 3 weeks after insertion, the use of intrauterine contraception should be avoided in patients with pyelonephritis, peritoneal dialysis and malformations [3].

No evidence of IUD failure in CKD patients has been reported [3]. It also seems that there is no higher incidence of infections. Caution should still be given to prevent infection at placement in at-risk patients. The LNG IUD, which induces a thickening of cervical mucus, did not show an increased risk of infection in a small retrospective case series of immune-suppressed renal transplant recipients [12].

Barrier Methods

Barrier methods (condoms, diaphragms, femidoms, cervical caps and sponges) have the advantage of a low rate of side effects. They are safe, do not interact with drugs and protect against sexually transmitted infections. The downside is their lower efficiency compared to other contraceptive methods. In CKD patients, especially those under immune suppression, particular care should be given to avoid barrier methods with an additional use of spermicide (i.e. diaphragms or cervical caps) as these promote urinary tract infections [13].

Surgical Sterilization

Surgical sterilization is a non-reversible contraceptive method. Options for surgical sterilization include female (tubal sterilization) and male surgical sterilization (vasectomy). The risks of these methods are linked to the surgical procedures (see Chapter 14).

Female sterilization is done by laparoscopy or by laparotomy, for example during caesarean section. It can be done by ligature or removal (salpingectomy) of the fallopian tubes. The latter procedure has a protective effect against certain forms of ovarian cancer [14]. Especially during caesarean section the removal of the fallopian trumps can be technically difficult and tubal ligation is done in that case.

Emergency Contraception

Emergency contraception is used to prevent an unintended pregnancy after unprotected or insufficiently protected sexual intercourse. It should be administered within 120 hours after the intercourse in order to be efficient. Options include the administration of a high dosage of progestin (Levonorgestrel 1.5 mg), a selective progestin receptor modulator (Ulipristal acetate 30 mg) or the placement of a copper-bearing IUD.

As these contraceptives do not contain oestrogens they can be administered in patients with CKD; caution is advised in severe chronic liver disease [3]. The WHO only gives a warning in case of venous thromboembolism. Repeated use of this form of contraception is not recommended [11]. A high dose of steroid hormones can interact with the metabolism of several drugs (e.g. calcineurin inhibitors) [3].

Recommendations for contraception in women with kidney disease include the following (see Table 30.1) [3, 15]. During most stages of the disease up to stage 3A, and if the patient does not suffer from hypertension or SLE with anti-phospholipid antibodies, basically all methods can be used with some exceptions. In patients with CKD in the context of hypertension or SLE with anti-phospholipid antibodies, CHC are contraindicated and CHC should be avoided in patients with proteinuria and diabetic nephropathy.

The vaginal ring and spermicides should be avoided in patients with recurrent infections or immunosuppressive therapy. The use of intrauterine contraceptives (copper IUD, LNG IUD) has a good efficacy/risk profile if measures are taken to prevent infection. Progestin-only contraceptives (progestin-only pill, implant) can be used in general.

Table 30.1 Elibility Criteria Kidney Diseases

- Stage 1-2-3A *(GFR ≥ 45 ml/min/1.73 m²)*[13]	No hypertension no SLE+aPL	All methods
- Hypertension, SLE, aPL - Stage 3B-4–5 *(GFR ≤ 44 ml/min/1.73 m²)*[13]		Avoid CHCs

Summary

Contraception in women with CKD needs to be highly effective in order to prevent an unplanned pregnancy which can induce a disease progression, exposure of the fetus to teratogenic substances and severe pregnancy complications like preeclampsia or preterm delivery. At the same time the methods used must consider contraindications related to the renal function and underlying diseases and drug treatment. Taking into account the balance between efficacy and health risks as well as additional factors to consider (comorbidities), it seems intrauterine contraception (copper IUD, LNG IUD) methods provide a good efficacy/risk profile. Care has to be taken during the insertion in immunosuppressed patients. Progestin-only contraceptives have a favourable risk profile with respect to cardiovascular complications, which is for most patients an important advantage. Combined hormonal contraceptives can be used in patients with stage 1–3a kidney disease without hypertension and without SLE with anti-phospholipid antibodies.

References

1. www.kidney.org/atoz/content/about-chronic-kidney-disease.

2. www.kidneyfund.org/all-about-kidneys/stages-kidney-disease.

3. Attini R, Cabiddu G, Montersino B et al. Contraception in chronic kidney disease: A best practice position statement by the Kidney and Pregnancy Group of the Italian Society of Nephrology. *J Nephrol.* 2020;**33**(6):1343–59.

4. Wiles KS, Nelson-Piercy C, Bramham K. Reproductive health and pregnancy in women with chronic kidney disease. *Nat Rev Nephrol.* 2018;**14**:165–84.

5. Ahmed SB, Vitek WS, Holley JL. Fertility, contraception, and novel reproductive technologies in chronic kidney disease. *Semin Nephrol.* 2017;**37**:327–36.

6. Burgner A, Hladunewich MA. Women's reproductive health for the nephrologist. *Am J Kidney Dis.* 2019;**74**:675–81.

7. Ahmed SB, Ramesh S. Sex hormones in women with kidney disease. *Nephrol Dial Transplant.* 2016;**31**:1787–95.

8. Nadeau-Fredette A-C, Hladunewich M, Hui D, Keunen J, Chan CT. End-stage renal disease and pregnancy. *Adv Chronic Kidney Dis.* 2013;**20**:246–52.

9. Lessan-Pezeshki M, Ghazizadeh S, Khatami MR et al. Fertility and contraceptive issues after kidney transplantation in women. *Transplant Proc.* 2004;**36**:1405–6.

10. Paulen ME, Folger SG, Curtis KM, Jamieson DJ. Contraceptive use among solid organ transplant patients: A systematic review. *Contraception.* 2010;**82**:102–12.

11. World Health Organization. Medical eligibility criteria for contraceptive use. 2015. https://bit.ly /3HxV1BB.

12. Ramhendar T, Byrne P. Use of the levonorgestrel-releasing intrauterine system in renal transplant recipients: A retrospective case review. *Contraception.* 2012;**86**:288–9.

13. Gupta K, Stamm WE. Pathogenesis and management of recurrent urinary tract infections in women. *World J Urol.* 1999;**17**:415–20.

14. Evans EC, Matteson KA, Orejuela FJ et al. Salpingo-oophorectomy at the time of benign hysterectomy. *Obstet Gynecol.* 2016;**128**:476–85.

15. Inker LA, Astor BC, Fox CH et al. KDOQI US commentary on the 2012 KDIGO clinical practice guideline for the evaluation and management of CKD. *Am J Kidney Dis.* 2014;**63**:713–35.

Chapter 31

Contraception in Women with Diabetes

Parivakkam S. Arunakumari and Charlotte Gatenby

Introduction

Diabetes mellitus (DM) is a major global public health concern affecting up to 10% of women of reproductive age in developed countries [1]. The number of affected individuals is steadily increasing globally [2].

Definition and Classification

Diabetes mellitus is a syndrome of hyperglycaemia that can broadly be classified into two types [1].

Type 1 diabetes (T1DM). Type 1 diabetes is a chronic, autoimmune condition with onset usually occurring before the age of 40 years. It accounts for approximately 10% of cases in adults and 98% of cases in children. Type 1 diabetes is caused by the primary beta cells of the pancreas failing to produce insulin, resulting in hyperglycaemia. Treatment involves careful glucose monitoring and administration of insulin in response to maintain good glycaemic control [1].

Type 2 diabetes (T2DM). Type 2 diabetes is caused by an insufficiency in the amount of insulin produced by the pancreatic beta cells, or it can be due to the development of resistance to the insulin produced. Approximately 90% of cases occur in adults. There is, however, an increasing number of cases in children. Type 2 diabetes is a condition associated with obesity, and, as such, treatment involves encouraging better diet and exercise regimes, oral medications and, occasionally, insulin [1].

Gestational diabetes mellitus (GDM). Gestational diabetes mellitus relates only to pregnancy and is not discussed in this chapter apart from postnatal considerations.

Significance of Contraception for Women with Diabetes Mellitus

Diabetes mellitus can result in numerous complications with long-term health implications for vascular,

neurological, renal and ophthalmic functions [1]. Poor glycaemic control, from a reproductive perspective, increases the risk of several adverse pregnancy outcomes, including intrauterine death, congenital abnormalities and maternal complications [3]. There is no evidence to suggest that DM impairs fertility [1]. Hence contraception is an important consideration for all diabetic women [4].

Medical Eligibility Criteria and Evidence

Medical eligibility criteria (MEC) were originally developed by the World Health Organization (WHO) in 1996 with the latest update in 2015 [5].

In 2005, the UKMEC guidelines were developed using best published evidence and knowledge from specialist consultants in the field of women's healthcare (Table 31.1). It has become a go-to reference for the safe provision of contraception across women's reproductive life course [6].

The Effect of Diabetes Mellitus on Contraceptive Choice

All women without diabetes-related complications are UKMEC 1 or 2 regardless of their insulin dependence, provided they have no diabetes-related sequelae of disease – neuropathy, retinopathy, neuropathy, other vascular disease or other contraindications [6].

Non-hormonal Methods

Fertility-awareness methods (FAM). Fertility-awareness methods involve monitoring changes in the woman's body during the menstrual cycle. They are as effective in the diabetic woman with regular menstrual cycles as in the non-diabetic woman. However, women with diabetes have a potentially increased risk of irregular menstrual cycles that may reduce the efficacy of FAM [1, 4].

Table 31.1 Summary of contraceptive methods with UK/WHO/USMEC scores [5, 6, 8]

Contraceptive method	Disease stage	UKMEC	WHOMEC	USMEC
POP	History of GDM	1	1	1
	Non-insulin dependent diabetes (NIDDM)	2	2	2
	Insulin dependent	2	2	2
	Neuropathy/retinopathy/nephropathy	2	2	2
	Other vascular disease or DM >20 years	2	2	2
IMP	History of GDM	1	1	1
	NIDDM	2	2	2
	Insulin dependent	2	2	2
	Neuropathy/retinopathy/nephropathy	2	2	2
	Other vascular disease or DM >20 years	2	2	2
DMPA	History of GDM	1	1	1
	NIDDM	2	2	2
	Insulin dependent	2	2	2
	Neuropathy/retinopathy/nephropathy	2	3	3
	Other vascular disease or DM >20 years	2	3	3
CHC	History of GDM	1	1	1
	NIDDM	2	2	2
	Insulin dependent	2	2	2
	Neuropathy/retinopathy/nephropathy	3	3–4	3–4
	Other vascular disease or DM >20 years	3	3–4	3–4
LNG-IUS	History of GDM	1	1	1
	NIDDM	2	2	2
	Insulin dependent	2	2	2
	Neuropathy/retinopathy/nephropathy	2	2	2
	Other vascular disease or DM >20 years	2	2	2
Cu-IUD	History of GDM	1	1	1
	NIDDM	1	1	1
	Insulin dependent	1	1	1
	Neuropathy/retinopathy/nephropathy	1	1	1
	Other vascular disease or DM >20 years	1	1	1

Barrier Methods

There is no evidence to suggest that diaphragms, cervical caps or male/female condoms are less effective in women with DM. There are no studies contraindicating spermicides from a diabetic perspective [1].

Intrauterine Contraception

Copper-bearing intrauterine device (Cu-IUD). Although there has been a theoretical concern that diabetes can worsen pelvic infection, this has not been substantiated in practical terms and IUC are UKMEC 1 for Cu-IUD [6].

Levonorgestrel intrauterine system (LNG-IUS). The levonorgestrel intrauterine system is UKMEC 2 for women with DM [6]. This applies even to women with retinopathy, nephropathy, neuropathy and vasculopathy [6]. Limited evidence on the use of the LNG-IUS among women with insulin-dependent or non-insulin-dependent diabetes suggests that these methods have little effect on short- or long-term diabetes control (e.g. glycosylated haemoglobin levels), haemostatic markers or lipid profile [6].

Progesterone-Only Contraception

Progesterone-only contraception (POC) has been demonstrated to have no adverse effects on serum lipid levels for women with GDM in two, albeit small studies [6]. Limited evidence is inconsistent regarding the development of non-insulin-dependent diabetes mellitus (NIDDM) amongst users of POC with a history of GDM. Further, the presence of end organ complications does not alter UKMEC status [6].

Depo medroxyprogesterone acetate (DMPA). There is some concern regarding DMPA's hypoestrogenic effect and its effect on high-density lipoproteins amongst users. The effects of DMPA can remain for some time following discontinuation [6].

Progestogen implant (IMP). The progestogen implant releases a constant dose of progesterone, reducing the potential for metabolic variations and maintaining steady-state blood-lipid ratios [1].

Progesterone-only pill (POP). The consensus view is that the effect of POP on carbohydrate metabolism is minimal. In general, diabetics have good pill compliance as they take regular medications to control their disease state. For younger diabetics, the extra efficacy and the 12-hour dosing period of desogestrel make it even more attractive [1].

Combined hormonal contraception (CHC). The use of CHC has a limited effect on daily insulin requirements for women with IDDM or NIDDM, and no effect on long-term diabetic control or progression to retinopathy [6]. Changes in lipid profile and haemostatic markers are limited and most remain within normal values [6]. The development of NIDDM in women with a history of GDM is not increased with the use of CHC; likewise lipid levels appear to be unaffected by use [6].

Although carbohydrate tolerance may change with CHC use, the major concerns are vascular disease due to diabetes and additional risk of arterial thrombosis due to use of CHC – including vaginal rings and transdermal patches [6].

The ideal candidate for the CHC would be young, with short duration of DM, without diabetic complications of the arterial, nervous, ophthalmic and renal systems and with no other risk factors for thrombosis and requiring maximal protection against pregnancy [4].

Sterilization

Women should consider permanent sterilization following completion of their family, especially when avoidance of pregnancy is essential for maternal health. Failure rate is estimated at 1 in 200. As sterilization is an operative intervention, glycaemic control needs to be addressed and perioperative antibiotics need to be considered [1].

Emergency Contraception

Three options for emergency contraception (EC) are in use in the United Kingdom with the addition of the Yuzpe method in the United States and where the WHO MEC is used. The Yuzpe method comprises a single dose 100 µg of ethinyl estradiol and 0.50 mg LNG, then a second dose of the same repeated 12 hours later [7].

Ulipristal acetate (UPA-EC)

Levonorgestrel (LNG-EC)

Cu-IUD

There are no MEC restrictions for any method of EC from a diabetic perspective as duration of use of medications provided for EC is reduced in comparison to that of regular use [7]. According to WHO MEC, the benefit of using EC outweighs the risk, even when there is severe vascular disease [5, 7].

Postnatal Contraception

The WHO recommends minimum inter-pregnancy intervals of 24 months following a live birth to reduce poor maternal, perinatal, neonatal and infant health outcomes associated with rapid repeat pregnancy rates [9]. Discussion and provision of postnatal contraception should be an essential part of antenatal and postnatal care for all women, especially those with DM. A woman's chosen method of contraception should be initiated immediately postpartum, if medically eligible [10]. The only contraceptive method that cannot be safely initiated following delivery is CHC. If other methods are not available or suitable for the patient immediately postpartum, 'bridging' contraception can be provided without the need for abstinence/condom use if commenced prior to day 21 postpartum [10].

Conclusion

The importance of avoiding unintended pregnancy should be an essential part of diabetes education. Taking a patient-centred, shared, non-judgemental approach will empower women to make healthy lifestyle choices.

References

1. Robinson A, Nwolise C, Shawe J. Contraception for women with diabetes: Challenges and solutions. *Journal of Contraception.* 2016;7:11–18.

2. UK Diabetes Prevalence 2019. Diabetes UK. 2020. http://bit.ly/3IlbRnp.

3. National Institute of Clinical Excellence. *Diabetes in pregnancy: Management from preconception to the postnatal period.* London: National Institute of Clinical Excellence, 2015, pp. 8–11.

4. Guillebaud J, MacGregor A. *Contraception: Your questions answered.* 7th edition. London: Elsevier, 2017.

5. World Health Organization. *Medical eligibility criteria for contraceptive use.* 5th edition. Geneva: World Health Organization, 2020, pp. 5, 111, 157, 186, 189, 211. https://bit.ly/3HxV1BB.

6. UK MEC 2016. Digital version. Ukmec. pagelizard.com. 2016. http://ukmec .pagelizard.com/2016.

7. World Health Organization. Emergency contraception factsheet. WHO International. 2018. https://bit.ly/3DFpUTh.

8. US Medical Eligibility Criteria (US MEC) for Contraceptive Use, 2016. Cdc.gov. 2016. http://bit.ly /3RhFASx.

9. World Health Organization. *Report of a WHO Technical report on birth spacing.* 1st edition. Geneva: World Health Organization, 2005. https://bit.ly /3EvtmAi.

10. Faculty of Sexual and Reproductive Healthcare. *Contraception after pregnancy.* 1st edition. London: Faculty of Sexual and Reproductive Healthcare, 2017. https://bit.ly/3SmTNhf.

Contraception in Women with Thyroid Dysfunction

Christina I. Messini, George Anifandis, Alexandros Daponte and Ioannis E. Messinis

Introduction

The thyroid gland is the largest endocrine gland in the human body, located in the anterior neck [1]. Its function is regulated by the anterior pituitary through the secretion of thyroid-stimulating hormone (TSH). The hypothalamic hormone that stimulates the secretion of TSH is thyrotrophin-releasing hormone (TRH). Three hormones are produced by the thyroid gland – that is, thyroxin or tetraiodothyronine (T4), triiodothyronine (T3) and calcitonin, which reduces the levels of calcium in blood. The production and secretion of T3 and T4, derived from the amino acid tyrosine, is controlled by TSH.

These two thyroid hormones via a feedback mechanism inhibit the secretion of TSH and TRH (Figure 32.1). Thyroid hormones stimulate cell metabolism and activity, increasing the metabolic rate. They play an important role in regulating the body's energy balance, maintaining energy homeostasis. Thyroxin, although more prevalent than T3, is weaker and at the level of cell receptors is converted to T3, which is the active form. Thyroid hormones induce glucogenolysis, lipolysis and proteolysis, increasing plasma levels of glucose, fatty acids and amino acids, respectively.

Ovarian Hormones and Thyroid Function

Oestrogen nuclear receptors α and β are expressed both in normal and pathological thyroid tissue [2]. The action of oestrogen is exerted via these two receptors, although non-genomic actions via membrane-associated oestrogen receptors have been noticed. Oestrogen exerts direct effects on the thyroid gland via the genomic receptors, stimulating the growth of thyroid cells and indirect effects related to the stimulation of increased synthesis of thyroxin-binding globulin (TBG) in the liver, which binds thyroid hormones in the circulation with high affinity [3]. As

such, it reduces the available thyroxin (free T4) for use by the cells. On the other hand, progesterone antagonizes the action of oestrogen and reduces the synthesis and secretion of TBG, thus increasing the available thyroxin in the cells (Figure 32.2).

Thyroid Dysfunction and Reproductive Health

The two main disorders of thyroid function are hyper- and hypothyroidism. Both of these disorders can affect a woman's reproductive function. Women suffering from hyperthyroidism experience menstrual disorders, mainly in the form of hypomenorrhea and polymenorrhea [4]. The exact mechanism is not clear, although increased sensitivity of the pituitary gland to gonadotropin-releasing hormone (GnRH) has been found to cause luteinizing hormone (LH) hyper secretion. Thyroxin also causes an increase in sex hormone-binding globulin (SHBG), which binds more oestrogen than normal. However, most women with

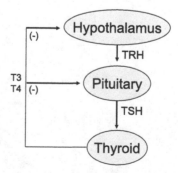

Figure 32.1 The hypothalamic-pituitary-thyroid axis. Hypothalamic thyrotrophin-releasing hormone (TRH) stimulates the secretion of thyroid-stimulating hormone (TSH) from the anterior pituitary and this in turn stimulates the secretion of thyroid hormones from the thyroid gland. Negative feedback mechanism of thyroid hormones on the hypothalamus and pituitary gland. T3: triiodothyronine; T4: tetraiodothyronine or thyroxin

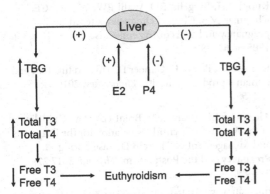

Figure 32.2 Effect of estradiol (E2) and progesterone (P4) on thyroid hormone homeostasis. Oral E2 stimulates the production of thyroxin-binding globulin (TBG) by the liver, which binds more thyroid hormones. As a result, the amount of free hormones decreases. On the other hand, P4 has the opposite effect. The combination of both, as in the oral contraceptive pill, ensures euthyroidism. T3: triiodothyronine; T4: tetraiodothyronine or thyroxin

hyperthyroidism remain ovulatory. In cases of hyperthyroidism, treatment is necessary for the homeostasis of the individual. It is recommended that the treatment is applied before pregnancy so the woman is euthyroid to ensure a good pregnancy outcome [5].

Hypothyroidism is due to many causes, but more often is primary hypothyroidism – that is, Hashimoto's thyroiditis. Subclinical hypothyroidism is more common than overt hypothyroidism and is characterized by elevated serum TSH. It may affect in several ways the reproductive function by changing oestrogen metabolism and the levels of SHBG leading to alterations in the feedback mechanisms and consequently to menstrual irregularities and anovulation. Hypothyroidism is also associated with increased rates of early pregnancy failure as well as pregnancy complications including preeclampsia and postpartum haemorrhage [4]. Elevated TSH levels may adversely affect treatment outcome through assisted reproduction. In the context of infertility management, it has been recommended that treatment should be able to maintain TSH levels below 2.5 mU/L before conception [6].

Contraception

There are two main questions about contraception and the thyroid gland, firstly, whether hormonal contraceptives affect normal thyroid function or the treatment for thyroid disease; and secondly whether such a treatment affects contraceptive effectiveness.

As already mentioned, oestrogen increases TBG production, leading to the binding of more T4 and T3 to this protein and increasing total T4 levels. The increase occurs during oral administration but not during transdermal administration as the latter avoids the first pass effect from intestine and liver [7].

The effects of combined oral contraceptive pills on thyroid function can vary depending on the composition of the formulation. The estrogenic component of the pill by increasing TBG can lead to the reduction of free thyroid hormones [8]. On the other hand, progesterone decreases TBG and increases the activity of thyroid hormones and the production of free T4 [9]. Nevertheless, the end result from their coexistence in combined oral contraceptive pills is not the same in all formulations. Some progestins have a higher anti-androgenic profile than others [10]. With some formulations containing various dosages of ethinylestradiol and either dynogest or levonorgestrel, an increase in T3 or T4 and possibly TSH has been shown, while with others free T3 and free T4 may only slightly increase or remain stable, although these two hormones in some cases may show opposite changes [10, 11].

A transient decrease in free T3 has been noted with levonorgestrel, which has slight anti-estrogenic properties. In addition, combined oral contraceptives containing desogestrel, cyproterone acetate, drospirenone or dienogest increased TBG but did not affect free T4 levels [12, 13]. Overall, although total T3 or T4 levels may increase due to increased binding to TBG, with the combined action of the estrogenic and progestogenic components, normal thyroid function does not seem to be impaired by the use of oral contraceptives (Figure 32.2). Nevertheless, rarely, an overproduction of T3 and T4 to compensate for the free hormone deficiency may persist after discontinuation of the pill, causing hyperthyroidism, as in a case report in which a woman developed Graves' disease after stopping the use of oral contraceptives [14].

Data on the effects of progestin-only contraceptives on thyroid function are limited. With the use of depot medroxyprogesterone acetate injections for contraceptive purposes, an increase in free T4 levels at 12 months has been reported, which was more than in women using an intrauterine contraceptive device [15]. However, a recent prospective randomized trial has demonstrated that the injectable contraceptive depot medroxyprogesterone acetate did not have any impact on thyroid function after 1 year of use [15].

Etonogestrel contained in a subdermal implant may induce minimal changes in thyroid function of no clinical importance [16]. Similarly, implants containing levonorgestrel do not seem to alter free T4 levels [17].

Progestogen-only pills containing either desogestrel or levonorgestrel show no impact on thyroid function [18]. Regarding vaginal rings, they contain both steroids. In a study using a ring delivering 15 µg ethinylestradiol plus 120 µg etonogestrel, TSH levels were increased after 3 cycles, but thyroxin levels were not affected [19]. Skin patches are also used for contraceptive purposes. In a study in Mexican women, using patches containing 6 mg norelgestromin plus 600 µg ethinylestradiol, it was shown that after 4 months of use there was no change in TSH and T4 levels, but there was a significant increase of T3 compared to baseline. Nevertheless, hormone values remained within the normal range [20].

Although, as mentioned, in the case of women with normal thyroid function the use of combined oral contraceptives does not seem to disrupt euthyroidism, in cases of hypothyroidism the dose of T4 needs to be adjusted based on monitoring of thyroid hormones and TSH levels. If the necessary dose of T4 cannot be adjusted while being treated with contraceptives, or if the woman wants to feel safer for proper replacement, then she may be offered progestogen-only pills, also explaining the lower contraceptive effectiveness.

The woman may also be offered a non-hormonal method of contraception. Animal experiments have shown that thyroidectomy in female mice reduces the expression of hepatic oestrogen receptors by 70%, a change which was reversed after administration of T3 to the animals [21]. Although thyroxin replacement therapy does not seem to affect the effectiveness of birth control medication, euthyroidism is required for a successful action of oral contraceptives. Combined oral contraceptives show no significant effect on autoimmune thyroid disease [22].

References

1. Broughton C, Ahmad B. Thyroid anatomy and physiology. In Llahana S, Follin C, Yedinak C, Grossman A (eds.). *Advanced practice in endocrinology nursing.* Cham: Springer, 2019, 497–503. https://doi.org/10.1007/978-3-319-99817-6_26.

2. Santin AP, Furlanetto TW. Role of estrogen in thyroid function and growth regulation. *J Thyroid Res.* 2011:875125.

3. Knopp RH, Bergelin RO, Wahl PW, Walden CE, Chapman MB. Clinical chemistry alterations in pregnancy and oral contraceptive use. *Obstet Gynecol.* 1985;66:682–90.

4. Krassas GE, Poppe K, Glinoer D. Thyroid function and human reproductive health. *Endocr Rev.* 2010;31:702–55.

5. Alexander EK, Pearce EN, Brent GA et al. Guidelines of the American Thyroid Association for the Diagnosis and Management of Thyroid Disease during Pregnancy and the Postpartum. *Thyroid.* 2017;27:315–89.

6. Busnelli A, Somigliana E, Benaglia L et al. In vitro fertilization outcomes in treated hypothyroidism. *Thyroid.* 2013;23:1319–25.

7. Chetkowski RJ, Meldrum DR, Steingold KA et al. Biologic effects of transdermal estradiol. *N Engl J Med.* 1986;314:1615–20.

8. Westhoff CL, Petrie KA, Cremers S. Using changes in binding globulins to assess oral contraceptive compliance. *Contraception.* 2013;87:176–81.

9. Sathi P, Kalyan S, Hitchcock CL, Pudek M, Prior JC. Progesterone therapy increases free thyroxine levels: Data from a randomized placebo-controlled 12-week hot flush trial. *Clin Endocrinol (Oxf).* 2013;79:282–7.

10. Torre F, Calogero AE, Condorelli RA et al. Effects of oral contraceptives on thyroid function and vice versa. *J Endocrinol Invest.* 2020;43:1181–8.

11. Wiegratz I, Kutschera E, Lee JH et al. Effect of four oral contraceptives on thyroid hormones, adrenal and blood pressure parameters. *Contraception.* 2003;67:361–6.

12. Sänger N, Stahlberg S, Manthey T et al. Effects of an oral contraceptive containing 30 mcg ethinyl estradiol and 2 mg dienogest on thyroid hormones and androgen parameters: conventional vs. extended-cycle use. *Contraception.* 2008;77:420–5.

13. Raps M, Curvers J, Helmerhorst FM et al. Thyroid function, activated protein C resistance and the risk of venous thrombosis in users of hormonal contraceptives. *Thromb Res.* 2014;133:640–4.

14. Ali S, Abbara A, Comninos A et al. A case of Graves' disease occurring following cessation of the oral combined contraceptive pill. *Endocrine Abstracts.* 2015;38:P124. https://doi.org/10.1530/endoabs.38.P124.

15. Quintino-Moro A, Zantut-Wittmann DE, Silva Dos Santos PN et al. Thyroid function during the first year of use of the injectable contraceptive depot medroxyprogesterone acetate. *Eur J Contracept Reprod Health Care.* 2019;24:102–8.

16. Biswas A, Viegas OA, Bennink HJ, Korver T, Ratnam SS. Effect of Implanon use on selected parameters of thyroid and adrenal function. *Contraception*. 2000;**62**:247–51.

17. Olsson SE, Wide L, Odlind V. Aspects of thyroid function during use of Norplant implants. *Contraception*. 1986;**34**:583–7.

18. Kivelä A, Ruuskanen M, Agren U, Dieben T. The effects of two progrestogen-only pills containing either desogestrel (75 microgram/day) or levonorgestrel (30 microgram/day) on carbohydrate metabolism and adrenal and thyroid function. *Eur J Contracept Reprod Health Care*. 2001;**6**:71–7.

19. Duijkers I, Killick S, Bigrigg A, Dieben TO. A comparative study on the effects of a contraceptive vaginal ring NuvaRing and an oral contraceptive on carbohydrate metabolism and adrenal and thyroid function. *Eur J Contracept Reprod Health Care*. 2004;**9**(3):131–40.

20. Hernandez-Juarez J, Garcia-Latorre EA, Moreno-Hernandez M et al. Metabolic effects of the contraceptive skin patch and subdermal contraceptive implant in Mexican women: A prospective study. *Reprod Health*. 2014;**11**:33.

21. Stavreus-Evers AC, Freyschuss B, Eriksson HA. Hormonal regulation of the estrogen receptor in primary cultures of hepatocytes from female rats. *Steroids*. 1997;**62**:647–54.

22. Benagiano G, Benagiano M, Bianchi P, D'Elios MM, Brosens I . Contraception in autoimmune diseases. *Best Pract Res Clin Obstet Gynaecol*. 2019;**60**: 111–23.

Contraception in Women with Polycystic Ovary Syndrome

Christina I. Messini, George Anifandis, Alexandros Daponte, Ioannis E. Messinis

Introduction

Polycystic ovary syndrome (PCOS), also known in the past as Stein–Leventhal syndrome, is a multifactorial disorder affecting 5–15% of all women of reproductive age, involving both the reproductive and endocrine systems. Polycystic ovary syndrome usually begins at puberty. In adolescent girls, diagnosis of PCOS is difficult, although hirsutism and oligomenorrhea are strongly associated with the presence of biochemical hyperandrogenism and polycystic ovaries [1]. According to the criteria of Rotterdam (2003), the diagnosis of PCOS requires the presence of at least two of the following three criteria, after excluding other diseases [28]:

1. Oligoovulation and/or anovulation.
2. Biochemical or clinical hyperandrogenism.
3. Polycystic ovary morphology and exclusion of other aetiologies (congenital adrenal hyperplasia, androgen-secreting tumours, Cushing's syndrome).

Pathophysiology

Up to now, there is no comprehensive pathophysiological explanation for PCOS. Its heterogeneity may reflect multiple mechanisms which in individual women are not necessarily involved simultaneously but help explain the close relation of metabolic–reproductive circuitry. Ovarian androgen excess and anovulation are key features of the disorder.

Several factors seem to be involved in the pathophysiology of PCOS [3]:

a. A disrupted balance between androgens and gonadotropins leads to an increased growth of small antral follicles and subsequent arrest of follicle growth creating the typical polycystic ovarian morphology.
b. A unique defect in insulin action, leading to hyperinsulinaemia and insulin resistance, reflects the interaction of genetic influences and environmental factors.
c. Multiple genetic and epigenetic factors have also been described.
d. High androgen levels disrupt the capability of ovarian steroid hormones to regulate GnRH/LH secretion via the classical feedback pathways. This results in diminished negative feedback mechanism of oestrogen and progesterone, contributing to luteinizing (LH) hyper secretion, which is observed in several women with PCOS.
e. An alteration in cortisol metabolism has also been described, resulting in enhanced adrenal androgen production.

Signs, Symptoms, Complications and Long-Term Sequelae

In women with PCOS, there is an imbalance of reproductive hormones with excessive production of androgens, associated with increased prevalence of serious clinical issues such as reproductive implications and metabolic dysfunction. Due to the complexity of the syndrome, there are various manifestations and long-term consequences for women's health [2], as described in Table 33.1.

Contraception

Contraception is essential in many women with PCOS. The use of hormonal contraception is the basis of the intervention, but because the syndrome is characterized by a variety of manifestations, which are usually treated with the use of ovarian hormones, these two issues – that is, contraception and treatment of the syndrome – will be discussed together. The importance of this is reinforced by the fact that many women with PCOS need treatment while they do not need contraception, but it is an important advantage for those who need both. In this case

Table 33.1 Characteristics, complications and potential risks in women with polycystic ovary syndrome

Clinical and biochemical characteristics

Menstrual disorders	Oligo/amenorrhea
Metabolic syndrome	Insulin resistance, large waist circumference
Weight gain	
Hyperadrogenism	Hirsutism located in face, chest, back or buttocks
	Acne or oily skin
	Thinning hair and hair loss

Complications

Infertility	
Pregnancy complications	Miscarriage, gestational diabetes, preterm delivery and pre-eclampsia

Long-term sequelae

Type 2 diabetes mellitus	
Depression	
Sleep apnoea/Sleep-disordered breathing	Overweight
Cardiovascular disease	Hypertension, dyslipidaemia, obesity
Endometrial cancer	

hormonal preparations provide benefits beyond contraception.

Polycystic ovary syndrome cannot be cured, but different symptoms associated with PCOS can be managed. Lifestyle changes can improve obesity and irregular menstruation. Aerobic exercise has shown moderate evidence in improving body mass index (BMI) of women with PCOS [6]. Diet seems to improve not only BMI, but also insulin resistance, and the longer the duration, the greater the improvement [7]. Compared with metformin, diet showed no significant difference in the improvement of BMI, insulin regulation and menstrual disorders [9].

Metformin is widely used in women with PCOS, particularly in those who are overweight. Although it is not approved by the United States Food and Drug Administration (FDA) for PCOS treatment, it is considered first-line treatment of type 2 diabetes. Studies have shown that metformin has many benefits in women with PCOS. When combined with lifestyle changes, it lowers BMI and subcutaneous adipose tissue and improves menstruation [19]. It also reduces insulin,

blood glucose and androgen levels and improves insulin resistance and acne [8]. In the long term metformin reduces cholesterol levels and the risk of heart disease [5]. Nevertheless, treatment up to 1 year with combined oral contraceptives (COCs) was more effective than metformin in improving the pattern of the menstrual cycle and reducing androgen levels [12]. Metformin in combination with COCs may be more useful for management of metabolic disorders [26].

Treatment for hirsutism and acne aims to block the effect of androgens alongside with the suppression of their production from the ovaries. Therapy of these manifestations includes oestrogen-progestin oral contraceptive pills (mainly those containing cyproterone acetate, desogestrel, levonorgestrel or drospirenone) and anti-androgens (such as spironolactone, flutamide and finasteride) [20]. For women treated only with anti-androgens, it is recommended to be covered with effective contraception in order to avoid potential risks of anti-androgens to a male fetus in case of unintended conception [24]. From all COCs, those containing cyproterone acetate seem to be more effective in improving hirsutism [17]. Although the first options in acne therapy are topical antiseptics and antibiotics, COC pills are an alternative whereas the progestin-only pill or the contraceptive implant can sometimes worsen acne [4].

In order to normalize menstruation in women with PCOS, oral contraceptives, contraceptive skin patches or contraceptive vaginal rings are recommended [23]. All provide effective contraception and can be used unless there are contraindications to taking hormones (Table 33.2). Both COC pills and progestin-only pills, also known as mini-pills, constitute an effective option in the management of PCOS symptoms [21]. A contraceptive vaginal ring is suggested in PCOS women who are overweight or who have moderate insulin resistance that does not require metformin administration [27]. On the other hand, limited evidence suggests that, in women weighing more than 90 kg, a contraceptive skin patch may have reduced efficacy [29].

The oestrogen component of hormonal contraceptives reduces free testosterone by increasing the synthesis of sex hormone-binding globulin (SHBG) that binds this steroid. Studies have shown that ethinylestradiol (EE) is more effective than natural oestrogen and that the use of 20–35 μg EE is associated with a higher SHBG production and a greater reduction of free testosterone levels. On the other hand, although the use of COCs may increase the relative

Table 33.2 Contraceptive options in women with polycystic ovary syndrome. COC: combined oral contraceptives; IUD: intrauterine device

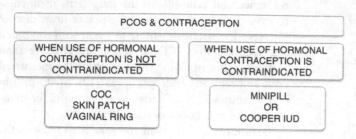

risk of venous thromboembolism (VTE) [13], especially in obese women with BMIs of more than 30 kg/m^2 [29], the risk is higher with higher doses of EE as, for example, when this steroid is combined with cyproterone acetate [24]. Also, the risk is increased for other adverse effects and therefore such formulations should be used after consideration [24]. Preparations with low-dose EE are therefore preferable. Polycystic ovary syndrome appears to be an independent risk factor for VTE. This should be taken into account in the management of PCOS or when contraception is also needed [10].

Most progestogens reduce ovarian production of androgens through a negative feedback mechanism, while some act directly to the androgen receptor. Drosperinone, when compared to chlormadinone acetate, has shown a stronger anti-androgenic effect [14]. Cyproterone acetate and drospirenone seem to be more effective than desogestrel in suppressing gonadotropin secretion and increasing SHBG levels in women with PCOS [15, 22]. Nevertheless, due to lack of clear evidence, a specific type of COC, dose of progestin/oestrogen or COCs cannot be currently recommended [25].

The risk of endometrial cancer is increased in PCOS women and many factors, such as early menarche, late menopause, nulliparity and unopposed oestrogen have been implicated. However, there is accumulated evidence that the use of COCs plays a protective role in endometrial cancer [11].

Depending on the duration of therapy (from 3 to 12 months), the use of all COC pills is associated with an increase in the levels of high- and low-density lipoprotein-cholesterol (HDL-C, LDL-C) and an increase in triglycerides (TG). Concerning BMI, fasting blood glucose, insulin resistance and blood pressure, no changes have been observed after long-term use of COCs [16]. Between dienogest, cyproterone acetate and levonorgestrel, the first two show the most favourable metabolic profile [18]. Because of the possible worsening in

lipid profile, factors such as BMI, hyperlipidaemia and hypertension need to be considered before the administration of COC [24]. Nevertheless, limited evidence shows no difference in acute myocardial infarction in obese women using COCs when compared to non-obese women using them.

Concerning contraception in PCOS women who are overweight, there is no recommendation different from that of general population. Obese women (BMI ≥ 30 kg/m^2) can use COCs without restriction because contraceptive effectiveness is maintained. However, if BMI is very high, COCs may not provide the required contraceptive protection [29].

There seems to be no difference in the effectiveness of contraceptive pills between women with PCOS and the general population. Therefore, any preparation given to women without the syndrome could be administered to women with it. However, due to the variety in the phenotype, it is recommended to choose compounds that, in addition to contraception, could address the predominant clinical manifestations of the syndrome. That is, individualization is suggested in order to minimize side effects and obtain the preferable result in both therapy and contraceptive effectiveness. Finally, non-hormonal contraceptive methods such as intrauterine devices can be also used effectively in women with PCOS, particularly when there are contraindications to hormonal contraception (Table 33.2).

References

1. Villarroel C, López P, Merino PM et al. Hirsutism and oligomenorrhea are appropriate screening criteria for polycystic ovary syndrome in adolescents. *Gynecol Endocrinol.* 2015;**31**:625–9.

2. http://bit.ly/3Y0jGpe.

3. Ibáñez L, Oberfield SE, Witchel S et al. An international consortium update: Pathophysiology, diagnosis, and treatment of polycystic ovarian syndrome in adolescence. *Horm Res Paediatr.* 2017;**88**:371–95.

4. www.nhs.uk/conditions/acne/treatment.

5. https://bit.ly/40qrtyn.

6. Dos Santos IK, Ashe MC, Cobucci RN et al. The effect of exercise as an intervention for women with polycystic ovary syndrome: A systematic review and meta-analysis. *Medicine (Baltimore)*. 2020;**99**:e19644.

7. Shang Y, Zhou H, Hu M, Feng H. Effect of diet on insulin resistance in polycystic ovary syndrome. *J Clin Endocrinol Metab*. 2020;**105**:dgaa425.

8. Yen H, Chang YT, Yee FJ, Huang YC. Metformin therapy for acne in patients with polycystic ovary syndrome: A systematic review and meta-analysis. *Am J Clin Dermatol*. 2020.

9. Kim CH, Chon SJ, Lee SH. Effects of lifestyle modification in polycystic ovary syndrome compared to metformin only or metformin addition: A systematic review and meta-analysis. *Sci Rep*. 2020;**10**:7802.

10. Gariani K, Hugon-Rodin J, Philippe J, Righini M, Blondon M. Association between polycystic ovary syndrome and venous thromboembolism: A systematic review and meta analysis. *Thromb Res*. 2020;**185**:102 8.

11. Ignatov A, Ortmann O. Endocrine risk factors of endometrial cancer: Polycystic ovary syndrome, oral contraceptives, infertility, Tamoxifen. *Cancers (Basel)*. 2020;**12**:1766.

12. Costello M, Shrestha B, Eden J, Sjoblom P, Johnson N. Insulin-sensitising drugs versus the combined oral contraceptive pill for hirsutism, acne and risk of diabetes, cardiovascular disease, and endometrial cancer in polycystic ovary syndrome. *Cochrane Database Syst Rev*. 2007;(1):CD005552.

13. Domecq JP, Prutsky G, Mullan RJ et al. Adverse effects of the common treatments for polycystic ovary syndrome: A systematic review and meta-analysis. *J Clin Endocrinol Metab*. 2013;**98**:4646–54.

14. Menshawy A, Ismail A, Abdel-Maboud M et al. *J Gynecol Obstet Hum Reprod*. 2019;**48**:763–70.

15. Amiri M, Ramezani Tehrani F, Nahidi F, Kabir A, Azizi F. Comparing the effects of combined oral contraceptives containing progestins with low androgenic and antiandrogenic activities on the hypothalamic-pituitary-gonadal axis in patients with polycystic ovary syndrome: Systematic review and meta-analysis. *JMIR Res Protoc*. 2018;7:e113.

16. Amiri M, Ramezani-Tehrani F, Nahidi F, Kabir A, Azizi F. Effects of oral contraceptives on metabolic profile in women with polycystic ovary syndrome: A meta-analysis comparing products containing cyproterone acetate with third generation progestins. *Metabolism*. 2017;**73**:22–35.

17. Amiri M, Kabir A, Nahidi F, Shekofteh M, Ramezani–Tehrani F. Effects of combined oral contraceptives on the clinical and biochemical parameters of hyperandrogenism in patients with polycystic ovary syndrome: A systematic review and meta-analysis. *Eur J Contracept Reprod Health Care*. 2018;**23**:64–77.

18. Silva-Bermudez LS, Toloza FJK, Perez-Matos MC et al. Effects of oral contraceptives on metabolic parameters in adult premenopausal women: A meta-analysis. *Endocr Connect*. 2020;**9**:978–98.

19. Naderpoor N, Shorakae S, de Courten B et al. Metformin and lifestyle modification in polycystic ovary syndrome: Systematic review and meta-analysis. *Hum Reprod Update*. 2015;**21**:560–74.

20. Barrionuevo P, Nabhan M, Altayar O et al. Treatment options for hirsutism: A systematic review and network meta-analysis. *J Clin Endocrinol Metab*. 2018;**103**:1258–64.

21. Conway G, Dewailly D, Diamanti-Kandarakis E et al. The polycystic ovary syndrome: A position statement from the European Society of Endocrinology. *Eur J Endocrinol*. 2014;**171**:P1–29.

22. Bhattacharya SM, Jha A. Comparative study of the therapeutic effects of oral contraceptive pills containing desogestrel, cyproterone acetate, and drospirenone in patients with polycystic ovary syndrome. *Fertil Steril*. 2012;**98**:1053–9.

23. Legro RS, Arslanian SA, Ehrmann DA et al. Diagnosis and treatment of polycystic ovary syndrome: An Endocrine Society clinical practice guideline. *J Clin Endocrinol Metab*. 2013;**98**:4565–92.

24. Teede HJ, Misso ML, Costello MF et al. Recommendations from the international evidence-based guideline for the assessment and management of polycystic ovary syndrome. *Fertil Steril*. 2018;**110**:364–79.

25. http://bit.ly/3X8i9vX.

26. Teede H, Tassone EC, Piltonen T et al. Effect of the combined oral contraceptive pill and/or metformin in the management of polycystic ovary syndrome: A systematic review with meta-analyses. *Clin Endocrinol (Oxf)*. 2019;**91**:479–89.

27. Mendoza N, Simoncini T, Genazzani AD. Hormonal contraceptive choice for women with PCOS: A systematic review of randomized trials and observational studies. *Gynecol Endocrinol*. 2014;**30**:850–60.

28. Rotterdam ESHRE/ASRM-Sponsored PCOS consensus workshop group. Revised 2003 consensus on diagnostic criteria and long-term health risks related to polycystic ovary syndrome (PCOS). *Hum Reprod*. 2004;**19**:41–7.

29. World Health Organization. *WHO guidelines: Medical eligibility criteria for contraceptive use*. 5th edition. Geneva: World Health Organization, 2015. www.who.int/publications/i/item/9789241549158.

Chapter 34

Contraception in Women with Special Needs
Life-Course Approach

Johannes Bitzer

Definitions

Different definitions and timelines are given for the various life phases.

Adolescence. The United Nations uses the term 'adolescence' for people aged 10–19 years, but the World Health Organization (WHO) defines adolescence from 10 years up to 21 years [1, 2]. In cultures where adolescent girls become mothers from the time their periods begin, adolescence is very short. Adolescence is thus at the same time a biological and a psychosocial definition.

Midlife. Midlife is from age 21 to age 40 (45 years). This is the life phase during which many developmental, professional and personal events occur: family building, pregnancies, childbirth, transition from dyad to triad and choice of profession or career.

Perimenopause, Menopausal Transition. Perimenopause is from the ages of 45 to 60 years. This is the end of the fertile phase. Many individuals are at the top of their professional careers and have responsibility for younger generations and for the elderly.

Each life phase is characterized by specific changes and challenges which vary from individual to individual but have common features or characteristics that are important for contraception. Contraceptive counselling should combine the general recommendations based on Medical Eligibility Criteria (MEC) with the patient's life-phase-related needs [1–5].

Adolescence

Several biological and psychosocial characteristics of this life phase are important for contraceptive counselling and care [6–8].

Biological Factors

In adolescence the hypothalamo-pituitary-ovarian (HPO) axis gradually develops into fully ovulatory cycles. As a consequence, adolescents may experience phases of prolonged or shortened cycles or irregular bleeding and some of them may develop heavy bleeding symptoms with acute haemorrhage.

Primary dysmenorrhea is a frequent symptom among adolescent girls and may be the first sign of developing endometriosis. Irregular cycles combined with hyper-androgenic skin systems may be the clinical manifestations of polycystic ovary syndrome, which is the most frequent endocrine disorder in young women and has a significant impact on the present and future health of the adolescent (metabolic syndrome, increased risk of endometrial carcinoma, anovulation and infertility).

During adolescence the young woman builds up her peak bone mass, which serves as the basis for her future bone health which becomes important at an older age regarding the risk of osteoporosis and fracture. The immune system is in a process of maturation and is still vulnerable to infection, including sexually transmitted infections (STIs). Many adolescents have difficulties with their weight and they may develop eating disorders which manifest as obesity or anorexia. Both manifestations can have a long-term impact on health.

Psychosocial Factors

Most adolescents start their sexual life and experience their first intimate and sexual encounter, which can have a long-standing impact on their future sexual health. They may also have several partners and thus increase their risk for attracting an STI.

Many adolescents have difficulties regulating their emotions, which are frequently very strong and fluctuating, and thus special behavioural patterns arise like mood swings, abrupt changes in behaviour, difficulties in concentrating and so forth. Mood instability and life challenges may lead to alcohol and drug abuse.

Another part of the development of an identity concerns the body. Many adolescents have body image concerns regarding beauty and attractiveness in an environment in which ideals are propagated by the media that are far from reality.

Contraceptive Needs of Adolescents

Efficacy. Adolescents need a highly effective method with a very low ideal and typical Pearl Index. Taking into account differences in adherence in diverse adolescent populations, this points to the necessity of long-acting methods independent of user adherence.

Health risks. Healthy adolescents are a low-risk population. At the same time health risks and complications have a very high negative impact in this age group. Adolescent contraception must not impair future fertility and not increase long-term health risks. Adolescent contraception should not impair organ development (musculoskeletal system, bone development).

Side effects. Contraceptive methods can exert negative effects on physical and psychological well-being. Adolescents are very sensitive to side effects because in this life phase many changes occur and there is an increased awareness towards signals from the body which may increase anxiety and insecurity. Subjectively experienced side effects like mood swings, decline in sexual desire or weight gain may lead to discontinuation of the method or inappropriate use, thereby reducing efficacy.

Additional benefits. Having the first intimate sexual contacts and intercourse means people in this age group need protection against STIs and HIV. For many adolescents it is difficult to maintain over a long period of time the regular use of a method. Methods independent of adherence and compliance overcome this difficulty. Not living in a steady relationship, adolescents need access to methods which are independent of the partner and under their control. Some adolescents are in need of help regarding specific complaints and symptoms. For these adolescents benefits are an important additional motivation to use the method.

Combined Hormonal Contraceptives during Adolescence [3, 4, 6–8]

See also Chapter 11.

Efficacy. The theoretical efficacy of combined hormonal contraceptives (CHCs) is high, but effectiveness varies strongly between countries, social strata and different adolescent populations.

Health risks. The main immediate health risks during use are thromboembolic events. The absolute risk is very low but, depending on the severity of the disease, even singular cases can contribute to a negative social image and scare adolescents. There is no risk regarding future fertility. There are even indications that CHCs preserve fertility. There is no evidence of long-term health risks. Indirect indication from a large long-term follow-up study is that CHC users have less long-term cardiovascular and oncologic morbidity and mortality. The risk regarding a reduction in the attainment of the individual peak bone mass is still controversial and there are no indications that adolescent users of CHC have a higher risk later in life to suffer from osteoporosis or osteoporotic fractures.

Side effects. Combined hormonal contraceptives may have a number of side effects like irregular bleeding, especially at the beginning of intake. Some adolescents report weight gain. There is no clear explanation of this symptom. There are reports of negative mood changes and loss of sexual desire and/or vaginal symptoms of dryness and pain. The relation to CHCs as causative factors is difficult to ascertain because of the lack of randomized clinical trials.

Additional characteristics. Combined hormonal contraceptives are independent of the partner and under the control of the adolescent. They offer a therapeutic effect on symptoms frequently found in the adolescent population like dysmenorrhea, acne or cycle irregularities. The effect is even more pronounced when CHCs are taken in a continuous regimen. Their efficacy depends on the user's adherence, which differs slightly between oral, transdermal and intra-vaginal applications. Intra-vaginal applications seem to facilitate adherence but this is not well studied.

Counselling

Advantages. The method profile corresponds to several important needs of this age group, especially concerning the regulatory of the menstrual cycle, use being under the control of the adolescent without intervention and having a therapeutic potential against existing symptoms and complaints like irregular or heavy bleeding, dysmenorrhea, hyper-androgenic skin symptoms and premenstrual syndrome, all of which are frequent conditions in this life phase.

Disadvantages. The disadvantages are user dependence and there is very low, albeit real risk of thromboembolic events. This needs good counselling about risk using absolute numbers and showing and discussing the pros and cons with the adolescent in a patient-centred way (see also contraceptive counselling).

Counselling in this age group is a challenge because there are many myths and misconceptions coming from the media, leading to what can be called hormonophobia, an irrational fear of hormones. This may need an open dialogue which on one hand takes these concerns seriously but on the other hand tries to inform and educate, putting the risks into perspective and showing the risk/benefit balance in an understandable way using appropriate language and eventually visual material. Another important aspect of counselling refers to the risk of STIs, which should be discussed in the context of sexual health in general. Prevention by concomitant use of condoms should be advised.

Progestogen-Only Pill during Adolescence

See also Chapter 12.

Efficacy. The theoretical efficacy of ovulation inhibiting preparations is high, but effectiveness varies strongly between countries, social strata and different adolescent populations. Effectiveness is much lower in older preparations which do not inhibit ovulation and where the contraceptive effect is based on changes in the cervical mucus

Health risks. The main advantage is that progestogen-only pills (POPs) do not carry cardiovascular risks, which makes them suitable for those adolescents who are afraid of thromboembolic complications or for those have an increased risk by combinations of family risk, smoking and obesity or those who have a personal history of VTE. There are no reports about long-term health risks. Regarding bone health, studies indicate that the maintenance of endogenous oestrogen levels is sufficient

Side effects. The main side effects are cycle irregularities with unexpected bleeding episodes. Although this is not a 'medical problem', it may be unacceptable for adolescents who want to see their regular monthly bleeding. Progestogens are known to interact with brain neuropeptides and Gaba receptors. It seems that in vulnerable young women this can have a negative impact on mood. A history of depression or low mood could be an indication to reconsider other options.

Additional characteristics. They offer some therapeutic effects on dysmenorrhea (primary or related to endometriosis).

Counselling

Advantages. The main advantage is that there is no increased risk of thromboembolic events neither on the venous nor on the arterial side. The method is under the control of the user and independent of the partner.

Disadvantages. The two most important disadvantages are cycle irregularity and user dependence. Another important aspect of counselling refers to the risk of STIs. There is no protection when using this method. Prevention of STIs by concomitant use of condom should be advised.

Depo Medroxyprogesterone Acetate [9]

Efficacy. The method itself has a high efficacy which is, however, still dependent on three monthly applications, which may be a challenge in this age group.

Health risks. No major short-term health risks are known. There is some controversy regarding VTE risk but not yet convincing evidence indicating an increased risk and the possible slightly increased risk for cervical carcinoma. The main health issue is the loss of bone mineral density due to suppression of endogenous oestrogen production, but this is considered reversible based on longitudinal and cross-sectional evidence [9]. There are no high-quality data to determine whether DMPA use in adolescence increases risk of bone fracture during adolescence or later in life, but there are no sufficient data.

Side effects. Taking all progestogen-only contraceptive methods together, this method has the strongest progestogenic effect and therefore can produce the general progestogen-associated side effects in a more pronounced way. Like with all progestogen-only methods, cycle irregularity and amenorrhea can be experienced in this age group as unwanted or desired side effect. The probability to induce amenorrhea is highest with this method. Some users observe weight gain, which is a problem in all age groups but may be especially problematic in a patient with eating problems. The possible prolonged period to regain full fertility is also a special issue in this age group.

Additional characteristics. Therapeutic effect on menstrual migraine and on catamenial epilepsy are additional benefits.

Counselling

Advantages. The main indication for Depo-Provera use in this age group is facilitating and supporting adherence, especially in adolescents who do not want or cannot have LARCs (e.g. uterine malformations, fear of implant). For some adolescents with irregular prolonged bleeding amenorrhea may be considered an advantage.

Disadvantages. The issue of possible weight gain is an important disadvantage as well as the possibly prolonged period to regain full fertility. The negative impact on metabolism is not something that adolescent takes notice of but it is of importance in this age group because in this life phase peak bone mass is acquired. At the moment the advice is to use DMPA in women under the age of 18 only after consideration of other methods and every 2 years a reassessment should be made. Another important aspect of counselling refers to the risk of STI infections in this age group. Prevention by concomitant use of condom should be advised.

Long-Acting Reversible Contraceptives during Adolescence

Efficacy. These are the most effective methods being user independent. Many national and international societies recommend these methods as first choice for adolescents.

Health risks. Copper IUDs and LNG IUS hold no major method-related short- or long-term health risks for this age group apart from the possible complications of these intrauterine contraceptives including rare incidences of expulsion, perforation and pregnancy (intrauterine, tubal pregnancies). The main issue for adolescents is the pain related to the insertion procedure coexisting with anxiety and aversion towards a foreign body inside the uterus.

No reports of long-term health risks from the implant exist. The main problem of the implant is migration accompanied by the necessity of invasive procedures to remove it. The incidence of these complications depends on the competence and training of the healthcare provider.

Side effects. For copper IUDs the main side effects are in rare cases hypermenorrhea, dysmenorrhea and lower abdominal pain. It is unclear whether tolerability varies with age. For the LNG-IUD some reports indicate that progestogen-only contraceptives have a negative impact on mood in the younger age groups. There is however still lack of good evidence (see

Chapter 17). The tolerability of bleeding irregularities, including amenorrhea, may be lower in this age group.

Counselling

Advantages. LARCs present the most effective contraceptive methods for this group with an optimal efficacy and safety profile.

Disadvantages. The main issues are insertion and removal and complications of these procedures. It is therefore very important that adolescents are well informed and care is taken to reduce pain during these procedures through good communication and different techniques and preparations (misoprostol, mefenamic acid, relaxation techniques, ultrasound etc.). There is no clear evidence which procedure is the most effective to reduce pain, but good communication during the procedure is a major element of pain reduction. Healthcare professionals should get appropriate training to make the procedure as painless as possible and reduce complications of insertion and removal. Another important aspect of counselling refers to the risk of STI infections. Prevention by concomitant use of condom should be advised.

Barrier Methods Use in Adolescents

See also Chapter 13.

Efficacy. The theoretical efficacy of male and female condoms is high. In real-life conditions there is, however, inconsistent use, leading to medium or even low effectiveness.

Health risks. There are no major health risk or side effects. Very rarely the use of spermicides can provoke an allergic reaction in the partner.

Additional characteristics. The most important additional benefit of these methods when properly used is protection against most STIs (see also Chapter 13). Male and female condom decrease the risk of transmission of STI associated with vaginal discharge (chlamydia, gonorrhoea, trichomoniasis and HIV). A lesser level of protection is provided for STI associated with genital ulcer or human papilloma virus (HPV). From incidence estimates, consistent use of condoms can decrease AIDS/HIV transmission by 85%.

Counselling. Counselling about STI risk is very important in this age group. Education about proper use of condoms or diaphragms should be part of contraceptive counselling (see also Chapter 13).

Fertility Awareness Methods

As the methods are based on prediction of ovulation, effectiveness is strongly influenced by cycle regularity and consistent monitoring of the parameters. There are no health risks or side effects.

Counselling. These methods are interesting for adolescents to get to know their body better and understand their cycle pattern, cycle-related complaints and so forth. They should be used together with another method, including consistent and permanent use of condoms.

The Middle-Aged Woman [9–12]

In this phase of life again biological and psychosocial changes and challenges have an impact on contraceptive counselling, decision-making and care.

Biomedical factors. After the increase of fertility in the late teens and 20s there is a decline of fertility starting around 35 and increasing dramatically towards the fourth decade. Women go through pregnancies and birth with a variety of outcomes having an impact on their physical and emotional health. The incidence and prevalence of benign gynaecological disorders increases like:

- Endometriosis, chronic pelvic pain.
- Ovarian cysts, functional and endometriotic.
- Development of fibromas.
- Early stages of malignant disease may manifest themselves.
- Cervical dysplasia and neoplasia.
- In some women metabolic risks increase (metabolic syndrome).

Psychosocial Factors

Stress, smoking, drug abuse and alcohol increase cardiovascular and mental health risks. Establishing a stable relationship and creating an environment to care for children needs knowledge and skills and represents a constant stress with possible impact on the endocrine system. For some women the reproductive life plan is interrupted and unfulfilled with the potential of not having a child. Women and men may experience separation, divorce and breaking up of relationship and family structures which gave stability of life and they have to rebuild their life.

Contraceptive Needs of Middle-Aged Women

Efficacy. Many women want to change contraception and others wish for a child. Some women do not want

the responsibility of short-acting methods and welcome methods which do not depend on regular intake.

Health risks. Although the relative risk increase regarding thromboembolic events remains the same as during adolescence, the age-related background increase in cardiovascular risks contributes to an increase in the absolute risk. At the same time additional risk factors like obesity and smoking have to be taken into account to protect women from complications. The increase of comorbidities in this age group (cardiovascular, oncologic, metabolic, endocrine) has to be integrated into the decision-making about use of methods. Existing symptoms and benign conditions (PMS, PMDD, bleeding problems) present opportunities to consider benefits of hormonal methods.

Side effects. Women in this age group are more familiar with their body and its reactions and signals. Side effects are therefore for many of them less alarming compared to adolescence and the acceptability of side effects may be higher.

Benefits. Protection against STI and HIV is important, but for many women it is not a priority. Gynaecologic comorbidities play an important role in this age group. Existing symptoms and benign conditions should be taken into account when deciding about methods. Therapeutic effects on endometriotic pain, ovarian cyst formation, skin changes in the context of polycystic ovary syndrome (PCOS), bleeding irregularities and dysmenorrhea are possible desired additional effects of contraceptives.

Combined Hormonal Contraceptives in Middle-Aged Women

Efficacy. The difference between efficacy and effectiveness is less than in the younger age group.

Health risks. The absolute thromboembolic risk increases with age. Nonetheless women without additional risk factors from the use of CHC are eligible according to the international guidelines and MEC. There is a small absolute risk increase in breast and cervical cancer among users which disappears 5 years after stopping. There are no major long-term cardiovascular or oncologic risks.

Side effects. Reported side effects do not seem to be different in different age groups. Subjective tolerability may be higher.

Additional characteristics. Combined hormonal contraceptives do not protect against PID and HIV. Taking into account the rate of divorce and separation in this age group, it remains, however, important to keep this risk in mind. Combined hormonal contraceptives have therapeutic potential for patients with endometriosis, functional ovarian cysts, hyper-androgenic skin symptoms and bleeding irregularities.

Counselling

Advantages. Combined hormonal contraceptives are highly effective when correctly used and the method is under the control of the woman. There is no need for an intervention. The long-term protection against endometrial and ovarian cancer is of importance in women with familial and genetic risks. Combined hormonal contraceptives are valuable methods for pregnancy spacing by women. The most important aspect is therapeutic potential, including typical benign conditions in this age group like endometriotic pain, irregular or heavy menstrual bleeding, hyper-androgenic skin symptoms, PMS and PMDD, ovarian cysts, PID or ectopic pregnancy.

Disadvantages. Age-related increase in cardiovascular problems, especially thrombotic risk, is potentiated by additional risk factors found in this age group. There is a small increased risk for breast and cervical cancer which disappears after stopping. The large spectrum of possible physical and psychological side effects varies from individual to individual and cannot be predicted but have to be reviewed in follow-up visits. There is no protection against STIs, which remain a risk in this age group.

Progestogen-Only Pill in Middle-Aged Women

See progestogen-only pill in adolescence regarding efficacy, health risks, side effects and special characteristics.

Counselling

The method profile corresponds to the needs of midlife women to have a low-dose, oestrogen-free contraceptive without thromboembolic risk. This is especially true for women with additional risk factors who want to have the method under their control and do not want interventions. The main disadvantage for this age group are cycle irregularity and dependence on user adherence.

Depo Provera in the Middle-Aged Woman

See earlier in this chapter.

Counselling

In this age group the delay of full fertility is an important disadvantage in women who want to space pregnancy and have a clear reproductive life plan. In long-term users intermittent evaluation of the estrogen levels and reevaluation of other options take into account possible health problems.

Long-Acting Reversible Contraceptives in Middle-Aged Women

The efficacy, health risks, side effects and special characteristics are the same as described about the use in adolescents.

Counselling

The LARCs present the most effective contraceptive methods with an optimal efficacy and safety profile independent of age. Submucous fibroma formation may limit use of intrauterine contraceptives in this age group. For long-acting intrauterine contraceptives (copper IUD, LNG IUD) immediate postpartum, post-miscarriage and post–termination of pregnancy insertion is an opportunity of serving women with a well-tolerated intervention in the context of another reproductive event. The implant can also be inserted immediately after birth, miscarriage or TOP. Menstrual irregularities, including heavy menstrual bleeding, are an indication for the therapeutic use of LNG IUDs.

Sexual history taking is important, including STI protection with a condom, and questions about sexual well-being should be addressed especially before and during pregnancy and in the postpartum period. These events can have a negative impact on sexual function (see Chapter 51). An important aspect of counselling refers to the age-related decline of fertility to increase awareness with respect to reproductive decision-making

Barrier Methods

See earlier in this chapter.

Counselling

Routine assessment of STI risk is still advised.

Fertility-Awareness Methods

See earlier in this chapter.

Counselling

Women with regular cycles and intention to delay the next desired pregnancy can be suitable for this method if interested to learn about it and practise regular monitoring, which could be facilitated by fertility trackers.

The Menopausal Transition

This life phase includes specific changes, having an impact on contraceptive counselling and care [13–15].

Biomedical Factors

Ovarian ageing leads to a strong decline in fertility, which confronts women with the decision about continuing contraception or trying to get pregnant. Pregnancy itself is associated with greater risks, including miscarriage, chromosomal abnormalities and pregnancy complications. Progesterone decline and oestrogen fluctuation lead in many women to bleeding irregularities including heavy menstrual bleeding. Climacteric symptoms like hot flushes, irritability and sleeping disorders may occur. Bone demineralization is observed due to the decline of oestrogen. There is an increase in the risk of age-related morbidity, including cardiovascular, oncologic, metabolic, neurologic and psychiatric diseases, and in the context of increased morbidity many women are under drug treatment.

Psychosocial Factors

Many women are confronted with ambivalence about family planning and have to decide about different options regarding their reproductive future.

Individuals and couples. Women and men have to care for their elderly parents. Many individuals have reached the top of their professional career with additional distress to maintain the position when at the same time they may experience a decline in energy and motivation. They may experience symptoms of burnout and depression as the result of the imbalance between the life stressors and the age-related decline in resources and coping capacity depending on the individual resilience. In this context women, men and couples may experience changes in sexual health and function with loss of interest, arousal and orgasmic difficulties and/or painful sex.

Contraceptive Needs of Women during the Menopausal Transition

Contraception should be continued until menopause, defined as 2 years after the last natural menstrual period in women under age 50 and until 1 year after the last natural menstrual period in women over age 50. If menopause cannot be confirmed, contraception should be continued until age 55.

Efficacy. These women need a highly effective method to protect against unintended high-risk pregnancy.

Health risks. The age-related rather dramatic increase in the risk for cardiovascular diseases is an important condition which has to be taken into account in the choice of methods as well as the increase in all types of chronic morbidity. Contraception should not aggravate symptoms and increase risk of the pre-existing disease and contraception should not interfere with treatment of diseases.

Side effects. Women in this phase of life may suffer from various physical and mental symptoms which impair general health. This may increase their susceptibility to side effects and decrease tolerability towards side effects which may aggravate pre-existing symptoms.

Additional characteristics. Contraceptives should if possible reduce or even have a therapeutic effect on frequent symptoms like bleeding irregularities, climacteric symptoms, perimenopausal depression and sexual dysfunction and protect against age-related disease like osteoporosis and cancer. Protection against STI and HIV is important but for many women not a priority; however, in several countries chlamydia, gonorrhoea, HIV and other STIs are on the increase in women in their 40s and 50s.

Combined Hormonal Contraceptives in Women during the Menopausal Transition

Efficacy. There is a high effectiveness also in typical use due to the reduced fertility.

Health risks. See the earlier section in this chapter on middle-aged women. Very important is the age-related increased absolute risk in thromboembolic diseases (venous and arterial) and the prevalence of health conditions which limit the use of CHCs (see the section on Medical Eligibility Criteria earlier in this chapter).

Side effects. Reported side effects do not seem to be different in different age groups. Subjective tolerability may be lower or higher.

Benefits. Combined hormonal contraceptives have a therapeutic potential regarding frequent symptoms like bleeding irregularity, climacteric symptoms, perimenopausal depression and sexual dysfunction.

They reduce the risk of ovarian and endometrial cancer

Counselling

Advantages. There is no intervention necessary and the method is under the control of the woman. The various preparations carry with them a therapeutic potential with regard to frequent symptoms like bleeding irregularity, climacteric symptoms, depressive mood and irritability, as well as sexual dysfunction.

Disadvantages. The most important disadvantage is the age-related absolute risk increase in cardiovascular especially thrombotic diseases. If this risk is potentiated by additional risk factors frequently found in this age group CHCs should not be prescribed. In women without these risk factors who have been for previous years using CHCs without complications there is some controversy taking into account the aforementioned beneficial effects (see also the section in this chapter on Medical Eligibility Criteria WHO, FSRH, CDC).

Progestogen-Only Pill and Depo Provera for Women in the Menopausal Transition

Counselling. The same counselling recommendations apply as given for the other age groups.

Long-Acting Reversible Contraceptives for Women in the Menopausal Transition

Efficacy. These are the most effective methods which are user and age independent.

Health risks. See the section earlier in this chapter on middle-aged women.

Side effects. There are no age-related differences in the side effect profile.

Special characteristics. See earlier in this chapter with other age groups.

Counselling

Advantages. The methods combine high effectiveness with a very good safety profile which from a medical point of view makes them first-choice methods. In addition the LNG IUD is considered the first choice for the treatment of heavy menstrual bleeding (HMB) and has some therapeutic effect on pain from endometriosis.

Disadvantages. There is a need for intervention which can limit the use due to uterine disease (intrauterine methods) or unacceptability of an implant in the arm. These methods provide no protection against STI and HIV.

Barrier Methods

See earlier in this chapter.

Fertility-Awareness Methods

Fertility-awareness methods are not advised due to the irregularity of cycles and the unpredictability of ovulation.

Summary

The life-course approach in contraception takes into account the different biological and psychosocial changes which typically occur from adolescence across midlife to the menopause. These changes lead to different needs and demands with respect to contraception in general but also for the individual woman in the respective life phase. These needs have an impact on the choice of the method by the woman. Counselling should help to make this choice to find the best method for the individual woman.

References

1. World Health Organization. *Health at key stages of life: The life-course approach to public health.* Updated. Copenhagen: WHO Regional Office for Europe, 2015. www.euro.who.int/__data/assets/pdf.

2. unfpa.org/sites/default/files/resource-pdf/One pager on youth demographics GF.pdf.

3. World Health Organization. *Medical eligibility criteria.* 5th edition. Geneva: World Health Organization, 2015. https://bit.ly/3kTOzNk.

4. FSRH Faculty of Sexual & Reproductive Healthcare (FSRH). UK Medical Eligibility Criteria for Contraceptive Use (UKMEC). 2016. https://bit.ly/3l9Vi6c.

5. U.S. Medical Eligibility Criteria for contraceptive use, 2016 Recommendations and Reports / Vol. 65 / No. 3.

6. World Health Organization Department of Reproductive Health and Research (WHO/RHR) and Johns Hopkins Bloomberg School of Public Health/Center for Communication Programs (CCP), Knowledge for Health Project. *Family planning: A global handbook for providers* (2018 update). Baltimore, MD and Geneva: Center for Communication Programs and World Health Organization, 2018.

7. Bitzer J. Oral contraceptives in adolescent women. *Best Pract Res Clin Endocrinol Metab.* 2013;27(1):77–89. https://doi.org/10.1016/j.beem.2012.09.005.

8. Bitzer J, Abalos V, Apter D, Martin R, Black A for Global CARE Group. Targeting factors for change: Contraceptive counselling and care of female adolescents. *European Journal of Contraception & Reproductive Health Care*. 2016;**21**(6):417–30. doi.org/10.1080/13625187.2016.1237629.

9. FSRH Clinical Guideline: Progestogen-only Injectable (December 2014, amended October 2020).

10. Mahmood T (Chair). EBCOG Standards of Care for Women's Health in Europe: Gynaecology Services. 2014. https://bit.ly/3l4ntDs.

11. Curtis KM, Jatlaoui TC, Tepper NK et al. U.S. selected practice recommendations for contraceptive use. *MMWR Recomm Rep*. 2016;**65**(No. RR–4): 1–66. http://dx.doi.org/10.15585/mmwr. rr6504a1.

12. Dehlendorf C, Krajewski C, Borrero S. Contraceptive counseling: Best practices to ensure quality communication and enable effective contraceptive use. *Clinical Obstetrics and Gynecology*. 2014;**57**(4): 659–73. https://doi.org/10.1097/GRF .0000000000000059.

13. https://bit.ly/3HF4GaA.

14. https://bit.ly/3HX3Kyu.

15. Bitzer J. Overview of perimenopausal contraception. *Climacteric*. 2019;**22**:44–50.

Male Contraception

Gideon A. Sartorius and Yacov Reisman

General Aspects: Physiology of Sperm Production

The adult testis has two main functions: production of male gametes and production of male sex hormones. The androgen production occurs in the interstitium between the seminiferous tubules, where Leydig cells are stimulated by luteinizing hormone (LII), which is secreted in a pulsatile manner by the pituitary. The production of spermatozoa, the spermatogenesis, occurs within the seminiferous tubules, where production and maturation of sperm is coordinated by Sertoli cells. The production of mature sperm starts with puberty and takes approximately 64 to 72 days. This process can be separated into four distinct phases:

- Mitotic proliferation of the testicular stem cells (spermatogonia) into diploid spermatocytes.
- A meiotic phase during which spermatocytes first double their chromosome number and the tetraploid spermatocytes then undergo two cell divisions, leading to haploid spermatids.
- Spermiogenesis, the phase when spermatids are transformed into testicular sperm with a condensed nucleus and a flagellum.
- Spermiation, when spermatozoa are released into the tubular lumen.

After release into the tubular lumen spermatozoa are transported through the rete testis in the epididymis for further maturation and storage before ejaculation. The process of sperm production is stimulated by the secretion of follicle-stimulating hormone (FSH) from the pituitary gland – and by high intratesticular concentrations of testosterone. However, it is essential to understand that exogenous testosterone inhibits spermatogenesis via suppression of FSH secretion in the pituitary [1].

About 100 million sperm are produced every day, and each ejaculation contains up to 200 million sperm, with a concentration of $> = 15$ million/ml, which is considered normal. Unused sperm are either resorbed or passed out of the body in urine [2].

General Aspects: Male Contraception

Worldwide, 41% of pregnancies were unplanned and 20% of these pregnancies resulted in abortion [3, 4]. These high rates of unintended pregnancy are the result of inadequate use of or access to modern methods of contraception. Contraception is the intentional avoidance of conception.

Male contraceptives work by 1) prevention of sperm production, 2) by disturbing the conceptive capacity of spermatozoa or 3) by preventing spermatozoa to reach the ovum – the so-called barrier methods. The male contraceptive methods that are available today are limited. Only two are feasible worldwide, the male condom (barrier) and vasectomy (sterilization). Nevertheless, both condoms and vasectomy have significant disadvantages. On the positive side, condoms do provide some protection against sexually transmitted infections (STI), but they have a suboptimal contraceptive efficacy and depend on discipline and availability of the condom at the time of intercourse [5]. Vasectomy requires surgery and can be expensive. Furthermore, vasectomy might cause chronic pain and is considered a definitive method [6].

The ideal male contraceptive should be safe (no adverse side effects), effective, acceptable (to men and their partners), and affordable (to programmes and potential users). While the majority of men are aware of and approve the use of family-planning methods, the use of current male contraception methods is poor, with regional and country variations. Low levels of use may be related to a low acceptance of the existing methods, as, for example, shown in a study conducted in Fiji, Iran, India and Korea, where men considered a male pill or injection more acceptable than a vasectomy. The available data suggest women in stable relationships will trust their partner to use a

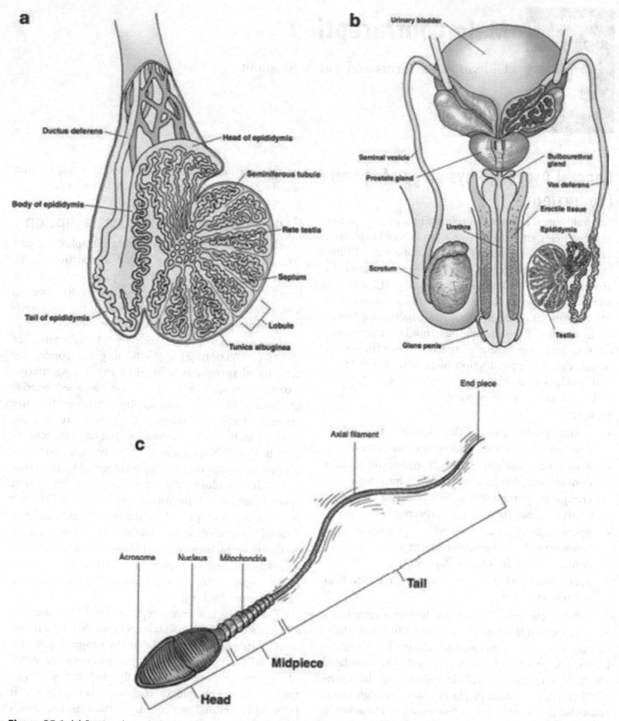

Figure 35.1 **(a)** Section through the testis showing the organization of how the tubules form a U-shape at the periphery. Note: that means that any peripheral testis biopsy or TESE procedure will not cause obstruction to the seminiferous tubules. But a deep biopsy will cause obstructive damage. **(b)** Male sex organs: overview showing the whole system. **(c)** Anatomy of a single normal mature spermatozoon (sperm). Note the importance of the acrosome at the head like a battering ram for egg penetration and the intense condensation of mitochondria at the mid-piece to provide energy for sperm mobility

male contraceptive if one is available [7]. A positive attitude towards the male pill does not inherently mean the person is confident about its effective use. Once the male pill is readily available, advertising efforts will target not only men, but also their female partners, as they appear important in the effective use of contraceptive methods and come into contact with healthcare services more frequently [6, 8].

Approaches to male contraception include targeting the sperm through inhibition of production (spermatogenesis), interrupting transport, blocking semen deposition and disrupting function and preventing fertilization. Inhibiting sperm production could be done through hormonal contraception (androgen alone, progestin + androgen, GnRH agonists or antagonists, FSH antagonists and vaccines).

Non-hormonal male contraception targets sperm production, maturation and/or function, without interrupting the hormonal pathway. Non-hormonal targets in the spermatogenesis and fertilization process have been identified, and contraceptive opportunities are currently being tested and in development [9].

Available Male Contraception Methods

Withdrawal and Natural Family Planning

Withdrawal or coitus interruptus is sometimes considered a male method of contraception and is mentioned as the primary method of contraception by 3–5% of couples. The medical community does not endorse withdrawal as an effective method of contraception. In couples using withdrawal as a sole method of contraception the stated one-year failure rate is 20–30% for typical use (real-life use) [10]. Another male-related method of contraception is fertility awareness (also known as 'natural family planning'). This method is driven by a female partner's knowledge of the timing of her ovulation. The contraceptive efficacy of this option with typical use has a failure rate similar to that of withdrawal [11]. However, both methods seem strongly dependent on diligence and training of users – the withdrawal method shows a failure rate with perfect use of 4% and the symptothermal method (the most elaborate method of fertility-awareness-based methods) even comes close to hormonal methods with a 0.4% failure rate with perfect use [10].

Condoms

Men have used condoms for contraception for several hundred years. Originally produced out of animal intestines, condoms have mostly been made from latex rubber since the 1920s. Condoms prevent pregnancies by blocking the route of semen to the cervix. With perfect use, the failure rate is 2% [10]. An added benefit of condoms is protection against STIs and HIV. On the other hand, failure rates are as high as 12–18% for typical use [10, 12]. The correct use of condoms refers to the application of condoms before vaginal penetration, preferably before any penetration. On application, the tip of the condom must be pressed to release trapped air and consequently provide space for semen. The shortcoming of this method apart from its failure rates is the possibility of latex allergies, the possibility of breakage and decreased sexual pleasure for some couples [12].

In general, men may use a condom if they are confident with their ability to use condoms correctly, with the way condoms fit or feel and in sex within a stable relationship. Men who don't experience confidence with the use of a condom may experience condom-associated erection loss. Furthermore, men who have perceived a larger decrease in pleasure with condom use are less likely to use condoms again then men with no decrease or lower decrease in pleasure [13].

Vasectomy

Vasectomy is a procedure in which the vasa deferentia are divided and ligated to prevent the flow of sperm from the testis. This is an outpatient procedure, conducted under local anaesthesia with minimal side effects. Vasectomy/sterilization is performed worldwide in 42–60 million men (5–8% of married couples) annually with a wide variety of prevalence across different parts of the world – for example, the prevalence in New Zealand is 23%, in the United States and the Netherlands 11%, in China 8% and in Brazil 1.6%. All other developing countries have less than 1% prevalence of use [11]. The "no-scalpel technique," developed in China, which uses scissors to create a single midline puncture in the scrotal raphe, has been widely adopted [14].

The patient's history should provide details on his marital status, number of children and reasons for the procedure. Medical and surgical records should also be checked, including a previous history of surgical or anaesthetic complications. The patient should receive detailed information about the procedure and post-operative care. Vasectomy is intended to be a permanent form of contraception and its benefits and potential complications should be explained as well. It should be emphasized that vasectomy does not produce immediate sterility and that another type of contraception is needed before vas occlusion is verified by a post-vasectomy semen analysis. Men should be always informed about the small possibility of vasectomy failure. The risk of pregnancy after vasectomy is approximately 1 in 2,000 for men who have post-vasectomy azoospermia [15].

Following vasectomies, pregnancy rates drop to clearly below 1% [10]. However, vasectomy is only appropriate for men who do not wish for any future fertility. Approximately 3–5% of men who have a vasectomy eventually request reversal, usually due to remarriage or the death of a child. Reversibility rates after vasectomy are only 50–75%, depending mainly on the interval between vasectomy and vaso-vasostomy [14].

A disadvantage of vasectomy is the delay in the onset of azoospermia and hence contraceptive efficacy of 3–4 months as sperm in the vas distal to the site of surgery still appear in the ejaculate. Vasectomy is associated with a low frequency of complications such as hematoma, infection and sperm granuloma. Post-operative pain can also be an issue. While most surgical pain is quickly resolved, 10–15% of men have chronic testicular discomfort following vasectomy [16]. Some of these men are relieved from their discomfort with the reversal of the vasectomy, indicating that the obstruction of the vases may cause their pain. Some men remain concerned about the detrimental effects of vasectomy on sexual activity; however, there is no proof of such an association [17]. All available data indicate vasectomy is safe and is not associated with increased risk of serious, long-term side-effects or diseases like testicular cancer, prostate cancer or heart disease [17].

Future Developments

Non-hormonal Contraceptives

The application of low-intensity ultrasound to the scrotum can increase the temperature of the tissue in the testes. Spermatogenesis cannot occur at core body temperature, which is why human testes are suspended in a scrotal sac with a network of blood vessels to facilitate cooling. Studies show that heat stress on the testicles contributes to the apoptosis of germ cells. No side effects are noted in ultrasound treatments; however, there is concern that heat treatment may cause DNA damage in consecutive sperm productions [18].

Reversible inhibition of sperm under guidance (RISUG) is a method of contraception directed at the destruction of sperm as it passes through the vas deferens. It is applied by injection of steric maleic anhydride (SMA) and dimethyl sulfoxide (DMSO) into the vas deferens. Within the next 72 hours, RISUG forms electrically charged precipitates in the lumen, with positive charges dominating. This forms an acidic environment. Sperm that pass through the RISUG-injected vas deferens suffer ionic and pH stress, causing acrosomal damage and rendering them unable to fertilize oocytes. The RISUG can be flushed out with intra-vasal injections of sodium bicarbonate, which will reverse its infertility effects, as has been shown in mice [19]. Phase I and II studies have confirmed its efficacy for at least 1 year, but duration of effect is probably much longer [20]. A variation of this technique is the intra-vas device (IVD). It involves injecting a 'plug' into the vas deferens which can be removed later. The IVD filters out the sperm as it passes through the vas deferens.

Contraceptive vaccines are designed to target the specific antigens of sperm. Vaccination with these sperm antigens (recombinant / synthetic peptide / DNA) has been shown to cause reversible contraceptive effects in animals through the formation of systemic and local anti-sperm responses. [21]. Other substances such as iodopyridines, adjudging, gamendazole, calcium channel blockers and gandarusa which interfere with the spermatogenesis or the Sertoli cell function are being tested as possible future non-hormonal contraceptives in males [22].

An orally effective contraceptive pill for men has been approved in Indonesia. The pill, taken 30–40 minutes before coitus, prevents the spermatozoa from penetrating the ovum extracellular coat (zona pellucida) and prevents fertilization by inhibiting multiple enzymes on the sperm head. The pill contains an agent from the leaves of the gandarusa plant. The pill became available to Indonesian men by prescription in 2014, but the exact compound and clinical data are not known [23].

Hormonal Contraceptives

The idea of hormonal contraception in men is to interrupt spermatogenesis by changing the hormonal pathway. Gonadotropin-releasing hormone (GnRH) from the hypothalamus is released in a pulsatile manner and stimulates the pulsatile secretion of luteinizing hormone (LH) and follicle-stimulating hormone (FSH) from the pituitary. The FSH stimulates Sertoli cells to induce spermatogenesis, while the LH stimulates Leydig cells to produce testosterone. Testosterone then provides negative feedback to the hypothalamus and pituitary, suppressing their activity and subsequently sperm production. Male hormonal contraception focusses on suppressing the hypothalamus and the pituitary action to inhibit spermatogenesis. This has been done by the provision of testosterone alone as well as testosterone in combination with progestins [21]. The defined goal of hormonal contraception is to reduce sperm counts to a concentration below 1 million sperm per millilitre, which reduces the chance of a pregnancy to below 1% per year [24].

Testosterone as a long-acting preparation that requires weekly administration through intramuscular injections is a possibility [22]. In a study by the World Health Organization (WHO), azoospermia was achieved within an average of 3 months in 70% of men receiving 200 mg T weekly. Once azoospermia is reached, testosterone can be effectively used alone as a contraceptive with a 0.8% failure rate. Reversibility occurs within an average of 4 months after discontinuation. However, this method has a few disadvantages: the efficacy of hormonal contraception is different to the ethnic background of study participants, with Asian participants showing higher efficacy than European, North American or Australian men [25]. Not all men receiving this therapy will become azoospermic; weekly injections are required and there were worrying side effects regarding HDL levels and testicular volume, albeit reversible after cessation of use. This method requires a few months to achieve azoospermia, therefore requiring another form of contraceptive until azoospermia is achieved [22]. Testosterone formulated in long-acting depot preparations with a half-life of 70 days that can be administered intramuscularly in intervals of 4–8 weeks is also being tested [23]. However, trials were stopped due to reports of side effects such as mood swings.

7α-Methyl-19-nortestosterone (MENT) is a synthetic androgen five times more potent than testosterone. It was developed to replace testosterone for contraceptive use because of the large amount of testosterone required to achieve long-term infertility. In addition, it is resistant to 5α-reductase and therefore shows less prostate stimulation. However, substituting testosterone with MENT led to a decrease in bone density. In addition, men receiving MENT and etonogestrel experienced loss of libido [4].

Exogenous progestins combined with testosterone provide better suppression of gonadotropins and are thus more effective at producing azoospermia at lower doses [19]. Several research projects have combined various progestins with androgens for a male contraceptive. An important disadvantage of using synthetic testosterone is that sperm production is suppressed at different rates in men of different ethnic origins. These differences may be due to genetic, dietary or environmental factors, but the exact reasons are unknown. Understanding the reasons may lead to new ways of providing effective contraception for all men of diverse ethnic backgrounds [23].

Conclusions

Contraception differs from most drugs in that healthy individuals use it for prevention rather than cure, therefore tolerance of side effects is low. It seems the time has come for the implementation of a novel, safe, effective and affordable male contraception. Contributions to the development of male contraception have been made. There are several potential methods for male contraception in which non-hormonal approaches are undergoing clinical trials and may be available in the near future. There is still no hormonal contraceptive ready to use for men. Improvement of our understanding of the molecular basis of the reproductive mechanism may reveal new possibilities and allow men to contribute more equally to the prevention of unintentional pregnancy.

References

1. Nieschlag E, Behre HM, Nieschlag S, eds. *Andrology, male reproductive health and dysfunction*. 3rd completely revised and updated edition. Berlin: Springer, 2010.

2. Gilbert SF. *Developmental biology*. 6th edition. Sunderland: Sinauer Associates, 2000. Spermatogenesis. www.ncbi.nlm.nih.gov/books/NBK10095.

3. Shah I, Ahman E. Unsafe abortion in 2008: Global and regional level and trends. *Reprod Health Matters* 2008;**18**:90–101.

4. Gava G, Meriggiola MC. Update on male hormonal contraception. *Ther Adv Endocrinol Metab*. 2019;**10**:1–9.

5. Trussell J, Vaughan B. Contraceptive failure, method-related discontinuation and resumption of use: Results from the 1995 National Survey of Family Growth. *Fam Plann Perspect*. 1999;**31**:64–72.

6. Heinemann K, Saad F, Wiesemes M, White S, Heinemann L. Attitudes towards male fertility control: Results of a multinational survey on four continents. *Human Repro*. 2005;**20**:549–56.

7. Glasier AF, Anakwe R, Everington D et al. Would women trust their partners to use a male pill? *Human Repro*. 2000;**15**:646–9.

8. Eberhardt J, Van Wersch A, Meikle N. Attitudes towards the male contraceptive pill in men and women in casual and stable sexual relationships. *J Fam Plann Reprod Health Care* 2009;**35**:161–5.

9. Nya-Ngatchou JJ, Amory JK. New approaches to male non-hormonal contraception. *Contraception* 2013;**87**:296–9.

10. Trussell J. Contraceptive efficacy. In Hatcher RA, Trussell J, Nelson AL et al. (eds.), *Contraceptive technology*. 20th revised edition. New York: Ardent Media, 2011, pp. 65–112.

11. Daniels K, Daugherty J, Jones J, Mosher W. Current contraceptive use and variation by selected characteristics among women aged 15–44: US, 2011–2013. *Natl Health Stat Report* 2015;**86**:1–14.

12. Roth MY. Male hormonal contraception. *Virtual Mentor* 2012;**14**(2):126–32.

13. Randolph ME, Pinkerton SD, Bogart LM et al. Sexual pleasure and condom use. *Arch Sex Behav*. 2007;**36**:844–8.

14. Li S-Q, Goltein M, Shu J, Huber D. The no-scalpel vasectomy. *J Urol*. 1991;**145**:341–4.

15. Cook LA, Van Vliet HAAM, Lopez LM, Pun A, Gallo MF. Vasectomy occlusion techniques for male sterilization. *Cochrane Database of Systematic Reviews* 2007;(2):Art. No.: CD003991. https://doi.org/10.1002/14651858.CD003991.pub3.

16. Myers SA, Mershon CE, Fuchs EF. Vasectomy reversal for treatment of the postvasectomy pain syndrome. *J Urol* 1997;**157**:518–20.

17. Campbell AD, Turok DK, White K. Fertility intentions and perspectives on contraceptive involvement among low-income men aged 25 to 55. *Perspect Sex Reprod Health* 2019;**51**:125–33.

18. Tsuruta JK, Dayton PA, Gallippi CM et al. Therapeutic ultrasound as a potential male contraceptive: Power, frequency and temperature required to deplete rat testes of meiotic cells and epididymites of sperm determined using a commercially available system. *Reprod Biol Endocrin*. 2012;**10**:7. https://doi.org/10.1186/1477-7827-10-7.

19. Jha RK, Jha PK, Guha SK. Smart RISUG: A potential new contraceptive and its magnetic field-mediated sperm interaction. *Int J Nanomedicine* 2009;**4**,55–64.

20. Guha SK, Singh G, Ansari S et al. Phase II clinical trial of a vas deferens injectable contraceptive for the male. *Contraception* 1997;**56**:245–50.

21. Mathew V, Bantwal G. Male contraception. *Ind J Endo Metab*. 2012;**16**:910–17.

22. Reynolds-Wright JJ, Anderson RA. Male contraception: Where are we going and where have we been? *BMJ Sex Reprod Health* 2019;**45**:236–42.

23. Tulsiani DRP, Abou-Haila A. Biology of male fertility control: An overview of various male contraceptive approaches. *Minerva Ginecol*. 2015;**67**:169–83.

24. Aalronen P, Amor JK, Anderson R et al. 10th summit meeting consensus: Recommendations for regulatory approval for hormonal contraception. *J Androl* 2007;**28**:362–3.

25. WHO Task Force on Methods for the Regulation of Male Fertility. Contraceptive efficacy of induced azoospermia and oligozoospermia in normal men. *Fertil Steril* 1996;**65**:821–9.

Chapter

36

Termination of Pregnancy
Overview

John J. Reynolds-Wright, Sharon T. Cameron

Introduction

Every woman has the recognized human right to decide freely and responsibly without coercion and violence the number, spacing and timing of their children and to have the information and means to do so, and the right to attain the highest standard of sexual and reproductive health. Access to legal and safe abortion is essential for the realization of these rights.

WHO statement on abortion

Prevalence of Abortion

Abortion is the most common gynaecological procedure worldwide and on average 56 million abortions are performed globally each year. One third of women will experience an induced abortion in their lifetime and most of them will have a single abortion [1]. When abortion is performed safely in a legal setting the complication rate is low and long-term morbidity and mortality are virtually non-existent [2] and 14 times lower than for childbirth [3]. However, less safe and least safe abortions are responsible for 31,000 maternal deaths and 7 million hospital admissions for complications globally each year [1].

Prohibiting abortion does not prevent abortion. There is no significant difference in abortion rates between countries that restrict abortion access and countries where abortion is broadly legal [1]. In the European context the majority of countries have legislation providing safe abortion, however there are notable exceptions, where abortion can be considered only in order to save a woman's life. As a result, women are forced to travel to neighbouring countries from areas with high abortion restriction to areas with less restriction.

Official statistics on abortion rates vary throughout Europe, from 0.1 per 1000 women aged 15–49 in Poland up to 20.8 per 1000 women aged 15–49

in Sweden [4]. This variation is due to differences in legal status, ease of access and robustness of methods of reporting abortion statistics between European nations.

Pre-abortion Assessment

Requesting an Abortion

When a woman requests an abortion, she should receive information on her options and be able to commence the abortion as soon as possible. Delays in access to abortion care result in greater gestational ages at abortion and therefore increased risk of a complication. If a clinician objects to the provision of abortion, it is his or her responsibility to direct the woman to another clinician willing to facilitate it without delay.

Abortion services should always be woman-centred and based on human rights. In addition, it should be appreciated that women who have sex with women, trans men and non-binary-assigned-female-at-birth patients may present to abortion services. A respectful, non-judgemental approach should be taken at all times and assumptions should not be made about an individual's circumstances. Rather, open and frank communication should take place.

Different jurisdictions have varying legislation and policies regarding the care of young girls who present to abortion services. There may be a requirement to involve social services or child protection services for girls below a certain age. It is essential that clinicians are familiar with their local, regional and national policies.

Pre-abortion Counselling

Women should not be subjected to mandatory or unrequested pre-abortion counselling as this only causes distress and adds delay to care. There may be women who present to abortion services who are undecided or uncertain of their decision to end the pregnancy. There should be provisions within a service for these women to access unbiased and non-judgemental counselling to support their decision-making if they wish to do so.

Furthermore, the majority of women will not require professional support or therapeutic counselling following an abortion. Again, there are certain groups who may be more likely to need support with decision-making or post-abortion support such as those with a previous history of mental ill health; those who belong to a religious group opposed to abortion; those who feel abortion is morally wrong but still wish to undergo it; and those who are ambivalent about their decision.

All women should receive high-quality information on abortion and the methods of treatment available to them. This information should ideally be available in advance of their appointment in order for it to be assimilated and so any areas of uncertainty can be raised at their consultation. Information should be available in multiple formats, including audiovisual, and in multiple languages [5]. Decision aids can be used to help women select a method of abortion if they are uncertain [6].

Medical History

Medical history should include reproductive history and previous contraceptive use. Complex medical conditions may warrant the involvement of other specialists – for example, a woman with cardiac disease may need the input of a cardiologist or anaesthetist and may require a particular method or location for her abortion care. Likewise, a previous history of caesarean section is important to elicit as this is a risk factor for uterine rupture, a rare complication in second-trimester medical abortion. Women should have an assessment for venous thromboembolism (VTE) and mechanical or pharmacological thromboprophylaxis should be available. Contraceptive history can identify any problems with previous methods and help to reach a woman-centred plan for future contraception.

Determining Gestational Age

Gestation can be reliably assessed using a woman's last menstrual period (LMP) either alone or in combination with clinical examination. When using LMP, it is important to elicit whether this was a true menstrual period and not bleeding related to contraception – if conceiving while using the contraceptive pill, for example.

If there is uncertainty over the accuracy of the LMP or significant discrepancy between LMP and clinical examination, an ultrasound scan should be arranged. Ultrasound is also necessary if there is bleeding and pain in early pregnancy in order to exclude an ectopic pregnancy. Routine ultrasound imaging in assessment for abortion is not essential and no national or international guidance mandates its use. However, ultrasound is often used to accurately date the gestational age. Women should never be forced to look at the ultrasound image but should not be prevented from doing so if they so wish.

Post-abortion Contraception

During the initial consultation for abortion a sensitive discussion around a woman's plans for post-abortion contraception should be made. Women value planning the method at this stage as it minimises the risk of further unplanned pregnancy. Most women will ovulate within 2 weeks following the abortion and many resume sexual intercourse by that time as well. Virtually all methods of contraception can be initiated immediately following an abortion.

Examination

Physical examination is not routinely required in patients attending for abortion unless this is the method of dating gestational age. On bimanual examination, a 7-week pregnancy will be approximately the size of a hen's egg and a 10-week pregnancy will be the size of an orange. Once a pregnancy is 12 weeks, it will be palpable above the symphysis pubis. A 20-week pregnancy is usually palpable at the level of the umbilicus.

Investigations

Haemoglobin testing is not routinely required but should be evaluated if the woman presents with a history or clinical symptoms or signs suggestive of anaemia. Rhesus status does not need to be checked for all patients. Guidelines on testing and use of anti-D prophylaxis following abortion vary throughout Europe. In many European countries Anti-D is not administered to women who are rhesus negative if they are having an early medical abortion (up to 10 weeks' gestation). A routine assessment should be made for risk of sexually transmitted infections (STIs). Chlamydia and gonorrhoea testing should be offered to all women and testing for HIV and syphilis is possible.

Methods of Abortion

Medical Abortion

Medical abortion is abortion using a combination of medications: mifepristone and misoprostol. Mifepristone is given orally as a single dose. This is followed 24–48 hours later by misoprostol. Under 10 weeks' gestation, a single dose of misoprostol is usually enough but, after 10 weeks' gestation, multiple doses may be required and are often given in a clinical setting such as a hospital or a standalone community facility.

In early pregnancy the trophoblast generates human choriogonadotropic hormone (hCG), which sustains the corpus luteum and in turn produces progesterone. After 10 weeks the placenta takes over the production of progesterone. Progesterone maintains the myometrium in a quiescent state.

Mifepristone is a potent progesterone receptor antagonist [7]. Mifepristone blocks the progesterone receptor, which allows an increase in the number of gap-junctions in myometrial cells, leading to greater propagation of electrical impulses. Simultaneously, mifepristone inhibits the action of prostaglandin dehydrogenase in the decidua, leading to increased concentrations of endogenous prostaglandins (see Figure 36.1).

Further, mifepristone increases the sensitivity of the myometrium to exogenous prostaglandins such as misoprostol. The net effect of these changes are an increase in contractility of the myometrium, which reaches its peak effect at 36 hours following administration of mifepristone.

In the cervix mifepristone recruits leukocytes which release collagenases and lead to softening of cervical tissue. Misoprostol also acts to soften and dilate the cervix. The combined action on the cervix and contraction of the myometrium following administration of misoprostol leads to detachment and expulsion of the fetus through the open cervix. Once the trophoblast has detached, levels of hCG decrease sharply and so the corpus luteum degenerates (known

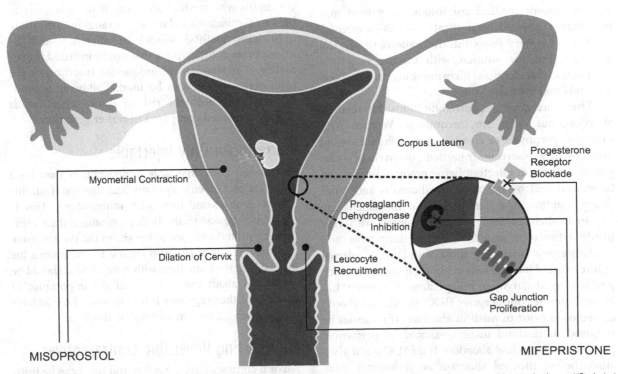

Figure 36.1 Mechanism of action for mifepristone and misoprostol during medical abortion. CCBY4.0 John Reynolds-Wright. https://flic.kr/p/2jVZMrt

as 'luteolysis'). Once this occurs progesterone levels decline further and the decidua is shed with bleeding.

Surgical Abortion

Surgical abortion is abortion facilitated by dilating the cervix and removing the fetus using suction evacuation, at later stages combined with forceps. Dilation of the cervix is achieved firstly by pharmacological preparation of the cervix with misoprostol (under 14 weeks). From 14 weeks preparation involves mifepristone, misoprostol, osmotic dilators or a combination of these. Preparation can be initiated between 1 and 24 hours pre-procedure depending on method and gestation. At the time of procedure the cervix is mechanically dilated to accommodate a suction catheter (under 14 weeks) or specialised forceps (over 14 weeks) and the pregnancy is removed piecemeal. Sharp curettage is outdated and contributes to intrauterine adhesions and so should not be used.

Choice of Method

Choice of method (see Table 36.1) should be based upon the woman's preference following a discussion of risks and benefits of methods available according to gestational age [8]. The decision may also be affected by any concurrent medical conditions the patient may have that may pose contraindications to either method.

There are very few contraindications to surgical abortion, but for women with uterine structural anomalies – for example, bicornuate uterus – medical methods may be more suitable.

There are several contraindications for medical abortion, but these are uncommon. Women with inherited porphyria or chronic adrenal failure should avoid medical abortion. Inherited porphyria is a rare genetic condition affecting heme production that can be exacerbated by hormonal medications and other drugs. Caution and careful clinical judgement are required when assessing whether women with very brittle asthma or women requiring long-term oral corticosteroids (including those with chronic adrenal failure) should have a medical abortion due to the anti-glucocorticoid activity of mifepristone. If a patient has an intrauterine contraceptive (IUC) in situ, this should be removed prior to medical abortion. If it cannot be removed, ultrasound imaging should be performed pre- and post-medical abortion. If the IUC is not visualised before medical abortion an abdominal x-ray should be considered to exclude perforation.

Post-abortion Contraception

Post-abortion contraception is an essential component of comprehensive abortion care [10].

Initiation

All methods of contraception can be initiated immediately following an abortion. Women who choose the most effective methods known as long-acting reversible methods of contraception (LARC) – that is, implant or intrauterine contraceptives to commence immediately after abortion – are less likely to experience unintended pregnancy in the subsequent year compared to women who choose less effective methods of contraception.

Progestogen-Only Implant

Subdermal contraceptive implants can be inserted at the time of surgical abortion or at administration of mifepristone for medical abortion. There is good evidence that initiation of an implant at this time does not affect the efficacy of medical abortion.

Intrauterine Methods

Intrauterine contraception can be inserted immediately after surgical abortion or after expulsion of the conceptus with medical abortion. If there is likely to be a significant delay in arranging insertion, a bridging method should be offered – that is, a temporary contraceptive that can be initiated immediately. The standard technique for insertion of the intrauterine device can be used. Following second-trimester abortion, the risk of device expulsion is slightly increased compared to earlier gestations.

Progestogen-Only Injectable

Progestogen-only injectable contraception may have a small impact on efficacy of medical abortion if administered at the same time with mifepristone. This is thought to be due to the high progestogen dose competing with mifepristone at the site of the progesterone receptor [11]. Women who choose to commence the injectable at the same time with mifepristone should be counselled about this risk and of the importance of confirming the pregnancy is terminated. The injectable can be given on the day of surgical abortion.

Short-Acting Reversible Contraceptives

All oral contraceptives, patches and rings can be initiated on the day of surgical abortion, the day of

Table 36.1 Methods of abortion at different gestations

Medical Abortion [9]		Surgical Abortion	
Gestation: Under 10 weeks	Mifepristone 200 mg orally followed 24–48 hours later by misoprostol 800 micrograms sublingually, buccally or vaginally	Gestation: Under 14 weeks	Manual or electric vacuum aspiration Performed under local anaesthetic Prepare cervix with sublingual misoprostol 400 micrograms 1 hour before
Gestation: 10+0 – 21+6 weeks	Mifepristone 200 mg orally followed 24–48 hours later by Misoprostol 800 micrograms sublingually, buccally or vaginally. Then 400mcg every 3 hours until fetus is expelled	Gestation: Over 14+0 weeks	Dilatation and evacuation Performed under conscious sedation or general anaesthetic Prepare cervix with mifepristone or osmotic dilators 24 hours in advance. Misoprostol can also be considered as above.
After 22+0 weeks	Consider feticide with ultrasound-guided intra-cardiac injection of potassium chloride, or intra-amniotic /intra-fetal digoxin, before medical abortion.		

mifepristone or expulsion of the pregnancy. Women should receive good information about what to do if they miss pills/patch/ring and when emergency contraception should be considered.

Sterilization

Female sterilization is generally not recommended at the time of either surgical or medical abortion as it is associated with a greater likelihood that the woman will regret having chosen a permanent procedure and that the risk of failure of the method is higher compared to an interval sterilization.

However, women should not be pressured into choosing a different method and the discussion should be clearly documented in her notes if she wishes to proceed to sterilization at the time of abortion.

Male sterilization is a highly effective method of contraception, but there is a significant lag time between procedure and confirmation of successful vasectomy with semen analysis (12–16 weeks) and so women should be counselled regarding the need for a bridging method.

Complications

Complications are not common with either method of abortion.

Uterine Perforation

Uterine perforation occurs between 1 and 4 in 1,000 cases of surgical abortion. This is more likely to occur in cases with advanced gestation and in those who have

had previous cervical surgery. The overall risk of perforation is low and occurs only in surgical methods. If perforation during surgical abortion is suspected, diagnostic laparoscopy should be considered to confirm and assess the extent of injury or need for laparotomy. If damage and bleeding are minimal, usually only antibiotic prophylaxis and observation are required. If the surgical abortion is not completed at the point of perforation, it can be completed under direct laparoscopic vision or the procedure can be abandoned and medical treatment initiated instead.

Uterine Rupture

There is a 1 in 1,000 risk of uterine rupture during medical abortion. The risk appears to be for those who have had a previous caesarean section. Almost all reported cases have occurred in second-trimester abortions. There is no evidence that reducing the dose or frequency of misoprostol reduces this risk. Clinicians must be alert to the signs and symptoms of rupture such as severe pain and shock. If there is evidence of uterine rupture, an emergency laparotomy to assess the injury or an emergency hysterectomy may be required.

Haemorrhage

Haemorrhage requiring transfusion (> 500 ml blood loss) occurs between 1 and 4 in 1,000 cases of medical or surgical abortion. This risk increases with gestational age. With medical abortion haemorrhage may occur at a delayed interval, indicating that admission for this procedure does not mitigate this risk. In the event of haemorrhage, blood transfusion may be required and emergency surgical evacuation of the uterus should be considered.

Cervical Trauma

Cervical trauma occurs in fewer than 1 in 100 cases of surgical abortion. Cervical preparation reduces the risk and depending on the extent of the injury, suturing of a cervical laceration may be required.

Infection

Infection is estimated to occur in approximately 1 in 100 cases. The risk is lower after medical than surgical abortion. Antibiotic prophylaxis reduces the risk after surgical abortion, but rates are low for both methods. Doxycycline is commonly used as it is broad spectrum and has anti-chlamydial activity.

Retained Products of Conception

Following both medical and surgical abortion, it is possible for pregnancy tissue to remain in the uterus, leading to persistent or heavy bleeding and/or become a focus of infection. Often this tissue will pass spontaneously but may need further medical treatment (additional doses of misoprostol) or surgical re-intervention.

References

1. Singh S, Remez L, Sedgh G, Kwok L, Onda T. *Abortion worldwide 2017: Uneven progress and unequal access.* New York: Guttmacher Institute, 2018. www .guttmacher.org/report/abortion-worldwide-2017.

2. Raymond EG, Grossman D, Weaver MA, Toti S, Winikoff B. Mortality of induced abortion, other outpatient surgical procedures and common activities in the United States. *Contraception.* 2014;90(5):476–9. www.ncbi.nlm.nih.gov/pubmed/25152259.

3. Raymond EG, Grimes DA. The comparative safety of legal induced abortion and childbirth in the United States. *Obstet Gynecol.* 2012;119(2 Pt 1):215–19. www .ncbi.nlm.nih.gov/pubmed/22270271.

4. Exelgyn. European abortion data. France: Exelgyn, 2019. https://abort-report.eu/europe.

5. Reynolds-Wright JJ, Belleuvre F, Daberius A et al. Information on early medical abortion for women using an audiovisual animation versus face-to-face consultation: A consortium randomized and quasi-randomized trial. *Acta Obstet Gynecol Scand.* 2020;99(12):1611–17. https://doi.org/10.1111/aogs .13944.

6. National Institute for Health and Care Excellence. *NICE abortion care guideline: Patient decision aids.* London: National Institute for Health and Care Excellence. 2019. http://bit.ly/3DGI6Mp.

7. Baird DT, Rodger M, Cameron IT, Roberts I. Prostaglandins and antigestagens for the interruption of early pregnancy. *J Reprod Fertil* Suppl. 1988;36:173–9. www.ncbi.nlm.nih.gov/pubmed/3193407.

8. National Institute for Health and Care Excellence. *Abortion care.* NG140 edition. London: National Institute for Health and Care Excellence, 2019. www .nice.org.uk/guidance/NG140.

9. World Health Organization. *Medical management of abortion.* Geneva: World Health Organization, 2018.

10. Faculty of Sexual and Reproductive Healthcare. Contraception after pregnancy. 2017. http://bit.ly /3DFyBwT.

11. Raymond EG, Weaver MA, Louie KS et al. Effects of depot medroxyprogesterone acetate injection timing on medical abortion efficacy and repeat pregnancy: A randomized controlled trial. *Obstet Gynecol.* 2016;128(4). https://bit.ly/3Y4uBy8.

Chapter 37

Termination of Pregnancy
Medical Methods

John J. Reynolds-Wright, Sharon T. Cameron

Introduction

Medical abortion is the use of medications, rather than surgical means to induce an abortion. The World Health Organization (WHO) recommends the use of a combination of mifepristone (a progesterone-receptor antagonist) followed by misoprostol (a synthetic prostaglandin) [1].

Mifepristone has several mechanisms of action in medical abortion – it blocks progesterone receptors, which in turn leads to a proliferation of gap junctions between myometrial cells. This results in greater conduction of electrical impulses across the myometrium and so greater contractility. At the same time, mifepristone inhibits the action of prostaglandin dehydrogenase in the decidua, resulting in a higher concentration of endogenous prostaglandins. Further, mifepristone recruits leucocytes to the cervical tissue which release collagenases and begin the process of cervical softening and dilation. At 36 to 48 hours following mifepristone, these effects are maximal and render the uterus highly sensitive to exogenous prostaglandins such as misoprostol [2].

Misoprostol has the effect of softening and dilating the cervix further and causing regular uterine contractions which lead to detachment and expulsion of the conceptus through a dilated cervix. In the second trimester the window of 36 to 48 hours between mifepristone and misoprostol becomes more important to facilitate the passage of a larger fetus. Misoprostol can be administered sublingually, buccally or vaginally with high efficacy, but oral administration should be avoided as it has a higher incidence of side effects and lower efficacy [3]. In the first trimester misoprostol can be given up to 72 hours after mifepristone, but intervals less than 24 hours are associated with higher failure rates.

Medical Abortion before 12 Weeks

Medical abortion before 12 weeks is highly effective and acceptable to patients, and the WHO recommend that it can be performed safely in a clinical setting or home setting. Bleeding and pain commence approximately 1–2 hours following misoprostol administration, reaching their peak at expulsion of the pregnancy. The majority of women will pass the pregnancy within 6 hours and will have bleeding that will be heavier than a period but then get progressively lighter. After 9 weeks further doses of misoprostol (400 micrograms) may be required if the pregnancy has not expelled within 4 hours of the first dose [1]. Home treatment means women can have their abortion at times that are convenient to them, allowing them to be with a supportive friend, their family or their partner.

Outcomes

Medical abortion at less than 12 weeks' gestation is highly effective with a complete abortion rate without surgical intervention of greater than 94% [4] Approximately 1% will have a continuing pregnancy after receiving medical abortion treatment and will require repeat medical or surgical treatment [5]. Treatment failure is slightly more likely for gestations over 8 weeks and if a lower than recommended dose of misoprostol is used.

Follow-Up

There is no need for routine in-person follow up after medical abortion before 12 weeks' gestation. Women should be given clear and consistent advice on the signs and symptoms of incomplete abortion, failed abortion, infection and haemorrhage. There should be clear directions on how to access emergency advice via telephone and emergency care if required [6]. In particular women should seek urgent medical attention if they experience very heavy bleeding (soaking more than two sanitary towels per hour), fever and chills or severe pain not controlled by analgesia.

If expulsion of the pregnancy has not been witnessed by a healthcare provider who can confirm complete abortion, this can instead be done using a low-sensitivity pregnancy test (that turns positive above 1,000 IU human chorionic gonadotropin (hCG)) 14 days after treatment [7]. An alternative option to exclude continuing pregnancy is serial hCG levels. Some clinical protocols compare baseline hCG (day of mifepristone administration) with a further hCG 7 days later, with a decrease of more than 80% indicating success.

Whilst ultrasound will accurately exclude continuing pregnancy, it can often identify material in the uterus that is clinically unimportant but can lead to unnecessary intervention. There is no endometrial thickness that predicts need for intervention following abortion [8]. Rather, incomplete abortion is a clinical diagnosis based upon bleeding and examination findings.

Medical Abortion after 12 Weeks

For pregnancies greater than 12 weeks' gestation, the same combination of drugs is used (mifepristone followed by misoprostol) except that further doses of misoprostol (400 µg) every 3 hours (buccal, sublingual or vaginal) are administered until expulsion of the pregnancy. Ninety-seven per cent of women will abort within 24 hours of the initial dose of misoprostol and median time from induction to complete abortion is 7.5 hours [9]. As multiple doses are required and in more advanced pregnancies pain and bleeding increases, abortion after 12 weeks' gestation should be carried out in a clinical facility. The fetal remains should be sensitively disposed by the facility where the abortion takes place or by the woman, and clinics should have policies in place for either eventuality and in accordance with national guidance.

Feticide at the End of the Second Trimester

Guidelines differ throughout the European Union but, in the United Kingdom, the Royal College of Obstetricians and Gynaecologists (RCOG) advise that after 21 weeks and 6 days gestation feticide is performed so there are no signs of life upon expulsion of the fetus [10]. Ultrasound-guided intra-cardiac potassium chloride to arrest cardiac activity is the most effective method but is technically difficult. Alternatively, intra-fetal or intra-amniotic digoxin can be used. While less effective than intra-cardiac potassium chloride, this is easier to administer and broadens the range of healthcare providers able to perform this activity.

Pain Management

Medical abortion is a painful process; however, the pain reported by women is influenced by many factors. Nulliparity, previous history of dysmenorrhoea and more advanced gestation are associated with greater pain at medical abortion. Adequate pain relief makes medical abortion more acceptable for women but evidence is limited on the best regimens to use, particularly in early pregnancy.

Non-steroidal anti-inflammatory drugs (NSAIDs) have the best evidence of pain relief for medical abortions in the first 12 weeks of pregnancy [11, 12]. In clinical practice these are often supplemented with paracetamol and weak opiates such as codeine or dihydrocodeine. Non-pharmacological methods such as a hot water bottle or heating pad applied to the abdomen may be useful adjuncts. Being in a familiar environment with a supportive person can improve a patient's ability to manage the pain they are experiencing. Not all patients require antiemetics, but those who are feeling particularly nauseated at assessment may benefit from a supply of antiemetic medication.

There is evidence that, after 12 weeks' gestation, NSAIDs can reduce opiate requirements and are associated with a shorter induction to abortion interval [13]. However, as gestation advances, analgesia requirements may increase and so clinical facilities providing medial abortion at this gestation should be able to administer strong opiates, such as morphine. Regional anaesthesia (in the form of epidural or spinal) can be considered to manage severe pain but is rarely used in clinical practice [14].

Complications

There are few complications associated with medical abortion and patients should be counselled about the risk of these if choosing medical abortion.

Uterine Rupture

Uterine rupture occurs in approximately 0.1% of cases during medical abortion. The risk of this appears to increase with gestation and seems to occur predominately in those who have had a previous caesarean delivery. Almost all reported cases occurred during second-trimester abortions. Previous caesarean delivery is not a contraindication for medical abortion, rather these women need to be counselled of this rare risk and clinical staff should be aware of their past obstetric history should they exhibit signs of rupture during their treatment. There is no evidence that reducing the dose or frequency of misoprostol reduces this risk.

Haemorrhage

Haemorrhage with blood loss greater than 500 ml and requiring transfusion is also rare and occurs in 0.1–0.4% of cases of medical abortion. As with uterine rupture, the risk of haemorrhage increases with gestation. Haemorrhage may occur at an interval of several days following medical abortion, which indicates that admission for medical abortion does not necessarily mitigate the risk of haemorrhage.

Infection

Infection, including endometritis, occurs in approximately 1% of cases of medical abortion. The risk of infection is lower after medical abortion compared to surgical abortion. Women should be offered screening for chlamydia and gonorrhoea prior to abortion and given treatment if positive. If testing for sexually transmitted infection is not available, a course of prophylactic antibiotics such as doxycycline can be considered, particularly if there are risk factors for infection such as a new partner.

References

1. World Health Organization. *Medical management of abortion*. Geneva: World Health Organization, 2018.

2. Baird DT, Rodger M, Cameron IT, Roberts I. Prostaglandins and antigestagens for the interruption of early pregnancy. *J Reprod Fertil Suppl*. 1988;**36**:173–9. www.ncbi.nlm.nih.gov/pubmed/3193407.

3. Akin A, Dabash R, Dilbaz B et al. Increasing women's choices in medical abortion: A study of misoprostol 400 microg swallowed immediately or held sublingually following 200 mg mifepristone. *European Journal of Contraception and Reproductive Health Care: Official Journal of the European Society of Contraception*. 2009;**14** (3):169–75. https://bit.ly/3Y4dRHh.

4. Kapp N, Eckersberger E, Lavelanet A, Rodriguez MI. Medical abortion in the late first trimester: A systematic review. *Contraception*. 2019;**99**(2):77–86. www.ncbi.nlm.nih.gov/pubmed/30444970.

5. Raymond EG, Shannon C, Weaver MA, Winikoff B. First-trimester medical abortion with mifepristone 200 mg and misoprostol: A systematic review. *Contraception*. 2013;**87**(1):26–37. www.sciencedirect.com/science/article/pii/S0010782412006439.

6. National Institute for Health and Care Excellence. *Abortion care*. NG140 edition. London: National Institute for Health and Care Excellence, 2019. www.nice.org.uk/guidance/NG140.

7. Cameron ST, Glasier A, Dewart H, Johnstone A, Burnside A. Telephone follow-up and self-performed urine pregnancy testing after early medical abortion: A service evaluation. *Contraception*. 2012;**86**(1):67–73. https://bit.ly/3HVuH5w.

8. Reeves MF, Fox MC, Lohr PA, Creinin MD. Endometrial thickness following medical abortion is not predictive of subsequent surgical intervention. *Ultrasound in Obstetrics and Gynecology*. 2009;**34**(1):104–9. https://doi.org/10.1002/uog.6404.

9. Ngoc NTN, Shochet T, Raghavan S et al. Mifepristone and misoprostol compared with misoprostol alone for second-trimester abortion: A randomized controlled trial. *Obstetrics and Gynecology*. 2011;**118**(3):601–8. https://bit.ly/3jvGIW8.

10. Royal College of Obstetricians and Gynaecologists. *The care of women requesting induced abortion: Evidence-based clinical guideline number 7*. London: Royal College of Obstetricians and Gynaecologists, 2011. http://bit.ly/3l9NnWr.

11. Avraham S, Gat I, Duvdevani N-R et al. Preemptive effect of ibuprofen versus placebo on pain relief and success rates of medical abortion: A double-blind, randomized, controlled study. *Fertility and Sterility*. 2012;**97**(3):612–15. https://bit.ly/3HTInhC.

12. Livshits A, Machtinger R, David LB et al. Ibuprofen and paracetamol for pain relief during medical abortion: A double-blind randomized

controlled study. *Fertility and Sterility*. 2009;**91**(5):1877–80. https://bit.ly/3wWhSla.

13. Fiala C, Swahn ML, Stephansson O, Gemzell-Danielsson K. The effect of non-steroidal anti-inflammatory drugs on medical abortion with mifepristone and misoprostol at 13–22 weeks

gestation. *Hum Reprod*. 2005;**20**(11):3072–7. www.ncbi.nlm.nih.gov/pubmed/16055455.

14. Jackson E, Kapp N. Pain control in first-trimester and second-trimester medical termination of pregnancy: A systematic review. *Contraception*. 2011;**83**(2):116–26. https://bit.ly/3wUEnHe.

Chapter 38

Termination of Pregnancy
Surgical Methods

Barbara Salje, Michelle Cooper

Introduction

Surgical termination of pregnancy was the first wide-spread method of abortion available. However, rates have declined in recent decades across Western Europe due to the increasing popularity of medical methods. In 2018 in England, 29% of abortions were performed surgically and most of these (24%) were by vacuum aspiration (VA)[1]. Vacuum aspiration is the principal technique used for surgical abortion at gestations under 14 weeks. Later surgical abortion is generally achieved by the distinct procedure of dilatation and evacuation (D&E). Sharp curettage in surgical abortion (where the uterine lining is scraped with a metal instrument) is now considered obsolete [2, 3].

Women should be given a choice of medical or surgical abortion across all gestations for which abortion is legally offered. However, the range of methods available in any region is often influenced by available expertise and local service arrangements. Whether performing the procedure directly or facilitating access to services elsewhere, knowledge of available surgical abortion procedures and how to counsel women appropriately is an important aspect of abortion care.

Methods of Surgical Termination

The method used to achieve surgical abortion largely depends on gestational age, provider expertise and local service arrangements. In many countries (such as in parts of the United Kingdom), access to surgical abortion in the second trimester is limited and may require travel to neighbouring regions. A summary of the available surgical methods is shown in Table 38.1.

Table 38.1 Technique appropriate for gestational age [2]

Less than 7 weeks	Early vacuum aspiration (special consideration)
7–14 weeks	Standard vacuum aspiration
14–24 weeks	Dilatation and evacuation

Vacuum Aspiration

This technique involves the trans-cervical passage of a plastic cannula connected to a source of vacuum to empty the contents of the uterine cavity. The suction pump may be either manual (MVA) or electric (EVA). It is a safe and quick procedure which can be performed throughout the first trimester and provides an alternative to previously used dilatation and curettage, which was associated with a higher complication rate [3].

It can be performed in a traditional theatre or ambulatory care setting and its efficacy is comparable to early medical abortion with success rates in the region of 96–98%. Failure is more likely to occur at early gestations (below 7 weeks) due the small size of the gestation sac, which may be missed. As such, inspection of aspirated tissue should be performed or followed up with serum human choriogonadotropic hormone (hCG) levels. With these safeguarding procedures in place the failure rate is highly acceptable at 0.13% [2].

Previously cervical preparation (ripening/priming) was reserved for later surgical procedures; it is now frequently recommended prior to all procedures as it has been shown to reduce the risk of uterine perforation, cervical trauma, haemorrhage and incomplete abortion [2, 4]. In Europe a single dose of vaginal misoprostol 2–3 hours before the procedure is most frequently used for this purpose (Table 38.2).

Electric Vacuum Aspiration

Traditional EVA can be performed in either a clinic or theatre setting. Following pre-procedure cervical preparation, pelvic examination and gentle cervical dilatation, a plastic suction cannula is passed into the uterine cavity. The cannulae may be rigid or flexible and come in a range of diameters (see Figure 38.1). The most appropriate size is selected based on the pregnancy gestation, degree of cervical dilatation and operator preference.

Table 38.2 Cervical priming [2, 7]

Pharmacological	Up to 14 weeks (considered up to 18 weeks)	Misoprostol 400 mg vaginally or sublingually 3 hours pre-op Repeated doses may be required at later gestations
Mechanical	Second trimester onwards	Osmotic dilators placed for 4–6 hours or overnight. After 18 weeks Mifepristone 200 mg orally can be given in addition.

Electrically driven suction is then connected and the uterine contents aspirated via continuous, low level suction (60–800 mmHg negative pressure). A combination of circular and gentle forward and back movement of the cannula is used until the uterus is empty. This is characterised by a 'gritty' sensation as it moves across the walls of the now contracted uterus and by the absence of further pregnancy tissue. The procedure is usually complete in under 10 minutes (depending on the gestational age). Occasionally the use of sponge forceps is necessary to remove tissue obstructing the opening at the distal tip of the cannula. Continuous ultrasound is not required during routine EVA; however, it has the potential to reduce the risk of retained products of conception requiring re-intervention (0% vs. 4.7%) [2].

Manual Vacuum Aspiration

Alternatively MVA is a convenient and low-cost means of achieving suction aspiration in office-based or low resource settings (see Figure 38.2). It has similar efficacy to EVA and is equally acceptable to women and providers [5]. A handheld 60 ml syringe is connected to a rigid or flexible cannula and suction generated by the syringe plunger and release of valves. The same approach just described is used to empty the uterine contents, which collect in the syringe chamber, allowing for later inspection. Once the syringe is full the procedure may need to be paused in order to empty the contents of the syringe before continuing. As the procedure can be performed in office-based settings without the need for general anaesthesia or

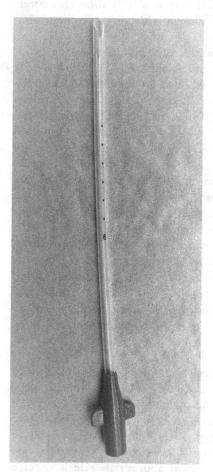

Figure 38.1 Example of flexible cannula. Size 6 mm Ipas Easy Grip® Cannula by WomanCare Global

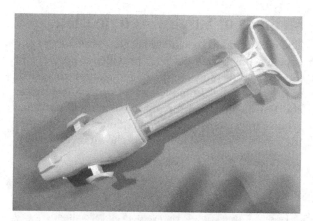

Figure 38.2 Ipas MVA Plus® by WomanCare Global

sedation, it can provide increased access to abortion. Intra- or para-cervical local anaesthetic can be used if required, which allows for faster recovery and discharge.

Dilation and Evacuation

Dilation and evacuation is now the most commonly used technique for achieving surgical abortion in the second trimester. With improved access to safe abortion care and advancements in training and technology, D&E now provides a safe and acceptable alternative to medical abortion at later gestations.

Following cervical preparation and aspiration of amniotic fluid, fetal extraction is achieved by inserting specialised forceps trans-cervically into the uterus. Cervical preparation can be achieved using osmotic dilators, pharmacological agents or a combination of the two. Osmotic dilators (such as laminaria or Dilapan-S) are placed into the cervix and gradually increase in size, causing the mechanical dilatation (see Figure 38.3). These can be placed overnight or the same day (over a period of 4–6 hours) depending on the type used and the degree of dilatation required.

Osmotic dilators may be used in conjunction with pharmacological agents to further increase cervical dilatation and reduce surgical time. Pain relief in the form of either a para-cervical block or lidocaine gel can be used to reduce the discomfort associated with insertion of osmotic dilators. Alternatively, pharmacological agents alone may be used for cervical preparation; however, this is associated with the need for greater mechanical dilatation during the procedure.

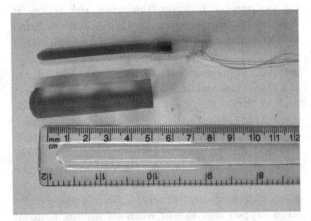

Figure 38.3 Osmotic dilator pre and post insertion. Dilapan – S®

When dilatation and evacuation for higher gestations is performed continuous ultrasound is recommended along with an experienced practitioner [2]. Uterine perforation is a considered a significant risk at this gestation and intra-operative ultrasound can reduce this from 1.4% to 0.2% [6].

Procedural Considerations

Analgesia

Analgesic options are local anaesthetic, sedation or general anaesthetic [7]. Services should be able to provide surgical abortion without the need for general anaesthetic with some patients accepting short-term pain over the disadvantages of general anaesthetic (drowsiness, slower recovery and fasting requirement) [2]. If requesting the procedure under local anaesthetic a pre-operative non-steroidal anti-inflammatory drug (NSAID) and para-cervical block is recommended [2]. Familiarity comes with experience and often practitioners will initially use local anaesthetic techniques for lower-gestation procedures [2].

Cervical Priming

As discussed earlier, cervical priming is an important aspect of surgical abortion to reduce the rate of complications [4, 7, 8]. It should be considered in all cases of surgical abortion but especially where there is an increased risk of cervical trauma or uterine perforation such as second-trimester procedures [7]. A summary of cervical priming agents and their use in surgical abortion is shown in Table 38.2.

Misoprostol can be administered either vaginally or sublingually. Although sublingual administration of misoprostol achieves superior dilatation, it is associated with increased gastrointestinal disturbance and may be less acceptable [2]. Other side effects of prostaglandins involve abdominal cramping, bleeding and potential expulsion of pregnancy tissue [2].

Infection Prevention

Antibiotic prophylaxis is recommended following surgical abortion to prevent upper genital tract infection [7, 9]. Commonly used antibiotics are doxycycline or metronidazole, with no additional benefit seen in the combination of these [7]. Adherence may be improved with a 3-day course of broad spectrum doxycycline with fewer side effects seen, rather than the traditional 7-day course of metronidazole [7].

Rhesus Alloimmunization

Surgical abortion is considered a potential 'sensitising event' for rhesus (Rh) alloimmunization. This can be prevented by the prophylactic administration of Anti-D immunoglobulin within 72 hours of the procedure [2]. Country-specific guidance may vary, but most regions recommend Anti-D administration for women undergoing surgical abortion, particularly at advanced gestations with higher exposure to fetal cells [7]. The Royal College of Obstetricians and Gynaecologists (RCOG) recommends [2]:

- 250IU for abortion at gestations below 20 weeks.
- 500IU for abortion at gestations after 20 weeks (with an additional Kleihauer test to assess for feto-maternal haemorrhage).

Venous Thromboembolism Prophylaxis

Although surgical abortion does not necessitate routine venous thromboembolism prophylaxis, the need for this should be individualised. Risk factors include personal history, body mass index (BMI) and gestation at time of procedure [2]. If required, low-molecular-weight heparin (LMWH) is given for at least 7 days post procedure. If deemed higher risk, LMWH could be started prior to the procedure and continued after termination is complete [7].

Risks of Surgical Termination

Complication rates for both medical and surgical abortions are relatively low but the risk profile differs. Incomplete termination requiring intervention and haemorrhage is higher in medical termination; however, complications requiring surgical intervention are seen more commonly in surgical termination [2]. Infection rates and serious morbidity are equal between the two groups [2]. Maternal mortality is extremely low at 0.32/100 000 maternities for all terminations of pregnancy [2]. There is no evidence of an association between termination of pregnancy and subsequent miscarriage or pre-term labour [2, 3]. Table 38.3 shows a summary of the recognised risks of surgical abortion, which should be discussed prior to procedure.

Table 38.3 Complications

Haemorrhage	0.2%
Perforation	0.4–0.5%
Cervical injury	0.2%
Ongoing pregnancy	0.23%
Retained tissue	2%
Infection	4.9%

Haemorrhage

Haemorrhage is defined as a blood loss greater than 500 ml or when blood transfusion is required. Quoted rates of 0.2% are given with less than this requiring blood transfusion [2]. Evidence suggests a trend towards higher rates in medical abortion; however, this was not statistically significant. As the uterus enlarges with advancing gestation it follows suit that the risk of haemorrhage increases (0.88/1000 at less than 13 weeks rising to 4/1000 when greater than 20 weeks) [2].

The cause of haemorrhage may come from retained tissue, trauma of the cervix, uterine perforation, infection or coagulopathy [3]. The management depends on the cause of bleeding. Uterotonic medications can be considered, especially at later gestations, but their prophylactic use in routine procedures is not required. Intravenous fluids and blood products should be utilised until definitive management is attained [3]. A Foley's catheter or intrauterine balloon tamponade can also be used to control bleeding.

Perforation

Surgical termination is the commonest cause of uterine perforation; however, the actual risk is low at 0.40–0.52%. Those requesting a surgical termination at later gestations are at increased risk. Additionally those with uterine anomalies, previous uterine surgery, recent pregnancy (last 6 months) or fibroids are at a higher risk and additional safeguarding measures such as ultrasound or experienced surgeon should be considered [10].

The majority are in the body of the uterus anteriorly and do not tend to cause significant haemorrhage. If a perforation has been identified at the dilatation stage (up to 5 mm) the patient can be given antibiotics and observed. Should the perforation happen after this or when attempting removal of pregnancy tissue, prompt laparoscopy should be performed with the potential need for laparotomy and colorectal surgeons input if bowel injury is suspected [10].

If perforation occurs in the cervical canal, lower segment or laterally, the perforation may include branches of the uterine vessels and can lead to a broad ligament haematoma or intra-abdominal haemorrhage. Prompt recognition is important in uterine perforation to limit further complications. Suction cannula cause 51.3% of perforations, dilators 24.4% and curettes 16.2% [10]. There is a risk of uterine rupture in subsequent pregnancies in the latter half of pregnancy and labour [10]. An earlier suspicion of rupture in labour should be considered when given a history of uterine perforation.

Cervical Injury

Cervical injury from dilatation is a rare but serious complication of surgical termination of pregnancy. It can lead to excessive bleeding or formation of false passages. The recommended use of cervical priming has reduced this risk and more recent studies quote a rate of less than 0.2%. At later gestation this rises to 1.16%, which is in keeping with the greater need for cervical dilatation [2].

Failed Procedure

Ongoing pregnancy can occur but is more common after medical terminations with rates of 0.9% compared to 0.5% for VA of early abortion [2, 3]. When suction aspiration is used the risk is higher at less than 6 weeks' gestation, for multiparous women, for women with uterine abnormalities, when performed by an inexperienced surgeon or when a small cannula is used [2]. In these situations it is important to observe pregnancy tissue on the aspirate to ensure completion of the procedure. Overall continuing pregnancy rates for surgical abortion is 0.23% [2].

Retained Tissue

Surgical abortion allows improved confirmation of complete uterine emptying through technical skills and experience and, occasionally, the use of ultrasound. As such, there are lower rates of failed or incomplete procedure compared to medical abortion and a lower re-intervention rate (2% vs. 5%, respectively) [2].

In the presence of retained tissue, women may report ongoing vaginal bleeding and/or persistently positive pregnancy test [3]. If infected, there may be associated abdominal pain, offensive vaginal discharge or fever. Uterine evacuation for retained tissue can be achieved either medically or with repeat vacuum aspiration. If the patient is clinically stable with no signs of infection, expectant management can be considered with the understanding that resolution will take longer [3].

Infection

Current rates of infection following surgical abortion is 4.9% [11]. Infection following termination of pregnancy is usually caused by presence of pre-existing genital tract organisms [2]. Prophylactic antibiotics at the time of surgical termination of pregnancy can reduce the risk of upper genital tract infection by around 40% [2, 3, 12]. If post-procedure there is clinical suspicion of infection, antibiotics should be given and re-evacuation of the uterus if retained tissue suspected [2, 3].

Adhesions

Development of intrauterine adhesions is rare following modern surgical abortion techniques, but more common after sharp curettage due to damage to the basal endometrial layer. This can lead to the rare condition of Asherman's syndrome, which is associated with pain and secondary infertility. Although rare, the actual incidence in women undergoing abortion is largely unknown but there may be a higher rate if re-evacuation is required [13, 14].

Aftercare

Formal routine follow-up is generally not required but women should be aware of how to access further support, particularly women with a history of mental health problems who are at increased risk [16].

Bleeding Pattern

Women should be counselled to expect light menstrual-like bleeding for up to 2 weeks [3]. Compared to medical abortion they will experience less pain and GI symptoms in the first 2 weeks following the procedure [2].

Contraception

Any method of contraception can be safely initiated at the time of surgical abortion, including the insertion of an intrauterine device (copper or levonorgestrel), if there is reasonable certainty the pregnancy has been removed [2]. Infection rates were not higher in women who chose to have immediate insertion [15], however, expulsion rates are noted to be higher in second-trimester termination with immediate insertion (up to 30%) [17].

Conclusions

Surgical abortion is a safe, effective and acceptable procedure for women who choose this method after careful counselling about their options. Vacuum aspiration is the most commonly used technique in the first trimester, whereas D&E is preferred for second-trimester procedures. Routine use of cervical preparation should be considered to reduce the risk of complications and is particularly important at later gestations. Skilled providers are central to providing this service and preserving women's choice of abortion method at all gestations.

References

1. *Abortion statistics, England and Wales*. 2018. http://bit.ly/3DBgIPS.

2. The care of women requesting induced abortion. 40 B 3270 RCOG Abortion guideline.qxd:3270 RCOG Abortion guideline.qxd 11/11/11.

3. World Health Organization. *Safe abortion: Technical and policy guidance for health systems*. 2nd edition. Geneva: World Health Organization, 2011.

4. Meirik O, Huong NT, Piaggio G et al. Complications of first-trimester abortion by vacuum aspiration after cervical preparation with and without misoprostol: a multicentre randomised trial. *Lancet*. 2012;**379** (9828):1817–24.

5. Dean G, Cardenas L, Darney P, Goldberg A. Acceptability of manual versus electric aspiration for first trimester abortion: A randomized trial. *Contraception*. 2003;**67**(3):201–6.

6. Darney PD, Sweet RL. Routine intraoperative ultrasonography for second trimester abortion reduces incidence of uterine perforation. *Journal of Ultrasound in Medicine*. 1989;**8**(2):71–5.

7. National Institute for Health and Care Excellence. *Abortion care. NICE guideline [NG140]*. London:

National Institute for Health and Care Excellence, 2019. www.nice.org.uk/guidance/ng140.

8. Kapp N, Lohr PA, Ngo TD, Hayes JL. Cervical preparation for first trimester surgical abortion. *Cochrane Database Syst Rev*. 2010(**2**): Art. No.: CD007207. https://doi.org/10.1002/14651858 .CD007207.pub2.

9. Low N, Mueller M, Van Vliet HA, Kapp N. Perioperative antibiotics to prevent infection after first-trimester abortion. *Cochrane Database Syst Rev*. 2012(**3**):CD005217. https://doi.org/10.1002/1465185 8.CD005217.pub2.

10. Shakir F, Diab Y. The perforated uterus. *Obstetrician and Gynaecologist*. 2013;**15**:256–61.

11. Carlsson I, Breding K, Larsson PG. Complications related to induced abortion: A combined retrospective and longitudinal follow-up study. BMC Womens Health. 2018;**18**(1):158–64. https://doi.org/ 10.1186/s12905-018-0645-6.

12. Sawaya GF, Grady D, Kerlikowske K, Grimes DA. Antibiotics at the time of induced abortion: The case for universal prophylaxis based on a meta-analysis. *Obstetrics and Gynecology*. 1996;**87**(5):884–90.

13. Hooker A, Fraenk D, Brölmann H, Huirne J. Prevalence of intrauterine adhesions after termination of pregnancy: A systematic review. *European Journal of Contraception & Reproductive Health Care*. 2016;**21**(4):329–35.

14. Mentula, M, Männistö, J, Gissler, M, Heikinheimo, O, Niinimäki, M. Intrauterine adhesions following an induced termination of pregnancy: A nationwide cohort study. *BJOG*. 2018;**125**:1424–31.

15. Grimes DA, Lopez LM, Schulz KF, Stanwood NL. Immediate postabortal insertion of intrauterine devices. *Cochrane Database Syst Rev*. 2010;(**6**): CD001777.

16. National Collaborating Centre for Mental Health. *Induced abortion and mental health: A systematic review of the mental health outcomes of induced abortion, including their prevalence and associated factors*. London: Academy of Medical Royal Colleges, 2011.

17. Reeves MF, Smith KJ, Creinin MD. Contraceptive effectiveness of immediate compared with delayed insertion of intrauterine devices after abortion: A decision analysis. Obstet Gynecol. 2007;**109**:1286–94.

Termination of Pregnancy at Different Gestational Phases

39

John J. Reynolds, Sharon T. Cameron

Introduction

Compassionate, non-judgemental abortion care should be provided to women seeking to end a pregnancy at the earliest gestation as possible and as late as necessary. Laws that prohibit abortion do not prevent abortion, but merely result in more unsafe abortions [1]. The legal requirements to access abortion vary significantly across Europe, and it is important for clinicians to be aware of their own country's regulations but also those of their close neighbours, as it is common for women who live in areas of greater restriction to travel to nearby countries with less restrictive legislation.

Abortion can be provided medically or surgically at any gestation of pregnancy. Medical and surgical abortion are equally safe and effective, with low rates of complications and continuing pregnancies or incomplete abortion. Successful abortion is achieved in more than 96% of cases of both medical and surgical abortion, so patients should be offered both options in most situations. Abortion can be safely performed by a wide cadre of trained healthcare providers in the first trimester [2]. At more advanced gestations, the setting of the abortion and the provider become more specialised in order to provide the safest care possible.

Medical Abortion

Under 12 Weeks

At less than 12 weeks' gestation, medical abortion can be safely performed in a womans' own home or in a clinical facility.

The recommended regimen for medical abortion at this gestation is mifepristone (a progesterone-receptor antagonist) 200 mg taken orally, followed 24–48 hours later by misoprostol (a synthetic prostaglandin) 800 mg taken sublingually, buccally or vaginally [3]. Misoprostol is significantly less effective when taken orally and has greater side effects, so oral administration is not recommended.

Women should be advised that medical abortion at this gestation is associated with bleeding similar to a heavy period (median blood loss at 8 weeks' gestation is 72 ml). Pain is cramping in nature and increases with gestation. Greater pain is reported by women who are nulliparous and those who experience dysmenorrhoea. There is evidence that non-steroidal anti-inflammatory drugs are effective to manage the pain [4, 5]. Weak oral opiates, such as dihydrocodeine, are usually advised for additional pain relief. Non-pharmacological therapies such as a hot-water bottle/pad to the abdomen, being in a relaxing environment and having a sympathetic friend, relative or family member may also help manage pain.

Women having abortions between 9 and 12 weeks' gestation use the same regimen as those under 9 weeks' gestation; however, they should be supplied with additional doses of misoprostol 400 mg to be used every 3 hours after the initial dose of 800 mg, until the pregnancy has been expelled [3]. The number of doses of misoprostol required is a median of 2.3 at this gestation band, so women who are having this procedure at home should be advised that, if the pregnancy has not been expelled after they have used three doses, they should contact the abortion provider for advice [6, 7].

Between 9 and 12 weeks' gestation there may be more pain and bleeding and the fetus will be visible – women should be made aware of what tissue they can expect to pass as this will prepare them psychologically and also prompt them to contact care if they have not passed appropriate tissue with the medical abortion treatment.

12–22 Weeks

Between 12 and 22 weeks' gestation medical abortion is usually conducted in a clinical facility, where nurses or midwives who are experienced in providing medical abortion in the second trimester and doctors with experience of complications of second trimester abortion are available.

As with medical abortion at earlier gestations, mifepristone 200 mg is administered and the woman is then admitted 48 hours later for misoprostol. Misoprostol is given in an initial dose of 800 mg and a dose of 400 mg is repeated every three hours until expulsion of the pregnancy. As with earlier gestations, there is a choice of route through which to administer misoprostol – sublingual, buccal or vaginal. However, once bleeding has started, the vaginal route should be avoided as this may affect absorption [8].

Serial doses of misoprostol can result in nausea, vomiting and diarrhoea. Anti-emetic and anti-diarrhoeal medications should be available and can be given prophylactically, particularly if the woman is nauseated prior to misoprostol administration.

There is evidence that regular dosing with non-steroidal anti-inflammatory medications reduces pain, decreases the need for opiates and reduces the time until expulsion of the fetus [9]. Strong opiates should be available to manage pain if required. Epidural pain relief could be considered but is rarely required [10].

Over 22 Weeks

As gestation advances beyond 22 weeks, the fetus is approaching viability, so feticide with ultrasound-guided intracardiac injection of potassium chloride should be considered before medical abortion prevent delivery of a viable fetus [11]. An alternative method of feticide is intra-fetal or intra-amniotic injection of digoxin [12, 13]. This is less effective than intracardiac potassium chloride, however, it is less technically difficult and so increases the number of staff who can perform it.

Contraception after Medical Abortion

All methods of contraception can be initiated immediately after medical abortion [14]. If the medical abortion is performed as an outpatient procedure, then subdermal implants and injectable methods can be given at the same time as mifepristone. Oral methods of contraception can commence the day of expulsion of the fetus. For intrauterine methods, these should be initiated once it has been confirmed that the pregnancy has been terminated. For women who expel a pregnancy at home, the exclusion of a continuing pregnancy (and therefore insertion of an intrauterine method) is usually made on the basis of a negative self-performed low-sensitivity urinary pregnancy test. If expulsion of the fetus has taken place in a clinical facility and this been visually confirmed by clinical staff, all methods, including intrauterine contraception, can be immediately started. If the abortion was performed in the second trimester, the woman should be counselled about the slightly higher chance of expulsion of intrauterine contraception at this stage.

Surgical Abortion

Under 14 Weeks

Surgical abortion for pregnancies less than 14 weeks' gestation are generally performed using manual vacuum aspiration (MVA) or electric vacuum aspiration (EVA) [15]. They can be performed in a wide range of settings including operating theatres, outpatient clinics and ward procedure rooms. The World Health Organization (WHO) recommend that VCA in the first trimester can be performed by a range of cadres of healthcare provider, including medical staff and allied healthcare professionals with appropriate training and depending on legislation surrounding abortion [2]. Both MVA and EVA can be performed under local anaesthetic, with or without light sedation. General anaesthetic is not required and carries inherent risks; however, this may be preferred by some women who do not want to be aware of what is happening during the procedure.

In both MVA and EVA, the woman should receive misoprostol before treatment to soften and dilate the cervix. A single dose of 400 mg given sublingually 1 hour prior to the procedure is as effective as the same dose administered vaginally 3 hours prior to the procedure [16]. Pre-treatment reduces the risk of incomplete abortion and may be an important strategy to prevent damage to the internal cervical os and subsequent cervical incompetence in future pregnancies.

At the time of procedure, the cervix should be visualised using a vaginal speculum and local anaesthetic administered. The cervix should then be gently dilated to a diameter in millimetres that equates to the number of weeks gestation – that is, 10 mm for a 10-week pregnancy. An equivalently sized plastic curette should be introduced through the cervix and then connected to method of suction. For MVA this is usually a plastic handheld syringe and for EVA this is usually an electrical pump device. The pregnancy tissue is then removed using suction and the curette removed once the uterus has been evacuated.

Over 14 Weeks

Surgical abortion beyond 14 weeks' gestation is performed using a method known as dilatation and evacuation (D&E). This process is more technically difficult than VCA and should be performed by appropriately trained medical staff. Dilation and evacuation can be performed in an operating theatre or outpatient setting in a procedure room. General anaesthesia can be used, but a combination of local anaesthetic and conscious sedation allows D&E to be performed in a broader variety of settings and without the need of an anaesthetist.

As with EVA/MVA, cervical preparation is needed in order to reduce damage from dilatation. Preparation can be achieved using either a single dose of mifepristone 200 mg and/or insertion of osmotic dilators into the cervix 24 hours pre-procedure [17]. At the time of procedure, these dilators are removed and the cervix further dilated to allow passage of instruments and removal of fetal parts.

The amniotic fluid is removed using suction evacuation. Specialised forceps are then introduced into the lower portion of the uterus and the fetus is then removed under ultrasound guidance. The placenta may need to be removed using the suction catheter at the end of the procedure.

Contraception after Surgical Abortion

All methods of contraception, including intrauterine methods, can be initiated immediately following surgical abortion and will be effective immediately. If an intrauterine method is inserted following D&E there is a higher chance of expulsion than in the first trimester due to greater dilatation of the cervix.

References

1. Singh S, Remez L, Sedgh G, Kwok L, Onda T. *Abortion worldwide 2017: Uneven progress and unequal access.* Vol. **2019**. New York: Guttmacher Institute, 2018. www .guttmacher.org/report/abortion-worldwide-2017.

2. World Health Organization. *Expanding health worker roles for safe abortion in the first trimester of pregnancy.* Geneva: World Health Organization, 2019. Report No.: WHO/RHR/16.02. https://bit.ly/3XTKt5U.

3. World Health Organization. *Medical management of abortion.* Geneva: World Health Organization, 2018.

4. Avraham S, Gat I, Duvdevani N-R et al. Pre-emptive effect of ibuprofen versus placebo on pain relief and success rates of medical abortion: A double-blind, randomized, controlled study. *Fertil Steril.* 2012;**97** (3):612–15. https://bit.ly/3HTInhC.

5. Livshits A, Machtinger R, David LB et al. Ibuprofen and paracetamol for pain relief during medical abortion: A double-blind randomized controlled study. *Fertil Steril.* 2009;**91**(5):1877–80. https://bit.ly /3wWhSla.

6. Hamoda H, Ashok PW, Flett GMM, Templeton A. A randomised controlled trial of mifepristone in combination with misoprostol administered sublingually or vaginally for medical abortion up to 13 weeks of gestation. *BJOG* 2005;**112**(8):1102–8. https://doi.org/10.1111/j.1471-0528.2005.00638.x.

7. Faúndes A, Fiala C, Tang OS, Velasco A. Misoprostol for the termination of pregnancy up to 12 completed weeks of pregnancy. *Int J Gynecol & Obstet.* 2007;**99**: S172–7. www.sciencedirect.com/science/article/pii/ S0020729207005097.

8. Tang OS, Schweer H, Lee SWH, Ho PC. Pharmacokinetics of repeated doses of misoprostol. *Hum Reprod.* 2009;**24**(8):1862–9. https://doi.org/10 .1093/humrep/dep108.

9. Fiala C, Swahn ML, Stephansson O, Gemzell-Danielsson K. The effect of non-steroidal anti-inflammatory drugs on medical abortion with mifepristone and misoprostol at 13–22 weeks gestation. *Hum Reprod.* 2005;**20**(11):3072–7. www .ncbi.nlm.nih.gov/pubmed/16055455.

10. Jackson E, Kapp N. Pain control in first-trimester and second-trimester medical termination of pregnancy: A systematic review. *Contraception.* 2011;**83**(2):116–26. https://bit.ly/3wUEnHe.

11. Pasquini L, Pontello V, Kumar S. Intracardiac injection of potassium chloride as method for feticide: Experience from a single UK tertiary centre. *BJOG: An International Journal of Obstetrics & Gynaecology* 2008;**115**(4):528–31. https://doi.org/10.1111/j.1471-0 528.2007.01639.x.

12. Molaei M, Jones HE, Weiselberg T et al. Effectiveness and safety of digoxin to induce fetal demise prior to second-trimester abortion. *Contraception.* 2008;**77** (3):223–5. www.sciencedirect.com/science/article/pi i/S0010782407005112.

13. Sharvit M, Klein Z, Silber M et al. Intra-amniotic digoxin for feticide between 21 and 30 weeks of gestation: A prospective study. *BJOG: An International Journal of Obstetrics & Gynaecology.* 2019;**126**(7):885–9. https://doi.org/10.1111/1471-052 8.15640.

14. Faculty of Sexual and Reproductive Healthcare. Contraception after pregnancy. 2017. https://bit.ly/3DFyBwT.

15. World Health Organization. Preventing unsafe abortion. 2019. http://bit.ly/3kh4R37.

16. Sääv I, Kopp Kallner H, Fiala C, Gemzell-Danielsson K. Sublingual versus vaginal misoprostol for cervical dilatation 1 or 3 h prior to surgical abortion: A double-blinded RCT. *Hum Reprod.* 2015;**30**(6):1314–22. www.ncbi.nlm.nih.gov/pubmed/25840429.

17. National Institute for Health and Care Excellence. Abortion care. NG140 ed. 2019. www.nice.org.uk/guidance/NG140.

Post-abortion Care

Dominique Baker, Chu Chin Lim, Tahir Mahmood

Introduction

The aftercare provided to a patient following an abortion, or a termination of pregnancy, can improve the safety and the patient's experience. The content and amount of aftercare required will depend on the patient's circumstances, method of abortion and whether it was safe or unsafe [1]. Here we aim to discuss the basic principles of abortion aftercare such as what and how to provide information to patients. We go on to discuss reduction of complications and how to manage those that do arise. Furthermore, the importance of contraception within post-abortion care mustn't be neglected as it reduces future unwanted pregnancies and therefore abortions.

General Principles

The patient should be provided with verbal and written – or pictorial if unable to read – information about the procedure they have had and how to access help if required. Advice and help should be available 24 hours a day to ensure safe management of any complications. In addition, there should be information on what signs and symptoms the patient should look out for such as persistent pregnancy symptoms, increasing pain, fever or heavy bleeding [1, 7]. Patients should be advised to avoid vaginal intercourse and the use of tampons until their bleeding has stopped [1]. Furthermore, before discharge pre-emptive medications such as analgesia, anti-emetics and iron tablets should be provided if required [7]. Patients can be advised that most people recommence routine activities of daily living within a few days of an abortion [1]. Depending on the individual circumstances, the patient may require additional support from outside agencies and these referrals should be promptly made. This could include sexual health, domestic violence or sexual violence support services [7].

A follow-up appointment should be provided if a misoprostol only schedule for medical abortion is used; however, it isn't routinely required for a surgical procedure or a medical abortion using mifepristone and misoprostol in combination. At this appointment the well-being of the patient should be assessed along with any risk of ongoing pregnancy [7]. The majority of patients prefer not to attend the clinic for face-to-face follow-up and there is evidence that there is no difference in concordance with follow-up regimes when patients follow an algorithm at home. The evidence as to whether in-person or remote follow-up alters the rate of unsuccessful abortions is inconclusive [18].

Patients who have had a medical abortion should be advised to take a urinary pregnancy test 3 weeks after the treatment to ensure no gestational trophoblastic disease is present and the procedure was successful. Although the rate of gestational trophoblastic disease is low at 1 in 20,000 abortions, a urinary pregnancy test is easy to carry out and can reduce the associated morbidity and mortality. The Royal College of Obstetricians and Gynaecologists have advised that there is no requirement to send products of conception for histology from surgical abortions as long as a fetus was identified prior to or during to the procedure [8].

Anti-D Immunoglobulin

There is currently a range in practices regarding anti-D immunoglobulin (anti-D) administration for medical or surgical abortions. The World Health Organization advises that rhesus status testing or administration of anti-D isn't a requirement for abortion provision, but, if it is available, it should be given to rhesus-negative patients. An abortion shouldn't be delayed while awaiting anti-D [1]. The Royal College of Obstetricians and Gynaecologists advise that all rhesus negative patients should receive anti-D, regardless of their gestation at the time of abortion. This differs from the National

Institute of Clinical Excellence, who advise that only surgical procedures and medical procedures over 10 weeks require anti-D administration [2, 12].

Contraception

Ideally, counselling regarding contraception should take place prior to an abortion as it improves uptake after the procedure [9]. If contraception is started immediately after an abortion, it has been shown to improve concordance and reduce future unplanned pregnancy rates. Some patients may prefer to discuss their options after their procedure or decline contraception altogether, both of these preferences should be respected [7].

Contraceptive options include oral contraceptives, barrier methods, injectables, patches, a vaginal ring, implants and intrauterine contraceptives. All of these methods can be started at the time of abortion, but patients should be informed that there is a higher expulsion rate of intrauterine contraceptives if fitted after a second-trimester abortion. In addition, a medical abortion should be confirmed as successful prior to insertion of an intrauterine contraceptive, while insertion is contraindicated in the presence of a septic abortion [1, 7].

Patients should be informed that long-acting reversible contraceptives such as the implant or intra-uterine contraceptives are more effective at preventing pregnancy and are recommended as first-line contraception in adolescents by the European Board and College of Obstetrics and Gynaecology [19]. Patients wishing to use injectable medroxyprogesterone acetate should be informed that administration at the same time as a medical abortion may increase the chance of an unsuccessful procedure and therefore an ongoing pregnancy. However, the absolute risk of this is low [2].

The cervical cap and diaphragms shouldn't be initiated until 6 weeks after a second-trimester abortion due to the increase in failure rates and infection. Similarly any person wanting to use the fertility awareness method should wait until their menstruation has resumed a predictable pattern [1]. Although it is technically possible to perform sterilization at the time of abortion, patients should be counselled that there are higher rates of failure and regret when performed at this time [12].

Patients should also be informed regarding emergency contraception regardless of their chosen method of contraception; this will help them to identify events when they may be at risk of pregnancy and require additional emergency contraception. Some patients may benefit from having a supply of emergency contraception at home, especially those using a barrier method or declining contraception [1]. However, care should be taken to ensure patients are fully informed regarding the most effective method of emergency contraception being the copper coil. Any unprotected intercourse 5 days after an abortion would require emergency contraception.

Venous Thromboembolism Prophylaxis

Deep vein thrombosis and pulmonary embolism are estimated to occur in 30.1 per 100,000 patients after an abortion. Although this rate is very low, it is nonetheless higher than in a cohort of matched non-pregnant patients, and therefore patients should have a risk assessment to determine the likelihood of them developing a venous thromboembolism after an abortion. Consideration should be given to starting high-risk patients on low-molecular-weight heparin before and after an abortion. The evidence is limited on when to start prophylaxis and for how long, but the National Institute for Health and Care Excellence has advised at least 7 days post procedure in those deemed high risk [2, 21].

Mental Health

Each patient will have a different reaction to having an abortion and should be referred to counselling if she requests it. However, it is important to emphasise that having an abortion is not associated with an increased risk of developing mental health conditions in the future. In addition, healthcare providers should be aware of local support groups and how patients can access these if desired [2]. Patients experiencing mental health symptoms after an abortion are most commonly found to have pre-existing conditions that predate the abortion [1].

Unsafe Abortions

Worldwide, 45% of abortions are carried out in unsafe conditions and this leads to the associated maternal mortality of between 4.7% and 13.2%. An unsafe abortion is any procedure performed by someone without relevant training or in a location that doesn't meet clinical standards [3]. Most European countries provide safe abortion within their legal structure dependent on the reason for abortion [4]. However, there were still an estimated 360,000 unsafe abortions within Europe in 2008 [5]. Therefore, knowledge of the management of unsafe abortions is an essential skill for anyone practising obstetrics and gynaecology as it reduces maternal mortality and morbidity [6, 20].

Potential complications of unsafe abortions include trauma, sepsis, retention of foreign bodies or overdoses of medications [1]. Furthermore, clinicians should be aware of signs and symptoms that an abortion may have occurred in unsafe conditions. This is to tailor aftercare to the individual, as the risks of complications are much higher in unsafe abortions. Signs of an unsafe abortion include 'vaginal laceration, cervical injury, uterine enlargement equivalent to a pregnancy of more than 12 weeks' of gestation and products of conception visible at the cervix' [10].

Complication Management

Ongoing Pregnancy

An unsuccessful abortion is more common with medical than surgical abortion, and reported failure rates of medical abortion vary between countries [1]. A recent Cochrane review found that success rates for self-administered and healthcare professional–administered medical abortion are similar. Success rates were found to range from 78% to 98%; however, the Royal College of Obstetricians and Gynaecologists advises that less than 1% of medical and surgical abortions result in an ongoing pregnancy [11, 12]. Several factors increase the risk of an unsuccessful procedure. These include the level of experience of the practitioner, congenital uterine anomalies, gestations less than 6 weeks and parous patients [14].

An ongoing pregnancy should be suspected if there is minimal bleeding after misoprostol administration, ongoing pregnancy symptoms or a positive follow-up pregnancy test. Ultrasound can be used to detect an ongoing pregnancy; however, measuring endometrial thickness alone is not a reliable method of identifying unsuccessful abortions. Patients diagnosed with an ongoing pregnancy after a medical abortion should be offered a surgical or repeat medical procedure as soon as available. If a patient chooses to continue the pregnancy, she should be informed there are limited data on the effects of misoprostol and mifepristone on pregnancy [1]. However, a prospective study from 2013 found the major congenital malformation rate to be similar to the background risk when exposure is during the first 12 weeks of pregnancy – 4.2% versus 1–3% [13].

The diagnosis of an ectopic pregnancy should be considered if the patient didn't have an intrauterine pregnancy confirmed on ultrasound prior to the abortion. This would be further reinforced if the uterus is small on palpation or an adnexal mass was present [10]. Patients having an abortion without an ultrasound-confirmed intrauterine pregnancy should be informed of the symptoms of an ectopic pregnancy and should be able to access advice if they develop any of these symptoms.

Incomplete Abortion

An incomplete abortion occurs when there are retained products of conception after the fetus has been expelled. Rates vary depending on abortion method, but a Swedish follow-up study showed that 4.1% of medical abortions at less than 12 weeks' gestation resulted in an incomplete abortion. After 12 weeks' gestation the rates from surgical and medical abortions were 1.7% and 4.6%, respectively. An incomplete abortion was defined as products of conception with placental appearances on ultrasound that measured more than 15 mm. However, the authors concluded that, although an incomplete abortion was the most common complication after a first-trimester medical procedure, their rates of surgical and second-trimester abortions were too low to draw conclusions regarding complication rates [22].

An incomplete abortion should be suspected if a patient has ongoing bleeding, fever, offensive discharge, pain or the products of conception retrieved at a surgical procedure do not correspond with gestation [1]. In any patient presenting with ongoing vaginal bleeding after an abortion a urine pregnancy test should be carried out to ensure ongoing pregnancy or gestational trophoblastic disease has been considered [8]. An ectopic pregnancy should also be considered if an intrauterine pregnancy wasn't confirmed by ultrasound prior to the abortion.

If a patient has retained products of conception she can be managed expectantly unless she is experiencing heavy bleeding. Some patients may wish to have a repeat dose of misoprostol or a vacuum aspiration; there is no demonstrable difference in success rates between these two options. However, if a patient is over 12 weeks' gestation the procedure should be confirmed as complete prior to discharge as they are more at risk of complications from retained products of conception [1].

Infection

Before an abortion patients should be assessed and offered testing for sexually transmitted infections to provide opportunistic screening and reduce the incidence of post abortion ascending infection. Chlamydia has been found to occur in 2.3% of patients requesting an abortion, whereas a lower prevalence of gonorrhoea is seen at 0.02% [22]. A Cochrane review found that antibiotic prophylaxis was effective at reducing the incidence of genital tract infections after both medical and surgical first-trimester abortions. No established regime of antibiotics has proven superior but commonly used antimicrobials include doxycycline, amoxicillin and metronidazole. It has been suggested that local infection and resistance patterns need to be taken into account when antibiotic recommendations are made [15]. However, the World Health Organization and the National Institute for Health and Care Excellence advise that antibiotics should only be offered to patients having a surgical abortion but not a medical abortion. This is because the incidence of severe infection after a medical procedure is low and the quality of the evidence to guide on the recommendation for prophylaxis before medical treatment was lacking. Furthermore, there were concerns about antibiotic resistance and low patient concordance with antibiotics [1, 2].

Signs and symptoms of infection include fever, ongoing vaginal bleeding, pain, offensive discharge and cervical motion tenderness. Patients reporting these symptoms should be reviewed and screened for sepsis. At examination high vaginal swabs for microscopy, culture and sensitivity should be taken, along with screening for chlamydia and gonorrhoea, if not already done prior to the abortion. Antibiotics should be provided and if there are signs of sepsis the patient should be admitted for intravenous treatment and a sepsis protocol. If there are any concerns regarding retained products of conception a surgical evacuation of the uterus should take place as source control for the infection [1].

Haemorrhage

The risk of significant haemorrhage during or after an abortion varies depending on method, country and whether it is safely performed or not. However, in a developed country it is estimated to occur in less than 1% of abortions, more commonly in medical procedures. By ascertaining the cause of the haemorrhage the clinician can appropriately direct their management. Possible causes include retained products of conception, uterine perforation, cervical trauma, atony, abnormal placentation or disseminated intravascular coagulopathy [16].

Clinicians should be aware of the emergency management of gynaecological haemorrhage working in a stepwise method. The patient will require large-bore intravenous access, fluid replacement and possibly blood products. Abdominal and vaginal examination will help to determine the cause and therefore the treatment of the haemorrhage. Emergency measures including bimanual compression can be initiated at examination.

Uterotonic medications such as misoprostol, carboprost, oxytocin or ergometrine can be used. There is a debate as to whether oxytocin is useful in first- and second-trimester haemorrhage management as the uterus has minimal oxytocin receptors at this gestation. Therefore, if these measures fail to control bleeding consideration should be given to manual compression with a balloon tamponade or a Foley catheter. This would be an off-label use of a Foley catheter, but it has been shown to be safe in the management of uterine atony. It can be filled with 30–80 ml of normal saline and consideration should be given to prophylactic antibiotics while a balloon tamponade is in situ [16].

Surgical management needs to be considered early if the aforementioned medical measures fail. This would include uterine artery embolization, laparotomy for brace sutures, uterine artery ligation and finally hysterectomy. Uterine artery embolization with interventional radiology will not be available in all clinical settings but has been shown to have a lower morbidity and mortality then laparotomy to treat haemorrhage. Hysterectomy after an abortion is rare, estimating to occur in 1.4 per 10,000 abortions [16]. The decision should ideally be made by two senior clinicians and once the decision has been made the procedure should be expedited as soon as possible to reduce further complications such as disseminated intravascular coagulopathy.

Perforation and Rupture

Perforation is estimated to occur in 1 out of every 1,000 uterine evacuations [17]. The World Health Organization advises that most perforations are small and require only observation and antibiotic treatment. However, it should be noted that perforation is the most common cause for a hysterectomy due to haemorrhage after an abortion [16]. A laparoscopy should be performed if possible to assess the extent of any intra-abdominal visceral damage and perform a repair if required [1]. Rupture is a rare occurrence but has been found to occur in 0.28% of misoprostol induced second trimester medical abortions [1]. This would require emergency management similar to that of a haemorrhage, but early laparotomy is required for repair or hysterectomy.

Discussion

Abortion is one of the most commonly performed gynaecological procedures and knowledge of how to care for a patient after the procedure is as important as the preparation prior to the procedure. An awareness of the potential complications of safe and unsafe abortions will help reduce the maternal mortality and morbidity associated with abortion. Aftercare needs to be tailored to each individual's needs and circumstances and practitioners should be aware of the additional requirements of patients requesting abortions, such as sexual health referrals and the need to screen for domestic abuse. Finally contraception care should be integrally combined with abortion services as it helps to prevent future unwanted pregnancies. By helping patients access ongoing contraception we can further reduce the morbidity and mortality associated with abortion by preventing its occurrence in the first instance.

References

1. World Health Organization. *Safe abortion: Technical and policy guidance for health systems.* 2nd edition. Geneva: World Health Organization, 2012.

2. National Institute for Health and Care Excellence. *Abortion care.* London: National Institute for Health and Care Excellence, 2019.

3. World Health Organization. Preventing unsafe abortion. September 2020. http://bit.ly/3HjI4uQ.

4. World Health Organization. Abortion in Europe. *Entre Nous: The European Magazine for Sexual and Reproductive Health.* 2005;59–72.

5. World Health Organization. *Unsafe abortion incidence and mortality: Global and regional levels in 2008 and trends during 1990–2008.* Geneva: World Health Organization, 2012.

6. Themmerman M. Missed opportunities in women's health: Post-abortion care. *Lancet Global Health.* 2019;7(1):e12–e13.

7. World Health Organization. *Clinical practice handbook for safe abortion.* Geneva: World Health Organization, 2014.

8. Tidy J, Seckl, M, Hancock BW. Management of gestational trophoblastic disease. Green-Top Guideline No. 38. *BJOG.* 2021;**128**(3): e1–e27.

9. Yassin AS, Cordwell D. Does dedicated pre-abortion contraception counselling help to improve post-abortion contraception uptake? *J Fam Plann Reprod Health Care.* 2005;31(2):115–16.

10. Royal College of Obstetricians and Gynaecologists. Best practice in comprehensive abortion care. Best practice paper No. 2. June 2015.

11. Gambir K, Kim C, Necastro KA, Ganatra B, Ngo TD. Self-administered versus provider-administered medical abortion (review). *Cochrane Database of Systematic Reviews.* 2020;**3** (3):CD013181.

12. Royal College of Obstetricians and Gynaecologists. The care of women requesting induced abortion. Evidence-Based Clinical Guideline Number 7. November 2011.

13. Bernard N, Elefant E, Carlier P, et al. Continuation of pregnancy after first-trimester exposure to mifepristone: An observational prospective study. *BJOG.* 2013;**120**:568–75.

14. Scott A, Glasier A. Failed medical and surgical termination of pregnancy. *Obstetrician and Gynaecologist.* 2002;4:217–21.

15. Low N, Mueller M, Van Vliet HAAM, Kapp N. Perioperative antibiotics to prevent infection after first-trimester abortion (review). *Cochrane Database of Systematic Reviews.* 2012;3.

16. Kerns J, Steinauer J. Management of post abortion hemorrhage. *Society of Family Planning. Contraception.* 2013;87:331–42.

17. Royal College of Obstetricians and Gynaecologists. Surgical management of miscarriage and removal of persistent placental or fetal remains. Consent Advice No. 10 (Joint with AEPU) January 2018.

18. National Institute for Health and Care Excellence. Abortion care: Follow-up after medical abortion up to 10+0 weeks. NICE guideline NG140, Evidence reviews. September 2019.

19. Mahmood T, Benefetto C. European Board and College of Obstetrics and Gynaecology position paper: EBCOG call for action for the prevention of unintended pregnancies. 2015.

20. Oppegaard KS. European Board and College of Obstetrics and Gynaecology. EBCOG position paper on medical abortion. 2015.

21. Liu N, Vigod SN, Farrugia MM, Urquia ML, Ray JG. Venous thromboembolism after induced abortion: A population-based, propensity-score-matched cohort study in Canada. *Lancet Haematol*. 2018;5(7):e279–e288.

22. Carlsson I, Breding K, Larsson PG. Complications related to induced abortion: A combined retrospective and longitudinal follow-up study. *BMC Women's Health*. 2018;18:158.

Infertility

Ioannis E. Messinis, Christina I. Messini, George Anifandis,
Alexandros Daponte

Definition

Infertility is defined as the inability of a couple to conceive after at least 1 year of regular unprotected sexual intercourse. According to the World Health Organization (WHO), infertility is a disease of the reproductive system [1]. In the literature other terms such as *subfertility* or *sterility* have been used at times. The latter, however, is no longer used as it implies almost permanent inability of conception, whereas today there are opportunities for treatment in almost all cases of infertility. Infertility is defined as primary when the woman has never been pregnant before and secondary, when the woman has had at least one clinical pregnancy regardless of whether it was full-term.

Prevalence

There is today no consensus on the prevalence of infertility. This is because most data come from individual clinics and their numbers are not representative of an area's total population of an area. However, most studies report a frequency of 10–20%. The lack of valid data gives an impression that the incidence of infertility has increased in recent years. This, however, does not seem to be true, as an analysis of several studies has shown that the incidence of infertility has remained constant with only small fluctuations for almost a complete century [2]. In these studies the problem is referred to as a childlessness rate. In women attempting spontaneous conception, the pregnancy rate is 20–25% per cycle and, over a period of 12 months, the percentage of pregnant women aged under 40 is about 80–85% with a small further increase to 90% at 24 months [3]. It is clear that the remaining 10–15% of women who do not conceive during this period of time is equal to the incidence of infertility (Figure 41.1).

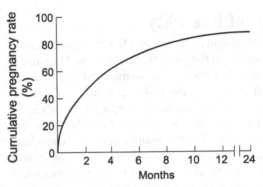

Figure 41.1 Estimated cumulative pregnancy rate in the normal population. After 24 months 10–15% will remain without pregnancy (frequency of infertility).

Prerequisites for Normal Conception

Many factors may affect the likelihood of conception. These include frequency of sexual intercourse, a woman's age, duration of infertility, smoking, exercise, body weight, psycho-emotional condition, general illness and drug use [2]. Although sexual intercourse two to three times a week is quite often recommended for infertile couples, the chance of conception increases with the increase in the frequency of intercourse and reaches a maximum (> 80%) when intercourse takes place more than four times a week.

The time of intercourse in relation to ovulation is also important. The closer the contact is, the greater the chance of conception, which reaches its maximum (33%) when intercourse occurs on the day of ovulation [4]. The age of the woman is also an important factor. It has been considered that the possibility of conception is maximum around the age of 25, decreasing linearly thereafter and more abruptly after the age of 38. The duration of infertility is an independent factor with the chance of conception decreasing significantly each month after 3 years. Different habits such as smoking or exercise can negatively affect fertility via different mechanisms. Weight loss or significant deviations from the ideal body weight play an important role in reducing fertility [2]. In order for a couple to achieve a pregnancy three appropriate conditions for normal conception must be met – normal ovarian function with ovulatory cycles, normal anatomy of the genital tract with patent fallopian tubes and semen with normal characteristics.

Causes of Infertility

Several conditions can cause infertility, which lead to the disruption of the physiological process. The cause is shared equally between the woman and the man [5]. Causes from the woman make up roughly 40%, causes from the man also make up roughly 40%, while the remaining 20% of causes are from both or are unknown. Overall, four main causes are considered responsible at a rate of about 25% each. These include disorders of ovulation, damage of the fallopian tubes, disorders of spermatogenesis and/or the male reproductive system and unexplained infertility (Figure 41.2).

Anovulation is related to disorders of the hypothalamo-pituitary-ovarian axis, dysfunction of other endocrine glands (adrenal, thyroid) and hyperprolactinaemia [6]. Causes of fallopian tube damage include inflammation of the genital tract resulting mainly from sexually transmitted infection, pelvic surgeries and endometriosis, while smoking can disrupt tubal function. Causes that disrupt spermatogenesis include congenital abnormalities of the male reproductive system, inflammation of the genitalia, endocrine disorders, neurological and psycho-emotional disorders,

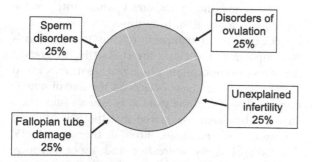

Figure 41.2 Main causes of infertility. Rough estimate of frequency. The rate of unexplained infertility also includes the small percentage (5–10%) of other causes (endometriosis, uterus, cervix)

chromosomal abnormalities, various toxic substances and varicose veins.

Nevertheless, in many cases male infertility is idiopathic. Uterine disorders can also contribute to infertility but in a very small percentage. Congenital abnormalities of the uterus or related to the use of diethylstilboestrol by the woman's mother during pregnancy, fibroids, endometrial polyps and endometrial adhesions are the most important, although their role has not been fully clarified and is evaluated only after other causes have been ruled out.

Diagnostic Workup

There is a variation in when infertility investigations should begin [5]. Usually the diagnostic workup begins after 1 year of unprotected intercourse. However, after the patient reaches the age of 35 and up to 40, the diagnostic process starts after 6 months. For patients older than 40 years the diagnostic process starts immediately. The same applies to the following cases – when there is a known infertility problem, menstrual disorders, diagnosed endometriosis, pelvic inflammatory disease, a history of more than one induced abortion and previous cancer treatment.

The diagnostic investigation of infertility includes taking a detailed history from the couple, clinical and gynaecological examination, ultrasound examination of the ovaries and uterus, assessment of ovulation and fallopian tubes with hysterosalpingography, semen analysis and basic hormonal testing for both men and women, including monitoring of ovarian reserves. The presence of regular menstrual cycles in the medical history and an increased progesterone value on day 21 of a 28-day cycle confirm ovulation. The inclusion of laparoscopy in the routine diagnostic workup of infertility is questionable unless there is an obvious disorder such as endometriosis or fallopian tube problems in hysterosalpingography.

The same applies to hysteroscopy, which is indicated when there are abnormal ultrasound findings in the endometrium – for example, polyps or fibroids – or there is suspicion of endometrial adhesions from the medical history or in hysterosalpingography. Post-coital or Huhner tests, often used in the past, are not used today as they have a low predictive value. When no specific cause is found during the diagnostic workup, the infertility is characterized as unexplained. However, the extent of the scrutiny has not been determined by a consensus and therefore several cases may not fall into this category. Certainly full investigation of the couple is required, although several diagnostic methods are insufficient. In general, to diagnose unexplained infertility, there must be normal findings from at least the following tests – blood progesterone, hysterosalpingography and/or laparoscopy/hysteroscopy and semen analysis [7].

Prognostic Biomarkers

During recent years, the concept of an ovarian reserve has emerged, for which there seems to be wide variations in the different age groups of women. Clinical laboratory research has shown some indicators such as various hormones and number of follicles as predictors of ovarian reserve. Thus it is recommended these indices are evaluated in infertile women of all ages as they can highlight those who will have a poor ovarian response to possible ovarian stimulation. Several such indicators have been investigated in recent years, but the top three in terms of reliability are antimullerian hormone (AMH), antral follicle count (AFC) and follicle-stimulating hormone (FSH).

Antimullerian hormone and AFC are currently equally important in clinical practice, showing a positive correlation between their values, while FSH follows with a lower predictive value [8]. Regarding AMH, an attempt has been made to investigate whether, in addition to ovarian reserves, it can predict other issues – for example, the outcome of infertility treatment. In the case of women undergoing in vitro fertilization (IVF), it is still unclear whether AMH levels can predict blastocyst formation or the achievement of pregnancy, while very low levels cannot rule out a successful outcome [9].

Treatment

The most appropriate treatment is aetiology based unless the cause of infertility is not known, in which case treatment is based on the application of the most effective methods according to evidence-based medicine. When the cause is anovulation, the most appropriate treatment is induction of ovulation provided that the fallopian tubes are patent and the semen analysis is normal [6]. It is not clear whether in older women or those with reduced ovarian reserve IVF should be the method of choice. There are two main categories of anovulation – hypogonadotropic hypogonadism and polycystic ovary syndrome (PCOS). In the first category (WHO group 1) ovulation is induced with the use of human gonadotropins

(FSH plus luteinizing hormone), while in PCOS clomiphene citrate or letrozole are used as a first-line treatment [10]. In case of failure or resistance to clomiphene, low-dose FSH protocols are used as a second-line treatment. Laparoscopic ovarian diathermy (LOD) is also used as a second-line treatment, but under certain conditions. Finally, upon failure of all these methods, IVF is the third line of treatment. Metformin may also be useful in cases of glucose intolerance or clomiphene resistance, whereupon it is administered in combination with clomiphene [11]. In women with anovulatory infertility and more advanced age (> 40 years), the first line may be skipped.

In women with tubal factor infertility, treatment is either laparoscopic salpingectomy (hydrosalpinx) or IVF. Fallopian tube surgery to open the lumen or create a new orifice is currently limited unless it is a young woman and the lesion is characterized as filmy adhesions. Salpingectomy due to hydrosalpinx improves the outcome of subsequent IVF treatment [12]. It should be noted that hysterosalpingography during the investigation of infertility can by itself resolve small adhesions in the fallopian tube and help spontaneous conception, especially when oily versus aqueous solution is used [13].

Treatment of endometriosis in infertile women depends on the stage of the disease [14]. In the early stages electrocautery of the foci can increase the chance of pregnancy, while, when there are endometriomas, the effort is as far as possible to avoid their removal because an operation reduces ovarian reserves with negative consequences for female fertility. Nevertheless, the role of surgery is still controversial. In the majority of cases treatment is provided in the context of assisted reproductive technology (ART). In the early stages the condition is initially treated as unexplained infertility but, soon after, IVF is the most appropriate option.

There does not seem to be a significant difference in the outcome of IVF treatment between endometriosis and other causes of infertility. In unexplained infertility intrauterine insemination (IUI) can be the first approach as long as there is no age limit for the woman; otherwise IVF is applied. Nevertheless, treatment is still largely empirical today based on individualization [15, 16].

From the uterus, cases of interest are the presence of submucosal fibroids (category 0–3) or endometrial polyps. The presence of endometrial adhesions may also play a role. In all such cases hysteroscopy should be performed for the removal of the lesions or the adhesions [17]. Unfortunately, in cases of congenital uterine anomalies, surgery has a limited role since only in a septate uterus can removal of the septum enhance the chances of a pregnancy. Recently the role of endometrial microbiota in the uterine cavity, which was thought to be sterile, has been investigated. It has been found that the microbial flora can significantly reduce implantation and pregnancy achievement by affecting the receptivity of the endometrium [18].

If there is a male factor, treatment should be aimed at addressing the cause – for example, in case of infection, treatment with antibiotics may be useful. However, most cases of oligo- or azoospermia are idiopathic for no apparent reason so treatment can be either IUI or IVF by intracytoplasmic sperm injection (ICSI) [19]. If azoospermia is related to hypogonadotropic hypogonadism, treatment with a combination of FSH and LH plus human chorionic gonadotropin (HCG) is recommended. Varicocele is a special condition with promising surgical results [20].

Prevention

Infertility is a global problem whose prevention is unpredictable [21]. However, avoiding certain procedures or situations may reduce the risk – for example, avoiding many sexual partners can reduce the risk of genital infection. Also, advising women to avoid abortions and to undergo only the absolutely necessary operations on their internal genitalia can prevent their damage. For example, small endometriomas may not be necessary to remove as the procedure may reduce ovarian reserve without improving the IVF outcome. In addition, in pelvic surgeries, an effort must be made to maintain the integrity and blood perfusion of internal genitalia. Of note is that a good and healthy diet is important while smoking and excessive alcohol as well as exposure of the body to a toxic environment should be avoided. It is also important to treat endocrine abnormalities – for example, of the thyroid gland or diabetes mellitus – before attempting conception.

Impact on Physical Health

Infertility may impact the health of the couple, especially the woman [22]. Although this condition usually affects the mental health of the individual, physical health problems can also arise. These problems are related either to the causes of infertility or to the diagnostic and/or therapeutic interventions. An example of a condition that can affect a person's physical activities is endometriosis, which can cause specific symptoms such as dyspareunia and dysmenorrhea. Although these symptoms may also be present in fertile individuals, infertility itself can exacerbate them through the psychic sphere.

On the other hand, dyspareunia reduces the frequency of sexual intercourse and hence favours infertility. In the case of conditions that can cause general health disorders, such as PCOS, which has long-term effects on women's health, infertility may delay some efforts to improve the phenotype such as, for example, weight reduction in obese women with the syndrome. It has further been suggested that infertility per se may predispose to serious illnesses, such as malignancies, but also increase the risk of early mortality [23].

Impact on Mental Health

Infertility can also affect the mental health of the couple [24]. Many aspects of the psychic sphere can be affected by a possible disruption in the couple's marital relationship and the risk of divorce. Although both partners are affected, the whole situation creates more intense stress in the woman than in the man. One factor that exacerbates stress is the age of the woman, as today's lifestyle leads many couples to decide to start childbearing quite late when ovarian reserve has been significantly reduced. Human reproduction is characterized by a gradual reduction in the likelihood of pregnancy with age. Unfortunately, many couples are not aware of this information or that IVF cannot exceed normal success rates. In fact, IVF results follow the same pattern with those of normal fecundity; as the conception rate decreases with age and above a certain limit, usually 45 years, the success rate is extremely low (Figure 41.3) [25, 26]. In recent years, with the improvement of fertility preservation techniques, young women are given the opportunity to freeze their eggs, which they will use at an older age when the conditions of their career will allow it. Indeed, the emergence of very effective cryopreservation methods for freezing eggs holds great promise in this regard, although legislative barriers may not reinforce this in young women [27].

An important parameter is the perception that women and men have about fertility/infertility. For many years, and possibly even still today, mainly in underdeveloped societies, the man believes he is not the cause of the problem, while the woman admits she

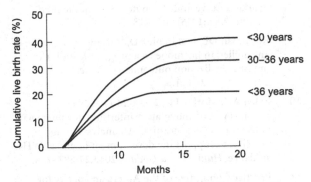

Figure 41.3 Cumulative live birth rate from IVF treatment. The effectiveness decreases with the age of the woman. The diagram is based on data presented in [26].

is. Certainly in developed societies the man is taking his share of responsibility for not achieving pregnancy. However, the inability to conceive calls into question the couple's ability to become parents and their role in society as successors to the human species. A variety of emotions emerge which create guilt and disturb the mental balance. In particular, a poor outcome of an infertility treatment, which before it begins raises serious hopes of success, causes maximum frustration [28].

In cases of unexplained infertility, the inability to find a cause sometimes creates a greater psychological burden. The condition is even worse after achieving a pregnancy that results in a miscarriage, especially when the cause of the miscarriage is unknown and the woman considers herself responsible. Additionally, stress itself increases the likelihood of pregnancy failure after IVF [29].

An infertile couple may experience a variety of psychological manifestations such as depression, anger, mood swings, anxiety, guilt and isolation [30]. It is clear that the severity of the psychological disorder depends on the psychological background of the woman and the man. Stress, anxiety and frustration are emotions of everyday life, but, when they are intense and persistent, the situation is more serious and beyond its characterization as a simple expected reaction. Many studies published in the literature in recent years have examined the psychological behaviour of women suffering from infertility or the impact this may have on treatment outcome but the results are varied with unclear conclusions [31]. In case of depression the feeling can be that of constant sadness or despair, tearing, sleep disorders with insomnia or

physical and mental fatigue, while the patients show negativity for even daily activities. In extreme cases the condition may require psychiatric treatment. Anger is another emotion infertile couples can show for even the least of reasons. This can happen during contact with other members of their family or even between the couple and is disastrous for the relationship. Although infertility can negatively affect the mental health of the couple, especially the woman, no convincing conclusions have been drawn on the marital relationship and quality of life [32].

In many couples the inability to have children creates a feeling of isolation and leads them to avoid participating in ceremonies such as baptism. This can gradually lead to social isolation with unpredictable consequences [30]. Guilt is another emotion created more in women than in men. The woman can blame herself for her bad past – for example, many sexual partners, induced abortions and so forth. Men feel less guilty, especially when the diagnostic process shows that there is a male factor. The problem of guilt is exacerbated when the family environment pressures the couple to have children. Today, of course, with the advancements in IVF, there are many potential treatments that did not exist in the past which can get couples out of this difficult position. However, some procedures, such as the need to use donor sperm or eggs, also make it difficult for many couples to accept this, as they consider it the genetic material of a stranger and not their own.

Infertility can be the first life crisis two people have to face together in their marriage and for which they were not prepared. Depending on their perception, the two individuals may never be able to cope and their communication may break down, leading to separation. In many cases sexual intercourse is imposed by other parameters such as ovulation, which makes reunion even more difficult. In addition, some women experience pain during intercourse, which is based on bad psychology (vaginismus). Lack of sexual desire leads the couple to avoid sexual intercourse. This can lead to the ruin of a treatment – for example, during induction of ovulation when the rupture of the follicle is timely scheduled.

Problems also arise when a man needs to ejaculate in order to perform insemination or IVF. Many men have such a problem or it takes them a long time, which may disrupt the function of the unit but can also affect the outcome of the treatment. Many of these treatments are costly and the couple may end up spending a large amount of money without achieving the goal of a healthy baby. The loss of money without benefit is an additional psychological burden on the couple. It should be noted that psychological problems can also occur in the case of secondary infertility, even if the couple already has a healthy child. These manifestations may be the same as those described earlier since the desire for pregnancy is the same or even greater.

Psychological interventions can decrease psychological stress and increase the success of a treatment [33]. Mental health professionals with knowledge in the field of infertility and special training in counselling offer support and encouragement so couples accept the situation as much as possible. This support helps to reverse the negative mood caused by anxiety, stress and depression. This is done using various tools such as cognitive behavioural strategies, positive coping skills training and communication skills training [24, 34].

References

1. Zegers-Hochschild F, Adamson GD, de Mouzon J et al. The International Committee for Monitoring Assisted Reproductive Technology (ICMART) and the World Health Organization (WHO) Revised Glossary on ART Terminology, 2009. *Hum Reprod.* 2009;24:2683–7.

2. Strickler RC. Factors influencing fertility. In Keye Jr WR, Chang RJ, Rebar RW and Soules MR (eds.) *Infertility evaluation and treatment.* Philadelphia, PA: W. B. Saunders 1995, pp. 8–18.

3. National Institute for Health and Care Excellence (NICE). *Fertility problems: Assessment and treatment. Clinical guideline 2013.* London: National Institute for Health and Care Excellence, 2013.

4. Wilcox AJ, Weinberg CR, Baird DD. Timing of sexual intercourse in relation to ovulation. Effects on the probability of conception, survival of the pregnancy, and sex of the baby. *N Engl J Med.* 1995;333:1517–21.

5. Thurston L, Abbara A, Dhillo WS. Investigation and management of subfertility. *J Clin Pathol.* 2019;72:579–87.

6. Messinis IE. Ovulation induction: A mini review. *Hum Reprod.* 2005;20:2688–97.

7. Gelbaya TA, Potdar N, Jeve YB, Nardo LG. Definition and epidemiology of unexplained infertility. *Obstet Gynecol Surv.* 2014;69:109–15.

8. Broekmans FJ, Kwee J, Hendriks DJ, Mol BW, Lambalk CB. A systematic review of tests predicting ovarian reserve and IVF outcome. *Hum Reprod Update.* 2006;12(6):685–718.

9. Reichman DE, Goldschlag D, Rosenwaks Z. Value of antimüllerian hormone as a prognostic indicator of in vitro fertilization outcome. *Fertil Steril.* 2014;101:1012–8.e1.

10. Balen AH, Morley LC, Misso M et al. The management of anovulatory infertility in women with polycystic ovary syndrome: An analysis of the evidence to support the development of global WHO guidance. *Hum Reprod Update.* 2016;22:687–708.

11. Practice Committee of the American Society for Reproductive Medicine. Electronic address: ASRM@asrm.org; Practice Committee of the American Society for Reproductive Medicine. Role of metformin for ovulation induction in infertile patients with polycystic ovary syndrome (PCOS): A guideline. *Fertil Steril.* 2017;108:426–41.

12. Johnson N, Van Voorst S, Sowter MC, Strandell A, Mol BW. Surgical treatment for tubal disease in women due to undergo in vitro fertilisation. *Cochrane Database Syst Rev.* 2010;1:CD002125.

13. Dreyer K, Van Rijswijk J, Mijatovic V et al. Oil-based or water-based contrast for hysterosalpingography in infertile women. *N Engl J Med.* 2017;376:2043–52.

14. Tanbo T, Fedorcsak P. Endometriosis-associated infertility: Aspects of pathophysiological mechanisms and treatment options. *Acta Obstet Gynecol Scand.* 2017;96:659–67.

15. Gunn DD, Bates GW. Evidence-based approach to unexplained infertility: A systematic review. *Fertil Steril.* 2016;105:1566–74.e1.

16. Practice Committee of the American Society for Reproductive Medicine. Evidence-based treatments for couples with unexplained infertility: A guideline. *Fertil Steril.* 2020;113:305–22.

17. Bosteels J, Van Wessel S, Weyers S et al.Hysteroscopy for treating subfertility associated with suspected major uterine cavity abnormalities. *Cochrane Database Syst Rev.* 2018;12(12):CD009461.

18. Benner M, Ferwerda G, Joosten I, Van der Molen RG. How uterine microbiota might be responsible for a receptive, fertile endometrium. *Hum Reprod Update.* 2018;24:393–415.

19. Tournaye H. Male factor infertility and ART. *Asian J Androl.* 2012;14:103–8.

20. Jensen CFS, Østergren P, Dupree JM et al. Varicocele and male infertility. *Nat Rev Urol.* 2017;14:523–33.

21. Inhorn MC, Patrizio P. Infertility around the globe: New thinking on gender, reproductive technologies and global movements in the 21st century. *Hum Reprod Update.* 2015;21:411–26.

22. Bakhtiyar K, Beiranvand R, Ardalan A et al. An investigation of the effects of infertility on women's quality of life: A case-control study. *BMC Womens Health*. 2019;**19**:114–22.

23. Senapati S. Infertility: A marker of future health risk in women? *Fertil Steril*. 2018;**110**:783–9.

24. Ezzell W. The impact of infertility on women's mental health. *N C Med J*. 2016;**77**:427–8.

25. De Geyter C, Calhaz-Jorge C, Kupka MS et al. ART in Europe, 2015: Results generated from European registries by ESHRE. *Hum Reprod Open*. 2020;**1**: hoz038.

26. Toftager M, Bogstad J, Løssl K et al. Cumulative live birth rates after one ART cycle including all subsequent frozen-thaw cycles in 1050 women: Secondary outcome of an RCT comparing GnRH-antagonist and GnRH-agonist protocols. *Hum Reprod*. 2017;**32**:556–67.

27. Calhaz-Jorge C, De Geyter CH, Kupka MS et al. Survey on ART and IUI: Legislation, regulation, funding and registries in European countries. The European IVF-monitoring Consortium (EIM) for the European Society of Human Reproduction and Embryology (ESHRE). *Hum Reprod Open*. 2020;**1**:hoz044.

28. Verhaak CM, Smeenk JM, Evers AW et al. Women's emotional adjustment to IVF: A systematic review of 25 years of research. *Hum Reprod Update*. 2007;**13**:27–36.

29. Zhou FJ, Cai YN, Dong YZ. Stress increases the risk of pregnancy failure in couples undergoing IVF. *Stress*. 2019;**22**:414–20.

30. Hart VA. Infertility and the role of psychotherapy. *Issues Ment Health Nurs*. 2002;**23**:31–41.

31. Purewal S, Chapman SCE, Van den Akker OBA. A systematic review and meta-analysis of psychological predictors of successful assisted reproductive technologies. *BMC Res Notes*. 2017;**10**:711.

32. Luk BH, Loke AY. The impact of infertility on the psychological well-being, marital relationships, sexual relationships, and quality of life of couples: A systematic review. *J Sex Marital Ther*. 2015;**41**:610–25.

33. Rooney KL, Domar AD. The relationship between stress and infertility. *Dialogues Clin Neurosci*. 2018;**20**:41–7.

34. Frederiksen Y, Farver-Vestergaard I, Skovgård NG, Ingerslev HJ, Zachariae R. Efficacy of psychosocial interventions for psychological and pregnancy outcomes in infertile women and men: A systematic review and meta-analysis. *BMJ Open*. 2015;**5**(1): e006592.

Hormones and Female Sexuality

Elisa Maseroli, Linda Vignozzi

Historical Overview

It has been known since the time of Aristotle that the ovaries are involved not only in reproduction but also in regulating female sexual behavior. In the late nineteenth century French physician Roberts reported that Indian women who suffered ovariectomy before puberty had no menstruation or sex drive. Subsequently Knauer restored estrous cyclicity and sexual behavior in ovariectomized dogs, rabbits, and guinea pigs by grafting ovaries into their abdominal cavity, and Brown-Séquard claimed multiple injections of rodent ovarian extracts could re-feminize ovariectomized women.

At the beginning of the twentieth century the vaginal epithelial cycle and its cytological changes were described and linked with different phases of sexual behavior, and, with the identification of estradiol and progesterone structure, steroid biochemistry was born. Since the 1930s oral estrogens were used to treat hot flashes in menopause and oral contraceptives were developed during the 1950s. Boling and Blandau pioneered research into hormone-driven sexual behavior demonstrating that injections of estradiol, followed by progesterone 48 hours later, could induce receptive behaviors in ovariectomized female rats. In the late 1960s estradiol receptors were found in the hypothalamus and limbic system by Pfaff, Sar, and Stumpf, while their molecular actions would be characterized 20 years later [1].

Meanwhile sexual medicine was taking its first steps with the publication of *Sexual Behavior in the Human Male* (1948) and *Sexual Behavior in the Human Female* (1953) by the American biologist Kinsey, followed by *Human Sexual Response* by Masters and Johnson (1966). These novel works raised controversial reactions and accompanied the sexual revolution of the 1960s and 1970s, when traditional sex roles were questioned, especially for women [1].

Since then, despite the technological progress that allowed us to examine brain activation following sexual or pharmacological stimuli in animal (i.e., microdialysis, cellular techniques) and human models (i.e., functional magnetic resonance imaging), our knowledge of the biological underpinnings of the sexual response has remained fairly superficial, especially in women. Women's sexuality is still considered a basically mental issue. Although many compounds have entered clinical trials in recent decades, hormonal options to treat female sexual dysfunction (FSD) are very limited. The neurobiology of female sexual behavior and its influence by sex hormones remains an underexplored field.

Physiology of Sex Steroids in Women

Biosynthesis and Regulation

Sex hormones are steroid compounds, which in women are synthesized from cholesterol mainly in the ovaries and in the *zona reticularis* of the adrenal cortex (Figure 42.1). In the mitochondria of steroidogenic cells, cholesterol is converted into pregnenolone by the P450 side-chain cleavage enzyme (P450scc). Soluble pregnenolone diffuses into the cytosol, where it is further metabolized into progesterone by the type II isozyme of 3β-hydroxysteroid dehydrogenase (3β-HSD). Progesterone is the principal secretory product of the corpus luteum in the luteal phase of the menstrual cycle and is required for implantation of the fertilized ovum and maintenance of pregnancy. Progesterone is hydroxylated through the activity of CYP 17β-hydroxylase to 17-OHP, which has little biologic activity. CYP17 also possesses 17,20-lyase activity, which results in the production of the C19 androgen precursors, dehydroepiandrosterone (DHEA) and androstenedione; DHEA is an important source of peripheral androgen production [2, 3].

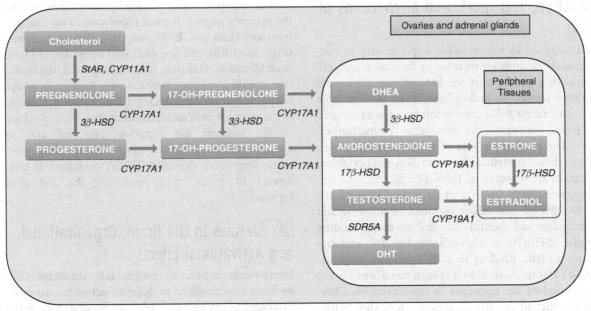

Figure 42.1 Synthesis of the main sex steroids in women. CYP = cytochrome P450; DHEA = dehydroepiandrosterone; DHT = dihydrotestosterone; HSD = hydroxysteroid dehydrogenase; SDR = short-chain dehydrogenase/reductase; StAR = steroidogenic acute regulatory protein. Reproduced with permission from [4]

In the ovary androgens are produced by the thecal cells and to a lesser degree by the stroma. Part of androstenedione is secreted directly into plasma, with the remainder converted to estrogen by granulosa cells. Androstenedione is a weak androgen and can also be converted to testosterone, the most potent secreted androgen, in the ovary and in extraglandular tissues by 17β-hydroxy steroid dehydrogenase (17β-HSD) [2].

Androgens are also the precursors of estrogens: estrone and 17β-estradiol are derived from Δ4-androstenedione and testosterone, respectively, through the action of aromatase. Aromatase production in the ovary is regulated primarily by FSH. 17β-estradiol is the principal and most potent estrogen secreted by the ovary; it regulates gonadotropin secretion controlling the menstrual cycle and fertility and promotes development and maintenance of female secondary sexual characteristics. During the menstrual cycle estrogens are produced by the granulosa cells of developing follicles, and dominate the follicular phase. Estrone is partly secreted by the ovary and partly derives from the extraglandular conversion of androstenedione. Estriol, the weakest natural estrogen, is mainly a metabolic product of estradiol and estrone [2].

Dihydrotestosterone (DHT) is the most potent androgen, derived from testosterone by the enzyme

5α-reductase (type 1 and type 2) in peripheral tissues (i.e., the pilosebaceous unit), and mediates some testosterone-induced effects. While androgen precursors and testosterone are aromatizable to estradiol, DHT is a non-aromatizable androgen.

Ovarian production of sex steroids is orchestrated in the follicle and corpus luteum in a cell-specific manner under the control of gonadotropins, luteinizing hormone (LH) and follicle-stimulating hormone (FSH), together with intraglandular paracrine and autocrine mechanisms. Luteinizing hormone and FSH are two polypeptide hormones produced by the gonadotropic cells of the anterior pituitary gland. Specifically, LH mediates androstenedione production in theca cells and FSH mediates estradiol production in granulosa cells.

During fetal life the gonadotropin-releasing hormone (GnRH) secretory system activates and has been described as playing a role in the masculinization of the brain and the development of sex behavior. After the first year of postnatal life, the hypothalamic-pituitary-gonadal axis remains quiescent until reactivation occurs to prompt pubertal onset following pulsatile GnRH secretion [2]. Adrenal androgen production, on the other hand, is stimulated by adrenocorticotropic hormone (ACTH).

Production, Transport, and Mechanisms of Action

When not used as substrate for a specific step in steroidogenesis, steroids are secreted by the synthetizing cell of endocrine glands into the bloodstream. In several peripheral tissues, including liver, brain, skin, adipose tissue, and target cells, conversion between androgens and from androgens to estrogens (aromatization) occurs. The production rate of sex steroids in women and the relative contribution of secretion and peripheral conversion are reported in Table 42.1 [5].

Approximately 40–65% of circulating testosterone and 20–40% of circulating estradiol circulate within the bloodstream bound to sex hormone-binding globulin (SHBG), a high-affinity but low-capacity binding protein. Binding to SHBG prevents hormone binding to its intracellular receptors; therefore only the free fraction of the hormone is considered bioactive. As a product of hepatic secretion, circulating SHBG levels are particularly influenced by first-pass effects of drugs: in fact, SHBG is increased by administration of estrogens (including those contained in combined hormonal contraceptives) and thyroxin, and decreased by androgens and glucocorticoids. Other modifiers of SHBG include upregulation by acute or chronic liver disease and downregulation by obesity. Because of the higher affinity of SHBG for DHT and testosterone compared to estradiol, its levels also affect the balance between bioavailable androgens and estrogens [2].

Sex steroids can act through two mechanisms: the classical genomic mechanism, mediated by specific nuclear receptors, and the non-genomic one, where the primary target is the cell membrane. Two estrogen receptors (ERα and ERβ), two progesterone receptors (PRA and PRB), and one androgen receptor (AR) have been identified. Diffusing into the target cell, the ligand (sex steroid hormone) interacts with its cognate receptor in the cytoplasm, inducing a conformational change of the receptor itself and its translocation to the nucleus. In the nucleus the ligand-receptor set acts as a transcriptional factor and can recognize specific hormone-responsive elements (HREs) contained in promoters of genes, thus modifying the cell gene expression [6].

Sex Steroids in the Brain: Organizational and Activational Effects

Interestingly, in neurons and glial cells, sex steroids can be further metabolized to different neurosteroids or be produced anew, and they play an essential role in the sexual differentiation of the central nervous system. During fetal life exposure to these hormones guides neuronal growth, synaptogenesis and cytoarchitecture, shaping sexually dimorphic neural structures and circuits related to cognitive, emotional, and sexual functions ("organizational effect"). In male rodents circulating testosterone is aromatized locally into estrogens and binds to ERs to masculinize the developing brain, whereas in females alpha-fetoprotein binds circulating estrogens, thus preventing them from crossing the blood-brain barrier. This mechanism protects the female brain from defeminization by estrogens. In

Table 42.1 Blood production rate and relative contribution (%) of glandular secretions and peripheral conversion to blood production of sex steroids in young adult women. Reproduced with permission from [5]. DHEA = dehydroepiandrosterone.

Hormone	Production rate (mg/24 h)	% from adrenals	% from ovary	% from conversion
Progesterone	0.8–2.5	50–70	10–25	20–55
(follicular)	15–50	5	90	1
(luteal)	230–310	mostly from placental origin	mostly from placental origin	mostly from placental origin
(pregnant)				
Testosterone	0.25–0.3	15–20	25–30	50–60
4Δ-androstenedione	2–5	30–45	45–60	10
DHEA	7–15	60–70	10–25	15
Estrone	0.6–0.8	1–2	60–70	30–40
17β-estradiol	0.01–0.1	0	85–90	10–15

primates and humans more complex processes occur, probably involving a direct action of testosterone upon ARs in the developing male brain [7].

In postnatal life, in particular during the pubertal transition, exposure to variations in gonadal hormones "activates" neural circuits in order to promote the expression of relevant gender-typical behaviors ("activational effect"). Functional neuroimaging studies reported an association between changes in sex steroids levels, activation of specific brain regions, and visual sexual stimulation in adult women. These data suggest the human brain shows a dramatic plasticity also during adulthood, maintaining the ability to respond to sex steroids [7].

Sex Steroids Levels across Women's Life Span

Females are exposed to dramatic fluctuations in sex steroids levels, both during the menstrual cycle and across the life span (Table 42.2). The female rodent is sexually receptive only near ovulation ("proestrus") since it conserves energetic resources by mating only when maximally fertile; in humans the influence of gonadal hormones on different behaviors is more subtle but still present. Emotional and cognitive cycle-dependent changes have been described in women, with improved verbal and impaired visuospatial tasks displayed during the luteal phase, when circulating estrogen and progesterone are elevated [8]. More importantly, the cyclic actions of estradiol and testosterone modulate the perception of male attractiveness and sexual responsiveness. In fact, a preference toward more masculine traits and odor cues of genetic dissimilarity and an increase in arousal have been reported around the time of ovulation, when testosterone peaks, whereas estradiol begins to rise a few days earlier [9]. It is believed that, during the fertile phase, such hormonal milieu contributes to alter the processing of sexual stimuli, leading to a shift toward an incentive value of sex.

Hormones, aging and sexual function are inextricably related in women. Estradiol levels range from 68 to 180 pg/ml through the menstrual cycle, decreasing to 12 pg/ml in menopause (Table 42.2). This fall has detrimental consequences on many systems, including not only the genitourinary tract, but also musculoskeletal tissue, bone mass, fat distribution, and energetic metabolism. On the other hand, the progressive decline of androgens is related to aging and starts earlier than menopause. During both pre- and postmenopausal years androgens circulate at higher concentrations than estradiol, despite being traditionally considered "male" hormones (Table 42.2) [10, 11].

In menopausal women about 80% of the serum DHEA is of adrenal origin and 20% of ovarian origin, while ovaries increase testosterone production. However, final testosterone decreases with age due to the inability of ovaries to compensate for the decrease of DHEA adrenal production. As expected, surgical menopause results in an abrupt decrease of all ovarian hormones. As well as estrogen deficiency, androgen insufficiency is associated with deleterious effects on overall quality of life and sexuality [10, 11].

The Physiologic Female Sexual Response

Historically the sexual response cycle was divided into four successive phases: desire (libido), arousal (excitement), orgasm, and resolution. This framework has

Table 42.2 Blood levels of the main sex steroids at different periods of reproductive life. 1 pg/ml = 0.1 ng/dl. Reproduced with permission from [5]. DHEA = dehydroepiandrosterone

Hormone	Early Follicular phase	Late follicular phase	Mid-luteal phase	Post-menopausal	Pregnancy third trimester
Progesterone (ng/dl)	56 ±10	56 ± 10	1350 ± 490	25 ± 8	12361 ± 3394
Testosterone (ng/dl)	22 ± 5	37 ± 9	35 ± 6	25 ± 12	67 ± 46
4Δ-androstenedione (ng/dl)	77 ± 28	220 ± 45	149 ± 43	75 ± 20	166 ± 111
DHEA (ng/dl)	515 ± 107	515 ± 107	515 ± 107	220 ± 80	363 ± 233
Estrone (pg/ml)	49 ± 8	75 ± 220	84 ± 8	29 ± 15	541 ± 278
17β-estradiol (pg/ml)	68 ± 14	180 ± 500	123 ± 11	12 ± 4	16640 ± 2375

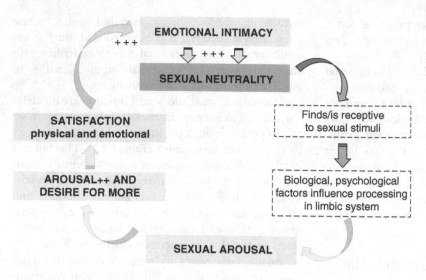

Figure 42.2 Alternative model of women's sexual response proposed by R. Basson. Adapted and reproduced with permission from [13]

represented the basis for the *Diagnostic and Statistical Manual* (DSM IV) definitions of FSD [12]. However, it has long been argued that this model cannot be applied consistently to women's sexual response. In more recent years it has been suggested that sexual function should be viewed as a circuit with each domain possibly overlapping and feeding back negatively or positively upon the others (Figure 42.2) [13].

For example, desire may not be present prior to sex ("spontaneous desire"), but may occur together with arousal in response to pleasurable activity ("responsive desire"). Initiating factors for sex other than desire are also common in women, often motivated by the wish for emotional closeness and the need for relational intimacy. Furthermore, the different sexual phases may vary in sequence, repeat or be absent during some or all sexual encounters, without these variations representing a disorder. In this regard, sexual satisfaction should be considered a subjective construct and, especially in women, it may not require achieving all phases, including orgasm. Finally, it is important to consider that sexual pain may negatively affect all aspects of the sexual response.

Sexual Desire

Where does sexual motivation stem from? According to the dual control model, in both genders, the initiation of sex behavior may be the consequence either of a direct excitation, or of a process of disinhibition [14]. From an evolutionary perspective the adaptive nature of excitation would drive individuals to seek out sex partners for reproductive purposes, whereas the adaptive nature of inhibition would guard against threatening situations. Moreover, in each individual, the propensity for excitation or inhibition has been reported to represent a personality trait based on genetics and subsequently modulated by the environment and experience. Noteworthy, the tendency toward excitation or inhibition may influence vulnerability to sexual dysfunction (i.e., in those too prone to inhibition) and hypersexual/high-risk sexual behavior (i.e., in those too prone to disinhibition). The hormonal milieu, together with sensory inputs and lessons from previous sexual encounters, can activate excitatory and inhibitory neurochemical mechanisms in the brain and in the genital tissues, shifting the balance around a "Sexual Tipping Point" in a dynamic process (Figure 42.3) [15].

Brain dopamine circuits form the core of the excitatory system, with the contribution of melanocortins, oxytocin, and norepinephrine transmission. Specifically, the activation of incertohypothalamic and mesolimbic dopamine transmission in the medial preoptic area (MPOA) and nucleus accumbens (NAcc) focuses attention on incentive sexual stimuli and engages motor patterns of sexual approach. The excitatory pathway is stimulated by sex hormones and by the expectancy of sexual rewards (orgasm or other kinds of gratification). Conversely, opioid, endocannabinoid, and serotonin systems are activated during sexual inhibition and blunt the ability of excitation circuits to be activated [1].

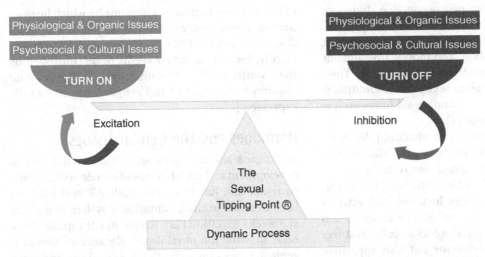

Figure 42.3 The Sexual Tipping Point® model. Adapted and reproduced with permission from the MAP Education & Research Foundation (mapedfund.org). The characteristic threshold for the expression of a sexual response for any person, that may vary within and between sexual experience. Adapted and reproduced with permission from [15].

Genital Arousal and Orgasm

As in men, the peripheral sexual response in women is a neurovascular event consisting in increased blood flow leading to swelling of genital tissues, clitoral engorgement and tumescence, and production of lubricating fluid transudate in the vagina. These hemodynamic mechanisms are regulated by the tone of the vascular and nonvascular smooth muscle [16].

The main arterial supply to the clitoris is via the iliohypogastric-pudendal arterial bed. The vagina is extensively irrorated throughout its length by an anastomotic network of blood vessels, with the main arterial supply arising from the vaginal branches of the uterine, pudendal, and ovarian arteries. Innervation to the corporal bodies of the clitoris and to the proximal two-thirds of the vagina is supplied by sympathetic and parasympathetic nerve fibers originating from the pelvic plexus, while somatic motor and sensory fibers travel within the pudendal nerve [17].

As in the penile corpora cavernosa, a high vasomotor tone of the arterial supply, through central sympathetic activation, keeps female genital blood flow at the minimal level in basal conditions. Following sexual stimulation, the decrease of central sympathetic tone and the release of vasodilator neurotransmitters such as nitric oxide (NO) rapidly increase blood flow to the genital tissues, which become fully vasocongested. Nitric oxide stimulates the formation of cyclic guanosine monophosphate (cGMP), which induces smooth muscle relaxation by multiple mechanisms, including stimulation of a cGMP-dependent protein kinase (protein kinase G). It has also been suggested that Ras homolog gene family member A (RhoA) and Rho-associated protein kinase (ROCK) signaling are involved in smooth muscle contraction/relaxant pathways in the clitoris [16].

The pelvic floor has also a critical role in these phases. Strong pelvic floor muscles, particularly the ischiocavernous muscle that attaches to the clitoral hood, and the *levator ani*, are crucial for adequate genital arousal and attainment of orgasm [17].

Hormones and Sexual Motivation

A great portion of knowledge concerning the regulation of sex behavior by gonadal steroids derives from laboratory animals, especially rats. Thanks to the easiness of its hormonal and pharmacological manipulation, the ovariectomized (OVX) female rat represents an excellent model of surgical menopause for the study of the female sexual response. Experiments in rodents conceptualized sex behaviors into two categories: appetitive and consummatory [1]. Consummatory behavior entails the act of mating itself and is highly sexually dimorphic; in female rodents it is expressed by the lordosis posture, a stationary flexion of the spine and deflection of the tail that allows penile intromission. Noteworthy, there is no human analog to the lordosis reflex since being "receptive" to vaginal penetration in women involves a conscious decision; this limits the clinical application of the neuroendocrine studies on lordosis in animals. On the other hand, appetitive behaviors aim at increasing the likelihood of mating, reflecting sexual motivation, and include investigation of a potential mate, approach, and solicitation. These behaviors are homologous to sexual interest/initiation in women and may be successfully used in research as surrogates of human desire [1].

Animal models have been shedding light on how fluctuations of steroids across the estrous cycle modulate female sexual motivation. In the absence of sex steroids administration, OVX animals do not display any sex behavior and actively reject mating attempts by males. The combination of estradiol and progesterone classically restores not only full lordosis behavior but also appetitive sexual behaviors [1]. Because either AR and ER are expressed abundantly in relevant brain regions, it is unclear whether testosterone positively modulates desire directly or through its conversion to estrogen [18].

Recently it has been reported that, in OVX rats primed with estradiol, the administration of the non-aromatizable androgen DHT enhanced sexual activity by significantly increasing both appetitive and receptive behaviors when compared to negative controls (oil vehicle only and oil + DHT), at comparable levels with the positive controls (treated with estradiol + progesterone). Furthermore, DHT enhanced appetitive behaviors when administered alone. These data support an independent role of androgens in the facilitation of female sexual desire [18].

The neurochemical mechanisms by which sex steroid stimulate engaging in sex have to be fully elucidated. Among hypothalamic centers, the MPOA and a recently identified ventral tegmental area (mPOA-VTA) circuit play a crucial role in sexual motivation in females and are regulated by ovarian hormones [19]. Estradiol augments the detection ability of male cues in the females' olfactory systems, modifying the vomeronasal sensory neuron (VSN) responses to pheromones, a process that involves kisspeptin/Kiss1 R signaling and triggers mate preference. In addition, estradiol facilitates the neuromodulatory control of information processing within the amygdala, a structure strongly implicated in the regulation of sex behavior [19].

Androgens seem to act as modulators of brain reward circuits, mediated by dopaminergic transmission [20]. Abnormal reward processing related to a blunted androgen signaling may constitute one of the neurobiological mechanisms by which hormonal fluctuations increase the risk of hypoactive sexual desire disorder (HSDD) in susceptible women. Finally, lordosis behavior seems to be controlled by the ventromedial hypothalamus (VMH), and requires both estradiol and progesterone to be fully expressed [1, 19].

Hormones and the Genital Tissues

Androgens and estrogens are critical modulators of development and maintenance of female genital tissue structure and function [21]. Both AR and ER have been detected in the genitourinary system as early as at 9 weeks' gestation [22]. Recent in vitro studies have been showing the physiologic relevance of steroidogenic enzymes, mainly those related to androgen rather than estrogen synthesis, in human vagina smooth muscle cells, thus indicating the vagina as an androgen synthesis organ [3].

Vaginal epithelium proliferation appears to be primarily under the control of estrogens. Indeed, menopause-associated estrogen deprivation results in vaginal atrophy, including thinning of the vaginal epithelium, decreased vaginal maturation index (VMI) and decreased smooth muscle, collagen, and elastin content. These structural changes undermine the functional properties of the epithelium, which appears friable, sensible, and less elastic, causing dryness and dyspareunia, and are restored by local estrogen administration [21].

Androgens also have a major role in regulating vaginal epithelial function, including mucin secretion from the vestibular glands and increased density of adrenergic nerves (Figure 42.4) [22]. Other mechanisms of positive regulation of vaginal function exerted by androgens include the maintenance of the integrity and thickness of the *muscularis* and the promotion of collagen fiber compactness in the *lamina propria* (Figure 42.4). In addition, in vagina smooth muscle cells, androgen signaling has been recently shown to activate a significant anti-inflammatory response, with a reduction of inflammatory mediators after stimulation with the cytokine interferon gamma [23]. Therefore, androgen deprivation could contribute to local chronic inflammation, a mechanism implicated in the genitourinary syndrome of menopause (GSM) and in particular in pain, discomfort, and recurrent urinary tract infections.

Genital perfusion is regulated by sex steroids in the context of baseline blood flow and during sexual

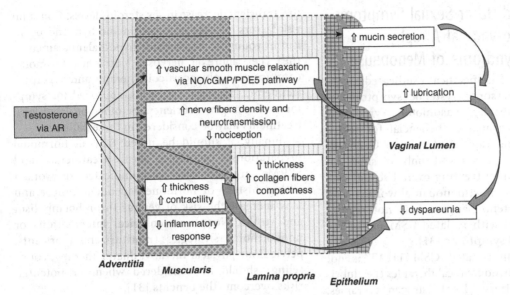

Figure 42.4 Potential mechanisms of regulation of vaginal function in the context of the female sexual response. Reproduced with permission from [22].
AR = androgen receptor. NO/cGMP/PDE5 = nitric oxide synthase/cyclic guanosine monophosphate/phosphodiesterase-5.

arousal. Specifically, testosterone and estradiol are both necessary to maintain a functional contractile and relaxant machinery in the clitoris and vagina [24, 25]. It has been observed that relaxation of vascular and nonvascular vaginal smooth muscle is facilitated by androgen priming and blunted by estrogens [25]. These observations are supported by increased synthesis and activity of nitric oxide synthase in the proximal vaginal tissues in response to androgens [25]. Accordingly, in the clitoris corpora cavernosa, testosterone improves the relaxation of vascular smooth muscle cells through the NO/cGMP pathway [24].

Hormonal Therapeutic Strategies for Female Sexual Disorders

Hypoactive Sexual Desire Disorder

Although low levels of androgens have been associated with low sexual desire [26], no cutoff level has been established to identify women with HSDD [5]. In contrast, compelling evidence consistently demonstrates that testosterone treatment improves the number of satisfactory sexual events, measures of sexual desire, pleasure, arousal, orgasm, responsiveness, and self-image, and reduces sexual concerns and distress in menopausal women [27]. Accordingly, a recent

global consensus position statement concluded that testosterone therapy, in doses that approximate premenopausal physiological concentrations, may be safely proposed for the treatment of HSDD in naturally or surgically postmenopausal women, with/or without concurrent hormonal replacement therapy (HRT) [28].

A 1% (10 mg/mL) testosterone cream is currently approved in Australia, whereas in other countries testosterone-based formulations (approved for hypogonadism in men or in galenic preparations) have to be used off-label. The transdermal route of administration is preferred because it has been associated with a neutral lipid profile. Serum testosterone levels should be measured at 3–6 months to prevent overdosing [29].

Although available data are promising, they are insufficient to make any recommendations regarding the use of testosterone in premenopausal women [28]. It should be noted that off-label testosterone treatment in women of reproductive age may be considered only in combination with safe contraception in order to prevent fetal virilization. In the United States central nervous system agents (flibanserin and bremelanotide) have been recently approved for the treatment of HSDD in premenopausal women only [5].

Dyspareunia and Other Sexual Symptoms Related to Vulvo-vaginal Atrophy/ Genitourinary Syndrome of Menopause

Estrogen-based HRT is specifically indicated for the treatment of bothersome systemic symptoms of menopause, specifically vasomotor symptoms. Although HRT may also be beneficial for sexual health by improving vaginal atrophy, a Cochrane review found that it showed only a small-to-moderate benefit when treating overall sexual dysfunction in peri- and postmenopausal women [30]. Accordingly, a systemic approach is not recommended in patients with isolated GSM or for the treatment of sexual symptoms [31].

For women with isolated GSM THAT is not responsive to nonhormonal local therapies (i.e., lubricants and moisturizers), local estrogen therapies, including tablets (natural estrogens), cream (estriol and promestriene), and ring (natural estrogens), are effective in restoring vaginal and urethral epithelium thickness and pH and microbiota composition, and improving genital arousal and orgasmic function [32]. Intravaginal DHEA (prasterone) has been also recently approved in Europe and in the United States, as a formulation of ovules to be inserted daily, for the management of moderate-to-severe menopausal dyspareunia. Recent studies have suggested that, within the vagina, DHEA is converted not only into estrogens, but also into androgens [3]. In placebo-controlled trials, prasterone improved dyspareunia and the other domains of sexual function [33].

Ospemifene is a selective estrogen receptor modulator (SERM) with an agonistic effect on vaginal epithelium. An FDA- and EMA-approved daily oral formulation is currently an option for postmenopausal women complaining of moderate-to-severe dyspareunia caused by GSM who are not eligible for local therapies. In phase III trials the improvement of GSM symptoms with ospemifene endured for up to 1 year. The most frequent adverse effect is increase in hot flashes; periodical ultrasound should also be performed to rule out endometrial hyperplasia. Finally, oral treatment with conjugated estrogen (CEE) combined with the SERM bazedoxifene (BZA) is approved for the treatment of VMS and vulvovaginal atrophy [29].

Women in reproductive age may also present vulvovaginal atrophy and other local symptoms related to a transient decrease in sex steroids levels. Common risk factors for hypoestrogenism and hypoandrogenism in young women include hypothalamic amenorrhea (i.e., anorexia nervosa), combined hormonal contraception, glucocorticoid therapy, and hyperprolactinemia [5]. Local estrogens, approved for symptoms of estrogen deficiency, or other off-label local treatments may be considered in these patients.

Finally, it should be noted that all hormonal preparations, including local treatments and SERMs, are generally contraindicated in women with a history of hormone-dependent cancer and may increase the risk of venous thromboembolism and stroke. Nonpharmacological interventions or nonhormonal strategies (moisturizers, lubricants, pelvic floor physical therapy, dilator therapy, counseling) should be considered whenever potential risks overcome the benefits [31].

References

1. Pfaus JG, Jones SL, Flanagan-Cato LM, Blaustein JD. Female sexual behavior. In Plant TM, Zeleznik AJ (eds.). *Knobil and Neill's physiology of reproduction*. 4th edition. Cambridge: Academic Press, 2015, pp. 2287–2370.

2. Bulun SE, Adashi E. The physiology and pathology of the female reproductive axis. In Kronenberg HM, Melmed S, Polonsky KS, Larsen PR (eds.). *Williams textbook of endocrinology*. Philadelphia, PA: Elsevier Health Sciences, 2007, pp. 587–663.

3. Cellai I, Di Stasi V, Comeglio P et al. Insight on the intracrinology of menopause: Androgen production within the human vagina. *Endocrinology*. 2020: bqaa219.

4. Maseroli E, Vignozzi L. Testosterone and vaginal function. *Sex Med Rev*. 2020;**8**(3):379–92.

5. Clayton AH, Vignozzi L. Pathophysiology and medical management of hypoactive sexual desire disorder. In Goldstein I, Clayton AH, Goldstein AT, Kim NN, Kingsberg SA (eds.). *Textbook of female sexual function and dysfunction*. Oxford: Wiley, 2018, pp. 59–100.

6. Wierman ME. Sex steroid effects at target tissues: Mechanisms of action. *Adv Physiol Educ*. 2007;**31** (1):26–33.

7. McEwen BS, Milner TA. Understanding the broad influence of sex hormones and sex differences in the brain. *J Neurosci Res*. 2017;**95**:24–39.

8. Pletzer B, Harris TA, Scheuringer A, Hidalgo-Lopez E. The cycling brain: Menstrual cycle related fluctuations in hippocampal and fronto-striatal activation and

connectivity during cognitive tasks. *Neuropsychopharmacology.* 2019;**44**(11):1867–75.

9. Slob AK, Ernste M, Van der Werff ten Bosch JJ. Menstrual cycle phase and sexual arousability in women. *Arch Sex Behav.* 1991;**20**(6):567–77.

10. Davison SL, Bell R, Donath S, Montalto JG, Davis SR. Androgen levels in adult females: Changes with age, menopause, and oophorectomy. *J Clin Endocrinol Metab.* 2005;**90**(7):3847–53.

11. Simon JA, Goldstein I, Kim NN et al. The role of androgens in the treatment of genitourinary syndrome of menopause (GSM): International Society for the Study of Women's Sexual Health (ISSWSH) expert consensus panel review. *Menopause.* 2018;**25**(7):837–47.

12. American Psychiatric Association. *Diagnostic and statistical manual of mental disorders.* 4th edition, text rev. Washington, DC: American Psychiatric Association, 2000.

13. Basson R. Rethinking low sexual desire in women. *BJOG.* 2002;**109**(4):357–63.

14. Carpenter D, Janssen E, Graham C, Vorst H, Wicherts J. Women's scores on the sexual inhibition/sexual excitation scales (SIS/SES): Gender similarities and differences. *J Sex Res.* 2008;**45**(1):36–48.

15. Perelman MA. Why the Sexual Tipping Point® Model? *Curr Sex Health Rep.* 2016;**8**:39–46.

16. Traish AM, Botchevar E, Kim NN. Biochemical factors modulating female genital sexual arousal physiology. *J Sex Med.* 2010;**7**(9):2925–46.

17. Salonia A, Giraldi A, Chivers ML et al. Physiology of women's sexual function: Basic knowledge and new findings. *J Sex Med.* 2010;**7**(8):2637–60.

18. Maseroli E, Santangelo A, Lara-Fontes B et al. The non-aromatizable androgen dihydrotestosterone (DHT) facilitates sexual behavior in ovariectomized female rats primed with estradiol. *Psychoneuroendocrinology.* 2020;**115**:104606.

19. Jennings KJ, de Lecea L. Neural and hormonal control of sexual behavior. *Endocrinology.* 2020;**161**(10): bqaa150.

20. Domínguez-Salazar E, Camacho FJ, Paredes RG. Prenatal blockade of androgen receptors reduces the number of intromissions needed to induce conditioned place preference after paced mating in female rats. *Pharmacol Biochem Behav.* 2005;**81** (4):871–8.

21. Traish AM, Vignozzi L, Simon JA, Goldstein I, Kim NN. Role of androgens in female genitourinary tissue structure and function: Implications in the genitourinary syndrome of menopause. *Sex Med Rev.* 2018;**6**(4):558–71.

22. Maseroli E, Vignozzi L. Testosterone and vaginal function. *Sex Med Rev.* 2020;**8**(3):379–92.

23. Maseroli E, Cellai I, Filippi S et al. Anti-inflammatory effects of androgens in the human vagina. *J Mol Endocrinol.* 2020;**65**(3):109–24.

24. Comeglio P, Cellai I, Filippi S et al. Differential effects of testosterone and estradiol on clitoral function: An experimental study in rats. *J Sex Med.* 2016;**13** (12):1858–71.

25. Traish AM, Kim N, Min K, Munarriz R, Goldstein I. Role of androgens in female genital sexual arousal: Receptor expression, structure, and function. *Fertil Steril.* 2002;**77**(Suppl 4): S11–S18.

26. Zheng J, Islam RM, Skiba MA, Bell RJ, Davis SR. Associations between androgens and sexual function in premenopausal women: A cross-sectional study. *Lancet Diabetes Endocrinol.* 2020;**8**(8):693–702.

27. Islam RM, Bell RJ, Green S, Page MJ, Davis SR. Safety and efficacy of testosterone for women: A systematic review and meta-analysis of randomised controlled trial data. *Lancet Diabetes Endocrinol.* 2019;**7** (10):754–66.

28. Davis SR, Baber R, Panay N et al. Global consensus position statement on the use of testosterone therapy for women. *J Clin Endocrinol Metab.* 2019;**104** (10):4660–6.

29. Scavello I, Maseroli E, Di Stasi V, Vignozzi L. Sexual health in menopause. *Medicina (Kaunas).* 2019;**55** (9):559.

30. Nastri CO, Lara LA, Ferriani RA et al. Hormone therapy for sexual function in perimenopausal and postmenopausal women. *Cochrane Database Syst Rev.* 2013;(6):CD009672.

31. The 2017 hormone therapy position statement of the North American Menopause Society. *Menopause.* 2018;**25**(11):1362–87.

32. Stuenkel CA, Davis SR, Gompel A et al. Treatment of symptoms of the menopause: An Endocrine Society clinical practice guideline. *J Clin Endocrinol Metab.* 2015;**100**(11):3975–4011.

33. Labrie F, Derogatis L, Archer DF et al. Effect of intravaginal prasterone on sexual dysfunction in postmenopausal women with vulvovaginal atrophy. *J Sex Med.* 2015;**12**(12):2401–12.

Chapter

43

Vulvovaginitis

Gilbert G. G. Donders, Werner Mendling, Francesco de Seta,
Henry J. C. de Vries

Physiological Changes of Vaginal Secretions

The thickness and health of the squamous epithelium of the vagina is strongly influenced by the presence of oestrogen during puberty, the reproductive period and particularly during pregnancy. At maturation the flaking off of dead cells at the surface and the subsequent release of glycogen from these cells is the power supply of Döderlein lactobacilli, which converts it into lactic acid and creates a low (acid) pH between 4 and 4.5. In children and after the menopause the pH is higher than 4.7, but during the fertile period it falls to less than 4.5 in healthy conditions.

This acid environment is important for the maintenance of the normal vaginal flora and to protect it against pathogenic germs. A change in the pH or the flora can lead to a disturbance of the balance. This can be due to the use of antibiotics, local antiseptics, application of vaginal rinses with hygienic products or foreign objects such as forgotten tampons, but also uterine bleeding, sexual contact, use of hormonal medications or after the transmission of sexually transmitted infections (STIs).

During the fertile period, in normal circumstances, a 1–4 ml secretion is produced by the vagina and the cervical glands in 24 hours. It is an odourless, translucent, white, but sometimes somewhat yellowish mucoid liquid which changes according to the phase of the menstrual cycle. Normally there is no itching, irritation or burning. In particular, during the pre-ovulatory phase, it may be very abundant and highly stretchy. During pregnancy the abundance of secretions is striking. The high content of glycogen is more likely to promote overgrowth of vaginal *Candida*. The use of combined oral contraceptives and progestins can change the cervical secretions into viscous mucus and in some women it can lead to vaginal dryness. Hypo-oestrogenaemia as in postmenopause phase or lactation leads to atrophy and a near absence of vaginal secretions. After the menopause vaginal secretions are usually minimal and can be brownish-yellow and sticky.

In order to discern such normal physiologic secretions from vaginal infections, it is of the utmost importance to establish an accurate and complete diagnosis prior to initiating therapy. Unfortunately, often a treatment (e.g. antifungals) is initiated solely on the basis of complaints without investigation (syndromic treatment). Also antibiotics are often prescribed solely based on an antibiogram of a vaginal culture. Irresponsible use of antibiotics can lead to the development of bacterial resistance to antibiotics and to the emergence of difficult-to-treat, chronic and recurrent *Candida* infections.

Besides being useless in treating *C.* non-*albicans* infections, frequent use of antifungal azole drugs can also lead to reduced susceptibility of *C. albicans*, and may give rise to allergies and unforeseen reactions like vulvar burning. In addition, the diagnosis of the vaginal microflora is made more difficult by prior use of intra-vaginal hygienic agents such as ovules, creams, tablets and rinses. Women referred for specialist advice should be warned to refrain from any vaginal products at least a week prior to the office visit.

Diagnosis of Vulvovaginitis

Clinical examination usually points in the right direction: itching must increase awareness of *Candida*, but also *Trichomonas* vulvovaginitis, pinworms and non-infectious causes like lichen sclerosus and eczema should always be considered. Also external interlabial or paraclitorial deep, purple-red fissures, as well as oedema and redness of the vulva and vagina are very suggestive of *Candida* infection. A malodorous superfluous discharge, on the other hand, makes the diagnosis of bacterial vaginosis (BV) or trichomoniasis more likely, but also a foreign object like a forgotten tampon and vaginal ulcerations, like in aerobic vaginitis or lichen planus may cause malodorous discharge.

A red vagina with a yellowish discharge and vaginal ulcers should suggest aerobic vaginitis (AV), but also *Trichomonas vaginalis* infection (TV), in the latter case especially when the secretion is abundant, yellowish green and frothy. A typical anaerobic odour, also described as a fishy smell, is suggestive of BV. In addition to these typical signs, we must, however, realize that a complete and correct diagnosis can rarely be settled solely on the basis of clinical findings. The typical textbook cases are more the exception than the rule, and most cases of vulvovaginitis require further investigation. Similarly, diagnoses made by patients themselves prove wrong in half of the cases, with the possible exception of patients with chronic recurrent infections, who can correctly identify their relapses after some time.

In the diagnosis of vaginitis the following tests can be used: pH measurement, potassium hydroxide test (odour test), wet mount microscopy, Gram stain, culture and enzymatic and molecular testing. Serology has no value for diagnosing vaginitis except when a sexually transmitted disease is suspected and co-infection has to be ruled out (detection of HIV, hepatitis B, or syphilis). PH measurements are suitable to detect an aberrant bacterial microflora such as BV, AV or TV (often with accompanying AV or BV, Figure 43.1). However, for the detection of *Candida*, pH measurement is not suitable: *Candida* has a slight preference for acidic pH, but can occur with all the possible types of microflora and pH values.

Cultivation of the vagina is rarely of value and should be used only to confirm a suspected diagnosis such as in suspected recurrent *Candida* vulvovaginitis. Except to detect group A or B streptococcus in pregnant or postpartum women, bacterial culture is seldom useful. Gram staining (known as the Nugent score) and wet mount examination of vaginal fluid are both adequate to detect BV and *Candida*, while the latter technique is superior for *Candida* and TV detection. If wet mount microscopy and specific culture media (e.g. Sulcovac) are not available, polymerase chain reaction (PCR) is advisable.

Candida Vulvovaginitis

Candida vaginitis or candidosis (American: candidiasis) is the most common type of vaginitis in Western Europe: about three out of four women will have to deal with it during their lifetime, and 5–8% of them will have recurrent relapses. Diabetes mellitus, pregnancy and the use of antibiotics are recognized factors contributing to the development of *Candida* vaginitis. The majority of cases are caused by *C. albicans*, although in the case of frequent relapses, and due to the abundant use of azole antifungals, there is a gradual upraise of non-albicans strains such as *C. glabrata*, *C. krusei* and *C. parapsilosis*.

The most common complaint is vulvar itching. Burning may occur but is atypical and should prompt further investigation for other diagnoses. Acute infection is characterized by redness and oedema of the

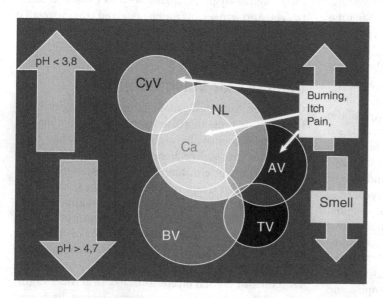

Figure 43.1 Relation of pH symptoms and preferential diagnosis of vulvovaginitis

vagina and vulva and by longitudinal inter-labial, clitoral, or para-perineal fissures. Sometimes you see scratch injuries that bleach and thicken the skin to make it look like lichen sclerosis (lichenification). The classically associated vaginal discharge (fluor vaginalis) is lumpy, white-yellow and adheres to the vaginal wall (like cottage cheese). Yet a watery discharge is also common and sometimes no discharge is seen. Typically the clinical findings are less pronounced in chronic relapsing patients.

The sexual partner may experience reactions such as redness and itching on the glans of the penis, typically a day after sexual contact. This usually heals quickly after application of azole and/or corticosteroid cream. Male partners should not be systematically treated with antifungal drugs because there is no evidence this decreases the recurrence rate in women. Although some recent studies seem to plead for caution in women with *Candida* vaginitis during pregnancy, there is no reason for general screening in pregnancy.

Diagnosis is clinical, confirmed by microscopy. Microscopy of a fresh specimen shows blastospores (ovoid structures), sometimes budding (snowman sign) and/or hyphae. The latter are typically absent in non-albicans infections. Also chronic, recurrent vulvovaginal infections more often present with numbers of difficult-to-discover blastospores. In case microscopy is unequivocal, a swab is taken from the upper third of the lateral vaginal wall and sent on an Amies/Stuart gel medium to the clinical lab for culture. Culture takes 24–48 hours and can be false negative, especially in women with chronic recurrent infections. To consolidate this diagnosis, self-testing at home with swabs that are sent in for cultures can substantially increase the sensitivity of the diagnosis.

Treatment

Primary treatment is a triazole, preferably applied vaginally or alternatively orally with identical results. For single, acute episodes, a one-dose treatment is sufficient, for example, locally in the form of vaginal ovules containing 200–1200 mg of miconazole, or orally 150–200 mg of fluconazole or 200 mg of itraconazole. In practice there is little difference in the operational efficacy of these various azoles, so it is rarely useful to switch from one product to another.

In women with suspected recurrent vaginal candidosis (four clinical exacerbations per year, of which at least one proven unambiguous microscopy or positive culture), other causes such as lichen sclerosus or eczema have to be considered and excluded. In case of recurrent vaginal candidosis, treatment can be commenced episodically when the symptoms appear, but most women nowadays prefer modern long-term treatments that prevent exacerbations. Many regimens such as taking oral fluconazole before and after menses, or once monthly before menses, can be tried, but are not validated.

Weekly treatment with 150 mg of fluconazole has been tried for 6 months, with fairly good results, but after stopping the prophylactic treatment recurrences were frequent. The most used and validated regimen in Europe to date prescribes 200 mg of fluconazole in a controlled, degressive manner (ReCiDiF regimen): first, weekly treatment for 2 months, followed by a pill every 2 weeks (for 4 months) and finally monthly (1 week prior to menses, for 6 months). Crucial and essential in this regimen is to conduct a full investigation at each therapy switch in which clinical examination, microscopy and culture have all three to be negative before proceeding to the next step. When clinical or microbial findings are still positive, continuation with the same regimen of treatment is recommended. In case of failure boric acid ovules and other non-triazole medications may then be applied (Figure 43.2). New potent azoles, adjunctive azole potentiators and probiotics are currently tested as treatment improvements. Finally, in case of recurrent vaginal candidosis, it is useful to exclude underlying triggers and risk factors such as diabetes mellitus, pregnancy and the use of oral contraceptives and antibiotics.

Bacterial Vaginosis

Bacterial vaginosis (BV) is a condition characterized by a decreasing lactobacillary microflora in favour of an overgrowth of numerous anaerobic bacteria. The terms 'Gardnerella vaginitis' and 'nonspecific vaginitis' are obsolete. Although BV is considered the most common form of vaginal infection, prevalence in Western Europe seems lower than the 15–35% sometimes reported in other countries. Women with frequent sexual contact, both with males and females, often suffer from BV. The disease recurs easily: 60% have at least one new recurrence within 1 year after successful treatment.

Bacterial vaginosis causes a malodorous vaginal discharge. Comparisons with the smell of rotting

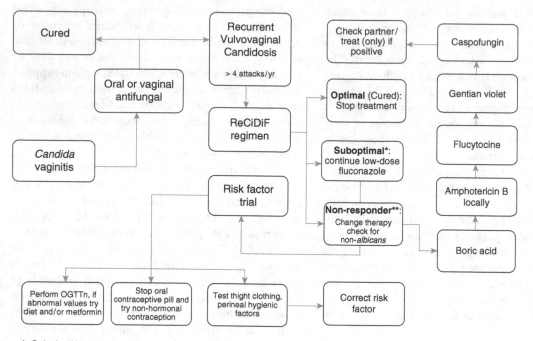

* Colonized but asymptomatic ** repetitive relapse despite maintenance therapy

Figure 43.2 Flow chart of treatment options of recurrent *Candida* vulvovaginitis [5].

fish are to be avoided since this is stigmatizing; rather let patients describe the smell. Frequent washing does not help, and even vaginal douching usually offers no more than momentary relief. Typically no inflammation is present, so redness, fissures, oedema and pain during sex are completely absent. The vaginal discharge is usually runny, watery and may be abundant. Despite these signs, the smell and discharge is normal in the view of many women. As a consequence, BV is thought to be asymptomatic in 50% of cases. The partner may temporarily take over the smell without other symptoms.

Although BV is restricted to the vagina, there is an association with an increased risk of infection with STIs such as HIV, *Trichomonas*, and herpes genitalis, and it is more often associated with ascending pelvic infection. There is also an increased risk of premature birth, although the mechanism is not yet fully unravelled. The increased production of enzymes that degrade fetal membranes like sialidase may play a crucial role. Furthermore, there are conflicting data about the reduction of the risk of preterm birth by its treatment with antibiotics.

A diagnosis of BV is confirmed by the presence of at least three of the following four Amsel's criteria: (1) homogeneous, whitish-grey discharge, (2) anaerobic

(fishy) smell, sometimes only after administration of potassium hydroxide solution, (3) increased vaginal pH above 4.5 and (4) typical 'clue cells' on fresh microscopy. In practice use of only the last-mentioned criterion is normally sufficient and very specific. The smell test is negative in 1 out of 10 women with BV and assessing the discharge is very subjective. Elevated pH points to impaired lactobacillary flora but is not specific for BV. Point-of-care tests based on pH (even if they have sialidase detection as an extra tool), are not very specific for BV as AV can also be sialidase and pH positive.

Nucleic acid amplification tests (NAATs) are being developed that detect a combination of BV-associated bacteria and are expected to be marketed soon as a point-of-care test. However, the speed and low cost of a microscopic examination by an experienced clinician is unbeatable. For those who have no wet mount preparation microscopy available, Nugent scoring on a Gram stain of a vaginal fluid smear can be an alternative, although in most practices this requires forwarding the sample to a microbiological laboratory with expertise, causing delay in diagnosis and treatment. Moreover, many laboratories do not apply the Nugent score system. Culture of vaginal fluid is not useful to detect BV, as harvesting *G. vaginalis* is insufficient prove of the presence of BV. Culture, however, can be helpful to detect an accompanying *Candida* co-infection, which occurs in up to 25% of BV cases.

Treatment

Bacterial vaginosis can be treated with: (1) metronidazole orally (1 g dd × 5 days) or vaginally (500 mg in the evening × 5 days), (2) clindamycin orally (300 mg 2d × 5 days) or vaginally (5 g clindamycin cream 2% × 5 days) or with 3) fluomyzin (100 mg vaginally in the evening × 6 days). In the United States a 0.75% metronidazole cream is approved for treatment while in Europe this low-dose treatment is not used or recommended. There is little difference in efficacy between all these forms of treatment, but it should be remembered that metronidazole can have side effects such as metallic taste, stomach upset and nausea. The alleged intolerance to alcohol ('antabuse effect') has not been confirmed in recent studies. Clindamycin has a higher risk to induce antibiotic resistance and can have dangerous side effects in association with QT interval-prolonging drugs such as fluconazole, heart medications and anticoagulants. A single dose of metronidazole 2 g orally is an appropriate therapy but leads to an increased risk of recurrence, so longer duration of treatment is advised. Since BV easily recurs, alternatives are being explored. Certain probiotics based on *L. acidophilus*, *L. rhamnosus* / *L. reuteri* and *L. plantarum* have proved useful in preventing relapses and as an adjuvant therapy to antibiotics, but are not effective enough to be used as treatment instead of antibiotics in acute cases. Products based on lactate or acidification (e.g. vitamin C) may be tried but the scientific evidence is scarce.

Aerobic Vaginitis and Desquamative Inflammatory Vaginitis

Aerobic vaginitis (AV) was described as a pathological condition in 2002. It was and is often confused with BV, but clearly has different characteristics and treatment needs and must therefore be distinguished from BV. The condition can vary greatly in severity and has since been detected worldwide in 7–12% of women, while during pregnancy it occurs in 3–5%.

Aerobic vaginitis may be asymptomatic in the majority of cases, but in moderate-to-severe AV a red, inflamed vagina with oedema (cobble stone vagina) and a mucoid, sticky yellow-brown discharge are often seen. There may be small ulcerations of the vaginal fornix, especially anteriorly. If these fuse together to form larger ulcers, a differential diagnosis with vaginal lichen planus should be considered. The introitus often looks blotchy with a tendency to be purplish red. Patients with AV have a painful, burning sensation and pain upon attempted coitus. Because AV, unlike BV, elicits a more or less pronounced inflammatory response, strongly increased pro-inflammatory cytokines and sialidases are present in the vagina. This explains why AV during pregnancy is associated with preterm birth, chorioamnionitis and fetal infection. Outside pregnancy AV is also associated with *Chlamydia*, *Trichomonas* and aggravation of HPV-induced cervical dysplasia.

To diagnose AV microscopic examination of wet mount vaginal fluid is required in symptomatic women (Figure 43.3). Scoring consists of five components, each given a score of 0, 1 or 2. The parameters to be evaluated are: (1) the number of lactobacilli, (2) the number of leukocytes per epithelial cell, (3) the proportion of leukocytes with an active, toxic view, (4) the presence of cocci or small bacilli and (5) the presence of parabasal epithelial cells. The sum of these scores provides an AV score ranging from 0 to 10. A score of 6 or more corresponds to moderate/severe AV. Severe AV has the most pronounced signs and is also known under the name of desquamative inflammatory vaginitis. As the name AV suggests, vaginal culture provides aerobic microorganisms, but vaginal cultures should in no way replace the microscopic diagnosis because the findings of aerobic microorganisms in the vagina can also be a part of a perfectly normal vaginal microflora. Recent research findings also raise hope for the future development of molecular tests to detect AV.

Treatment

Treatment of AV is ideally based on microscopy findings. Local antibiotics such as kanamycin were used in Italy with success, but are not available in most European countries. Oral moxifloxacin is effective but appears to be a radical treatment best reserved for severe and topical treatment-resistant infections. In general the use of antibiotics is not a good solution because of the short-lived effect. The use of probiotics can help to improve the microflora and prevent recurrences, but its direct action on moderate/severe AV has not yet been

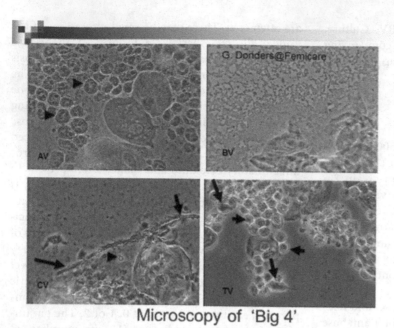

Microscopy of 'Big 4'

Figure 43.3 Typical images of aerobic vaginitis (AV), arrows pointing at toxic leukocytes, bacterial vaginosis (BV), *Candida* vaginitis (CV) with long arrows indicating hyphae and short arrow to blastospore, and *Trichomonas* vaginitis (TV), with long arrows showing the *Trichomonas* parasites and short arrows leukocytes

firmly proven. Local use of fluomyzin seems to have a beneficial effect. Topical formulations containing oestrogens, antibiotics and/or corticosteroids seem to have the most powerful effect.

Trichomonas vaginalis Vaginitis

T. vaginalis (TV) is an obligate parasite with four freely moving flagella and a fifth which is connected to the cell body and is perceived as an undulating membrane. The length of this movable parasite can vary from 7 to 23 microns, so it is twice as big as a leukocyte. The parasite usually resides across the squamous epithelium of especially the cervix, vulva and vagina. The urethra is less frequently infected. Other locations where the parasite can be isolated are the glands of Bartholin and Skene, and even the fallopian tubes. Invasion of the superficial epithelial cells takes place, but the deeper cell layer is not penetrated. Nonspecific inflammatory responses are seen with the increase in plasma cells in the subepithelial layer. There is an association between TV and the transmission of the HIV virus and it may harbour mycoplasma microorganisms.

Unlike candidiasis and BV, TV is conceived as an obligate STI and is often evident in the mostly asymptomatic sexual partner. With 250 million new infections each year, *Trichomonas* is the world's most frequently diagnosed treatable STI, although mainly in underdeveloped settings and much less frequently in Western settings. In European countries, despite the feeling it is less present, the prevalence is still estimated at 0.3–2%.

T. vaginalis is often asymptomatic. As a consequence, in Flanders, 0.4% of women express TV DNA in their cervical smears, mostly undiagnosed and untreated. Due to a lapse in attention, doctors have lost the expertise to properly detect and treat TV. Vaginal discharge is the main symptom of TV and is characterized by its yellow-green, foamy and smelly aspect. In severe infections the vaginal epithelium has a strawberry aspect caused by point-like haemorrhages and erosions. The cervix may show red lumps (strawberry cervix), but this symptom is often not present. Dysuria may also occur as a result of urethritis. Sexual contact is often painful or not possible. Pruritus is an less well known but often prominent symptom, which often gives rise to incorrect treatment with antifungal agents. Rarely TV can cause bartholinitis. Male partners of women with *Trichomonas* are mainly asymptomatic, yet urethritis or mucopurulent discharge can sometimes present in infected males.

Diagnosis is best done while the patient waits, using microscopic examination of a wet mount preparation of vaginal fluid. The causative *Trichomonas* parasites are easily detected by their typical shape and mobility. The parasites lose their mobility after 10–20 minutes, so care must be taken to carry out the investigation quickly after collection of the specimen and to use 0.9% NaCl for dilution, otherwise TV parasites die and become difficult to detect. With a trained eye and use of phase contrast at least 7 out of 10 cases of TV will be detected. Sometimes parasites are found in PAP smears, although this is not a reliable means of detection, especially at an older age when atrophy is also present. Typically, a higher pH of the discharge of more than 4.5 is found.

When a microscope is not available or examination remains negative despite suspicion, culture or PCR can be requested. Cultivation of *T. vaginalis* has a higher sensitivity (80–90%) than wet mount preparation (50–80%). However, it should be emphasized that a simple swab on Amies (or other) transport medium in general does not enable detection of TV! Only specific liquid media can be used in close contact with your microbiological laboratory. Increasingly, therefore, confirmation of TV is reverted to PCR techniques. Such specific NAAT tests on cervical smears or self-collected vaginal samples are expensive yet have an even higher sensitivity and allow simultaneous screening for *N. gonorrhoeae* and *Chlamydia*.

Treatment

T. vaginalis should always be treated, irrespective of the symptoms, especially since TV can harbour and spread other infections such as viruses and mycoplasmas. Metronidazole or tinidazole (500 mg 2 dd × 5 days) orally are the preferred regimens. Sexual partners should also be treated. Refractory TV is very rare, and requires higher dosages. In rare cases switching to other products such as paromomycin is required.

Cytolytic Vaginosis

Often women with vulvovaginal complaints are barely or not investigated and for convenience treated with antifungal drugs in the form of vaginal creams or pessaries. This does not only have the disadvantage that patients are not relieved of their symptoms, but also that further diagnostic workup becomes more difficult. One common finding in such women is cytolytic vaginosis, which often involves a burning sensation and sometimes increased watery secretion, which may form layers that can peel off. The low pH values (less than 3.8) and a typical finding of epitheliolysis on microscopic examination confirm the diagnosis. Usually a normal lactobacilli dominant flora is present, often with *L. crispatus*.

Treatment

In older publications the use of clindamycin was advocated, but this is no longer recommended. Treatment consists of the alkalization of the vagina, by local use of NaHCO$_3$ containing fluids. In some Scandinavian countries estriol has been used, allegedly with some success, although this treatment seems paradoxical and is not generally accepted.

Other and Differential Diagnosis

Sometimes an adequate explanation for the vulvovaginal symptoms cannot be found. In such cases it is always necessary to revise the diagnosis of 'infection' and to look for other reasons to explain the symptoms. For example, patients may suffer from vulvodynia (introital pain), or there is a skin disease such as lichen sclerosus, lichen planus, psoriasis or eczema. Also take into account the possibility of cervicitis and urethritis.

References

1. Donders GG. Definition and classification of abnormal vaginal flora. *Best Pract Res Clin Obstet Gynaecol.* 2007;**21**:355–73.

2. www.cdc.gov/mmwr/preview/mmwrhtml/rr6403a1.htm.

3. Donders GG, Bellen G, Byttebier G et al. Individualized maintenance regimen using individualised decreasing: Dose of fluconazole for recurrent vulvo-vaginal Candidiasis (ReCiDiF trial). *Am J Obstet Gynecol.* 2008;**199**:613–19.

4. Sherrard J, Wilson J, Donders G, Mendling W, Jensen JS. 2018 European (IUSTI/WHO) International Union against sexually transmitted infections (IUSTI) World Health Organisation (WHO) guideline on the management of vaginal discharge. *International Journal of STD & AIDS.* 2018:956462418785451.

5. Donders GG, Bellen G, Mendling W. Management of recurrent vulvovaginal candidosis as a chronic illness. *Gynecol Obstet Invest.* 2010;**70**(4):306–21.

Chapter 44

Sexually Transmitted Genital Infections
HPV, Tricho, Herpes, Chlamydia

Gilbert G. G. Donders, Henry J. C. de Vries

Summary

Sexually transmitted infections (STIs) impose a lifelong threat and a large burden for sexually active women. Chlamydia, gonorrhoea and trichomoniasis can lead to irreversible infertility, pelvic inflammatory disease (PID) and life-threatening conditions such as ectopic pregnancy. Current risk groups for STIs especially include adolescents and young adults who have recently become sexually active. In this phase of life sexual partner change occurs more frequently and these young people may be inexperienced regarding safer-sex techniques. Obstetrician-gynaecologists need to have special attention for this age group.

The asymptomatic nature of many STIs can delay diagnosis, increasing the risk of long-term sequelae. Selection of women at high risk of STIs, low threshold of screening and vast knowledge about the proper treatment of the index patient and her partner are crucial in the proper management of STIs. For PID or other infections where *C. trachomatis*, *N. gonorrhoea* or *M. genitalium* could be involved, empiric antibiotic treatment is advised in order to minimize long term sequelae such as infertility due to severe or recurrent ascending infections. Use of nucleic acid amplification tests (NAATs) for diagnosis offers a high sensitivity of detection for these organisms, allowing a switch to specific drugs once results are known. With NAATS self-sampling is optional, although for cervicitis/PID diagnosis proper endocervical swabs are preferable. Also for HPV self-sampling is getting a bigger role in STI management, increasing screening efficacy in hard-to-reach populations in remote and underserved settings. Current developments focus on point-of-care tests that can generate test results while the patient waits, further improving screening opportunities. The availability of HPV vaccination has a potential impact in the prevention of cervical and other HPV-induced cancers.

Introduction

Sexually transmitted infections are usually transmitted through contact between mucosal membranes but can also be transmitted via oral and anal sex, or even by mutual masturbation and sharing sex toys. For this reason condom use does not fully protect against all STIs. Even though many STIs are asymptomatic, severe disease consequences such as chronic pelvic pain, infertility, and pregnancy complications can occur, so screening for STIs in vulnerable people is a must.

Getting an STI depends largely on the individual's sexual behaviour. Sex with multiple partners is a known risk factor, especially when sexual relations overlap each other in time (concurrent partnerships) and when condoms are not used consistently. Sex for money or goods, recreational drug use and sex with partners met via dating sites and chat rooms are also associated with an increased risk for STIs. This requires an unbiased and open-minded history taking and low-threshold-testing attitude of the caregiver. Sexually transmitted infections occur more frequently among groups with a low socio-economic status (SES) and are more frequent in urbanized areas as opposed to rural regions.

Ulcerative STIs such as genital herpes, syphilis and lymphogranuloma venereum make individuals more susceptible to blood-borne viruses such as HIV, hepatitis B and hepatitis C. Also, in a quarter of the individuals diagnosed with gonorrhoea, a *Chlamydia trachomatis* co-infection is found. This is why it is recommended to routinely screen for a number of STIs in patients with STI-related symptoms or in case of risk behaviour and syndromic treatment to cover undetected but frequently encountered infections can be advisable.

Genital Herpes

Genital herpes is caused by double-stranded DNA herpes simplex virus (HSV) type 1 and type 2. The

HSV-1 infections manifest especially in and around the mouth, whereas both HSV-1 and HSV-2 infections are localized on and around the genitals. Both symptomatic and asymptomatic recurrences can occur from dorsal ganglia along the spinal cord, where the virus hides from humoral and cellular immunity. Mechanical stimuli, physical stimuli as ultraviolet light, fatigue and stress, the suppression of cellular immunity, fever or hormonal changes in the menstrual cycle can all trigger viral reactivation. Typical blisters and erosions might occur in the same region where the primary infection occurred.

Genital HSV-2 infections reactivate more often than genital HSV-1 infections. The average number of HSV-2 recurrences is four or five times in the first year. After this the frequency usually decreases. Primary HSV-1 infection usually occurs at a younger age, yet this gives no protection against HSV-2 infection. However, a primary HSV-2 infection is more often asymptomatic in previously HSV-1 seropositive patients.

The primary infection usually causes severe pain, vesicles, erosions and oedema, both in the internal and external ano-genital area. A primary episode is usually accompanied by loco-regional lymphadenopathy and sometimes by dysuria, fever and general malaise. Urinary micturition can become so painful that urinary retention occurs. In rare cases neurogenic involvement (e.g. neck stiffness, headache and photophobia) with aseptic meningitis) may occur. Complications such as meningitis, transverse myelitis or radiculitis may occur with primary genital herpes. Lesions usually heal without scar formation. The total duration can vary from 3 to 10 days. During a primary episode of genital herpes symptoms are usually more severe than during a recurrent infection, but even primary infections may be asymptomatic.

Patients with frequent recurrent herpes can experience prodromal symptoms such as tingling, stinging and discomfort in the affected skin area before the recurrence becomes manifest. The recurrence rate in an HSV-2 infected patient is 9 in 10 and in a HSV-1 patient 1 in 2.

Pregnant women who contract a primary herpes infection in the last 6 weeks before birth are at risk of infecting their newborn, causing herpes neonatorum, a serious, potentially life-threatening infection, and hence necessitate a C-section. Earlier in pregnancy women will develop a humoral inflammatory response and share their protective antibodies with their child via the placenta, preventing herpes neonatorum. Always the newborn requires strict follow-up and, if necessary, prophylactic treatment with acyclovir. Some experts advise prophylactic acyclovir during the last month of pregnancy in a mother with frequent recurrences.

Currently most NAATs can distinguish between HSV-1 and HSV-2 and are preferred above viral cultures. Susceptibility testing on a viral culture can be of use in patients with immune disorders or severe, drug-resistant recurrences. Determination of HSV type-specific antibodies has little use in daily practice and is not recommended.

Oral nucleoside analogues (acyclovir derivatives) suppress the replication of the virus, but have no effect on latent virus incorporated in the host genome. Therefore these therapies are not curative and after discontinuation of treatment HSV reactivation can occur. However, if started within 48 hours after onset of symptoms, or during the prodromic phase, the duration and severity of symptoms can be reduced. For primary infections therapy with acyclovir 3 times 400 mg or valacyclovir 2 times 500 mg is usually started irrespective of the duration of symptoms. Severe cases require admission to the hospital with intravenous acyclovir, urinary catheter and pain medication. In case of infections recurring 6 times per year or more, prophylactic therapy (2 times 400 mg acyclovir dd) can be considered. Local application of acyclovir crème is obsolete.

Genital herpes places a huge psychosocial burden on patients due to its lifelong persistence, tendency to cause frequent clinical recurrences and potential transmissibility towards partners as well as newborn babies during birth. A non-judgemental approach is essential.

Trichomonas vaginalis vaginitis

With 250 million new infections each year, *Trichomonas* is the world's most frequently diagnosed treatable STI, although mainly in underdeveloped settings and much less frequently in Western settings. *T. vaginalis* (TV) is a parasite that typically resides on the squamous epithelium of the cervix and vagina and less often infects the urethra, the glands of Bartholin and Skene and even the fallopian tubes. The length of this movable parasite can vary from 7 to 23 microns, double the size of a leukocyte. Superficial invasion of the epithelium causes an inflammatory response with the presence of plasma cells in the sub-epithelial layer. There is an association between TV and the transmission of the HIV virus and it may harbour mycoplasma microorganisms.

T. vaginalis is often asymptomatic. As a consequence, in Flanders, 0.4% of women express TV DNA in their cervical smears, mostly undiagnosed. Due to a lapse in attention doctors have lost the expertise to properly detect and treat TV. Vaginal discharge is the main symptom of TV and is characterized by its yellow-green, foamy and smelly aspect. In severe infections the vaginal epithelium has a strawberry aspect caused by point-like haemorrhages and erosions. The cervix may show red lumps (strawberry cervix) but this sign is often lacking. Dysuria may also occur as a result of urethritis. Sexual contact is often painful or not possible. Pruritus is often prominent, which frequently gives rise to incorrect treatment with antifungal agents. Rarely TV can cause bartholinitis. Male partners of women with *trichomonas* are mainly asymptomatic, yet urethritis or mucopurulent discharge can sometimes be found.

Diagnosis is best done by microscopic examination of a wet mount preparation of vaginal fluid. The causative *trichomonas* parasites are easily detected by their mobility and, if seen, the diagnosis is certain (high specificity). The parasites lose their mobility after 10–20 minutes, so care must be taken to carry out the investigation quickly after removal of the specimen and to use 0.9% NaCl for dilution, otherwise TV parasites die and become difficult to detect. With a trained eye and use of phase contrast at least 7 out of 10 cases of TV will be detected. Sometimes parasites are found in PAP smears, although this is not a proper means of detection, and diagnostic confirmation is needed before treatment is installed. Typically a higher pH of the discharge of more than 4.5 is found.

When a microscope is not available or examination remains negative despite suspicion, culture or PCR can be requested. Cultivation of *T. vaginalis* has a higher sensitivity (80–90%) than wet mount preparation (50–80%). However, it should be emphasized that a simple swab on Amies (or other) transport medium in general does not enable detection of TV! A specific liquid media should be used in close contact with your microbiological laboratory. Today confirmation of TV is increasingly reverted to polymerase chain reaction (PCR) techniques. Such specific NAAT tests on cervical smears or self-collected vaginal samples are expensive yet have an even higher sensitivity and allow simultaneous screening for *N. gonorrhoeae*, *M. genitralium* and *C. trachomatis*.

T. vaginalis should always be treated, irrespective of the symptoms, especially since TV can harbour and spread other infections such as viruses and mycoplasmas. Metronidazole or tinidazole (500 mg 2 dd × 5 days) orally are the preferred regimens. Sexual partners should also be treated. Refractory TV is rare and requires higher dosages or switching to other products such as paromomycin.

Gonorrhoea

The gonococcus is only pathogenic to humans and has a preference for the epithelium of the urethra cervical epithelium and the para-urethral glands. The glands of Bartholin, rectal mucosa, throat and conjunctiva are other preferred locations. By means of filamentous protein structures on the surface of the bacterium (pili) the gonococcus first attaches to and then enters the epithelial cell to multiply in a phagosome, causing cell death and spread of the disease. In severe cases sepsis can occur or release of bacterial lipo-oligosaccharides and peptidoglycan, causing cell damage of the fallopian tube, leading to occlusion and infertility. Although gonorrhoea infections induce both cellular and humoral immune responses, these offer no more than partial protection because of the production of extracellular IgA1-protease and the changing antigenic properties of the pili. As a result, immunity cannot be achieved against the infection, even not after vaccination.

Mutations in genes encoding for penicillin-binding proteins transferred to other microbes through plasmids have led since 1976 to more strains with resistance to penicillin. Soon after this tetracycline-resistant strains emerged in the 1980s, followed by fluoroquinolones in the 1990s. For this reason ceftriaxone is the last-resort evidence-based option for the blind treatment of gonorrhoea. Even though resistance to ceftriaxone has started to be reported sporadically, there is no effective alternative for it, leading to the fear that this 'superbug' may gain in importance in the future unless new and powerful alternatives are developed. Current populations at risk of infection are men who have sex with men and youngsters (age < 20 years). Gonorrhoea prevalence is rising in most European countries.

In 60% of women gonorrhoea is asymptomatic. Cervicitis can be recognized by thick yellow pus from the cervix which is red, swollen and painful to the touch (by sex or examination). In cases of PID women can become really sick with vaginal discharge, dysuria, somnolence, fever and abdominal pain. As rectal mucosa and oropharynx can be affected, these locations require attention too. Peri-hepatitis (Fitz-Hugh-Curtis syndrome), rash, pustules and arthritis can occur. In neonates gonorrhoeal conjunctivitis due to inoculation during vaginal birth can cause blindness if left untreated.

Nucleic acid amplification tests are the standard diagnostic today and very sensitive for the detection of gonococci. An advantage of NAATs is that they can be performed on samples collected by the caregiver or the patient such as urine samples and vaginal and anal smears. Culture and light microscopy are less sensitive than NAAT. Many NAAT platforms test for both gonorrhoea and chlamydia infection in the same sample, which is useful as both bacteria can give a similar presentation and symptoms frequently occur simultaneously in the same patient. In women cervical swabs are more sensitive than urine samples. A disadvantage of NAAT is that they do not provide antimicrobial susceptibility profiles (antibiograms). Therefore, after positive PCR, and before treatment, cultures are still advised for susceptibility testing, especially in patients with persistent symptoms after treatment, pregnant women and PID cases.

For empiric treatment (before results are known) 500 mg intramuscular ceftriaxone (an extended spectrum cephalosporin) is the first choice. Other extended spectrum cephalosporins are not recommended due to their less favourable pharmacokinetic properties. Ceftriaxone will be combined with 1 g azithromycin or 7 days doxycycline unless a PCR has excluded chlamydia.

Chlamydia Infection

C. trachomatis has a preference for columnar epithelium and the transformation zone of the cervix, urethra and anus. The chlamydia bacteria can only replicate in the phagosome within epithelial cells (obligatory intracellular). The symptoms of a C. trachomatis infection are caused by a combination of the effects of bacterial replication (and subsequent cell lysis) and the immunological response of the host. C. trachomatis can prevent cell apoptosis and cause persistent infections in which the infected cells are not lysed.

C. trachomatis biovars A to C are the causative agent for hyperendemic and non-venereal trachoma, a chronic, inflammation of the conjunctiva and eyelids eventually/sometimes resulting in blindness (low-resource countries). The biovars L1, L2 and L3 are responsible for the invasive disease called lymphogranuloma venereum, while the more common D to K biovars induce the often asymptomatic urogenital and anorectal infections. A final stage of such chlamydia infection is scarring of the fallopian tube, this can lead to infertility and ectopic pregnancy.

C. trachomatis infections are the most common bacterial STIs in Western countries, with a prevalence of 2–8% in 15–25-year-old women, and fivefold higher in cities than in rural areas. Among female visitors to STI clinics the prevalence is 15% or more. Urogenital chlamydial infections are associated with low levels of education, multiple prior sex partners, unsafe sex and young people under the age of 25. Lymphogranuloma venereum occurs mainly in the tropics and subtropics and in Western countries among men who have sex with men.

Three quarters of urogenital C. trachomatis infections are asymptomatic. If symptoms occur they are often non-specific with vague abdominal pain, contact bleeding and vaginal discharge. Ascending infections may result in PID with peritonitis symptoms, malaise and peri-hepatitis (Fitz-Hugh-Curtis syndrome).

Lymphogranuloma venereum (LGV) has two specific clinical presentations – the classic inguinal syndrome and the anorectal syndrome. Initially genital ulcers characterize the inguinal syndrome, but they can easily be missed when located internally. Subsequently inguinal lymphadenopathy arises and buboes form. If no treatment is given inguinal LGV can lead to a chronic genital inflammation with the formation of fistulas and local obstruction of lymphatic vessels, resulting in genital lymphedema (elephantiasis) or esthiomene if it involves the female genitalia. The anorectal syndrome is characterized by proctitis (with tenesmus ani, pain, bleeding, rectal discharge and constipation), often without detectable lymphadenopathy. Furthermore, LGV can cause systemic symptoms such as weight loss and fever and give rise to irreversible strictures and fistulas.

C. trachomatis can cause an autoimmune syndrome known under the acronym SARA (sexually acquired reactive arthritis), with arthritis, conjunctivitis and tenovitis, and a characteristic skin eruption called keratoderma blennorrhagica. Individuals with HLA-B27 haplotype are more susceptible to SARA.

Currently NAAT tests are used for diagnosis of *C. trachomatis*, offering the advantage of self-sampling by vaginal and anal smears by the patient herself. Urine samples are not recommended for the diagnosis of chlamydia in women because ascending infections can be missed. Diagnosis of LGV requires LGV-type-specific NAAT tests. Serological tests have no place in the diagnosis.

C. trachomatis urogenital infections are sensitive to tetracyclines, macrolides, sulphonamides and certain fluoroquinolones. Currently azithromycin in single 1 g dose is the treatment of choice for uncomplicated *C. trachomatis* infection, with 7 days 200 mg doxycycline daily as a good alternative. The first-choice treatment for LGV is doxycycline for 3 weeks. Erythromycin is also effective but gives more gastrointestinal side effects. In case of pregnancy erythromycin is the drug of choice, but azithromycin is also not contraindicated.

Pelvic Inflammatory Disease

Pelvic inflammatory disease is defined as the occurrence of infection with inflammation of the female sexual organs above the cervix. The origin of PID is basically via the ascending route, necessitating careful examination of the vagina and cervix. The prevalence of PID is not exactly known as it is dependent on the diagnostic methods used. Classically *Neisseria gonorrhoeae* and *Chlamydia trachomatis* are the most notorious microorganisms causing PID, but *Mycoplasma genitalium*, vaginal aerobic commensals (e.g. streptococci, enterococci, staphylococci, *E. coli* and *H. influenzae*) and anaerobic bacterial vaginosis-associated bacteria are also often involved. *M. hominis* is occasionally recovered from the pelvic organs in women with PID, but other mycoplasmata such as *Ureaplasma urealyticum* and *U. parvum* are generally not considered causative agents.

Often the complaints of bilateral lower abdominal pain start after a menstrual period. Also recent abdominal dyspareunia, fever, abnormal vaginal bleeding and increased yellowish or green vaginal discharge can be signs. Clinical examination reveals tenderness of the lower abdomen upon palpation, and when adnexae or cervix are digitally examined. Long-term complications are correlated to the severity of the symptoms. Timely treatment is vital to prevent irreversible sequelae. A major concern is decreased fertility, which is correlated with the number of recurrences of PID.

Subsequent to a PID attack, ectopic pregnancies occur in 1% and chronic pelvic pain in 30% of women.

Excluding *N. gonorrhoeae* and *C. trachomatis* (and if available also *M. genitalium*) on an cervical swab is obligatory. While positive test results confirm the diagnosis, neither negative endocervical findings nor the absence of signs of inflammation of the cervix can rule out PID. Microscopic examination of endocervical smears containing palisaded leucocytes in mucoid structures or > 30 leucocytes at 400x magnification, especially in the absence of lactobacilli, is supportive of a PID diagnosis but is in itself not very specific. However, normal microflora and complete absence of mucoid leucocytes make the diagnosis of PID very unlikely.

Blood tests may reveal an elevated erythrocyte sedimentation rate, elevated white blood cell count and increased C-reactive protein. In postpartum patients one has to be extremely careful as the blood leucocytes can be normal or low despite the presence of imminent sepsis, often caused by *Streptococcus viridans*. If in doubt, or if there is no optimal response to therapy, laparoscopy and/or endometrial biopsy is warranted.

Before NAAT tests results are known empiric broad antibiotic coverage of *N. gonorrhoeae*, *C. trachomatis* and anaerobes is the first-line therapy. Different combinations are optional and usually depend on local guidelines. When *M. genitalium* is considered a potential pathogen azithromycin or moxifloxacin should be used. In cases where *N. gonorrhoeae* or *C. trachomatis* are detected treatment should include specific drugs as discussed earlier in this chapter. Partners have to be investigated and/or treated in such cases. Except for seriously ill patients, oral therapy can be started first but, if recovery is not seen after 24–48 hours, hospital admission for further diagnostic workup and intravenous antibiotic therapy is indicated. Antibiotic coverage is continued for 14 days. Unprotected sex is contraindicated during the full course of treatment. In case of tubo-ovarian abscesses, drainage under echography or during laparoscopy may be indicated.

Human Papillomavirus Infections

The human papillomavirus (HPV) is very contagious and, as a consequence, an estimated 70% of sexually active women contract it at least once in their lifetime. It transmits via sexual contact, which can be penile-vaginal, penile-anal, vagina-vaginal, or via oral sex, fingers or sex toys. Sporadic transmission to the throat via lase smoke during interventions on the infected genital mucosae or use of instruments has been reported but is extremely rare, as is transmission through towels or toilet seats.

Most infections, including the oncogenic ones, disappear within 12 months. Human papillomavirus lasting for more than 12 months carries an increased risk of latency and oncogenic transformation in the cervix, anus, vulva and throat. Although older age and HIV are risk factors for disease progression, it is currently unclear which types will progress to disease in which women. Human papillomavirus 16 and 18 are currently still the most widespread and pathogenic viruses but, due to increasing coverage of vaccination against HPV viruses worldwide, the prevalence is now declining in many parts of the world. Human papillomavirus 16 and 18 cause 50% of cervix cancers, 90% of anal cancers and 25% of throat cancers.

Other viruses, like HPV types 31, 33, 35, 39, 45, 51, 52, 56, 58, 59, 68, 73 and 82 are considered intermediate risk as disease progression is slower and less frequent. Furthermore, application of the modern 9-valent vaccine before infection has taken place decreases not only the HPV types 16 and 18 but also oncogenic types 31, 33, 45, 52 and 58, as well as the genital warts inducing HPV types 6 and 11. Still the HPV types causing some 10% of cervix cancers will be uncovered by vaccinations and even become more prominent in the future, necessitating continued cervix screening, even in vaccinated women.

Frequent change of sex partners is the most obvious risk factor, especially at a young age. In several studies of women the presence of anti-HPV antibodies, indicative of prior infection, has also been associated with a decreased risk of subsequent infection with HPV of the same type, particularly type 16, suggesting the potential for protective immunity following natural infection. However, the extent and duration of such protection is unknown and many women do not develop antibodies following infection. Still this results in a lower infection risk in elderly people. Correct and consistent condom use partially reduces the risk of HPV infection, as skin-to-skin contact still enables transmission of the virus. Although use of an intrauterine device has been associated with a lower risk of cervical cancer, it does not appear to be associated with either the acquisition or clearance of genital HPV infection. Concomitant presence of vaginal dysbiosis by bacterial vaginosis or aerobic vaginitis has been demonstrated as an increased risk factor.

Genital warts are single or multiple benign HPV-induced epithelial tumours spread over a large area of vulva, vagina, cervix and perineal and perianal area. Disease eradication can be painstakingly difficult as, despite destruction of the lesions with electrocautery, cryotherapy or laser, lesions may recur frequently. Imiquimod cream may reduce these recurrences but needs to be applied three times a week for several weeks or months and can cause a very severe reaction.

References

1. Holmes KK, Sparling PF, Stamm WE et al. (eds.). *Sexually transmitted diseases*. 4th edition. New York: McGraw-Hill, 2008.

2. Unemo M, Bradshaw CS, Hocking JS et al. Sexually transmitted infections: Challenges ahead. *Lancet Infect Dis*. 2017;**17**(8):e235–e279.

3. Gupta S, Kumar B. *Sexually transmitted infections*. 2nd edition. New Delhi: Reed Elsevier, 2012.

4. www.cdc.gov/mmwr/preview/mmwrhtml/rr6403a1.htm.

5. www.iusti.org/regions/europe/euroguidelines.htm.

6. https://bit.ly/3XTrvgm.

Chapter 45

Sexually Transmitted Genital Infections
Syphilis, Gonorrhoea, Hepatitis, HIV

Brigitte Maria Frey Tirri

Human Immunodeficiency Virus

Human immunodeficiency virus/acquired immunodeficiency syndrome (HIV/AIDS) is an infectious disease affecting the immune system [3–5]. It was first described in 1981 and has become over the years one of the most devastating diseases in humankind. The human immunodeficiency virus (HIV) is the causative agent of acquired immune deficiency syndrome (AIDS). Around the world, 38 million people were living with HIV at the end of 2019 (World Health Organization (WHO) Statement). About 33 million people have died.

The human immunodeficiency virus is a retrovirus (RNA-virus) targeting the $CD4^+T$ helper cells. Its replication takes place in the lymphoid tissue in $CD4^+T$ cells and macrophages through complex processes that include inserting its genes into cellular DNA. During this integration step the activation of a cellular enzyme called DNA-dependent protein kinase (DNA-PK) occurs. This enzyme normally coordinates the repair of simultaneous breaks that comprise DNA. As HIV integrates its genes into human cellular DNA, single-stranded breaks occur where viral and cellular DNA meet. These breaks activate DNA-PK, which then elicits a signal that causes the CD4+-T cell to die. This leads to a loss of cells needed to fight a viral infection and thus a gradual impairment of the body's defences.

The transmission of HIV occurs during unprotected sexual intercourse as well as through shared syringes and needles for injecting drugs, and via needle-sticks in clinical settings. Transmission from an infected mother to her child during pregnancy, labour or postnatally while breastfeeding is also possible.

The clinical picture depends on the stage of the infection. Shortly after transmission a massive viremia follows and disseminates widely to lymphoid organs. During this stage mild flu-like symptoms are common. These symptoms disappear after a few weeks. As a defence reaction, the body produces antibodies that are detectable in the blood. This is followed by a symptom-free phase lasting for months or years. Undiscovered, the virus continues to proliferate and destroy the immune system. With further progression non-specific symptoms of disease emerge such as colds, fever, coughs and swelling of the lymph nodes. Finally characteristic severe infections and tumours appear, characterizing the last stage of HIV infection. This is diagnosed as AIDS if certain criteria are met. Diseases that define AIDS include cervical cancer and Kaposi's sarcoma.

Diagnostics of HIV are evolving. Fourth-generation tests detect not only antibodies against HIV-1 and HIV-2, but also HIV-1-p24 antigen in the blood. This enables quicker testing at 6 weeks after exposure and should thus be adopted as the first method of choice when diagnosing HIV. This reduction in the window between exposure to diagnosis identifies patients with the highest risk of transmission, therefore enabling behaviour modification and earlier commencement of therapy. These tests are commonly used in laboratories, HIV checkpoints and emergency departments. Third-generation tests detect only HIV-1 and HIV-2 antibodies and can be done only 12 weeks after exposure. These are used in self-administered tests sold in pharmacies or supermarkets or on the Internet. Nucleic acid amplification test (NAATs), typically plasma HIV-1 RNA testing, are not recommended for initial HIV screening as they offer only a marginal advantage over fourth-generation screening assays, are costlier and can be associated with false-positive results. They can be useful in confirming infection and in circumstances where antibody production may be impaired.

Who should be tested? According to the International Union against Sexually Transmitted Infections (IUSTI) guidelines, the following indications warrant HIV testing (see Table 46.1):

How to interpret a negative test? Individuals with a negative result after initial HIV screening should be

Table 46.1 Indications for HIV testing according to the grading of recommendations

Strong recommendation (Grade 1)	Weaker recommendation (Grade 2)
Individuals	Individuals
• Who seek care in STI/GU/DV clinics regardless of clinical signs or symptoms or risk factors	• Who voluntarily seek testing, especially if they have never been tested before
• With symptoms compatible with acute retroviral syndrome	• Who are sexually active transgender men with casual partners
• With AIDS-defining conditions or indicator conditions	• Individuals reporting chemsex
• With a past or current history of STI	• With a new sexual partner
• Who have been sexually assaulted	• Who are known sexual contacts of patients with an STI
• Who are known sexual contacts of people infected with HIV	• Who are sexual contacts of people at recognized risk of HIV infection
• Who are sexually active men having sex with men (MSM), heterosexual men and women and transgender women with casual partners	• Who exchange sex for money or goods
• Who inject drugs and share needles	• Who are children of mothers with HIV who have no documented evidence of a previous negative test
• Reporting sexual contact with a partner from a country with a high HIV prevalence regardless where contact occurred	
• Individuals who received blood or other blood products before introduction of routine HIV screening (in most European countries this is before 1985)	
• Any pregnant woman regardless of risk factors	
• Who are using pre-exposure prophylaxis (PrEP) or post-exposure prophylaxis for sexual exposure (PEPSE).	

considered uninfected unless the patient presents with symptoms of primary HIV infection or has a history of recent high-risk exposure (≤ 6 to 12 weeks depending on the test). Individuals who remain at risk should be offered repeated testing. Individuals taking pre-exposure prophylaxis (PrEP), where there is a risk of impaired antibody development and simultaneous, microbiogically proven infection with another virus should have a repeat test. Individuals presenting for PrEP should also have a second test after they have completed their course of treatment. A first positive test needs to be confirmed with the use of a sensitive and highly specific test different from the screening test done by a laboratory with experience in HIV confirmation.

Every HIV-positive individual needs to start anti-retroviral therapy (ART) regardless of CD4 cell count. Starting treatment early has clear benefit for the patient. It reduces morbidity and mortality, prevents their partners from being infected and, from a public health perspective, it reduces community viral load and HIV transmissions. Lifelong treatment is necessary to remain healthy as this suppresses replication of the virus; however, there is no effective cure for HIV. Viral suppression is defined as having fewer than 200 copies of HIV per millilitre of blood. Antiretroviral therapy can reduce the viral load to undetectable levels of < 50 copies/ml. The significance of this is that an HIV-positive person with an undetectable viral load is essentially non-infectious to others as they have no viral shedding in their bodily fluids.

There are different classes of anti-HIV drugs including non-nucleoside reverse transcriptase inhibitors (NNRTIs), nucleoside or nucleotide reverse transcriptase inhibitors (NRTIs), protease inhibitors (PIs) and integrase inhibitors and entry or fusion inhibitors. Each class of drugs blocks the virus in different ways. Therapy is usually a combination of three or more medications from several different drug classes. Two drugs from one class and a third drug from a second class are typically used. This approach has the best chance of lowering the HIV viral load in the blood.

Today different classes are combined in one pill, thus reducing individual drug resistance, the formation of new drug-resistant strains of HIV and subsequent maximization of viral suppression. Treatment side effects include gastrointestinal symptoms – for example, nausea, vomiting, diarrhoea, cardiac disease, renal and hepatic damage, osteoporosis, abnormal cholesterol levels, hyperglycaemia and central nervous system disturbances, as well as sleep problems. Drug interactions with other medications is also common.

Various methods with differing effectiveness are available to prevent HIV infection. Following safer-sex rules by checking one's own sexual behaviour and using barrier methods – for example, male and female condoms – have an 80–90% effectiveness of reducing HIV transmission. Research with topical microbicides is ongoing. For people using injectable drugs it is important to have access to clean syringes and needles.

An effective prevention is HIV pre-exposure prophylaxis (PrEP), a combination of two antiretroviral HIV medications taken orally daily or intermittently (during high-risk exposure phases for HIV). The efficacy is 90% if the medication is taken as prescribed. The other highly effective therapy is HIV post-exposure prophylaxis (PEP) if taken as soon as possible but no later than 48 hours after exposure. Three different HIV medications have to be taken for 30 days.

Pregnant women need special attention as untreated pregnant women can transmit the infection vertically during pregnancy, birth and breast-feeding. Therefore every pregnant woman should be offered relevant information and HIV screening. Women engaging in high-risk behaviour should also be tested in the third trimester. If infected, women should be seen by specialists for HIV and be commenced on ART. If viral load is measurable then a caesarean section should be performed and breastfeeding avoided. If a woman is HIV positive with an undetectable viral load she can spontaneously conceive without in vitro fertilization, give birth naturally and, after careful consideration, also breastfeed.

To end the AIDS epidemic by 2030, WHO set a treatment target of 90–90–90 by 2020. This meant by the year 2020 90% of all people living with HIV would know their HIV status, 90% of all people with diagnosed HIV infection would receive sustained ART and 90% of those treated people would have viral suppression.

Hepatitis B and C

Hepatitis B (HBV, a DNA virus) and Hepatitis C (HCV, an RNA virus) have much in common, so both infections will be discussed in this section [6, 7]. Hepatitis B and C are the most dangerous chronic infections with a mortality rate higher than malaria, tuberculosis or HIV. Forty per cent of individuals worldwide are serologically positive for HBV. Across the globe 3.5% of people suffer from chronic HBV and 1% from chronic HCV infection. They live mostly in Asia, the Middle East, Africa and part of America. Only 9% of all HBV-infected individuals and 20% of all HCV-infected individuals know their diagnosis. In contrast to HBV, HCV can be cured.

The transmission of HBV and HCV occurs during unprotected sexual intercourse (via blood, semen, vaginal secretions or saliva), through shared syringes and needles for injecting drugs, via needle-sticks in clinical settings and through breast milk. Transmission of HBV is more common in heterosexual intercourse then homosexual intercourse then intravenous drug use (IVDU). Conversely, the incidence of HCV transmission is more common in IVDU then homosexual intercourse (MSM), especially when an individual is also HIV-positive. The transmission of HCV through heterosexual and homosexual intercourse between women (WSW) is very rare and therefore no barrier prophylaxis is recommended in stable sexual relationships. In countries with a high prevalence of HBV transmission of HBV from mother to child is the most frequent.

Prevention is similar to prevention in HIV – following safer-sex rules by checking one's own sexual behaviour and using condoms. For people using injectable drugs it is important to have access to clean syringes and needles. Screening of persons at risk for HBV aor HCV infection is also an important step to reduce transmission. The HBV vaccine effectively prevents HBV infection. Neonates of affected mothers and non-immune individuals at risk (single unprotected high-risk sexual exposure or parenteral exposure/needle-stick from an infectious source) need a combination of specific hepatitis B immunoglobulin (HBIG) and active vaccine.

Clinical manifestation with classic signs and symptoms of acute hepatitis (e.g. fever, malaise, absence of appetite, icterus, acholic faeces, amber urine, elevated liver enzymes and signs of cholestasis) are found only in 35% of HBV cases and 15% of HCV cases around 45–180 days after transmission. The mainstay of treatment is symptomatic. Other extra-hepatic manifestations such as glomerulonephritis and vasculitis may occur. Mother-to-child transmission is usually asymptomatic. An acute liver failure is rare with HBV (0.5%) and very rare with HCV infection. Ninety-five per cent of HBV infections in adults will resolve spontaneously, unlike in infants, where the majority (90%) develop a chronic infection. The recovery rate from HCV is around 25%.

Chronic HBV/HCV sufferers have long-term but treatable complications such as cirrhosis and liver cancer. Chronic HCV infection only leads to a hepatocellular carcinoma if chronic hepatitis (80%) and cirrhosis (15–20% in 20 years) occur. Hepatocellular carcinoma can also occur in chronic HBV infection without chronic hepatitis (30%) or cirrhosis (20% in 20 years). The risk of progression to cirrhosis depends on the HBV prevalence of the country, being male, having a double viral hepatitis infection or a hepatitis infection and another disease affecting the liver (e.g. obesity or alcoholism). Chronic hepatitis can also cause extrahepatic manifestations such as vasculitis, glomerulonephritis, Sjögren's syndrome and polyarthritis.

Screening should be offered to individuals at risk for HBV and HCV. Screening for HBV is done by measuring anti-hepatitis B core antigen (AHBC) levels and, if positive, hepatitis B surface antigen (HBsAg) levels. In pregnancy screening should be done by measuring HBsAg levels, as in asymptomatic women only a possible chronic HBV infection is of interest. If the vaccination status of a person is unknown then anti-HBs levels should be measured. Screening for chronic HCV infection is carried out by measuring anti-HCV levels. If positive, then assessment of hepatitis C virus core antigen (HCcAg) or HCV RNA via polymerase chain reaction (PCR) is necessary. If the two tests are positive serological testing and liver function tests are included. All individuals diagnosed with a hepatitis B or C infection should be counselled about avoiding risky behaviour and screening tests for other sexually transmitted infections (STIs) (HIV, chlamydia, gonorrhoea, syphilis etc.). Partner notification is also recommended.

Treatment of HCV infection is now possible with specific antiviral medication. It avoids risk of progression to cirrhosis and hepatocellular carcinoma, extrahepatic manifestations, risk of infecting others and improves quality of life while reducing mortality. The treatment blocks the reproduction of the virus in three different ways. The newest generation of the medication is useful in all genotypes. Side effects are rare (headache and fatigue).

Treatment of HBV infection is indicated in all patients who meet one of the following criteria: (1) HBV-DNA positive with cirrhosis, (2) have existing liver fibrosis with elevated liver enzymes and HBV-DNA levels greater than 2,000 IU/ml, (3) have HBV while receiving concomitant HCV treatment, (4) are immunosuppressed – for example, receiving chemotherapy – or (5) have HBV with extrahepatic manifestations. Entecavir and Tenofovir are the mainstays of treatment. Treatment often needs to be taken for several years but is effective in reducing the risk of cirrhosis (< 10% over 20 years). Another option is interferon alpha.

Pregnant women infected with HBV should continue therapy during pregnancy. It is recommended that women with newly diagnosed HBV infection (routine screening in the first trimester measuring HBsAg) and an HBV DNA > 200,000 IU/ml should start with Tenofovir at 24–28 weeks of pregnancy to reduce vertical transmission to the newborn and continue treatment until directly after birth. The newborn should be vaccinated with HBIG and active vaccine within 12 hours after birth. With this protocol a caesarean section is not necessary and breastfeeding is possible. Mother-to-child transmission can be avoided in more than 98% of the cases.

Syphilis (Lues)

Syphilis is caused by infection with the spirochete bacterium *Treponema pallidum* [1, 2]. It is transmitted by direct contact with an infectious lesion primarily through sexual contact (acquired syphilis) or by vertical transmission (transplacentally) during any stage of pregnancy (congenital syphilis). Worldwide syphilis is a highly prevalent infection among MSM and sex workers. Since 2000 there has been an increase of syphilis in the European Union (EU)/European Economic Area (EEA), mainly due to an increase among MSM.

Acquired syphilis is classified into early (infectious) and late syphilis. Early syphilis is defined as an infection acquired less than 1 year previously (as defined by the European Centre for Disease Prevention and control (ECDC) or less than 2 years (WHO definition). Early syphilis is subdivided into primary, secondary and early latent syphilis subgroups and late syphilis is subdivided into late latent and tertiary syphilis. Congenital syphilis is divided into early (infection in the first 2 years of life) and late, including stigmata of congenital syphilis.

Routine tests for syphilis should be carried out in all pregnant women, blood donors, blood products or solid organs and groups at higher risk of syphilis such as individuals with newly diagnosed STIs, individuals with HIV, persons on PrEP, patients with hepatitis B and/or C, MSM, sex workers and attendees at sexual health clinics (dermato-venerology/genitourinary medicine, STI clinics).

The classification of the different stages is based on clinical signs and symptoms. After an incubation period of 10–90 days, the disease starts with a chancre (ulcer or erosion) and lymphadenopathy. The chancre is a superficial, single, painless and indurated lesion, most often in the anogenital region. Sometimes it can be atypical in size and number. This stage is called primary syphilis. Thirty per cent of untreated patients develop secondary syphilis within the first year due to bacteraemia. Secondary syphilis involves the skin (roseola and papular syphilis) and causes mucocutaneous lesions. Both signs are seen in 90% of individuals with secondary syphilis. Other signs include fever, generalized lymphadenopathy, hepatitis, splenomegaly, periostitis, arthritis, aortitis and glomerulonephritis. Neurological symptoms (meningitis, cranial nerve palsies) can also occur in secondary syphilis.

Latent syphilis is diagnosed by a combination of positive serological tests without clinical symptoms or a positive serological test and unequivocal evidence that the infection was acquired in the past year. The division in early and late latent is not always evident and misclassification is common between the two groups.

The other subdivision of late syphilis is tertiary syphilis and clinical features are seen as gummatous syphilis. These consist of nodules/plaques or ulcers on the skin, mucosae or viscera. In addition there are neurological signs (late neurosyphilis) – for example, meningitis, cranial nerve dysfunction and so forth – or cardiovascular signs (cardiovascular syphilis). The diagnosis of syphilis is complex. Today PCR testing is the preferred method to detect *Treponema pallidum* in suspicious lesions. The dark field examination, previously the gold standard method for detection, is no longer recommended for routine diagnosis.

Serological testing for syphilis is used for screening as mentioned earlier in this chapter. These consist of different groups of tests. There are non-treponemal tests (NTT) such as venereal disease research lab tests (VDRL) and treponemal tests (TT) such as the Treponema pallidum hemagglutination (TPHA) test. Other tests include IgM antibody tests and rapid point-of-care tests (POCTs) using treponemal

antigens. The last two are not commonly used. For primary screening tests from the first two groups are used. Generally screening is done with a TT and confirmation should be followed by a quantitative NTT; NTTs are used not only for screening and for confirming screening tests, but also to monitor serological activity and effect of treatment. To confirm or exclude neurosyphilis serologic tests (NTT or TT) in cerebrospinal fluid are used.

The therapy of syphilis is dependent on the stage of syphilis. In early syphilis injection of 2.4 million units or two separate injections of 1.2 million units of penicillin G benzathine (BPG) in each buttock intramuscularly (IM) on day one is the preferred treatment. As a second-line therapy procaine penicillin 600,000 units IM daily for 10–14 days may be administered if BPG is not available. Patients with bleeding disorders or penicillin allergy may be prescribed doxycycline 200 mg daily orally for 14 days. The latter regimen does not have the same efficacy as penicillin, however.

In late syphilis the same medications administered as a multiple dosing regimen are suitable. Treatment of syphilis can provoke a Jarisch-Herxheimer reaction – an acute febrile illness with headache, myalgia, chills and rigors resolving within 24 hours. The reaction is common in early syphilis (10–25%) and, in the absence of neurological or ophthalmic involvement, is not dangerous. Prevention of a Jarisch-Herxheimer reaction can be effectively achieved with commencing a 3-day course of oral prednisolone 20–60 mg daily, 24 hours prior to starting syphilis treatment. A rare reaction known as procaine psychosis, procaine mania or Hoigné syndrome is associated with the use of procaine. Management of the reaction by providing the patient calm and verbal reassurance is the mainstay of treatment; however, diazepam 5–10 mg may be used if convulsions occur.

Special situations exist in pregnancy. Women with untreated early syphilis have a 70–100% chance of transmitting the infection to their unborn infant, leading to stillbirths in up to one third of cases. If TT is positive and NTT is negative the tests should be repeated 1 month later. Most transmissions to the fetus occur in late pregnancy (after 28 weeks) and treatment before this period will usually prevent congenital features. In women at increased risk and in settings with a high prevalence of syphilis, serology should be repeated ideally during third trimester at 28–32 weeks' gestation and at delivery. Treatment is the same as that in non-pregnant individuals. Follow-up and test of cure are important. Serological testing with an NTT (VDRL/rapid plasma reagin) at regular intervals are required to detect persistent infection or reinfection. A TT test may remain positive for life.

Congenital syphilis is confirmed by identifying *T. pallidum* in the placenta or autopsy material using PCR. Children with late congenital syphilis are diagnosed based on specific clinical features – interstitial keratitis, Clutton's joints, Hutchinson's incisors, high palatal arch, saddle nose deformity and other typical signs. Serological tests can initially be negative in infants infected in late pregnancy. When the mother is treated during the last trimester of pregnancy, the treatment can be inadequate for the child and the child may still develop congenital syphilis.

Pre-exposure prophylaxis (PrEP) for HIV results in an increase of frequency of condom-less sex and studies have shown an increase of STIs in general. Regular testing for syphilis (every 3 months) is advised in this population. Patients with syphilis as well as with other STIs should be seen for sexual contact notification. Depending on the stage of syphilis, partners in the last 3–24 months should be notified by the patient or the health department. Forty to sixty per cent of traced sexual contacts, including pregnant women, of patients with early syphilis are likely to be infected. Notification of syphilis (and most of the other STIs) to the relevant national authority is mandatory in most European countries.

References

1. Janier M, Unjemo M, Dupin N et al. 2020 European guideline on the management of syphilis. *JEADV*. 2021.**35**(3):574–88.

2. Kingston M, French P, Higgins S et al. UK national guidelines on the management of syphilis 2015. *Int J STD AIDS*. 2016;**27**(6):421–46.

3. Gökengin D, Wilson-Davies E, NAzli Zeka A et al. 2021 European guideline on HIV testing in genito-urinary medicine settings. *JEADV* 2021;**35**(5):1043–57.

4. Hampel B, Böni J, Vernazza P et al. Neues aus der HIV: Diagnostik. *Swiss Medical Forum*. 2021;**21**(3–4):52–4.

5. Tarr P, Boffi el-Amari E, Haerry D et al. HIV-Prä-Expositionsprophylaxe (PrEP). *Swiss Medical Forum*. 2017;**17**(26–7):579–82.

6. Brook G, Brockmeyer N, Van de Laar T. et al. 2017 European guideline for the screening, prevention and initial management of hepatitis B and C infections in sexual health settings. *Int J STD AIDS*. 2018;**29**(10):949–67.

7. www.bashh.org/guidelines: 2017 interim update of the 2015 BASHH National Guidelines for the Management of the Viral Hepatitides.

8. www.cdc.gov/hpeatitis/hbv/index.htm.

Chapter

46

Sexual Counselling
General Principles

Johannes Bitzer

Prevalence of Sexual Problems

The US National Health and Social Life survey, which was undertaken in people aged 18–59 years, reported that sexual dysfunction is more prevalent for women (43%) than men (31%) [1]. Another US study of 1,550 women and 1,455 men aged 57–85 years found that the prevalence of sexual activity declined with age (73% among respondents 57–64 years of age, 53% among respondents 65–74 years of age and 26% among respondents 75–85 years of age); women were significantly less likely than men at all ages to report sexual activity [2].

The most prevalent sexual problems among women were low desire (43%), difficulty with vaginal lubrication (39%) and inability to climax (34%). A very large US study of 31,581 women with a mean age of 49 years (range 18–102) also found that the most common sexual problem was low desire (38.7%), followed by low arousal (26.1%) and orgasm difficulties (20.5%), and their prevalence changed with age [3]).

The prevalence of any sexual problem was 44.2%. Age stratification revealed a sharp increase in the prevalence of all three sexual problems by age group. Only 27.2% of women aged 18–44 years reported any of the three problems, compared with 44.6% of middle-aged women and 80.1% of elderly women. Low desire was the most common of the three problems among all age groups. However sexual problems associated with personal distress were much less common, although reported by approximately 12% of women and peaking in women aged 50–59. Sexually related personal distress was lowest in elderly women (12.6%), and present in 25.5% and 24.4% of middle-aged and younger women, respectively.

What Is Sexuality? What Are the Challenges for Healthcare Professionals?

Sexuality is an internal experience. Each person has her or his individually grown concept or script of sexuality. Sexuality is closely linked to intensive emotions and self-image. Suffering from sexuality is subjective and is the result of a mismatch between the sexual life desired and the sexual life lived at present. This means for the healthcare professional that she/he should listen carefully and actively, be open to and interested in the patient's concept of love and sexuality, respond to complex emotions like shame and respect and handle the limitations of the patient in an empathic way, avoiding intrusion and even trauma.

Sexuality is a biopsychosocial phenomenon. Human sexuality is the result of a complex interaction between the body and the mind of the individual and the relationship and social context in which the individual lives. The 'sexual body' perspective includes the physiology and endocrinology of the human sexual response during the different phases of desire, arousal, orgasm and resolution. The brain, the endocrine and autonomous nervous system and the peripheral neurovascular and neuromotor response are interlinked with positive and negative feedback mechanisms

The 'sexual mind' perspective comprises the subjective experience during a sexual activity and encounter, from feelings of desire, feeling excited and the experience of the body to perception of the self and identity. The 'sexual relationship' and social perspective is about the interaction with the partner, the differences in needs, the possible conflicts and dynamics of the relationship. It includes the impact of the environment (personal and public) on an individual's sexual life (norms, ideals, media etc.).

It is important to realize that disturbances on one level will frequently also affect the other levels. This means for the healthcare professional that she/he has to assess at the same time the biological, psychological and social characteristics of the patient, learn how to communicate with a couple and integrate these findings into a comprehensive model of understanding the problem by developing a systemic perspective.

Sexuality is not static but part of the individual's biographical changes. Sexuality is subject to constant modifications due to biopsychosocial changes in life. The dynamics of change can be very different individually and between partners. This means for the healthcare provider that she/he has to adapt the communication to the life phase of the patient and get some insight into the sexual biography of the patient. Talking to adolescents about sex is different and needs a different language compared to addressing sexual health around menopause or in the elderly patient.

The transition from sexual health to sexual ill health is a continuum. There is no dichotomous difference between the two. Most men and women have sexual problems at least once in their life. Sexual health is not the absence of sexual problems but is related to the capacity to respond to problems and changes. Men and women experience threats to sexual health but they have also resources to address them. This means for the healthcare provider that she/he should know her or his own sexual problems, sexual needs and sexual fears, she/he should be open to the solutions found by the patients and she/he should be patient and not try to find a quick solution. Therapeutic modesty helps to avoid overreacting (like prescribing the immediate use of drugs and operations).

Difficulties Encountered by Patients and Physicians

Patients may have different barriers when it comes to talking about sexual issues [2]. Disclosing sexual difficulties may be embarrassing to patients because they may feel inferior and insecure about how the physician is viewing them. Shame arises when a person is exposing a usually hidden weakness. This feeling is especially strong when the patient is afraid of negative judgement by the physician.

Patients may feel that sexuality is not an issue for a medical consultation. Medicine is about diseases and sexuality may seem to them a luxury with which

they do not want to bother the physician. Some patients have the impression their physician will not have the time to talk about sexual issues and/or they may feel the physician is not interested or competent in this part of human life. Finally patients may be completely unaware of the specific treatments available for sexual dysfunction and they may believe nothing can be done for sexual problems.

Physicians also have barriers. Some feel addressing sexual issues creates too much closeness to the patient and they are afraid that they would hurt or embarrass the patient if they actively raise this issue. Some physicians report they do not feel adequately trained in sexual medicine. Finally, a reason which is not frequently mentioned but which may be quite important is the fact that talking about the patient's sexual problems touches on the physician's own sexual life and may remind him/her of difficulties and unresolved problems.

How to Overcome the Barriers and Have a Professional Talk about Sex in a Medical Consultation

The medical consultation in which sexual issues are discussed has to fulfil certain criteria [4].

- The consultation should be patient centred and at the same time well structured to collect biomedical and psychosocial data.
- The healthcare provider should proactively address intimate issues and at the same time not too invasively explore without permission of the patient.
- The counselling should give enough space and time and at the same time respect the time limits of a medical consultation.
- The consultation should combine biomedical, diagnostic and therapeutic procedures with verbal interventions that follow the principles of counselling.

Sexual Counselling As a Dialogue between the Healthcare Provider and the Patient (Couple)

The integration of these different elements can best be described as a stepwise dialogue between the healthcare provider and the patient or couple with questions and answers leading from clarifying and defining the problem to a diagnosis. From there the contributing factors can be explored, which then allows the healthcare provider to research and offer therapeutic options [4–6]. It is up to the patient or couple to decide which way to go. The following case illustrates this interaction.

A 52-year-old Gravida II, para II comes for a yearly check-up. She has no major complaints except for some vaginal dryness which is under treatment with local oestrogen. The healthcare provider has known her for many years and the woman has never mentioned any sexual problem. The healthcare provider wonders if she/he should address sexuality in the context of the local treatment of the vaginal dryness.

Step 1 Address sexuality

The physician can employ helpful communication techniques in order to give the patient an opportunity to talk about her sexuality if she wants.

'Are you sexually active?' If yes: 'Are you satisfied with your sexual life? Are there any problems?' If no: 'Is this because you want it so, or are there difficulties?'

Another invitation would be: 'Many women with vaginal dryness report pain during intercourse.'

Another more general invitation would be: 'I wanted to mention that, if you find yourself having any sexual problems at any point, don't be afraid to tell me.'

Step 2 Listen and encourage the patient to tell her story

The patient takes up the invitation.

Patient: 'The local treatment is fine. But is this normal? I have completely lost interest in sex. If it were not for my husband I could live without it.'

Healthcare provider: 'You said you have no more interest in sex. Tell me more about it. How does this lack manifest itself in your life?'

The healthcare provider should listen and encourage the patient to tell her story. She/he should not go directly into taking a history or asking direct questions but should invite the patient to tell more. The patient has thus the possibility to choose her own words and rhythm. This will give important indirect information to the physician about the patient's inner map of her sexuality. How does she feel? Is she anxious about losing the partner? Is this the main problem?

Patient answers: 'From time to time we have still intercourse. My husband is nice and tries his best. I do not feel much. It is a problem for him but I do not think he will look for another woman.'

Step 3 Ask direct questions

In the next step the healthcare provider asks direct questions.

- 'When did the problem start?'
- 'Has this lack of interest in sex always been there? Was it different before? When did you consider your desire for sex good for you?'
- 'Did the loss of desire develop gradually or occur abruptly?'
- According to your experience, is this lack of desire related to specific situations?'
- 'Is this lack related to your partner? For example, does your partner have sexual difficulties or specific behaviours (like lack of stimulation) that are unattractive to you? Is the issue related to your partner's appearance?'
- 'Have you experienced other sexual problems before like pain during intercourse or arousal difficulty?'

The patient answers: 'In the beginning of our relationship sex was quite okay, although sex was not the most important thing in our marriage. There was a decline of desire and interest after our first child was born. It has nothing to do with my husband. He is still attractive to me.'

Step 4 Discuss a typical episode

In the next step of the interview the patient is invited to talk about her last sexual experience (alone or with the partner).

Healthcare provider: 'Please remember the last time you were sexually active (masturbation, intercourse). What happened? Who started the activity? How did you react? What thoughts did you have? What were your feelings?'

The patient answers: 'It is usually at the weekend. My husband starts touching me. Being touched feels sometimes uncomfortable, sometimes not. It is not a problem of foreplay. It is just that my body does not respond.'

Step 5 Offer a descriptive diagnosis

With the information obtained the physician can establish what can be called a descriptive diagnosis in which she/he tries to summarize the answers to the following questions:

- Is it a problem of desire, arousal, orgasm or pain?
- Is there a combination of problems?
- Is this problem long-standing since the beginning of being sexually active?
- Is it secondary after a time when the problem did not exist (primary versus secondary)?
- Is the problem related to specific situations and/or the partner and are there situations when the problem disappears like on weekends or holiday (situational versus global)?
- Did the problem develop gradually or is it related to a specific event like menopause or drug treatment (abrupt versus gradually developing)?

In this case the descriptive diagnosis would be secondary desire and arousal disorder with personal distress and negative impact on the relationship leading to avoiding intimacy.

Step 6 Explore the contributing factors and ask for the patient's perspective

In the following part of the interview the physician wants to explore with the patient the factors contributing to the sexual dysfunctions and the belief of the patient. This follows the biopsychosocial concept of sexuality described earlier in this chapter.

The healthcare provider asks: 'Now I would like to look into possible factors that may contribute to the problem. It is important to acknowledge that there is usually not a single factor but a combination. What are your thoughts about the problem? Do you see any causes?'

The patient answers: 'I do not know. I love my husband. We could have a good life. Many think it is the menopause. I am not sure. Maybe it is also related to stress with my elder son.'

The healthcare provider then goes further in the exploration and at the same time informs and educates the patient about possible factors. 'Many diseases can have a negative influence on a woman's sexuality like dysfunctions of the thyroid, diabetes and operations, but also mental health problems and drugs like antidepressants and some antihypertensives.'

The patient answers: 'I am basically healthy. Sometimes I feel a bit depressed and then there is my continuous fight with my weight. I do not like my body as it is now.'

The healthcare provider answers: 'Another important cause is hormonal changes. Did you notice any changes in your sexual desire in relation to the menstrual cycle or under the pill or during the post-partum period? What about the time around your menopause?'

The patient answers: 'I noticed some changes while taking the pill but I thought this was normal. After the birth of my first child, yes, but I felt more depressed and overwhelmed like many women. My last period was 1 year ago. That might have added to the problem.'

The healthcare provider follows up: 'An important part in one's sexual experience now are former experiences and a person's sexual biography and sex education. How was the atmosphere around love and sexuality at home when you were a child? Did you live sexuality with other partners? What did you experience? Did you suffer any negative or traumatic events?'

The patient answers: 'We did not talk about sex at home. I do not know if there were any problems between my parents. They were a normal couple except for a short period when I was a teenager. We got some information in school about contraception and from listening to older girls. With my second partner I had problems. He was very jealous and aggressive, even violent. Sometimes these images come back.'

The healthcare provider responds: 'Our partners and family of course have an influence on our sexuality. Like in all relationships there are forces which bind us together and those which somehow tear us apart; there are strengths and weaknesses. Sometimes the man has a problem like not getting a hard enough erection or he comes too fast to orgasm, which will have a negative impact on the woman's sexuality. What about your relationship? What would you consider the strengths and weaknesses?'

The patient replies: 'I love my husband. He has a lot of work to do. After years, of course, love-making becomes routine and the excitement diminishes. I realized that when we have sex he comes rather fast. We do not talk about this. It is so difficult to talk. I do not want to hurt him. Our everyday life is going very well. We are a good team.'

The healthcare provider answers: 'Society, culture and especially the media can play a role in our sexual lives, especially regarding how the body should look and how sexy we should be. We also have stress at work and our living conditions must provide time and room for intimacy.'

The patient answers: 'There is sex everywhere but of course young people, young bodies. I feel sometimes old and ugly. This is not my world. I miss romance and tenderness.'

Step 7   Provide an explanatory diagnosis

After the exploration of the factors these answers can be summarized as a working hypothesis along the biopsychosocial model.

- Medical: Menopausal transition and ovarian hormone sensitivity of the brain (reaction to oral contraceptives, premenstrual syndrome, postpartum).
- Psychological: Lack of sexual education and repetitive negative experience (failure to respond with feeling of guilt).
- Relationship and Environment: Difficulties communicating with the partner (possible premature ejaculation in the partner). Alienation through culture regarding body image and sexuality.

Step 8   Define the aims of treatment

The next step in counselling is to define the aims of treatment. What does the woman or couple want to achieve? What should change and what should stay the same? What are realistic expectations and what can or must be accepted?

Patient: 'I understand we are not young anymore and it will not be like in the beginning but I want more intimacy, more talking to each other. I also want that my body gives me more pleasure, sexy feelings, more drive. I want to get out of the routine.'

Step 9   Discuss the options and share decision-making

The healthcare provider then presents different treatment options based on the understanding of the sexual problem:

- Lifestyle changes. When does your body signal well-being ? Walking in the woods, exercising, dancing, listening to music, enjoying a good meal.
- Hormonal treatment. Menopausal hormone therapy has proven to increase desire in women around menopause, especially as transdermal oestrogen therapy and eventually an androgenic substance.

- Individual counselling. Look more closely at the biography and how to find one's own sexual script (what do I want?).
- Couples counselling sessions. Help the couple to talk about emotions without being afraid of being hurt or hurting the other.

In the final stage the patient and the physician together will decide what type of treatment or treatment combination has the highest probability to be effective, the lowest risk for the patient and fits into the patient's value system and life situation.

Summary

Counselling patients with sexual problems can be challenging for both the patient and the healthcare provider due to insecurity and feelings of shame on the patient's side and feelings of helplessness and getting lost regarding time on the side of the healthcare provider. With this structured approach, combined with the tools of patient-centred communication (active listening, reflecting, summarizing), the physician can provide sexual counselling, a diagnostic workup and therapeutic planning in the time-limited frame of a medical consultation.

References

1. Laumann EO, Paik A, Rosen RC. Sexual dysfunction in the United States: Prevalence and predictors. *JAMA.* 1998;**281**:537–44.

2. Lindau ST, Schumm LP, Laumann EO et al. A study of sexuality and health among older adults in the United States. *N Engl J Med.* 2007;**357**:762–74.

3. Shifren JL, Monz BU, Russo PA, Segreti A, Johannes CB. Sexual problems and distress in United States women: Prevalence and correlates. *Obstet Gynecol.* 2008;**112**:970–8.

4. Brandenburg U, Schwenkhagen A. Sexual history. In Goldstein I, Meston CM, Davis SR (eds.). *Women's sexual function and dysfunction.* London: Taylor and Francis, 2006, pp. 343–9.

5. Bitzer J. *Sexuelle Dysfunktion der Frau: Ursachen und aktuelle Therapieoptionen.* London: Unimed Verlag Bremen, 2008, p. 40.

6. Brandenburg U, Bitzer J. The challenge of talking about sex: The importance of patient physician interaction. *Maturitas.* 2009;**63**:124–7.

Chapter 47

Disorders of Desire, Arousal and Orgasm in the Female

Rossella E. Nappi, Lara Tiranini and Giulia Stincardini

Introduction

Sexual dysfunction is a term used to describe various sexual problems with overlapping biological, psychological and relational aetiologies within the sociocultural context. Current definitions of sexual dysfunction in women reflect a change in our understanding of the functioning of the normal sexual response. Rather than the traditional view of sexual response progressing through discrete phases in sequence (desire, arousal, orgasm and resolution), it is now evident that each phase may overlap in a variable way according to a wide range of internal and external stimuli within a biopsychosocial framework. Moreover, sexual satisfaction associated with the subjective experience is of paramount importance to evaluate the distress associated with sexual symptoms in order to establish a diagnosis of female sexual dysfunctions (FSDs) [1].

Epidemiology

Historical data indicate that women (age range 18–59 years) report more sexual problems (43%) than men (31%) do and low desire is the most common symptom (32%) followed by infrequent orgasm (28%), lack of sexual satisfaction (27%) and sexual pain (21%) [2]. Sexual complaints are often comorbid and when distress is measured taking into account also other factors such as age, duration of sexual relationships, feelings for partners and so forth, epidemiology of FSDs is much lower, affecting around 1 out of 10 women across the lifespan [3]. The prevalence of FSDs, particularly low desire associated with distress, is higher in women aged 44–65 years, with a decline of distress, but not of sexual symptoms, at older ages [4]. Female sexual dysfunctions may be lifelong or acquired, generalized or situational. In daily practice consultation, they are very common in women of any age, especially during specific reproductive periods (adolescence, puerperium and menopause), when biopsychosocial adjustments take place. In addition, FSDs may affect women suffering from medical or gynaecological conditions, taking hormonal and non-hormonal drugs interfering with the sexual response or showing intrapersonal, interpersonal and sociocultural issues [5].

Disorders of Desire, Arousal and Orgasm in Women: An Evolving Field

The American Psychiatric Association (APA) and the World Health Organization (WHO) published independent compilations of psychiatric and medical-psychological nosology, known as *The Diagnostic and Statistical Manual* (DSM) and the International Classification of Disease (ICD), respectively. In addition, the International Society for the Study of Women's Sexual Health (ISSWSH), the International Consultation of Sexual Medicine (ICSM) and the American Foundation of Urologic Diseases (AFUD) have published evidence-based consensus guidelines on definitions, nomenclature, diagnostic criteria and classification systems of FSDs that go beyond those provided in the DSM psychiatric compendia [6].

Briefly, it is essential to understand the long road to reach the current view on FSDs that stems from the evolving models of sexual functioning over time. Starting from the linear model of human sexual response, Masters and Johnson [7] focussed on genital arousal (four stages: excitement, plateau, orgasm and resolution) and, thereafter, the linear model of Kaplan focussed on mental arousal (three stages: desire, arousal and orgasm) [8]. Nowadays the circular incentive-based model by Basson points to intimacy as a driver of sexual response [9]. Indeed, women may manifest responsive desire to sexually stimulating physical intimacy, moving from a state of sexual neutrality because of a variety of incentives (emotions, feelings, communicative needs, etc.) other than

3. Importance of foreplay, non-penetrative sexual activity and use of vibrators to assist with arousal and orgasm.
4. Assessing the patient's ability to talk with partner(s) and coaching for better communication.

As far as advanced management is concerned, there is general agreement that the therapeutic algorithm should be based on a multidisciplinary approach, including biomedical and psychosexual treatments [5]. Medical treatment strategies can target the urogenital system, mainly involved in GAD and sexual pain with poor orgasmic response, and those brain mechanisms governing desire, cognitive arousal, mental reward and satisfaction [30]. Hormonal treatments include local oestrogens (estradiol, estriol, promestriene, conjugated oestrogens) and androgens (dehydroepiandrosterone (DHEA) and testosterone) and systemic oestrogens, progestogens and testosterone, namely used in peri- and postmenopausal women to relieve GSM and HSDD.

Tibolone is a selective tissue estrogenic activity modulator to enhance desire and arousal, whereas ospemifene is a selective oestrogen receptor modulator used to relieve GSM [5, 20, 21, 26, 30]. Non-hormonal treatments may target the central response (flibanserin, bremelanotide, other psychoactive agents such as bupropion in combination with trazodone especially in women with comorbid depression, buspirone, apomorphine) or the peripheral response (PDE-5 inhibitors in special groups of patients (diabetes, spinal cord injury, multiple sclerosis, SSRI users, etc.), l-arginine, phentolamine).

Even blends of pro-sexual ingredients taken orally or topically are available on the market to help the sexual response [5, 30]. Non-pharmacologic treatments may include devices such as the clitoral vacuum or laser and the integration of sex therapy or pelvic floor physical therapy to improve genital arousal and orgasm [15, 21]. Psychosexual treatments include cognitive-behavioural interventions (cognitive-behavioural therapy (CBT), sensate focus/couple interventions, mindfulness and psychodynamic approaches) alone or combined with pharmacological strategies [5, 21]. In conclusion, FSDs are complex and multidimensional, but basic knowledge regarding screening, education, management and referral may help every clinician to provide better care for women.

References

1. Basson R, Leiblum S, Brotto L et al. Definitions of women's sexual dysfunction reconsidered: Advocating expansion and revision. *J Psychosom Obstet Gynaecol*. 2003;24:221–9.

2. Laumann EO, Paik A, Rosen RC. Sexual dysfunction in the United States: Prevalence and predictors. *JAMA*. 1999;281:537–44.

3. Nappi RE, Cucinella L, Martella S et al. Female sexual dysfunction (FSD): Prevalence and impact on quality of life (QoL). *Maturitas*. 2016;94:87–91.

4. Shifren JL, Monz BU, Russo PA, Segreti A, Johannes CB. Sexual problems and distress in United States women: Prevalence and correlates. *Obstet Gynecol*. 2008;112:970–8.

5. Kingsberg SA, Althof S, Simon JA et al. Female sexual dysfunction: Medical and psychological treatments, Committee 14. *J Sex Med*. 2017;14:1463–91.

6. Parish SJ, Cottler-Casanova S, Clayton AH et al. The evolution of the female sexual disorder/dysfunction definitions, nomenclature, and classifications: A review of DSM, ICSM, ISSWSH, and ICD. *Sex Med Rev*. 2021;9:36–56.

7. Masters WH, Johnson VE. *Human sexual response*. Boston, MA: Little, Brown, 1966.

8. Kaplan H. *Disorders of sexual desire and other new concepts and techniques in sex therapy*. New York: Brunner/Hazel, 1979.

9. Basson R. Using a different model for female sexual response to address women's problematic low sexual desire. *J Sex Marital Ther*. 2001;27:395–403.

10. Sand M, Fisher WA. Women's endorsement of models of female sexual response: The nurses' sexuality study. *J Sex Med*. 2007;4:708–19.

11. Derogatis LR, Sand M, Balon R, Rosen R, Parish SJ. Toward a more evidence-based nosology and nomenclature for female sexual dysfunctions: Part I. *J Sex Med*. 2016;13:1881–7.

12. Parish SJ, Goldstein AT, Goldstein SW et al. Toward a more evidence-based nosology and nomenclature for female sexual dysfunctions: Part II. *J Sex Med*. 2016;13:1888–1906.

13. Parish SJ, Meston CM, Althof SE et al. Toward a more evidence-based nosology and nomenclature for female sexual dysfunctions: Part III. *J Sex Med*. 2019;16:452–62.

14. McCabe MP, Sharlip ID, Atalla E et al. Definitions of sexual dysfunctions in women and men: A consensus statement from the Fourth International Consultation on Sexual Medicine 2015. *J Sex Med*. 2016;13:135–43.

spontaneous sexual desire. In this way mental and genital arousal coexist and may reinforce each other, leading to emotional and physical satisfaction with or without orgasm.

However, Basson's model seems to apply more to women with FSDs than to women without [10]. Moreover, the sexual response of women is highly heterogeneous and several biopsychosocial circumstances affect the clinical relevance of sexual symptoms across the lifespan. That being so, there is a certain amount of controversy around the new DSM-5 classifications based upon Basson's model that have significantly changed well-established definitions, nomenclature and diagnostic criteria for FSDs. Then, FSDs are still an evolving topic in both research and practice. In the DSM-5 female sexual desire disorder is merged with sexual arousal disorder in one new disorder named female sexual interest/arousal disorder (SIAD).

For teaching purposes, here we refer to the ISSWSH evidence-based guidelines [11–13] published by a multidisciplinary group of sexual medicine experts, which used the phrase 'sexual disorders associated with the distinct phases of the sexual response', working in conjunction with the ICSM committee [14]. According to these guidelines FSDs manifest as chronic sexual symptoms related to sexual pain and the three phases of the sexual response cycle: desire, arousal and orgasm.

Definitions

Extensive discussion is still ongoing into the diagnostic evaluation of desire and arousal disorders in women. In routine practice it is convenient to use the terminology of hypoactive sexual desire disorder (HSDD) and refer to subtypes of arousal disorder. Even subtypes of disorders of orgasm can be identified, to expand further on the DSM-5 definition of female orgasmic disorder (FOD) [11–13].

Hypoactive sexual desire disorder manifests as any of the following for a minimum of 6 months:

- Lack of motivation for sexual activity as manifested by either:
  - Reduced or absent spontaneous desire (sexual thoughts or fantasies)
  - Reduced or absent responsive desire to erotic cues and stimulation or inability to maintain desire or interest through sexual activity

- Loss of desire to initiate or participate in sexual activity, including behavioral responses such as avoidance of situations that could lead to sexual activity, that is not secondary to sexual pain disorders combined with clinically significant personal distress that includes frustration, grief, incompetence, loss, sadness, sorrow, or worry [12, 15].

Arousal difficulties have been classified as following:

1. female cognitive arousal disorder (FCAD) characterized by the distressing difficulty or inability to attain or maintain adequate mental excitement associated with sexual activity as manifested by problems with feeling engaged or mentally turned on or sexually aroused, for a minimum of 6 months [13, 15]
2. female genital arousal disorder (FGAD) characterized by the distressing difficulty or inability to attain or maintain adequate genital response, including vulvovaginal lubrication, engorgement of the genitalia, and sensitivity of the genitalia associated with sexual activity, for a minimum of 6 months [13, 15]
3. persistent genital arousal disorder/genito-pelvic dysesthesia (PGAD/GPD) is characterized by the persistent or recurrent, unwanted or intrusive, distressing feelings of genital arousal or being on the verge of orgasm (genital dysesthesia), not associated with concomitant sexual interest, thoughts, or fantasies with inconsistent evidence of genital arousal during symptoms, for a minimum of 6 months [15, 16].

Female orgasmic disorder is characterized by the persistent or recurrent, distressing compromise of orgasm frequency, intensity, timing or pleasure associated with sexual activity for a minimum of 6 months. It should not be diagnosed in women achieving a clitoral orgasm but not an orgasm with vaginal penetration, or in those not receiving adequate stimulation [12, 13, 15]. Female orgasmic illness syndrome (FOIS) is characterized by peripheral (diarrhea, constipation, muscle aches, abdominal pain, diaphoresis, chills, hot flashes, fatigue, akathisia and genital pain) and/or central (disorientation, confusion, decreased verbal memory, anxiety, insomnia, depression, seizures and headache) aversive symptoms that occur before, during or after orgasm not related per se to a compromise of orgasm quality [12, 13, 15].

Pathophysiology and Risk Factors

The neurobiology of HSDD is not fully understood but it certainly includes an imbalance between excitatory and inhibitory aspects of the sexual response. Sex hormones, namely testosterone and estradiol, influence the complex network of excitatory (dopamine, noradrenaline and melanocortin receptors (MC3 R and MC4 R)) and inhibitory (serotonin, the endocannabinoid and opioid systems) signals modulating sexual desire, arousal, orgasm and satisfaction. This array of molecules is produced by specific nuclei in the brain stem which maintain projections to various other brain areas and the spinal cord.

Other important neuromodulators include prolactin, a satiating hormone released following orgasm, and oxytocin and vasopressin, the so-called social neuropeptides. It is likely that HSDD involves either a predisposition towards inhibitory pathways in the brain or a neuro-adaptation of structures and functions resulting in decreased excitation and/or increased inhibition [17]. Intrapersonal (depression, anxiety, distraction, negative body image, childhood maltreatment, sexual abuse and emotional neglect) and interpersonal experiences and behaviours (habituation and lack of stimuli, relationship discord/maltreatment, partner sexual dysfunction, life-stage stressors, cultural or religious issues) may modulate such a neuroendocrine balance. Even medical (uro-gynaecological/pelvic, endocrine, cardiovascular, neurological, oncological, etc.) and/or psychiatric conditions, chronic pain syndromes, use of drugs (psychoactive agents, hormonal contraceptives, anti-hormones, etc.) and other organic factors (lifestyle, substance abuse, sleep quality, etc.) may impinge upon central and peripheral sexual threshold across the life cycle of the individual woman [18].

Cognitive engagement in response to a sexual stimulus (arousal) and the motivation to engage in a sexual activity (sexual interest) may overlap in some women because they share the same neurobiological basis, but may reflect distinct constructs. On the other hand women may experience FCAD and FGAD independently or in various combinations and such distinction reflects the evidence that subjective sexual arousal does not always coincide with genital arousal as measured by objective measures such as the vaginal photoplethesmography [19]. In the periphery, sex hormones interplay with adrenergic, cholinergic and non-adrenergic, and non-cholinergic (NANC) neurotransmitters and other vasoactive substances such as vasointestinal peptide (VIP) and nitric oxide (NO),

regulating genital vasocongestion, vaginal lubrication and clitoral engorgement.

Sex hormones are also crucial for the functional anatomy of urogenital tissues exerting a direct role on the neurovascular and neuromuscular response of clitoral and vaginal tissues to sexual stimulation. Following menopause, hypoestrogenism and androgen insufficiency significantly contribute to an impairment of genital arousal [20]. Subcategories of FGAD are related to vascular injury or dysfunction and/or neurologic injury or dysfunction. There is a common underlying neurologic basis attributable to spontaneous intense activity of the genito-pelvic region represented in the somatosensory cortex and its projections. Diverse biopsychosocial contributors (neuropathies, discontinuation of selective serotonin receptor inhibitors (SSRIs), catastrophization, shame, embarrassment) have been identified in the manifestation of PGAD/GPD [16]. On the other hand neurovascular conditions, drugs and other psycho-relational and sociocultural determinants commonly associated with HSDD and arousal disorders may variably impair orgasm, which stems from a combination of a peripheral reflex associated with a specific brain activation [12, 15].

Assessment

The ISSWSH convened a multidisciplinary, international expert panel to develop a process of care (POC) that outlines recommendations for identification of sexual problems in women and describes core and advanced competencies in FSDs [15]. Ideally, every clinician should be able to screen for FSDs and deliver basic counselling that represents a fundamental step of management [21]. Following a universal screening with the aim to uncover sexual concerns and make clear that they are common in daily practice, clinicians should provide care (assessment and treatment) according to their level of expertise, being able to refer to sexual medicine specialists if sexual concerns require specific competences. A basic screening algorithm [15] includes:

1. Legitimize importance of assessing sexual function; normalize as part of usual history and physical examination.
2. Ask in the context of discussing relationships; assess if the woman is sexually active.
3. Enquire about sexual behaviour (sexual concerns, lack of sex, orientation).

If sexual concerns are detected the four-step model provides a framework for engaging with the patient [15] and includes:

1. Elicit the patient's story (a narrative description of the problem in order to assess impact).
2. Name and (re)frame attention to the sexual concern or problem (collecting more details according to the level of expertise and putting into context).
3. Empathically witness (reflect and understand the sexual concern or problem; in some cases it helps the woman to have a better awareness of the reasons behind it).
4. Refer for assessment and treatment (time, skills, comfort levels, resources); patients should not feel dismissed.

Core-level assessment [15] includes:

1. Current sexual function for each sexual response domain (desire, arousal, orgasm).
2. Presence of sexual pain.
3. Sexual and romantic relationships (if applicable).
4. Distress about and impact of the sexual problem.

Patient should feel at ease in a private environment and confidentiality is essential. Validated screeners may be useful, even in the waiting room, in order to legitimize sexual problems in the consultation and to offer the possibility to discuss some items [15]. The Decreased Sexual Desire Screener is a useful tool [22] and it has been included in the standard POC for management of HSDD [23]. Several questionnaires and interviews may be helpful to obtain a comprehensive sexual and psychosocial history, and they are generally used in advanced diagnostic settings even to guide and monitor therapeutic interventions [23, 24]. Over the past 20 years the most widely used self-administered questionnaire in research and practice is the Female Sexual Function Index (FSFI), a 19-item brief, multidimensional instrument for assessing the key dimensions of sexual function in women (desire, arousal, lubrication, orgasm, pain, satisfaction) with an established cut-off score of 26.55 for FSDs [25]. In any case, at the core level, clinicians should be able to identify the most common sexual problems that cause distress, including low sexual desire, difficulty with sexual arousal and orgasm, sexual pain/genito-pelvic pain penetration dysfunction and relationship problems [15].

Medical history is essential both in core and advanced settings to make a proper diagnosis and to

establish an appropriate management of FSDs, which often requires multi-specialized approaches with a special interest in sexual medicine (gynaecologists, urologists, endocrinologists, mental care experts, pelvic floor physical therapists, psychotherapists, sex therapists, etc.) [15]. A comprehensive assessment should include the aforementioned risk factors for FSDs and medication history (SSRIs and other psychotropic drugs, anticonvulsants, cardiovascular medications, painkillers, etc.).

A focus on reproductive history, including pubertal development, menstrual abnormalities (periods of amenorrhea, polycystic ovarian syndrome, etc.), gynaecological conditions (endometriosis, pelvic masses, recurrent urogenital infections, incontinence, etc.), infertility, obstetric history (pregnancy loss, deliveries, complications, etc.), use of contraceptive methods and/or other hormonal agents and menopausal status, is essential. When indicated by the medical history a complete physical examination, including a focussed pelvic examination, may direct care by excluding clear conditions, especially genito-urinary syndrome of menopause (GSM) and other dermatological disorders affecting the vulvar skin and/or pelvic floor abnormalities [26]. Laboratory testing may contribute to clinical assessment by identifying metabolic and/or endocrine diseases (diabetes, thyroid dysfunction, hyperprolactinemia, etc.), helping to diagnose menopausal stages (hypoestrogenism, androgen insufficiency) and to rule out infection (pH, cultures) [23, 26]. Finally, assessment of physical and sexual health of partners, when present, should be part of the assessment of the sexual health of women, especially following menopause [27].

General Principles for Management

Core interventions before referral include [15]:

1. Education about the effects of ageing, sexually adverse effects of medication and so forth in women taking hormonal contraception prior to the switch to a different option may be helpful [28].
2. Prescription of personal lubricants, moisturizers and local hormone therapy for dyspareunia secondary to GSM; in postmenopausal women the early recognition of symptoms associated with vaginal atrophy is crucial to avoid the negative vicious circle of sexual pain-inducing desire, arousal and orgasm disorders with an impact on quality of life of elderly couples [29].

15. Parish SJ, Hahn SR, Goldstein SW et al. The International Society for the Study of Women's Sexual Health Process of Care for the Identification of Sexual Concerns and Problems in Women. *Mayo Clin Proc*. 2019;**94**:842–56.

16. Goldstein I, Komisaruk BR, Pukall CF et al. International Society for the Study of Women's Sexual Health (ISSWSH) review of epidemiology and pathophysiology, and a consensus nomenclature and process of care for the management of persistent genital arousal disorder/genito-pelvic dysesthesia (PGAD/GPD). *J Sex Med*. 2021 F:S1743-6095(21)00175–2. https://doi.org/10.1016/j.jsxm.2021.01.172.

17. Kingsberg SA, Clayton AH, Pfaus JG. The female sexual response: Current models, neurobiological underpinnings and agents currently approved or under investigation for the treatment of hypoactive sexual desire disorder. *CNS Drugs*. 2015;**29**:915–33.

18. Kingsberg SA, Simon JA. Female hypoactive sexual desire disorder: A practical guide to causes, clinical diagnosis, and treatment. *J Womens Health (Larchmt)*. 2020;**29**(8):1101–12.

19. Handy AB, Stanton AM, Meston CM. Understanding women's subjective sexual arousal within the laboratory: Definition, measurement, and manipulation. *Sex Med Rev*. 2018;**6**:201–16.

20. Simon JA, Goldstein I, Kim NN et al. The role of androgens in the treatment of genitourinary syndrome of menopause (GSM): International Society for the Study of Women's Sexual Health (ISSWSH) expert consensus panel review. *Menopause*. 2018;**25**:837–47.

21. Al-Azzawi F, Bitzer J, Brandenburg U et al. Therapeutic options for postmenopausal female sexual dysfunction. *Climacteric*. 2010;**13**:103–20.

22. Clayton AH, Goldfischer E, Goldstein I et al. Validity of the decreased sexual desire screener for diagnosing hypoactive sexual desire disorder. *J Sex Marital Ther*. 2013;**39**:132–43.

23. Clayton AH, Goldstein I, Kim NN et al. The International Society for the Study of Women's Sexual Health Process of Care for Management of Hypoactive Sexual Desire Disorder in Women. *Mayo Clin Proc*. 2018;**93**:467–87.

24. Meston CM, Derogatis LR. Validated instruments for assessing female sexual function. *J Sex Marital Ther*. 2002;**28**(Suppl **1**):155–64.

25. Meston CM, Freihart BK, Handy AB, Kilimnik CD, Rosen RC. Scoring and interpretation of the FSFI: What can be learned from 20 years of use? *J Sex Med*. 2020;**17**:17–25.

26. Simon JA, Davis SR, Althof SE et al. Sexual well-being after menopause: An International Menopause Society white paper. *Climacteric*. 2018;**21**:415–27.

27. Jannini EA, Nappi RE. Couplepause: A new paradigm in treating sexual dysfunction during menopause and andropause. *Sex Med Rev*. 2018;**6**:384–95.

28. Both S, Lew-Starowicz M, Luria M et al. Hormonal contraception and female sexuality: Position statements from the European Society of Sexual Medicine (ESSM). *J Sex Med*. 2019;**16**:1681–95.

29. Nappi RE, Martini E, Cucinella L et al. Addressing vulvovaginal atrophy (VVA)/genitourinary syndrome of menopause (GSM) for healthy aging in women. *Front Endocrinol (Lausanne)*. 2019;**10**:561.

30. Nappi RE, Cucinella L. Advances in pharmacotherapy for treating female sexual dysfunction. *Expert Opin Pharmacother*. 2015;**16**:875–87.

Sexual Pain Disorders in the Female

48

Francesca Tripodi

Introduction

Considerable evidence indicates sexual pain (SP) is a common concern in women of reproductive age (12–60%) despite findings suggesting that around 40% of women between the ages of 20 and 40 did not seek help for their condition [1]. Most women who suffer from SP struggle to understand and cope with this distressing problem, which negatively affects their identity, sexuality and romantic relationships. Nearly all healthcare professionals have seen a woman or a couple that suffers from SP, whether they know it or not. Evidence also indicates that healthcare providers poorly understand and often misdiagnose SP [2]. The broad range of prevalence estimates and poor understanding stem from differences between the populations involved in a study design and the inconsistent use of definitions.

The traditional sexual medicine definitions of female SP refer to the two diagnostic entities of dyspareunia (persistent or recurrent pain with attempted or complete vaginal entry or vaginal sexual intercourse) and vaginismus (persistent or recurrent difficulties to allow vaginal entry of a penis/finger/any object despite the woman's expressed wish to do so) [3, 4]. Sexual pain can also fall under the general term *vulvodynia*, a vulvar pain of at least 3 months' duration without a clear identifiable cause and potential associated factors [5]. The 2015 Consensus Terminology and Classification of Persistent Vulvar Pain and Vulvodynia further provides pain descriptors (location, triggers, onset, and temporal pattern). Some women report pain located deeper in the vaginal canal or in the lower pelvis, which is then categorized as deep dyspareunia [6].

In the latest edition of the *Diagnostic and Statistical Manual of Mental Disorders* (DSM-5) [7] dyspareunia and vaginismus have been collapsed into a single diagnostic entity called genito-pelvic pain/penetration disorder (GPP/PD) due to considerable overlap between the two conditions. The diagnostic criteria for this disorder refer to four symptom dimensions: (1) difficulty in experiencing vaginal penetration, (2) pain with vaginal penetration, (3) fear of vaginal penetration or pain during vaginal penetration and (4) pelvic floor muscle dysfunction. These criteria represent distinct phenomenological experiences yet a diagnosis can be made based on only one dimension. Symptoms must be present for at least 6 months, cause clinically significant distress in the individual and not be better explained by another problem such as relationship distress, individual vulnerability, medical condition or correlated factors.

On one hand, the DSM-5 definition emphasizes the multidimensional aspects of GPP; on the other, the GPP/PD umbrella seems to underestimate the peculiarities of the different conditions characterized by SP. Also, it is too strictly focussed on pain interference with sexual intercourse (regardless of the pain location) rather than the whole sexual experience and quality of life (QoL). Furthermore, the 6-month criteria might exclude a significant number of women suffering from SP without considering their distress and the possible effects of pain on the psychological status and QoL in the early period.

Without entering the debate, we think the International Classification of Diseases (ICD-11) [8] fits better both research and clinical practice when it comes to female SP as it distinguishes the diagnosis between the three main conditions that affect women and allows for adding associated factors such as biological, psychological, behavioural, relational and cultural variables. They are described as follows:

Dyspareunia

- Recurrent genital pain or discomfort that occurs before, during or after sexual intercourse, or superficial or deep vaginal penetration related to an identifiable physical cause, not including lack of lubrication. Confirmation is by medical assessment of physical causes.

Vulvodynia

- Chronic sensation of pain, burning or rawness of vulval skin which cannot be ascribed to any specific cause and persists for at least 3 months.
- Symptoms may be diffuse and unprovoked (dysaesthetic vulvodynia) or localized, usually to the vulval vestibule, and provoked by touch (vestibulodynia).
- Dysaesthetic vulvodynia characteristically occurs in postmenopausal women who are often not sexually active: pain is spontaneous and frequently occurs independently of touch.
- Vestibulodynia occurs typically in younger women and is characterized by vestibular tenderness to touch, erythema of the vestibular epithelium and secondary dyspareunia.

Sexual Pain-Penetration Disorder (Vaginismus)

- Difficulties with penetration, including due to involuntary tightening or tautness of the pelvic floor muscles during attempted penetration.
- Vulvovaginal or pelvic pain during penetration.
- Fear or anxiety about vulvovaginal or pelvic pain in anticipation of, during or as a result of penetration.
- The symptoms are recurrent during sexual interactions involving or potentially involving penetration, despite adequate sexual desire and stimulation; are not attributable to a medical condition that adversely affects the pelvic area; result in genital and/or penetrative pain or to a mental disorder; are not entirely attributable to insufficient vaginal lubrication or postmenopausal/age-related changes; and are associated with clinically significant distress.

This classification, however, has two problems: (1) it seems to perpetuate the dichotomy between organic and psychogenic GPP, bringing back the traditional view of dyspareunia as a somatic disease and vaginismus (sexual pain-penetration disorder) as a psychogenic disorder; and (2) it removes sexuality from the experience of vulvodynia. Nevertheless, it can orient clinicians on a better diagnosis, assessment and treatment plan by grouping women with different complaints, needs and profiles.

Assessment and Sexual Interview

Inquiring about sexual pain should be routine when a woman complains about a sexual problem, as it is known that sexual disorders can overlap. It should also be part of regular gynaecological consultation. Harlow et al. [9] found that only 60% of women who reported chronic genital pain seek treatment and about half of them never receive a diagnosis. Direct questions are often necessary, as women may not volunteer information about this problem for embarrassment or fear of stigmatization.

Many patients have been told for many years that their pain is not real, so meeting a clinician who trusts them and their symptoms can result in enormous relief. Therefore, creating an open, validating and non-judgemental context for the assessment is essential. When a woman is in a committed relationship her partner should be encouraged to attend and participate in the assessment.

As sexual medicine has slowly moved away from a biomedical model, the biopsychosocial model is now widely accepted as the most valuable and comprehensive approach that helps to understand, assess and treat SP [2, 10]. Yet a lack of knowledge regarding pathways and interactions rather than the relative influence of biological and psychosocial variables in predicting pain and its consequences have been reported [10]. Assessment and diagnosis of SP should include organic, cognitive, affective, behavioural, interpersonal and cultural factors that may be involved in the onset, persistence and exacerbation of the symptom. The sexual interview can be structured into three areas (Figure 48.1).

Step 1: Assessment of the Pain

Clinically relevant to evaluate SP in a woman are the following observations:

- Tightening of the vaginal muscle resulting in the inability to penetrate.
- Tension, pain or a burning sensation felt when penetration is attempted or completed.
- Tensing or tightening of the pelvic floor muscles when attempting vaginal intercourse.
- Significant fear or anxiety associated with the pain of intercourse. This fear may be present before, during or after vaginal penetration.
- A decrease in or no desire to have intercourse.
- Voluntary avoidance of sexual activity.

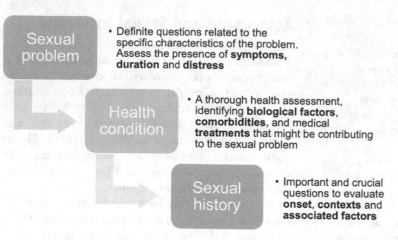

Figure 48.1 Three-step algorithm to conduct a sexual interview

The severity of the condition ranges from a total inability to experience vaginal penetration in any situation to the ability to experience penetration in one situation but not in another. For example, a woman might not feel pain when inserting a tampon but might experience intense discomfort with intercourse.

The assessment should begin with a detailed evaluation of the pain as it is experienced now with the following descriptors, most of which have been confirmed by a consensus of different scientific societies [11]:

- Location (superficial or deep).
- Generalized (involvement of the whole vulva/vagina).
- Localized (e.g., vestibulodynia, clitorodynia).
- Provoked (insertional, direct pressure).
- Unprovoked (the pain appears spontaneously and can be unrelenting).
- Onset (lifelong or acquired).
- Mild, moderate or severe.
- Temporal pattern: intermittent, persistent, constant, immediate, delayed.
- Duration.

Assessment of the pain should also include factors that may ameliorate or exacerbate the symptom: comorbid chronic pain conditions (fibromyalgia, irritable bowel syndrome, temporomandibular disorder, bladder pain syndrome); associated issues (e.g., other sexual problems, relationship and psychological distress); personal explanations for the pain; and previous treatment attempts and outcomes. Also, how the woman has dealt with this problem and if she continues to have sexual intercourse despite pain is

crucial information. In line with that, exploring masturbation, if any, could be informative about behavioural adjustments. Moreover, it is important to ask about genital pain during nonsexual activities (e.g., urination, tampon use, physical exercise), demonstrating an understanding of whether and how the pain influences other aspects of women's lives [6]. Given that the three conditions (dyspareunia, vulvodynia, vaginismus) may overlap, leading to the vicious circle of pain (Figure 48.2), we can still differentiate specific characteristics that can help the primary diagnosis.

Dyspareunia

Women with superficial dyspareunia will present with either tissue damage (inflammation, atrophy, dystrophy, etc.) that can explain nociceptive pain, or a previous history of infection or perineal trauma that can justify neuropathic pain. Deep dyspareunia is frequently associated with deep penetration and can be related to endometriosis and bladder/pelvic floor dysfunctions. Dyspareunia (superficial and deep) can also have a psychosomatic component, so it is worth checking for psychiatric comorbidities. The prevalence of dyspareunia mainly depends on the definition used and therefore the population sampled, but the prevalence estimates range are 7–46% in the general population [12, 13].

Vulvodynia

Women with vulvodynia can experience pain in only one area of the vulva, while others experience pain in multiple locations. The most commonly reported

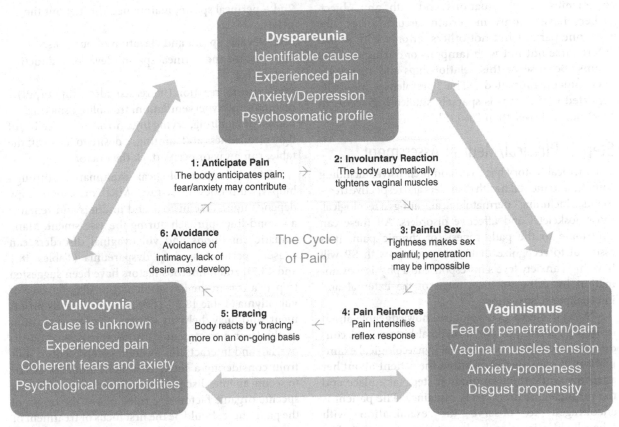

Figure 48.2 The vicious circle of pain and overlapping conditions

symptom in women with provoked vestibulodynia is burning, but descriptions of the pain vary: 'acid being poured on my skin', 'constant, knife-like pain', 'pinpricks'. It may be constant, intermittent or happen only when the vulva is touched, and the condition is usually defined as lasting for years. Pressure applied to the vestibule or the vulva exacerbates the symptoms. The most common situations that evoke the pain are vaginal penetration during sexual activity, gynaecological examinations and using internal feminine hygiene products.

Sufferers may be pain-free for much of their day, experiencing the pain only during activities that involve vaginal pressure or penetration. Lifetime estimates are 10–28% in reproductive-aged women in the general population [9]. Women showing dysaesthetic vulvodynia typically report a fairly constant burning or itching pain over a large region of their external genitals. It can occur at any time of day during various activities and spontaneously. The pain can be exacerbated by contact with the vulva during sexual activity. It has been found

that women with vulvodynia and other comorbid pain conditions are more likely to have a more severe natural history, difficulty in achieving remission from their vulvar pain and proneness to relapse [14].

Vaginismus

Vaginismus is commonly discovered among teenage girls and women in their early 20s when they first attempt to use tampons, have penetrative sex or undergo a Pap smear. Awareness of vaginismus may not happen until vaginal penetration is attempted. The condition is characterized by spasms and involuntary contractions of the vaginal muscles due to the uncontrolled tensing of the pelvic floor muscles, specifically the pubococcygeus group of muscles. The pain happens only with penetration and usually goes away after withdrawal.

Breathing cessation and general muscular spasms when attempting intercourse may appear. Women describe the pain as a tearing sensation or a feeling like the partner is 'hitting a wall'. Some women have vaginismus in all situations and with any object. Others have it only in certain circumstances, like with one partner but not others, or only with sexual intercourse but not with tampons or during medical exams. Because of this relationships and marriages stay unconsummated. The prevalence of self-reported vaginismus is sparsely studied but seems to be about or lower than 5% [15].

Step 2: Physical/Medical Assessment

The medical history has to be comprehensive, including somatic and mental health disorders and respective treatments, including dermatological, uro-gynaecological, musculoskeletal and affective disorders. All these can contribute to the pathogenesis of chronic pain. It is essential to recognize that many women with SP will have high anxiety levels in response to a physical examination involving an assessment of the external and internal pelvic structures.

A physician or gynecologist knowledgeable about genital pain should take a medical history and conduct an interactive, educational gynaecological examination. It consists of educating the patient about her anatomy while the examination steps take place and the rationale for the steps is explained. The patient is encouraged to observe the examination with a handheld mirror and ask questions if needed. The examination should include a cotton-swab test, which consists of palpating different areas of the vulva and asking the woman to rate the intensity of the pain (e.g., on a scale from 0–10), as well as vaginal and cervical cultures to exclude infection-related pain and serum hormonal testing for abnormalities [16]. If possible, careful palpation of the uterus and adnexae using a small speculum and/or a transvaginal sonographic assessment may be performed for deep genito-pelvic pain [4].

Finally, evaluating the pelvic floor, trunk and lower extremity musculature is advisable in patients presenting with SP; they may present an increase in pelvic floor muscle tone, especially at the superficial level, and inadequate pelvic floor muscle strength and control. Pelvic floor excursion testing (by assessing contraction, relaxation, and bulge) can demonstrate muscle overactivity [16].

Women with vaginismus can react in different ways to the physical examination, and these can elucidate the degree of the symptom [17]:

1st – perineal and levator spasm, relieved with reassurance.

2nd – perineal spasm, maintained throughout the pelvis.

3rd – levator spasm and elevation of buttocks.

4th – levator and perineal spasm, elevation; adduction and retreat.

5th – visceral reaction (increased adrenalin output): palpitations, hyperventilation, trembling, shaking, nausea or vomiting, crying uncontrollably, a feeling of light-headedness and fainting, a desire to jump off the table, run away or even attack the doctor.

Extended gynaecological examination through biopsy, ultrasound, X-ray, MRI or laparoscopy depends upon case history and findings and remains a second-line approach during the assessment. Many somatic conditions and vulvovaginal disorders can cause superficial or deep dyspareunia (Tables 48.1 and 48.2), and numerous factors have been suggested to play a role in the initiation and/or maintenance of vulvodynia (Table 48.3). They may be clinically prominent and may help to choose further evaluation methods or a treatment path. Factors can co-occur, overlap and interact; this awareness represents a shift from considering a single treatment modality as key to seeing an interdisciplinary approach as ideal. When specific organic factors are ruled out as the origin of the pain, these should be the first focus of treatment or adequately managed before diagnosing vulvodynia or vaginismus.

Step 3: Sexual History and Contributing Factors

A sexual history should include questions about both partnered and solo activities, prior sexual experiences – including any unwanted sexual experiences – the impact of the pain on sexual desire, arousal, orgasm, frequency of sexual activity/intercourse and sexual satisfaction. The quality of the sexual stimulation and arousal has to be investigated too. Any history of interpersonal trauma, in childhood or at present (physical or sexual abuse, intimate partner violence), must be assessed as it has important implications for treatment [19, 20]. Evaluating the associated factors that may have predisposed or maintained the symptom is an integral part of the sexual interview. Specifically, healthcare providers should explore:

- Partner factors, such as their health status or challenges with sexual intercourse and presence of sexual dysfunctions.

spontaneous sexual desire. In this way mental and genital arousal coexist and may reinforce each other, leading to emotional and physical satisfaction with or without orgasm.

However, Basson's model seems to apply more to women with FSDs than to women without [10]. Moreover, the sexual response of women is highly heterogeneous and several biopsychosocial circumstances affect the clinical relevance of sexual symptoms across the lifespan. That being so, there is a certain amount of controversy around the new DSM-5 classifications based upon Basson's model that have significantly changed well-established definitions, nomenclature and diagnostic criteria for FSDs. Then, FSDs are still an evolving topic in both research and practice. In the DSM-5 female sexual desire disorder is merged with sexual arousal disorder in one new disorder named female sexual interest/arousal disorder (SIAD).

For teaching purposes, here we refer to the ISSWSH evidence-based guidelines [11–13] published by a multidisciplinary group of sexual medicine experts, which used the phrase 'sexual disorders associated with the distinct phases of the sexual response', working in conjunction with the ICSM committee [14]. According to these guidelines FSDs manifest as chronic sexual symptoms related to sexual pain and the three phases of the sexual response cycle: desire, arousal and orgasm.

Definitions

Extensive discussion is still ongoing into the diagnostic evaluation of desire and arousal disorders in women. In routine practice it is convenient to use the terminology of hypoactive sexual desire disorder (HSDD) and refer to subtypes of arousal disorder. Even subtypes of disorders of orgasm can be identified, to expand further on the DSM-5 definition of female orgasmic disorder (FOD) [11–13].

Hypoactive sexual desire disorder manifests as any of the following for a minimum of 6 months:

- Lack of motivation for sexual activity as manifested by either:
  - Reduced or absent spontaneous desire (sexual thoughts or fantasies)
  - Reduced or absent responsive desire to erotic cues and stimulation or inability to maintain desire or interest through sexual activity

- Loss of desire to initiate or participate in sexual activity, including behavioral responses such as avoidance of situations that could lead to sexual activity, that is not secondary to sexual pain disorders combined with clinically significant personal distress that includes frustration, grief, incompetence, loss, sadness, sorrow, or worry [12, 15].

Arousal difficulties have been classified as following:

1. female cognitive arousal disorder (FCAD) characterized by the distressing difficulty or inability to attain or maintain adequate mental excitement associated with sexual activity as manifested by problems with feeling engaged or mentally turned on or sexually aroused, for a minimum of 6 months [13, 15]

2. female genital arousal disorder (FGAD) characterized by the distressing difficulty or inability to attain or maintain adequate genital response, including vulvovaginal lubrication, engorgement of the genitalia, and sensitivity of the genitalia associated with sexual activity, for a minimum of 6 months [13, 15]

3. persistent genital arousal disorder/genito-pelvic dysesthesia (PGAD/GPD) is characterized by the persistent or recurrent, unwanted or intrusive, distressing feelings of genital arousal or being on the verge of orgasm (genital dysesthesia), not associated with concomitant sexual interest, thoughts, or fantasies with inconsistent evidence of genital arousal during symptoms, for a minimum of 6 months [15, 16].

Female orgasmic disorder is characterized by the persistent or recurrent, distressing compromise of orgasm frequency, intensity, timing or pleasure associated with sexual activity for a minimum of 6 months. It should not be diagnosed in women achieving a clitoral orgasm but not an orgasm with vaginal penetration, or in those not receiving adequate stimulation [12, 13, 15]. Female orgasmic illness syndrome (FOIS) is characterized by peripheral (diarrhea, constipation, muscle aches, abdominal pain, diaphoresis, chills, hot flashes, fatigue, akathisia and genital pain) and/or central (disorientation, confusion, decreased verbal memory, anxiety, insomnia, depression, seizures and headache) aversive symptoms that occur before, during or after orgasm not related per se to a compromise of orgasm quality [12, 13, 15].

Pathophysiology and Risk Factors

The neurobiology of HSDD is not fully understood but it certainly includes an imbalance between excitatory and inhibitory aspects of the sexual response. Sex hormones, namely testosterone and estradiol, influence the complex network of excitatory (dopamine, noradrenaline and melanocortin receptors (MC3 R and MC4 R)) and inhibitory (serotonin, the endocannabinoid and opioid systems) signals modulating sexual desire, arousal, orgasm and satisfaction. This array of molecules is produced by specific nuclei in the brain stem which maintain projections to various other brain areas and the spinal cord.

Other important neuromodulators include prolactin, a satiating hormone released following orgasm, and oxytocin and vasopressin, the so-called social neuropeptides. It is likely that HSDD involves either a predisposition towards inhibitory pathways in the brain or a neuro-adaptation of structures and functions resulting in decreased excitation and/or increased inhibition [17]. Intrapersonal (depression, anxiety, distraction, negative body image, childhood maltreatment, sexual abuse and emotional neglect) and interpersonal experiences and behaviours (habituation and lack of stimuli, relationship discord/maltreatment, partner sexual dysfunction, life-stage stressors, cultural or religious issues) may modulate such a neuroendocrine balance. Even medical (uro-gynaecological/pelvic, endocrine, cardiovascular, neurological, oncological, etc.) and/or psychiatric conditions, chronic pain syndromes, use of drugs (psychoactive agents, hormonal contraceptives, anti-hormones, etc.) and other organic factors (lifestyle, substance abuse, sleep quality, etc.) may impinge upon central and peripheral sexual threshold across the life cycle of the individual woman [18].

Cognitive engagement in response to a sexual stimulus (arousal) and the motivation to engage in a sexual activity (sexual interest) may overlap in some women because they share the same neurobiological basis, but may reflect distinct constructs. On the other hand women may experience FCAD and FGAD independently or in various combinations and such distinction reflects the evidence that subjective sexual arousal does not always coincide with genital arousal as measured by objective measures such as the vaginal photoplethesmography [19]. In the periphery, sex hormones interplay with adrenergic, cholinergic and non-adrenergic, and non-cholinergic (NANC) neurotransmitters and other vasoactive substances such as vasointestinal peptide (VIP) and nitric oxide (NO), regulating genital vasocongestion, vaginal lubrication and clitoral engorgement.

Sex hormones are also crucial for the functional anatomy of urogenital tissues exerting a direct role on the neurovascular and neuromuscular response of clitoral and vaginal tissues to sexual stimulation. Following menopause, hypoestrogenism and androgen insufficiency significantly contribute to an impairment of genital arousal [20]. Subcategories of FGAD are related to vascular injury or dysfunction and/or neurologic injury or dysfunction. There is a common underlying neurologic basis attributable to spontaneous intense activity of the genito-pelvic region represented in the somatosensory cortex and its projections. Diverse biopsychosocial contributors (neuropathies, discontinuation of selective serotonin receptor inhibitors (SSRIs), catastrophization, shame, embarrassment) have been identified in the manifestation of PGAD/GPD [16]. On the other hand neurovascular conditions, drugs and other psycho-relational and sociocultural determinants commonly associated with HSDD and arousal disorders may variably impair orgasm, which stems from a combination of a peripheral reflex associated with a specific brain activation [12, 15].

Assessment

The ISSWSH convened a multidisciplinary, international expert panel to develop a process of care (POC) that outlines recommendations for identification of sexual problems in women and describes core and advanced competencies in FSDs [15]. Ideally, every clinician should be able to screen for FSDs and deliver basic counselling that represents a fundamental step of management [21]. Following a universal screening with the aim to uncover sexual concerns and make clear that they are common in daily practice, clinicians should provide care (assessment and treatment) according to their level of expertise, being able to refer to sexual medicine specialists if sexual concerns require specific competences. A basic screening algorithm [15] includes:

1. Legitimize importance of assessing sexual function; normalize as part of usual history and physical examination.
2. Ask in the context of discussing relationships; assess if the woman is sexually active.
3. Enquire about sexual behaviour (sexual concerns, lack of sex, orientation).

If sexual concerns are detected the four-step model provides a framework for engaging with the patient [15] and includes:

1. Elicit the patient's story (a narrative description of the problem in order to assess impact).
2. Name and (re)frame attention to the sexual concern or problem (collecting more details according to the level of expertise and putting into context).
3. Empathically witness (reflect and understand the sexual concern or problem; in some cases it helps the woman to have a better awareness of the reasons behind it).
4. Refer for assessment and treatment (time, skills, comfort levels, resources); patients should not feel dismissed.

Core-level assessment [15] includes:

1. Current sexual function for each sexual response domain (desire, arousal, orgasm).
2. Presence of sexual pain.
3. Sexual and romantic relationships (if applicable).
4. Distress about and impact of the sexual problem.

Patient should feel at ease in a private environment and confidentiality is essential. Validated screeners may be useful, even in the waiting room, in order to legitimize sexual problems in the consultation and to offer the possibility to discuss some items [15]. The Decreased Sexual Desire Screener is a useful tool [22] and it has been included in the standard POC for management of HSDD [23]. Several questionnaires and interviews may be helpful to obtain a comprehensive sexual and psychosocial history, and they are generally used in advanced diagnostic settings even to guide and monitor therapeutic interventions [23, 24]. Over the past 20 years the most widely used self-administered questionnaire in research and practice is the Female Sexual Function Index (FSFI), a 19-item brief, multidimensional instrument for assessing the key dimensions of sexual function in women (desire, arousal, lubrication, orgasm, pain, satisfaction) with an established cut-off score of 26.55 for FSDs [25]. In any case, at the core level, clinicians should be able to identify the most common sexual problems that cause distress, including low sexual desire, difficulty with sexual arousal and orgasm, sexual pain/genito-pelvic pain penetration dysfunction and relationship problems [15].

Medical history is essential both in core and advanced settings to make a proper diagnosis and to establish an appropriate management of FSDs, which often requires multi-specialized approaches with a special interest in sexual medicine (gynaecologists, urologists, endocrinologists, mental care experts, pelvic floor physical therapists, psychotherapists, sex therapists, etc.) [15]. A comprehensive assessment should include the aforementioned risk factors for FSDs and medication history (SSRIs and other psychotropic drugs, anticonvulsants, cardiovascular medications, painkillers, etc.).

A focus on reproductive history, including pubertal development, menstrual abnormalities (periods of amenorrhea, polycystic ovarian syndrome, etc.), gynaecological conditions (endometriosis, pelvic masses, recurrent urogenital infections, incontinence, etc.), infertility, obstetric history (pregnancy loss, deliveries, complications, etc.), use of contraceptive methods and/or other hormonal agents and menopausal status, is essential. When indicated by the medical history a complete physical examination, including a focussed pelvic examination, may direct care by excluding clear conditions, especially genitourinary syndrome of menopause (GSM) and other dermatological disorders affecting the vulvar skin and/or pelvic floor abnormalities [26]. Laboratory testing may contribute to clinical assessment by identifying metabolic and/or endocrine diseases (diabetes, thyroid dysfunction, hyperprolactinemia, etc.), helping to diagnose menopausal stages (hypoestrogenism, androgen insufficiency) and to rule out infections (pH, cultures) [23, 26]. Finally, assessment of physical and sexual health of partners, when present, should be part of the assessment of the sexual health of women, especially following menopause [27].

General Principles for Management

Core interventions before referral include [15]:

1. Education about the effects of ageing, sexually adverse effects of medication and so forth in women taking hormonal contraception prior to the switch to a different option may be helpful [28].
2. Prescription of personal lubricants, moisturizers and local hormone therapy for dyspareunia secondary to GSM; in postmenopausal women the early recognition of symptoms associated with vaginal atrophy is crucial to avoid the negative vicious circle of sexual pain-inducing desire, arousal and orgasm disorders with an impact on quality of life of elderly couples [29].

297

3. Importance of foreplay, non-penetrative sexual activity and use of vibrators to assist with arousal and orgasm.
4. Assessing the patient's ability to talk with partner(s) and coaching for better communication.

As far as advanced management is concerned, there is general agreement that the therapeutic algorithm should be based on a multidisciplinary approach, including biomedical and psychosexual treatments [5]. Medical treatment strategies can target the urogenital system, mainly involved in GAD and sexual pain with poor orgasmic response, and those brain mechanisms governing desire, cognitive arousal, mental reward and satisfaction [30]. Hormonal treatments include local oestrogens (estradiol, estriol, promestriene, conjugated oestrogens) and androgens (dehydroepiandrosterone (DHEA) and testosterone) and systemic oestrogens, progestogens and testosterone, namely used in peri- and postmenopausal women to relieve GSM and HSDD.

Tibolone is a selective tissue estrogenic activity modulator to enhance desire and arousal, whereas ospemifene is a selective oestrogen receptor modulator used to relieve GSM [5, 20, 21, 26, 30]. Non-hormonal treatments may target the central response (flibanserin, bremelanotide, other psychoactive agents such as bupropion in combination with trazodone especially in women with comorbid depression, buspirone, apomorphine) or the peripheral response (PDE-5 inhibitors in special groups of patients (diabetes, spinal cord injury, multiple sclerosis, SSRI users, etc.), l-arginine, phentolamine).

Even blends of pro-sexual ingredients taken orally or topically are available on the market to help the sexual response [5, 30]. Non-pharmacologic treatments may include devices such as the clitoral vacuum or laser and the integration of sex therapy or pelvic floor physical therapy to improve genital arousal and orgasm [15, 21]. Psychosexual treatments include cognitive-behavioural interventions (cognitive-behavioural therapy (CBT), sensate focus/couple interventions, mindfulness and psychodynamic approaches) alone or combined with pharmacological strategies [5, 21]. In conclusion, FSDs are complex and multidimensional, but basic knowledge regarding screening, education, management and referral may help every clinician to provide better care for women.

References

1. Basson R, Leiblum S, Brotto L et al. Definitions of women's sexual dysfunction reconsidered: Advocating expansion and revision. *J Psychosom Obstet Gynaecol*. 2003;24:221–9.

2. Laumann EO, Paik A, Rosen RC. Sexual dysfunction in the United States: Prevalence and predictors. *JAMA*. 1999;281:537–44.

3. Nappi RE, Cucinella L, Martella S et al. Female sexual dysfunction (FSD): Prevalence and impact on quality of life (QoL). *Maturitas*. 2016;94:87–91.

4. Shifren JL, Monz BU, Russo PA, Segreti A, Johannes CB. Sexual problems and distress in United States women: Prevalence and correlates. *Obstet Gynecol*. 2008;112:970–8.

5. Kingsberg SA, Althof S, Simon JA et al. Female sexual dysfunction: Medical and psychological treatments, Committee 14. *J Sex Med*. 2017;14:1463–91.

6. Parish SJ, Cottler-Casanova S, Clayton AH et al. The evolution of the female sexual disorder/dysfunction definitions, nomenclature, and classifications: A review of DSM, ICSM, ISSWSH, and ICD. *Sex Med Rev*. 2021;9:36–56.

7. Masters WH, Johnson VE. *Human sexual response*. Boston, MA: Little, Brown, 1966.

8. Kaplan H. *Disorders of sexual desire and other new concepts and techniques in sex therapy*. New York: Brunner/Hazel, 1979.

9. Basson R. Using a different model for female sexual response to address women's problematic low sexual desire. *J Sex Marital Ther*. 2001;27:395–403.

10. Sand M, Fisher WA. Women's endorsement of models of female sexual response: The nurses' sexuality study. *J Sex Med*. 2007;4:708–19.

11. Derogatis LR, Sand M, Balon R, Rosen R, Parish SJ. Toward a more evidence-based nosology and nomenclature for female sexual dysfunctions: Part I. *J Sex Med*. 2016;13:1881–7.

12 Parish SJ, Goldstein AT, Goldstein SW et al. Toward a more evidence-based nosology and nomenclature for female sexual dysfunctions: Part II. *J Sex Med*. 2016;13:1888–1906.

13. Parish SJ, Meston CM, Althof SE et al. Toward a more evidence-based nosology and nomenclature for female sexual dysfunctions: Part III. *J Sex Med*. 2019;16:452–62.

14. McCabe MP, Sharlip ID, Atalla E et al. Definitions of sexual dysfunctions in women and men: A consensus statement from the Fourth International Consultation on Sexual Medicine 2015. *J Sex Med*. 2016;13:135–43.

15. Parish SJ, Hahn SR, Goldstein SW et al. The International Society for the Study of Women's Sexual Health Process of Care for the Identification of Sexual Concerns and Problems in Women. *Mayo Clin Proc.* 2019;**94**:842–56.

16. Goldstein I, Komisaruk BR, Pukall CF et al. International Society for the Study of Women's Sexual Health (ISSWSH) review of epidemiology and pathophysiology, and a consensus nomenclature and process of care for the management of persistent genital arousal disorder/genito-pelvic dysesthesia (PGAD/GPD). *J Sex Med.* 2021 F:S1743–6095(21)00175–2. https://doi.org/10.1016/j.jsxm.2021.01.172.

17. Kingsberg SA, Clayton AH, Pfaus JG. The female sexual response: Current models, neurobiological underpinnings and agents currently approved or under investigation for the treatment of hypoactive sexual desire disorder. *CNS Drugs.* 2015;**29**:915–33.

18. Kingsberg SA, Simon JA. Female hypoactive sexual desire disorder: A practical guide to causes, clinical diagnosis, and treatment. *J Womens Health (Larchmt).* 2020;**29**(8):1101–12.

19. Handy AB, Stanton AM, Meston CM. Understanding women's subjective sexual arousal within the laboratory: Definition, measurement, and manipulation. *Sex Med Rev.* 2018;**6**:201–16.

20. Simon JA, Goldstein I, Kim NN et al. The role of androgens in the treatment of genitourinary syndrome of menopause (GSM): International Society for the Study of Women's Sexual Health (ISSWSH) expert consensus panel review. *Menopause.* 2018;**25**:837–47.

21. Al-Azzawi F, Bitzer J, Brandenburg U et al. Therapeutic options for postmenopausal female sexual dysfunction. *Climacteric.* 2010;**13**:103–20.

22. Clayton AH, Goldfischer E, Goldstein I et al. Validity of the decreased sexual desire screener for diagnosing hypoactive sexual desire disorder. *J Sex Marital Ther.* 2013;**39**:132–43.

23. Clayton AH, Goldstein I, Kim NN et al. The International Society for the Study of Women's Sexual Health Process of Care for Management of Hypoactive Sexual Desire Disorder in Women. *Mayo Clin Proc.* 2018;**93**:467–87.

24. Meston CM, Derogatis LR. Validated instruments for assessing female sexual function. *J Sex Marital Ther.* 2002;**28**(Suppl 1):155–64.

25. Meston CM, Freihart BK, Handy AB, Kilimnik CD, Rosen RC. Scoring and interpretation of the FSFI: What can be learned from 20 years of use? *J Sex Med.* 2020;**17**:17–25.

26. Simon JA, Davis SR, Althof SE et al. Sexual well-being after menopause: An International Menopause Society white paper. *Climacteric.* 2018;**21**:415–27.

27. Jannini EA, Nappi RE. Couplepause: A new paradigm in treating sexual dysfunction during menopause and andropause. *Sex Med Rev.* 2018;**6**:384–95.

28. Both S, Lew-Starowicz M, Luria M et al. Hormonal contraception and female sexuality: Position statements from the European Society of Sexual Medicine (ESSM). *J Sex Med.* 2019;**16**:1681–95.

29. Nappi RE, Martini E, Cucinella L et al. Addressing vulvovaginal atrophy (VVA)/genitourinary syndrome of menopause (GSM) for healthy aging in women. *Front Endocrinol (Lausanne).* 2019;**10**:561.

30. Nappi RE, Cucinella L. Advances in pharmacotherapy for treating female sexual dysfunction. *Expert Opin Pharmacother.* 2015;**16**:875–87.

Sexual Pain Disorders in the Female

Francesca Tripodi

Introduction

Considerable evidence indicates sexual pain (SP) is a common concern in women of reproductive age (12–60%) despite findings suggesting that around 40% of women between the ages of 20 and 40 did not seek help for their condition [1]. Most women who suffer from SP struggle to understand and cope with this distressing problem, which negatively affects their identity, sexuality and romantic relationships. Nearly all healthcare professionals have seen a woman or a couple that suffers from SP, whether they know it or not. Evidence also indicates that healthcare providers poorly understand and often misdiagnose SP [2]. The broad range of prevalence estimates and poor understanding stem from differences between the populations involved in a study design and the inconsistent use of definitions.

The traditional sexual medicine definitions of female SP refer to the two diagnostic entities of dyspareunia (persistent or recurrent pain with attempted or complete vaginal entry or vaginal sexual intercourse) and vaginismus (persistent or recurrent difficulties to allow vaginal entry of a penis/finger/any object despite the woman's expressed wish to do so) [3, 4]. Sexual pain can also fall under the general term *vulvodynia*, a vulvar pain of at least 3 months' duration without a clear identifiable cause and potential associated factors [5]. The 2015 Consensus Terminology and Classification of Persistent Vulvar Pain and Vulvodynia further provides pain descriptors (location, triggers, onset, and temporal pattern). Some women report pain located deeper in the vaginal canal or in the lower pelvis, which is then categorized as deep dyspareunia [6].

In the latest edition of the *Diagnostic and Statistical Manual of Mental Disorders* (DSM-5) [7] dyspareunia and vaginismus have been collapsed into a single diagnostic entity called genito-pelvic pain/penetration disorder (GPP/PD) due to considerable overlap between the two conditions. The diagnostic criteria for this disorder refer to four symptom dimensions: (1) difficulty in experiencing vaginal penetration, (2) pain with vaginal penetration, (3) fear of vaginal penetration or pain during vaginal penetration and (4) pelvic floor muscle dysfunction. These criteria represent distinct phenomenological experiences yet a diagnosis can be made based on only one dimension. Symptoms must be present for at least 6 months, cause clinically significant distress in the individual and not be better explained by another problem such as relationship distress, individual vulnerability, medical condition or correlated factors.

On one hand, the DSM-5 definition emphasizes the multidimensional aspects of GPP; on the other, the GPP/PD umbrella seems to underestimate the peculiarities of the different conditions characterized by SP. Also, it is too strictly focussed on pain interference with sexual intercourse (regardless of the pain location) rather than the whole sexual experience and quality of life (QoL). Furthermore, the 6-month criteria might exclude a significant number of women suffering from SP without considering their distress and the possible effects of pain on the psychological status and QoL in the early period.

Without entering the debate, we think the International Classification of Diseases (ICD-11) [8] fits better both research and clinical practice when it comes to female SP as it distinguishes the diagnosis between the three main conditions that affect women and allows for adding associated factors such as biological, psychological, behavioural, relational and cultural variables. They are described as follows:

Dyspareunia

- Recurrent genital pain or discomfort that occurs before, during or after sexual intercourse, or superficial or deep vaginal penetration related to an identifiable physical cause, not including lack of lubrication. Confirmation is by medical assessment of physical causes.

Vulvodynia

- Chronic sensation of pain, burning or rawness of vulval skin which cannot be ascribed to any specific cause and persists for at least 3 months.
- Symptoms may be diffuse and unprovoked (dysaesthetic vulvodynia) or localized, usually to the vulval vestibule, and provoked by touch (vestibulodynia).
- Dysaesthetic vulvodynia characteristically occurs in postmenopausal women who are often not sexually active: pain is spontaneous and frequently occurs independently of touch.
- Vestibulodynia occurs typically in younger women and is characterized by vestibular tenderness to touch, erythema of the vestibular epithelium and secondary dyspareunia.

Sexual Pain-Penetration Disorder (Vaginismus)

- Difficulties with penetration, including due to involuntary tightening or tautness of the pelvic floor muscles during attempted penetration.
- Vulvovaginal or pelvic pain during penetration.
- Fear or anxiety about vulvovaginal or pelvic pain in anticipation of, during or as a result of penetration.
- The symptoms are recurrent during sexual interactions involving or potentially involving penetration, despite adequate sexual desire and stimulation; are not attributable to a medical condition that adversely affects the pelvic area; result in genital and/or penetrative pain or to a mental disorder; are not entirely attributable to insufficient vaginal lubrication or postmenopausal/age-related changes; and are associated with clinically significant distress.

This classification, however, has two problems: (1) it seems to perpetuate the dichotomy between organic and psychogenic GPP, bringing back the traditional view of dyspareunia as a somatic disease and vaginismus (sexual pain-penetration disorder) as a psychogenic disorder; and (2) it removes sexuality from the experience of vulvodynia. Nevertheless, it can orient clinicians on a better diagnosis, assessment and treatment plan by grouping women with different complaints, needs and profiles.

Assessment and Sexual Interview

Inquiring about sexual pain should be routine when a woman complains about a sexual problem, as it is known that sexual disorders can overlap. It should also be part of regular gynaecological consultation. Harlow et al. [9] found that only 60% of women who reported chronic genital pain seek treatment and about half of them never receive a diagnosis. Direct questions are often necessary, as women may not volunteer information about this problem for embarrassment or fear of stigmatization.

Many patients have been told for many years that their pain is not real, so meeting a clinician who trusts them and their symptoms can result in enormous relief. Therefore, creating an open, validating and non-judgemental context for the assessment is essential. When a woman is in a committed relationship her partner should be encouraged to attend and participate in the assessment.

As sexual medicine has slowly moved away from a biomedical model, the biopsychosocial model is now widely accepted as the most valuable and comprehensive approach that helps to understand, assess and treat SP [2, 10]. Yet a lack of knowledge regarding pathways and interactions rather than the relative influence of biological and psychosocial variables in predicting pain and its consequences have been reported [10]. Assessment and diagnosis of SP should include organic, cognitive, affective, behavioural, interpersonal and cultural factors that may be involved in the onset, persistence and exacerbation of the symptom. The sexual interview can be structured into three areas (Figure 48.1).

Step 1: Assessment of the Pain

Clinically relevant to evaluate SP in a woman are the following observations:

- Tightening of the vaginal muscle resulting in the inability to penetrate.
- Tension, pain or a burning sensation felt when penetration is attempted or completed.
- Tensing or tightening of the pelvic floor muscles when attempting vaginal intercourse.
- Significant fear or anxiety associated with the pain of intercourse. This fear may be present before, during or after vaginal penetration.
- A decrease in or no desire to have intercourse.
- Voluntary avoidance of sexual activity.

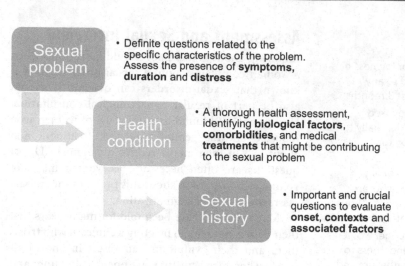

Figure 48.1 Three-step algorithm to conduct a sexual interview

The severity of the condition ranges from a total inability to experience vaginal penetration in any situation to the ability to experience penetration in one situation but not in another. For example, a woman might not feel pain when inserting a tampon but might experience intense discomfort with intercourse.

The assessment should begin with a detailed evaluation of the pain as it is experienced now with the following descriptors, most of which have been confirmed by a consensus of different scientific societies [11]:

- Location (superficial or deep).
- Generalized (involvement of the whole vulva/vagina).
- Localized (e.g., vestibulodynia, clitorodynia).
- Provoked (insertional, direct pressure).
- Unprovoked (the pain appears spontaneously and can be unrelenting).
- Onset (lifelong or acquired).
- Mild, moderate or severe.
- Temporal pattern: intermittent, persistent, constant, immediate, delayed.
- Duration.

Assessment of the pain should also include factors that may ameliorate or exacerbate the symptom: comorbid chronic pain conditions (fibromyalgia, irritable bowel syndrome, temporomandibular disorder, bladder pain syndrome); associated issues (e.g., other sexual problems, relationship and psychological distress); personal explanations for the pain; and previous treatment attempts and outcomes. Also, how the woman has dealt with this problem and if she continues to have sexual intercourse despite pain is

crucial information. In line with that, exploring masturbation, if any, could be informative about behavioural adjustments. Moreover, it is important to ask about genital pain during nonsexual activities (e.g., urination, tampon use, physical exercise), demonstrating an understanding of whether and how the pain influences other aspects of women's lives [6]. Given that the three conditions (dyspareunia, vulvodynia, vaginismus) may overlap, leading to the vicious circle of pain (Figure 48.2), we can still differentiate specific characteristics that can help the primary diagnosis.

Dyspareunia

Women with superficial dyspareunia will present with either tissue damage (inflammation, atrophy, dystrophy, etc.) that can explain nociceptive pain, or a previous history of infection or perineal trauma that can justify neuropathic pain. Deep dyspareunia is frequently associated with deep penetration and can be related to endometriosis and bladder/pelvic floor dysfunctions. Dyspareunia (superficial and deep) can also have a psychosomatic component, so it is worth checking for psychiatric comorbidities. The prevalence of dyspareunia mainly depends on the definition used and therefore the population sampled, but the prevalence estimates range are 7–46% in the general population [12, 13].

Vulvodynia

Women with vulvodynia can experience pain in only one area of the vulva, while others experience pain in multiple locations. The most commonly reported

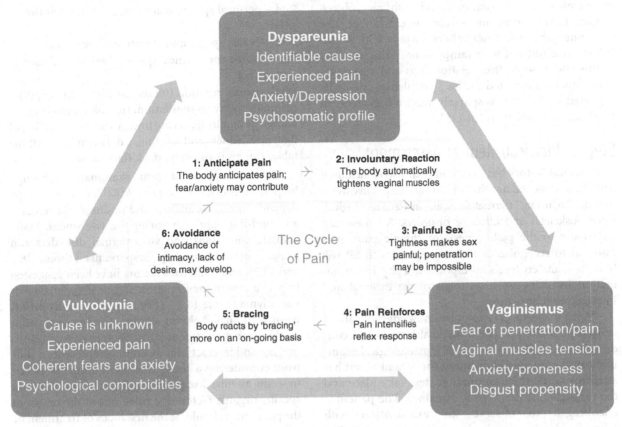

Figure 48.2 The vicious circle of pain and overlapping conditions

symptom in women with provoked vestibulodynia is burning, but descriptions of the pain vary: 'acid being poured on my skin', 'constant, knife-like pain', 'pinpricks'. It may be constant, intermittent or happen only when the vulva is touched, and the condition is usually defined as lasting for years. Pressure applied to the vestibule or the vulva exacerbates the symptoms. The most common situations that evoke the pain are vaginal penetration during sexual activity, gynaecological examinations and using internal feminine hygiene products.

Sufferers may be pain-free for much of their day, experiencing the pain only during activities that involve vaginal pressure or penetration. Lifetime estimates are 10–28% in reproductive-aged women in the general population [9]. Women showing dysaesthetic vulvodynia typically report a fairly constant burning or itching pain over a large region of their external genitals. It can occur at any time of day during various activities and spontaneously. The pain can be exacerbated by contact with the vulva during sexual activity. It has been found

that women with vulvodynia and other comorbid pain conditions are more likely to have a more severe natural history, difficulty in achieving remission from their vulvar pain and proneness to relapse [14].

Vaginismus

Vaginismus is commonly discovered among teenage girls and women in their early 20s when they first attempt to use tampons, have penetrative sex or undergo a Pap smear. Awareness of vaginismus may not happen until vaginal penetration is attempted. The condition is characterized by spasms and involuntary contractions of the vaginal muscles due to the uncontrolled tensing of the pelvic floor muscles, specifically the pubococcygeus group of muscles. The pain happens only with penetration and usually goes away after withdrawal.

Breathing cessation and general muscular spasms when attempting intercourse may appear. Women describe the pain as a tearing sensation or a feeling like the partner is 'hitting a wall'. Some women have vaginismus in all situations and with any object. Others have it only in certain circumstances, like with one partner but not others, or only with sexual intercourse but not with tampons or during medical exams. Because of this relationships and marriages stay unconsummated. The prevalence of self-reported vaginismus is sparsely studied but seems to be about or lower than 5% [15].

Step 2: Physical/Medical Assessment

The medical history has to be comprehensive, including somatic and mental health disorders and respective treatments, including dermatological, uro-gynaecological, musculoskeletal and affective disorders. All these can contribute to the pathogenesis of chronic pain. It is essential to recognize that many women with SP will have high anxiety levels in response to a physical examination involving an assessment of the external and internal pelvic structures.

A physician or gynecologist knowledgeable about genital pain should take a medical history and conduct an interactive, educational gynaecological examination. It consists of educating the patient about her anatomy while the examination steps take place and the rationale for the steps is explained. The patient is encouraged to observe the examination with a handheld mirror and ask questions if needed. The examination should include a cotton-swab test, which consists of palpating different areas of the vulva and asking the woman to rate the intensity of the pain (e.g., on a scale from 0–10), as well as vaginal and cervical cultures to exclude infection-related pain and serum hormonal testing for abnormalities [16]. If possible, careful palpation of the uterus and adnexae using a small speculum and/or a transvaginal sonographic assessment may be performed for deep genito-pelvic pain [4].

Finally, evaluating the pelvic floor, trunk and lower extremity musculature is advisable in patients presenting with SP; they may present an increase in pelvic floor muscle tone, especially at the superficial level, and inadequate pelvic floor muscle strength and control. Pelvic floor excursion testing (by assessing contraction, relaxation, and bulge) can demonstrate muscle overactivity [16].

Women with vaginismus can react in different ways to the physical examination, and these can elucidate the degree of the symptom [17]:

1st – perineal and levator spasm, relieved with reassurance.

2nd – perineal spasm, maintained throughout the pelvis.

3rd – levator spasm and elevation of buttocks.

4th – levator and perineal spasm, elevation; adduction and retreat.

5th – visceral reaction (increased adrenalin output): palpitations, hyperventilation, trembling, shaking, nausea or vomiting, crying uncontrollably, a feeling of light-headedness and fainting, a desire to jump off the table, run away or even attack the doctor.

Extended gynaecological examination through biopsy, ultrasound, X-ray, MRI or laparoscopy depends upon case history and findings and remains a second-line approach during the assessment. Many somatic conditions and vulvovaginal disorders can cause superficial or deep dyspareunia (Tables 48.1 and 48.2), and numerous factors have been suggested to play a role in the initiation and/or maintenance of vulvodynia (Table 48.3). They may be clinically prominent and may help to choose further evaluation methods or a treatment path. Factors can co-occur, overlap and interact; this awareness represents a shift from considering a single treatment modality as key to seeing an interdisciplinary approach as ideal. When specific organic factors are ruled out as the origin of the pain, these should be the first focus of treatment or adequately managed before diagnosing vulvodynia or vaginismus.

Step 3: Sexual History and Contributing Factors

A sexual history should include questions about both partnered and solo activities, prior sexual experiences – including any unwanted sexual experiences – the impact of the pain on sexual desire, arousal, orgasm, frequency of sexual activity/intercourse and sexual satisfaction. The quality of the sexual stimulation and arousal has to be investigated too. Any history of interpersonal trauma, in childhood or at present (physical or sexual abuse, intimate partner violence), must be assessed as it has important implications for treatment [19, 20]. Evaluating the associated factors that may have predisposed or maintained the symptom is an integral part of the sexual interview. Specifically, healthcare providers should explore:

- Partner factors, such as their health status or challenges with sexual intercourse and presence of sexual dysfunctions.

Table 48.1 Physical conditions causing genital sexual pain (adapted from [15])

Endometriosis	Predominant cause of deep dyspareunia in premenopausal women
Pelvic inflammatory disease	Abdominal adhesions with chronic pain, including deep dyspareunia
Oestrogen deficiency	Common cause of dyspareunia in postmenopausal women due to vulvovaginal atrophy
Pelvic organ prolapse, urinary incontinence	Do not seem to affect sexual function, but patients should be informed about potential deleterious impacts after surgery
Interstitial cystitis	Commonly reported in patients with dyspareunia
Female genital mutilation	Aside from dyspareunia, other severe adverse effects occur and for many women, lifelong suffering
Gynaecological cancer therapy	Pelvic radiation and chemotherapy cause fibrosis and atrophy of the lower genital tract, hampering lubrication and causing dyspareunia
Cancer chemotherapy	Causes atrophy of the vaginal mucosa; local oestrogen therapy is cautioned in women with breast cancer
Graft vs. host reaction	Reported adverse effect in the vagina after systemic immunosuppressive treatment
Malformations	Vaginal septum, congenital abnormalities
Hidradenitis suppurativa	Chronic scarring in severe cases
Uterine fibroid	Pressure pain of the bladder and intestine, mainly deep dyspareunia
Irritable bowel syndrome	Comorbid in women with localized provoked vulvodynia
Pelvic radiation	Causes atrophy, agglutination, decreased lubrication, and dryness, superficial as well as deep dyspareunia

Table 48.2 Vulvar pain caused by a specific disorder (adapted from [5, 11])

Infectious (e.g., recurrent candidiasis, herpes)

Inflammatory (e.g., lichen sclerosus, lichen planus, immunobullous disorders)

Neoplastic (e.g., Paget disease, squamous cell carcinoma)

Neurologic (e.g., post-herpetic neuralgia, nerve compression, or injury, neuroma)

Trauma (e.g., female genital cutting, obstetrical)

Iatrogenic (e.g., postoperative, chemotherapy, radiation)

Hormonal deficiencies (e.g., genitourinary syndrome of menopause (vulvovaginal atrophy), lactational amenorrhea)

Table 48.3 Potential factors associated with vulvodynia (adapted from [5, 11, 18])

Comorbidities and other pain syndromes (e.g., painful bladder syndrome, fibromyalgia, irritable bowel syndrome, temporomandibular disorder; level of evidence 2)

Genetics (level of evidence 2)

Hormonal factors (e.g., pharmacologically induced; level of evidence 2)

Inflammation (level of evidence 2)

Musculoskeletal (e.g., pelvic muscle overactivity, myofascial, biomechanical; level of evidence 2)

Neurologic mechanisms

Central (spine, brain; level of evidence 2)

Peripheral: neuroproliferation (level of evidence 2)

Psychosocial factors (e.g., mood, interpersonal, coping, role, sexual function; level of evidence 2)

Structural defects (e.g., perineal descent; level of evidence 3)

- Cultural and religious factors, such as attitudes towards sexuality, sexual scripts, stereotypes and wrong beliefs.

The final component of taking a sexual history is assessing the cognitive, affective, behavioural and interpersonal dimensions of the pain in both the woman and her partner if she is in a relationship. Several cognitive distortions may play a role in genital pain and treatment outcomes, including catastrophizing, hypervigilance and pain self-efficacy (i.e., the belief in one's ability to control the pain). Affective reactions such as fear of pain and increased anxiety or depression are also common. These responses likely contribute to the extensive avoidance, which can go beyond vaginal intercourse to other sexual activities and expressions of physical affection seen in many women and couples [2].

- Relationship factors, such as differences in sexual desire and lack of communication.
- Individual vulnerability factors, such as poor body image and self-confidence, psychological problems (anxiety) or personality traits.

It has been found that women experiencing genital pain show lower sexual function in general, higher levels of sexual distress, more negative emotions related to sexual experiences, lower scores in all QoL domains and higher levels of psychopathological symptoms when compared to asymptomatic women [1].

Moreover, it is helpful to assess how pain affects relationship dynamics and how relationship factors may predict pain and sexual satisfaction [10, 21]. Partners' responses to the pain can be solicitous (e.g., expressions of attention and sympathy), negative (e.g., expressions of hostility, frustration) and facilitative (e.g., affection and encouragement of adaptive coping), with the two former associated with more negative outcomes for the relationship and the latter with more positive results in alleviating vulvovaginal pain and improving sexual satisfaction [20, 22]. Mood and sexual motivation, specifically, sexual goals, sexual communal strength and unmitigated sexual communion seem to be other modulating factors in the experience of the pain [20]. The degree of emotional self-disclosure about the pain and subsequent validating and invalidating partner reactions count as well. These interpersonal factors may inhibit or promote more adaptive emotional processes, with consequent implications for the couple.

Treatment Approach

The patient's contextual situation, understood after a good case history and adequate physical examination, will build the base for the chosen treatment strategies. Reasons for SP are embedded in a sexual, somatic, psychological, relational and social context, all of which should be addressed before offering treatment and referrals. There is no 'one size fits all' approach and no 'or–or' approach, but an 'and–and' approach is recommended. Based on promising results from numerous studies, a multidimensional and multidisciplinary approach is increasingly being used [4, 10, 15, 16, 23–25]. The patient should be offered a tailored individualized treatment in which she feels accepted and understood, agrees to avoid any painful sexual activity and participates in the decision-making (Figure 48.3). Several treatment modalities are often combined, targeting different hypothesized etiological mechanisms. A multidisciplinary approach is crucial; the team may include a gynecologist, psychosexologist, pelvic floor physiotherapist and nursing staff, including a midwife. A management plan may contain education (pain management), pelvic floor exercises, prophylactic medication, and changes in sexual behaviours and patterns. Sometimes modified sensate focus therapy can be a valuable part of counselling.

Treatment interventions tend to be delivered beginning with less invasive, safer options, followed by second-line approaches such as medication or psychotherapy and ending with more risk-laden modalities such as surgery, depending on the primary diagnosis and factors involved, the subtype of genitopelvic pain and patient preference (Figure 48.4). This approach is based on clinical observations and, when possible, empirical evidence. In parallel with accumulating evidence suggesting the involvement of multiple etiological pathways, a multidisciplinary model of care has been espoused by most experts in the field, as per the Fourth International Consultation on Sexual Medicine for Women's Sexual Pain Disorders [16].

This model, applied in a combined rather than sequential fashion, includes a speedier treatment process, less resistance to any single modality, more engaged patients and healthcare professionals, increased coherence among the various physicians and therapists involved and, last but not least, targeting multiple dimensions of SP simultaneously. A key to the success of working in a multidisciplinary fashion lies in challenging patients' assumptions about their pain being entirely physical or psychological.

Until patients adopt a multifactorial view of their problem, it remains challenging to develop a strong therapeutic alliance and work collaboratively, irrespective of the type of treatment or healthcare professional. One way to achieve this is to provide education about the interdependency of biomedical, cognitive,

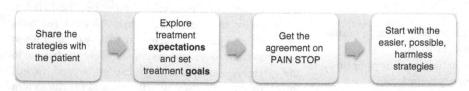

Figure 48.3 Tailoring the treatment strategy to the patient's needs, starting from the safer options

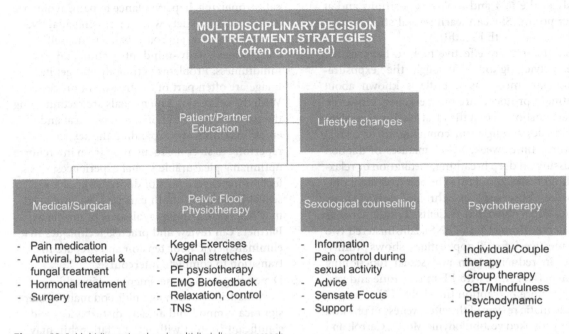

Figure 48.4 Multidimensional and multidisciplinary approach

affective, behavioural and relationship factors in the onset and maintenance of SP.

Education, Lifestyle Changes, and Pelvic Floor Exercises

The first therapeutic steps should aim to:

- Decrease pain.
- Decrease fear and anxiety.
- Decrease muscle tension.
- Improve active relaxation and proprioception.
- Increase the diameter of the comfortable vaginal opening.
- Desensitize vaginal vestibule/entry.
- Improve sexual function.

Education

Starting with the education of the patient and the partner (if present) is always important. Topics can include anatomy of the genitals, physiology and psychology of the sexual response, conditions for painless and satisfying sexual activity (motivation, adequate stimulation, sufficient lubrication, relaxation of the pelvic floor, time, intimacy, focalized attention to the erotic sensations), vicious circle of the pain, the different components of the pain

experience (sensory, affective, physiological, cognitive, behavioural), the influence of social/cultural factors and so forth.

Lifestyle

Lifestyle changes can also help the woman to take care of her needs and sexual well-being by learning coping measures to relieve symptoms and prevent further irritation. They can include clothing and laundry, hygiene, tips for safe physical activity and relaxation techniques. Patients with chronic vulvodynia and overlapping irritable bowel syndrome may benefit from dietary recommendations (low-oxalate diet, oral calcium citrate).

Physiotherapy

Pelvic floor interventions aim for progressive desensitization, myofascial trigger point release and facilitate the woman getting more comfortable with vaginal insertion. Kegel exercises are an easy way for a patient to familiarize herself with pelvic floor control and relaxation. Once the woman succeeds in squeezing and relaxing the right muscles, she can try inserting one finger while doing the exercises. Vaginal stretches can follow, teaching the woman to apply progressive pressure on the vaginal entrance, specifically at the 6, 4 and 8 o'clock positions and at her trigger points. She can learn several stretch manoeuvres combined with breathing.

Vaginal dilators are effective tools to help further eliminate pelvic tightness through the exposure-accommodation mechanism. Little is known about what treatment protocols are most effective. However, a recent review showed that the ideal dilation treatment routine includes a long-term commitment of over 3 months, three times/week, 11–15 minutes of dilation time, focussing on deep breathing, meditation or relaxation without distraction [26]. The best treatment outcomes were observed in chronic pelvic pain, vaginismus and vulvodynia patients. Transcutaneous electrical nerve stimulation (TENS), administered two to three times/week for 20 applications, shows promising results in reducing pain and sexual functioning improvements, together with PF muscle tone and vestibular nerve fibre perception threshold [27].

In a systematic review of the effectiveness of physical therapy for provoked vestibulodynia Morin, Carroll and Bergeron [28] concluded that, although the literature is plagued with methodological shortcomings such as non-standardized intervention and use of other ongoing treatments, multimodal physical therapy showed consistent effectiveness across studies with significant improvement of pain in 71–80% of women.

Sexological Counselling and Psychotherapy

Combining physical therapy and sex therapy as a first-line intervention in a multidisciplinary approach to treatment is promising [29–33]. Cognitive behavioural sex therapy and pain management generally focus on reducing pain, improving sexual function and well-being and increasing relationship satisfaction by targeting the thoughts, emotions, behaviours and couple interactions associated with the experience of SP. They can be delivered in group, couple or individual therapy formats.

a. The first phase of treatment typically involves psycho-education about a multidimensional view of pain and its negative impact on sexuality, including the role of psychological factors in the maintenance and exacerbation of the pain and ensuing sexual difficulties. Self-exploration of the genitals to localize the pain and the use of a pain diary are generally introduced at this stage; drawing, reading and web education may help.

b. The second phase focusses on reducing maladaptive coping strategies such as catastrophizing, hypervigilance to pain, avoidance and excessive anxiety while increasing adaptive strategies such as approach behaviours, self-assertiveness, body–mind integration and mindfulness. Problems with body and genital image are often part of the treatment process. With the couple, treatment goals are reconnecting the partners through nonsexual physical and emotional intimacy; expanding the sexual repertoire to steer the focus away from intercourse optimizing pleasurable sexual experiences; facilitating experiences of desire, arousal and sexual intimacy for both partners. Scheduled sex may help in disrupting avoidance of intimacy. Partners can review and practise techniques that eliminate pelvic floor tension and prepare to transition to complete intercourse.

c. Depending on the assessment and unfolding of treatment, issues such as childhood maltreatment, significant mood and anxiety disturbances and significant conflict within the relationship may need to be addressed if they are thought to be related to the SP or interfere with the targeted work on pain and sexuality, and if the patient wishes to do so.

Although there is still a pressing need for more randomized clinical trials, it is noteworthy that sex therapy/pain management is the most empirically validated intervention to date [6].

Medical Options

Medical treatment includes the therapy of underlying disorders, if any, such as infections, dermatological diseases, endometriosis, ovarian cysts, vulvovaginal atrophy or dystrophia. The second medical strategy is based on chronic pain medication like gabapentin combined with amitriptyline or serotonin and noradrenaline reuptake inhibitors (SNRIs), usually off-label [34]. Because women with genito-pelvic pain often consult their family physicians in their initial attempts to seek help, they often receive medical intervention, including topical applications and oral medications, the most common of which are topical lidocaine and tricyclic antidepressants. Specifically, medical options comprise [16]:

1. Antinociceptive agents.

    Local anaesthetics (level of evidence 2).

    Capsaicin (level of evidence 3).

    Botulinum type A (level of evidence 2).

2. Anti-inflammatory agents.

Corticosteroids (level of evidence 2).

Interferon (level of evidence 2).

Hormonal treatments (level of evidence 2–3).

3. Systemic medications.

Antidepressant (level of evidence 2).

Anticonvulsant (level of evidence 3).

4. Surgical options.

Vulvar vestibulectomy (level of evidence 2).

However, conclusions from the Fourth International Consultation on Sexual Medicine [16] indicate these are not recommended due to a lack of evidence supporting their efficacy; instead, the best treatment options are psychosexual interventions and pelvic floor physical therapy, with and without accompanying medication (especially in cases in which the neuropathic component in the onset of pain is essential). Centrally acting systemic medication may help initially provide patients with pain-free episodes, reducing the activation of the chronic pain centres in the limbic system.

Vestibulectomy, a minor day surgery involving the excision of about 2 mm of the lower part of the vulvar vestibule, has been the most studied treatment for provoked vestibulodynia. Some studies support the positive outcome of this surgical excision, with success rates of 65–70% or higher, although, at long-term follow-up, no better than cognitive behavioural therapy (CBT) [35]. Still, some clinicians and the authors of this chapter warn this surgery should be recommended only after the failure of more conservative options. Hence, within a multimodal treatment approach, non-surgical interventions are recommended first.

Acknowledgements

I thank Johannes Bitzer for his knowledgeable review; he is always a source of inspiration for a sensitive approach to women's distress.

References

1. Nimbi FM, Rossi V, Tripodi F et al. Genital pain and sexual functioning: Effects on sexual experience, psychological health, and quality of life. *J Sex Med.* 2020;**17**:771–83.

2. Bergeron S, Rosen NO, Morin M. Genital pain in women: Beyond interference with intercourse. *Pain.* 2011;**152**:1223–5.

3. Lewis RW, Fugl-Meyer KS, Corona G et al. Definitions/epidemiology/risk factors for sexual dysfunction. J Sex Med. 2010;**7** (4 Pt 2): 1598–1607. https://doi.org/10.1111/j.1743-6109.2010.01778.x. PMID: 20388160.

4. Van Lankveld JJ, Granot M, Weijmar Schultz WC et al. Women's sexual pain disorders. *J Sex Med.* 2010;**7**(1 Pt 2): 615–31. https://doi.org/10.1111/j.1743-6109.2009.01631.x. PMID: 20092455.

5. Bornstein J, Goldstein AT, Stockdale CK et al. 2015 ISSVD, ISSWSH, and IPPS consensus terminology and classification of persistent vulvar pain and vulvodynia. *J Sex Med.* 2016;**13**(4):607–12. https://doi.org/10.1016/j.jsxm.2016.02.167. Epub 2016 Mar 25. PMID: 27045260.

6. Bergeron S, Rosen NO, Pukall C, Corsini-Munt, S. Genital pain in women and men. In Hall KSK, Binik YM (eds.). *Principle and practice of sex therapy.* 6th edition. New York: Guildford Press, 2020, pp. 118–28.

7. American Psychiatric Association. *Diagnostic and Statistical Manual of Mental Disorders (DSM-5™).* Arlington, VA: American Psychiatric Association, 2013.

8. World Health Organization. *International statistical classification of diseases and related health problems.* 11th revision. Geneva: World Health Organization, 2018.

9. Harlow BL, Kunitz CG, Nguyen RH et al. Prevalence of symptoms consistent with a diagnosis of vulvodynia: Population-based estimates from 2 geographic regions. *Am J Obstet Gynecol.* 2014;**210**:40.e1–40. e8.

10. Dewitte M, Borg C, Lowenstein L. A psychosocial approach to female genital pain. *Nat Rev Urol.* 2018;**15**(1):25–41. https://doi.org/10.1038/nrurol.2017.187. Epub 2017 Nov 28. PMID: 29182603.

11. Bornstein J, Preti M, Simon JA et al. Descriptors of vulvodynia: A multisocietal definition consensus (International Society for the Study of Vulvovaginal Disease, the International Society for the Study of Women Sexual Health, and the International Pelvic Pain Society). *J Low Genit Tract Dis.* 2019;**23**(2):161–3. https://doi.org/10.1097/LGT.0000000000000461. PMID: 30768446.

12. Hill DA, Taylor CA. Dyspareunia in women. *Am Fam Physician.* 2021;**103**(10):597–604. PMID: 33983001.

13. Mitchell KR, Geary R, Graham CA et al. Painful sex (dyspareunia) in women: Prevalence and associated factors in a British population probability survey. *BJOG.* 2017;**124**(11):1689–97. https://doi.org/10.1111/1471-0528.14518.

14. Reed BD, Harlow SD, Plegue MA, Sen A. Remission, relapse, and persistence of vulvodynia: A longitudinal population-based study. *J Womens Health (Larchmt).*

2016;**25**(3):276–83. https://doi.org/10.1089/jwh
.2015.5397. Epub 2016 Jan 11. PMID: 26752153;
PMCID: PMC4790209.

15. Fugl-Meyer KS, Bohm-Starke N, Damsted Petersen C
et al. Standard operating procedures for female
genital sexual pain. *J Sex Med.* 2013;**10**:83–93.

16. Goldstein AT, Pukall CF, Brown C et al. Vulvodynia:
Assessment and treatment. *J Sex Med.* 2016;**13**
(4):572–90. https://doi.org/10.1016/j
.jsxm.2016.01.020. Epub 2016 Mar 25. PMID:
27045258.

17. Pacik PT, Cole JB. When sex seems impossible:
Stories of vaginismus and how you can achieve
intimacy. *Odyne*, 2010, pp. 40–7.

18. Pukall CF, Goldstein AT, Bergeron S, et al.
Vulvodynia: Definition, prevalence, impact, and
pathophysiological factors. *J Sex Med.* 2016;**13**
(3):291–304. https://doi.org/10.1016/j
.jsxm.2015.12.021. PMID: 26944461.

19. Corsini-Munt S, Bergeron S, Rosen NO et al.
Perspective on childhood maltreatment for women
with provoked vestibulodynia and their partners:
Associations with pain and sexual and psychosocial
functioning. *J Sex Res.* 2017;**54**(3):308–18. https://doi
.org/10.1080/00224499.2016.1158229. Epub 2016
Apr 21. PMID: 27100406.

20. Rosen NO, Bergeron S. Genito-pelvic pain through
a dyadic lens: Moving toward an interpersonal
emotion regulation model of women's sexual
dysfunction. *J Sex Res.* 2019;**56**(4–5):440–61. https://
doi.org/10.1080/00224499.2018.1513987. Epub 2018
Sep 25. PMID: 30252510.

21. Bergeron S, Corsini-Munt S, Aerts L. et al. Female
sexual pain disorders: A review of the literature on
etiology and treatment. *Curr Sex Health Rep.* 2015
(7):159–69. https://doi.org/10.1007/s11930-015-0053-y.

22. Rosen NO, Bergeron S, Glowacka M, Delisle I,
Baxter ML. Harmful or helpful: Perceived solicitous
and facilitative partner responses are differentially
associated with pain and sexual satisfaction in women
with provoked vestibulodynia. *J Sex Med.* 2012;**9**
(9):2351–60. https://doi.org/10.1111/j.1743-6109
.2012.02851.x. Epub 2012 Jul 19. PMID: 22812596.

23. Rosen NO, Dawson SJ, Brooks M, Kellogg-Spadt S.
Treatment of vulvodynia: Pharmacological and
non-pharmacological approaches. *Drugs.* 2019;**79**
(5):483–93. https://doi.org/10.1007/s40265-019-0108
5-1. PMID: 30847806.

24. Spoelstra SK, Dijkstra JR, Van Driel MF, Weijmar
Schultz WC. Long-term results of an individualized,
multifaceted, and multidisciplinary therapeutic
approach to provoked vestibulodynia. *J Sex Med.*
2011;**8**(2):489–96. https://doi.org/10.1111/j.1743-610
9.2010.01941.x. PMID: 20646179.

25. Vandyken C, Hilton S. Physical therapy in the
treatment of central pain mechanisms for female
sexual pain. *Sex Med Rev.* 2017;**5**(1):20–30. https://doi
.org/10.1016/j.sxmr.2016.06.004. Epub 2016 Aug 3.
PMID: 27498209.

26. Liu M, Juravic M, Mazza G et al. Vaginal dilators:
Issues and answers. *Sex Med Rev.* 2021;**9**:212e220.

27. Murina F, Bianco V, Radici G et al. Transcutaneous
electrical nerve stimulation to treat vestibulodynia:
A randomized controlled trial. *BJOG.* 2008;**115**
(9):1165–70. https://doi.org/10.1111/j.1471-0528
.2008.01803.x.

28. Morin M, Carroll MS, Bergeron S. Systematic review
of the effectiveness of physical therapy modalities in
women with provoked vestibulodynia. *Sex Med Rev.*
2017;**5**(3):295–322. https://doi.org/10.1016/j
.sxmr.2017.02.003. Epub 2017 Mar 28. PMID:
28363763.

29. Corsini-Munt S, Bergeron S, Rosen NO,
Mayrand MH, Delisle I. Feasibility and preliminary
effectiveness of a novel cognitive-behavioral couple
therapy for provoked vestibulodynia: A pilot study.
J Sex Med. 2014;**11**(10):2515–27. https://doi.org/10
.1111/jsm.12646. Epub 2014 Jul 24. PMID:
25059263.

30. Brotto LA, Yong P, Smith KB, Sadownik LA. Impact
of a multidisciplinary vulvodynia program on sexual
functioning and dyspareunia. *J Sex Med.* 2015;**12**
(1):238–47. https://doi.org/10.1111/jsm.12718. Epub
2014 Oct 30. PMID: 25354520.

31. Masheb RM, Kerns RD, Lozano C, Minkin MJ,
Richman S. A randomized clinical trial for women
with vulvodynia: Cognitive-behavioral therapy vs.
supportive psychotherapy. *Pain.* 2009;**141**(1–
2):31–40. https://doi.org/10.1016/j.pain.2008.09.031.
Epub 2008 Nov 20. PMID: 19022580; PMCID:
PMC2728361.

32. Bergeron S, Khalifé S, Dupuis M, McDuff P.
A randomized clinical trial comparing group
cognitive-behavioral therapy and a topical steroid for
women with dyspareunia. *Journal of Consulting and
Clinical Psychology.* 2016;**84**(3):259–68.

33. Sadownik LA, Seal BN, Brotto LA. Provoked
vestibulodynia: Women's experience of participating
in a multidisciplinary vulvodynia program. *J Sex Med.*
2012;**9**:1086–93.

34. Bitzer J, Kirana PS. Female sexual dysfunctions. In
Lew-Starowicz M, Giraldi A, Krüger, THC (eds.).
Psychiatry and sexual medicine. Cham: Springer
Nature Switzerland AG, 2021, pp. 109–34.

35. Landry T, Bergeron S, Dupuis MJ, Desrochers G. The
treatment of provoked vestibulodynia: A critical
review. *Clin J Pain.* 2008;**24**(2):155–71. https://doi.org
/10.1097/AJP.0b013e31815aac4d. PMID: 18209522.

Vulvodynia

Leonardo Micheletti, Gianluigi Radici, Chiara Benedetto

Introduction

Vulvodynia is a chronic painful condition with dramatic adverse effects on quality of life. A complex syndrome, it poses a diagnostic challenge for which interdisciplinary skills in several fields (vulvology, neurobiology, algology, psychology, sexology) are required. This chapter provides clinicians with an updated overview for correct diagnosis and management of vulvodynia in clinical practice.

Definition

Vulvodynia refers to chronic vulval pain without a clearly identifiable cause [1]. Chronic pain persists for a period of at least 3 months. It can arise secondary to disorders of infectious (e.g., recurrent candidiasis, genital herpes), inflammatory (e.g., lichen sclerosus, lichen planus, immunobullous disorders), or neoplastic origin (e.g., Paget's disease, squamous cell carcinoma) or from trauma (e.g., obstetric lacerations, female genital cutting), iatrogenic procedures (e.g., postoperative, chemotherapy, radiation), hormonal deficiencies (e.g., genitourinary syndrome of menopause, lactational amenorrhea), or neurologic disorders (e.g., postherpetic neuralgia, nerve compression or trauma).

When chronic vulval pain occurs as an idiopathic problem, it is termed vulvodynia. Vulvodynia is categorized by location, provocation, onset, and temporal pattern.

- Location. Vulvodynia can be generalized or localized. Generalized vulvodynia involves the whole vulva while localized vulvodynia means involvement of a part of the vulva such as the vaginal vestibule (vestibulodynia), clitoris (clitorodynia), or one side of the vulva (hemivulvodynia).
- Provocation. Vulvodynia is subdivided into provoked, spontaneous, or mixed (provoked and spontaneous) subtypes. Provoked refers to pain elicited by physical contact, sexual, nonsexual, or both – vaginal penetration, clothing, pressure during tampon insertion, cotton-tipped applicator pressure, and fingertip pressure. Spontaneous refers to pain that occurs in the absence of physical contact.
- Onset. Provoked vulvodynia is classified as primary or secondary depending on whether the onset of pain is triggered by physical contact.
- Temporal pattern. Vulvodynia can be constant or intermittent depending on whether the pain is always present.

Epidemiology

The exact prevalence and incidence of vulvodynia are unknown. In the United States questionnaire-based epidemiologic studies report a prevalence of 3.8–8.3% and an incidence of 4.2 cases per 100 person-years. The prevalence is similar in white and black women and higher in Hispanic women. It remains stable until age 70 years, after which it declines. It is similar across all age groups in sexually active women. Vulvodynia is uncommon in prepubertal girls. Provoked vestibulodynia is the most prevalent subtype, followed by spontaneous generalized vulvodynia. Overlap between the two subtypes is common, suggesting they are not different diseases but rather different pain phenotypes of the same condition.

Pathophysiology

By definition, the cause of vulvodynia is unknown. Most likely it is a multifactorial disorder. Etiologic factors include comorbid chronic pain conditions, genetic and hormonal factors, inflammation, and musculoskeletal, neurological, and psychosocial factors. From a neurobiological perspective, vulvodynia can be viewed as dysfunctional pain. In the next paragraphs we will explain the different forms of pain based on the current neurobiological pain classification system, which divides pain into nociceptive, inflammatory, neuropathic, and dysfunctional pain [2].

Nociceptive Pain

Nociceptive pain refers to high-threshold pain associated with the perception of noxious, tissue-damaging stimuli such as intense mechanical or thermal stimuli or chemical irritants. Nociceptive pain is both adaptive and protective because it helps prevent tissue damage by means of the withdrawal reflex and the unpleasantness of sensation, both of which serve as an alarm signal that warns against further contact with the noxious stimulus. Nociceptive pain results from activation of nociceptors, the primary afferent sensory neurons that respond only to intense stimuli. In the clinical context nociceptive vulval pain is not a clinical problem, except when it must be suppressed by anesthesia before surgery or other clinical procedures.

Inflammatory Pain

Inflammatory pain refers to a low-threshold pain associated with peripheral tissue damage and inflammation. It is characterized by spontaneous pain and pain hypersensitivity. Spontaneous pain describes the pain that arises in the absence of any peripheral stimulus. Pain hypersensitivity or tenderness refers to allodynia and hyperalgesia. Allodynia is pain provoked by a low-intensity stimulus such as a light touch that does not normally provoke pain. Hyperalgesia is exaggerated and prolonged pain caused by a stimulus such as a pinprick that normally provokes pain.

Like nociceptive pain, inflammatory pain is adaptive and protective because tenderness discourages physical contact with or movement of the damaged body part, thus minimizing further damage until healing occurs. Inflammatory pain is caused by inflammatory mediators released by damaged inflammatory cells. Most inflammatory mediators increase nociceptor excitability (peripheral sensitization). Sensitized nociceptors release neuropeptides and neurotrophins into the spinal cord, inducing a state of increased excitability of central nociceptive neurons (central sensitization). In the clinical context inflammatory vulval pain is associated with specific vulval disorders caused by tissue damage (e.g., erosions, excoriations, fissures, and ulcers).

Neuropathic Pain

Neuropathic pain is a low-threshold pain caused by a lesion in which there is structural damage to the somatosensory nervous system. The neural damage can produce negative (sensory deficits) or positive symptoms (gain of function) such as paresthesia, dysesthesia, spontaneous pain, allodynia, and hyperalgesia. Unlike nociceptive and inflammatory pain, neuropathic pain is maladaptive and devoid of protective function; it is generated by the nociceptive system but without adequate stimulation of its peripheral nociceptors.

The major mechanisms underlying neuropathic pain are ectopic activity in injured neurons, peripheral sensitization of uninjured afferents, and central sensitization. Ectopic activity is an action potential discharge arising from membrane hyperexcitability in damaged neurons at the site of injury and more proximal axonal sites.

In the clinical context neuropathic vulval pain most commonly results from a lesion of the peripheral nervous system. The peripheral nerves of the vulva are the pudendal nerve (S2–S4), the perineal branch of the posterior cutaneous nerve of the thigh (S1–S3), the ilioinguinal nerve (L1), and the genital branch of the genitofemoral nerve (L1–L2). Mechanical lesion of the peripheral nerves results from compression, stretching or transection usually caused by obstetric, surgical or other types of trauma to the pelvic floor. Compression, termed nerve entrapment, is the most common form of mechanical injury. Compression can be due to abdominal masses, deep infiltrating endometriosis or lumbar or sacral disc herniation in some cases. Bicycle riding can cause compression on the pudendal nerve in Alcock's canal. Surgery, radiotherapy, and chemotherapy can induce chronic pain due to nerve injury. The most frequent diseases associated with peripheral neuropathic pain are acute herpes zoster neuralgia and postherpetic neuralgia. Central neuropathic pain most commonly results from spinal cord injury, stroke, or multiple sclerosis.

Dysfunctional Pain

Dysfunctional pain is a low-threshold pain that arises consequent to abnormal function of the central nervous system in the absence of a noxious stimulus, active peripheral tissue inflammation or structural damage to the nervous system. Dysfunctional pain syndromes include fibromyalgia, tension-type headache, temporomandibular joint disease, chronic primary pelvic pain, irritable bowel syndrome, chronic primary bladder pain syndrome, and vulvodynia. The high comorbidity rate of these apparently different pain syndromes suggests they share a common pathophysiology.

Dysfunctional pain is a low-threshold pain characterized by spontaneous pain and pain hypersensitivity (allodynia and hyperalgesia). Like neuropathic pain, it is maladaptive and non-protective. It is triggered by acute peripheral precipitating events (peripheral tissue inflammation) in individuals with a "central" pain-prone phenotype. This phenotype includes genetic and epigenetic factors, family history of chronic pain and mood disturbances, female sex, personal history of multifocal pain, somatic symptoms (e.g., fatigue, sleep difficulties, memory deficits), psychological distress (e.g., anxiety, depression, post-traumatic stress disorder, catastrophizing), and hypersensitivity to non-painful sensory stimuli (e.g., bright light, loud noises, odors). Following exposure to a peripheral precipitating event, such individuals develop abnormal central sensitization characterized by more widespread spontaneous pain and pain hypersensitivity outside the inflamed area, with pain persisting beyond healed peripheral tissue.

Based on the current neurobiological pain classification system, vulvodynia can be regarded as dysfunctional pain caused by abnormal function of the central nervous system itself in the absence of peripheral tissue inflammation or neural damage [3, 4]. Studies utilizing quantitative sensory testing (QST) revealed a lower mechanical pain threshold in vulval and peripheral body regions. Also, functional magnetic resonance imaging (fMRI) showed augmented brain response to pressure stimuli at sites remote from the vulva in patients with vulvodynia. This abnormal central sensitization is triggered by peripheral precipitating events, most frequently a vulval infection or a dermatosis, in women a with "central" pain-prone phenotype, as described earlier in this chapter.

Symptoms

Pain is most often described as burning or sometimes as stinging, tearing, or pressure. Superficial dyspareunia is usually present in provoked vulvodynia. Pain is often associated with many other symptoms, including physical disability with impaired sitting or walking, sexual dysfunction, and psychological distress.

Diagnosis

The diagnosis of vulvodynia is made by exclusion of specific vulval or neurologic disorders associated with chronic vulval pain. The next step after diagnosis is to determine the vulvodynia phenotype.

History

Detailed history taking is the first diagnostic step. It will include data on family history, pain characteristics (location, elicitors, quality, intensity, onset, temporal pattern), history of trauma and surgery, concurrent diseases, mental health status, childhood emotional trauma, sexuality, and previous treatments and their outcomes.

Clinical Examination

Clinical examination is key to diagnose vulval disorders causing vulval pain. The clinician will examine the vulva either with the naked eye or with a 2- or 3-power magnifying lens. Higher-power magnification with a colposcope is not recommended. Colorimetric tests are useless and misleading. Dermoscopy can be useful for the evaluation of pigmented lesions. Biopsy may be necessary for histologic analysis in some circumstances. Speculum examination is essential to identify vaginal findings such as atrophy, erythema, erosions, ulcerations, abnormal discharge or synechiae. In the presence of vaginal discharge a specimen should be collected for microbiology laboratory analysis. Testing for human papillomavirus is useless.

Diagnosis of Neuropathic Pain

Diagnosis of neuropathic pain requires history of a somatosensory nervous system lesion and a neuroanatomically plausible distribution of the pain. On sensory examination, negative and positive sensory signs indicating involvement of the somatosensory nervous system should be confined to the innervation territory of the damaged nervous structure. In the clinical approach to vulval pain, gynecologists can perform a sensory examination with two simple tools: a wooden cotton swab and a dermatomal map of the vulval region (Figure 49.1). Neuroimaging or neurophysiological methods can be used to confirm the presence of nerve lesions [5].

Determination of Vulvodynia Phenotype

After establishing the diagnosis of vulvodynia, the clinician will classify the vulvodynia phenotype based on pain location, provocation, onset, and temporal patterns. The cotton swab test (Q-tip test) can be used to identify vulval areas of mechanical allodynia (provoked pain). Testing can be performed either in a clockwise direction or

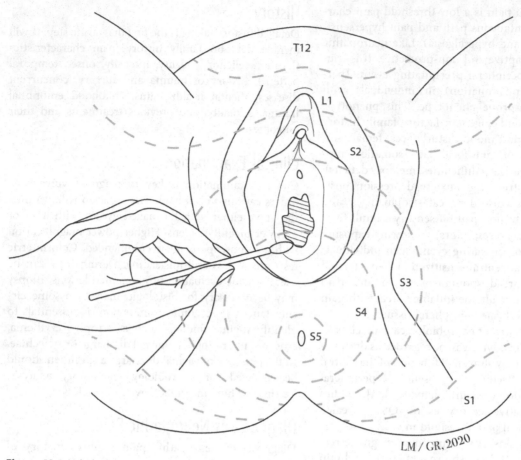

Figure 49.1 Vulval sensory examination

according to anatomical structures, including the medial tights, mons pubis, labia majora, labia minora, interlabial sulcus, clitoral hood, perineum, and vestibule. The vestibule is tested at the 2:00, 4:00, 6:00, 8:00, and 10:00 positions. The patient is asked to rate the provoked pain on a visual analog scale, a numerical rating scale, or a verbal categorical rating scale.

Intravaginal muscle palpation with a single, well-lubricated finger often reveals hypertonic pelvic floor muscle dysfunction. Hypertonicity is likely not a cause but rather a result of the pain and is maintained by ongoing mechanical allodynia.

Management

The literature describes a wide range of treatment options for vulvodynia; guidelines are available, although high-quality studies that inform them are lacking [6, 7]. Currently available treatment can provide many women with significant improvement in symptoms, though it can be slow, incomplete, and not definitive. Because vulvodynia is a multifactorial syndrome, an individually tailored, multimodal approach is recommended.

Counseling

Empathic interaction, patient education, and reassurance are effective therapeutic tools. Explaining treatment and its rationale can strengthen the placebo effect, a positive expectation of pain relief that increases the therapeutic efficacy of treatment. Counseling includes education for self-care. Use of vulval irritants, such as soap, over-washing, perfumed products, unnecessary topical medications, tight synthetic clothing, and panty liners should be avoided, as should engagement in activities such as cycling or horse riding. Washing with cool or warm water only is recommended. After washing, vegetable or olive oil can be used as an emollient to enhance skin moisture and barrier function.

Psychological Therapy

Psychological therapy is often effective. Both cognitive behavioral therapy and supportive psychotherapy can be recommended to reduce sexual pain and improve sexual function. Group cognitive behavioral therapy has fewer complications but can be as efficacious as surgery in improving psychological and sexual function. Individual and couple psychosexual therapy is often helpful for the woman and her partner alike.

Medical Treatment

The mainstay of medical treatment for vulvodynia is oral therapy with pain neuromodulators, which include tricyclic antidepressants (TCAs), serotonin-norepinephrine reuptake inhibitors (SNRIs), and calcium channel α2-δ ligand anticonvulsants. These drugs are prescribed as pain neuromodulators and not as antidepressants or anticonvulsants. Benefit may take several weeks (sometimes up to 12 weeks) to appear; side effects are more common at the beginning but then wane with continued use. Table 49.1 presents the mechanisms of action, dosage, and common side effects of pain neuromodulators.

In addition to oral therapy, lidocaine 2–5% gel or ointment is commonly used in localized provoked vulvodynia, both as long-term overnight use or 10–30 minutes before sex or physiotherapy. Its analgesic activity is mediated by the blockade of sodium channels on nociceptors. Lidocaine may cause a burning or stinging sensation for several minutes after application. Treatment should be stopped if it causes contact dermatitis. Male sexual partners may experience penile numbness. Oral contact should be avoided. Benzocaine is not advised because of its major potential for sensitization.

Various other topical treatments have been proposed, but evidence for benefit from their use is limited. Moreover, the vehicles in topical preparations can further irritate the vulva. Other topical treatments, including corticosteroids, testosterone, and antifungals, are ineffective. Evidence for the benefit of vaginal diazepam is limited, and its use cannot be recommended because of potential systemic absorption and depressant effects on the central nervous system.

There is insufficient evidence to recommended the use of local injectables such as corticosteroids, anesthetics, botulinum toxin A, and enoxaparin. Similarly, isolated or multilevel nerve blocks with a topical anesthetic, with or without corticosteroids, have shown variable efficacy; therefore, their use cannot be recommended.

Physiotherapy

Physiotherapy may be particularly helpful in patients with hypertonic pelvic floor muscle dysfunction. It includes manual therapy techniques, biofeedback, dilators, transcutaneous electrical nerve stimulation (TENS), and gentle exercise programs such as walking, swimming, yoga, stretching, and massage.

Surgery

Vestibulectomy, a surgical excision of all or part of the vaginal vestibule followed by covering of the resulting defect with vaginal mucosa, has been proposed in women suffering from provoked vestibulodynia. Long-term follow-up suggests, however, that the response by women with severe provoked vestibulodynia to vestibulectomy is comparable to conservative management. Moreover, surgery is an invasive procedure associated with complications including bleeding, hematoma, infection, inclusion cyst, Bartholin's cyst, wound dehiscence, and scar tissue formation. Women receiving surgery may also experience persistence, worsening, or recurrence of pain. Summarizing, vestibulectomy may be considered only in women suffering from provoked vestibulodynia after other conservative treatments have failed.

Vestibuloplasty, in which the vestibule is denervated, is ineffective. Laser vaporization of the vulval epithelium and other laser procedures are not supported by scientific evidence and lack biological plausibility; therefore, they cannot be recommended.

References

1. Bornstein J, Goldstein AT, Stockdale CK et al. 2015 ISSVD, ISSWSH, and IPPS consensus terminology and classification of persistent vulval pain and vulvodynia. *J Low Genit Tract Dis.* 2016;20:126–30.

Table 49.1 Mechanisms of action, dosage, and common side effects of pain neuromodulators

Medication	Mechanisms of action	Initial/maximum dosage	Titration	Common side effects
Tricyclic antidepressants				
Amitriptyline	Inhibition of monoamines reuptake Block of sodium channels	10 mg at bedtime / 150 mg at bedtime or in a twice daily regimen	Increase by 10 mg daily every 7–10 days up to the efficacy and side effects	Anticholinergic effects, orthostatic hypotension, tachycardia, sedation, somnolence, confusion, weight gain
Serotonin-Norepinephrine Reuptake Inhibitors				
Duloxetine	Inhibition of serotonin and norepinephrine reuptake	30 mg once daily / 60 mg twice daily	Increase to 60 mg once daily after 1 week, then to 60 mg twice daily after 1 week, up to the efficacy and side effects	Nausea, hypertension at high dosages
Venlafaxine		37.5 mg once daily / 225 mg daily, in a once or twice daily regimen	Increase by 37.5–75 mg daily every 7 days, in a once or twice daily regimen, up to the efficacy and side effects	
Calcium Channel α2-δ Ligands				
Gabapentin	Block of alpha-2-delta subunit of voltage-gated calcium channels	100–300 mg at bedtime / 1,200 mg 3 times daily	Increase to twice daily, then 3 times daily by 100–300 mg daily every 3–7 days up to the efficacy and side effects	Sedation, dizziness, peripheral edema, weight gain
Pregabalin		25–75 mg at bedtime / 300 mg twice daily	Increase to twice daily by 25–75 mg daily every 3–7 days up to the efficacy and side effects	

2. Woolf CJ. What is this thing called pain? *J Clin Invest.* 2010;**120**:3742–4.

3. Micheletti L, Radici G, Lynch PJ. Provoked vestibulodynia: Inflammatory, neuropathic or dysfunctional pain? A neurobiological perspective. *J Obstet Gynaecol.* 2014;**34**:285–8.

4. Micheletti L, Radici G, Lynch PJ. Is the 2003 ISSVD terminology and classification of vulvodynia up-to-date? A neurobiological perspective. *J Obstet Gynaecol.* 2015;**35**:788–92.

5. Haanpää M, Attal N, Backonja M et al. NeuPSIG guidelines on neuropathic pain assessment. *Pain.* 2011;**152**:14–27.

6. De Andres J, Sanchis-Lopez N, Asensio-Samper JM et al. Vulvodynia: An evidence-based literature review and proposed treatment algorithm. *Pain Pract.* 2016;**16**:204–36.

7. Stockdale CK, Lawson HW. 2013 Vulvodynia guideline update. *J Low Genit Tract Dis.* 2014;**18**:93–100.

Chapter 50

Disorders of Desire, Arousal and Orgasm in the Male

Yacov Reisman

Introduction

Since the publication of Masters and Johnson's *Human Sexual Inadequacy* in the 1970s, the general term *sexual dysfunction* became part of the vocabulary of clinical medicine and generally refers to sexual behaviour. Sexual functioning requires an integration of neurological, vascular and endocrine systems and interpretation in the brain. As a complex biopsychosocial process, in addition to the biological factors, including health and psychological status of the person/couple (mood, personality traits), and psychosocial factors like religious beliefs, personal experience, ethnicity and socio-demographic conditions play an important role in sexual functioning and satisfaction. It is important to keep in mind that sexual satisfaction does not always correlate with sexual function. Furthermore, partnered sexual activity involves interpersonal relationships and the unique attitudes, needs and responses of each of the partners. A problem in any of these areas may lead to sexual complaints or dysfunctions [1].

In the American Psychiatric Association's (APA) *Diagnostic and Statistical Manual of Mental Disorders, Fifth Edition* (DSM-5) sexual dysfunctions are defined as 'a heterogeneous group of disorders that are typically characterized by a clinically significant disturbance in a person's ability to respond sexually or to experience sexual pleasure' [2]. The male sexual dysfunctions include male hypoactive sexual desire disorder, arousal-erectile disorder and ejaculation disorders (in females classified as orgasmic disorder) such as premature (early) and delayed ejaculation. Furthermore, the DSM-5 categorizes substance/medication-induced sexual dysfunction, another specified sexual dysfunction, and unspecified sexual dysfunction. The dysfunctions are further assigned subtypes according to the onset of the sexual problem (lifelong vs. acquired) and situations in which the symptoms usually occur (generalized vs. situational) and specified severity (according to the clinical judgement as mild, moderate and severe) [2]. These categorizations help clinicians to focus on the relevant history.

As sexual dysfunctions involve biopsychosocial factors, it is recommended to assess during the diagnosis of male sexual dysfunctions the following issues: (1) medical factors relevant to prognosis, course or treatment, including previous surgical interventions and use of medications; (2) individual vulnerability factors (e.g., poor body image; history of sexual, physical or emotional abuse), psychiatric comorbidity (e.g., depression, anxiety) or stressors (e.g., job loss, migration, financial worries); (3) partner factors (e.g., partner's sexual problems; partner's health status); (4) relationship factors (e.g., poor communication; discrepancies in sexual desire); and (5) cultural or religious factors (e.g., inhibitions related to prohibitions against sexual activity or pleasure; attitudes towards sexuality) [1].

The World Health Organization (WHO) has also published a new classification system for sexual dysfunctions, the International Classification of Disease (ICD-11), in which the conditions related to sexual health present in an integrated (biopsychosocial) approach [3]. The ICD-11 for male sexual disorders separates delayed ejaculation and orgasmic dysfunction (subjective experience of orgasm). The topic of male sexual dysfunction is too broad to be tersely summarized. To understand in detail the specific dysfunctions, readers can refer to *The ESSM Manual of Sexual Medicine* [1].

Prevalence of Male Sexual Dysfunctions

The prevalence of male sexual dysfunction in the general population is high and even more prevalent in men with chronic conditions such as cardiovascular disease, endocrine dysregulation and psychiatric issues [4]. Epidemiological studies suggest that sexual dysfunction is a major public health problem.

A National Survey of Sexual Attitudes and Lifestyles (NATSAL) study found that at least one sexual disorder was identified by about 42% of males and 51% of females who had had sex in the previous year [4]. The most common male sexual dysfunction is premature ejaculation. However, epidemiological data cannot be translated into DSM-5 sexual dysfunction diagnoses because they do not always measure distress, which is a prerequisite for diagnosis [2].

Although sexual problems are quite prevalent, in clinical practice they are often under-recognized and under-diagnosed. Many clinicians lack understanding about how to identify and assess sexual problems. It is recommended that physicians need basic knowledge and an appropriate attitude towards human sexuality. It should be noted that male partners of female with sexual complaints can have sexual problems as well [5].

Evaluation of Male Sexual Dysfunctions

In accordance with international guidelines, the assessment of any patient with sexual dysfunction requires understanding of the type of sexual dysfunction and the variables associated with or contributing to it. Detailed history (sexual, medical and psychosocial), focussed physical examination, laboratory testing (when required), self-reported questionnaires and consultation with relevant clinicians are therefore included in the proper assessment. The existence of physical and psychological comorbidities, use of medication and substance abuse should always be given close consideration [6]. Organic and psychogenic factors can coexist in many cases, particularly in people or couples with long-standing sexual dysfunction.

Both the clinician and the patient could be uncomfortable to discuss sex-related problems. Patients could also have the perception of failure or of being abnormal. Clinicians should anticipate the patient's embarrassment and understand that such concerns could be difficult to discuss. Some patients do not necessarily have sexual dysfunction but, because of inadequate information and a negative attitude towards sex, they may perceive that they do. In addition, sexual problems in certain patients can be due to values and cultural traditions [1].

Before the start of treatment, the treatment goals should be established according to the patient/couple expectations, which need to be realistic. The choice of treatment should be made according to the preferences of the patient/couple. The clinician must educate the patient/couple about the treatment modalities available and assist them in making a reasoned decision.

Hypoactive Sexual Desire Disorder in Men

Definitions and Epidemiology

The manifestations of sexual desire are so diverse that research in the area has been difficult to generate. It incorporates both subjective and behavioural phenomena such as sexual dreams, sexual desires, initiation of a partner's sexual behaviour, responsiveness to sexual actions, self-stimulation initiation, genital stimuli and increasing responsiveness to eroticism in the environment.

Sexual desires are the product of a positive interplay between internal cognitive processes (thoughts, fantasy and imagination), neurophysiological mechanisms (central arousability) and affective components (mood and emotion). Dimensions of relationship, psychological adaptation and cognitive and biological factors are all linked to sexual desire. The biological basis for all is still not known in humans [6, 7].

Low sexual desire in men is one of the most difficult sexual disorders to define, assess and treat. The key issue is the lack of objective measurements and a description that is generally accepted. According to the DSM-5 classification, hypoactive sexual desire disorder (HSDD) is a sexual dysfunction characterized as a persistent or recurrent lack (or absence) of sexual fantasies and desire for sexual activity, as judged by a clinician taking into account factors that affect sexual functioning (e.g., age; general and sociocultural contexts of the individual's life). Symptoms need to persist for a minimum of 6 months. The complaints must cause marked distress or severe interpersonal difficulties, cannot be better accounted for by another major mental disorder (except another sexual dysfunction) and cannot be due solely to the effects of a substance or general medical condition [2].

Despite the fact that there are countless studies on HSDD in females, research on HSDD in men is scant. Besides, numerous men are treated for various sexual diagnoses such as erectile dysfunction (ED) and depression which often coexist while they are experiencing HSDD. Population-based studies report prevalence ranges of 3–50% of reduced sexual interest. A multicentre survey including 906 men (mean age

48.8 years) enrolled for a pharmaceutical study found that 30% met the DSM-5 criteria for HSDD.5 A survey involving 1,455 men aged 57–85 years indicated that 28% of men reported loss of desire and 65% of them felt bothered about it [8]. According to expert opinion, it seems that the most common types of HSDD in men are acquired and situational [7]. Interestingly, on the population level sexual interest appears quite stable from the late teens up to about 60 years; from there on it diminishes uniquely [8].

One of three subtypes of HSDD is diagnosed in men:

- Lifelong/generalized: The individual has little to no desire for sexual stimulation and has never had it (with a partner or alone).
- Acquired/generalized: The man had previously sexual desire but lost interest in partnered or solitary sexual activity.
- Acquired/situational: The man with his current partner was previously sexually attracted but now loses sexual interest in him/her yet has a need for sexual stimulation (i.e., alone or with someone other than his current partner). This is related to the relationship than to desire.

Pathophysiology

In the case of acquired/generalized HSDD, conceivable causes include low levels of androgens (testosterone), high levels of prolactin and various medical/health/psychiatric conditions, mainly chronic problems. It appears that, for a man to feel sexual desire, a minimum amount of testosterone is necessary. Androgens are not the only requisite for desire and women also need androgens, but in lower amounts. Supra-physiological blood testosterone levels do not correlate with higher sexual desire. Significant hyperprolactinaemia has a detrimental effect on sexual function, negatively affecting sexual desire as well as erectile function and testosterone production. Other endocrine disorders such as hypothyroidism are also associated with male HSDD. Depression is related to hypothyroidism and hypogonadism and may be the explanation for this connection [9].

In many chronic systemic diseases such as kidney failure, chronic liver diseases, haematological diseases and HIV, HSDD may also be present. In this situation the problem is multifactorial because of the presence of low physical condition, hormonal influences and intrapersonal and relational issues linked to the

deterioration of the quality of life. Men with prostatitis/chronic pelvic pain syndrome have been found to have substantially less sexual desire or feeling, fewer sexual activities, less excitement/erectile activity and orgasm and more sexual pain than men without any condition of pain.

It is well recognized that psychiatric illnesses, in particular depression and anxiety disorder, often trigger a decrease in sexual desire. This is also true of the medical treatments of these conditions [8]. However, depression can freeze many aspects of a couple's sexual activity, which can be regarded as the cause or consequence of serious emotional distress. On the other hand, depression-related psychological symptoms such as anhedonia, fatigue and low energy may impair sexual function. Libido, sexual arousal and orgasm/ejaculation can also be impaired by antidepressants. It is important to examine antidepressants' role in depressed patients' sexual dysfunction.

Studies on the role of psychological variables in male HSDD have shown that in assessing sexual desire, cognitive and emotional dimensions play an important role. Men with conservative sexual views and restrictive sexual attitudes, as well as men who tend to concentrate more on negative thoughts during sexual activity (such as erection issues) and less on romantic thoughts and who have fewer positive emotions, are more likely to have low sexual desire and to develop HSDD [10–12]. In the case of acquired/situational HSDD intrapersonal and relational issues (e.g., tension in the couple, negative feelings), cognitive and cultural influences (e.g., sexual values, automatic thinking during sexual activity), problems with intimacy, family problems or other stressful events in life are potential triggers.

Hypoactive sexual dysfunction disorder has apparent implications for sexual functioning. A decrease in sexual motivation may lead to ED or a decrease in sexual activity, and vice versa a decrease in sexual desire can result from ED. In this situation HSDD is potentially an evasive reaction that has been put in order to reduce the discomfort associated with sexual performance impairment [11].

Assessment

It can be difficult to diagnose HSDD in men. The clinician is recommended to ask about the need and wish for sexual activity, attraction or desire. A shift in normal routine is easily recognized by most patients and this is the manner in which the disorder is identified most of the time. The indicators of sexual desire, which may be a good clinical clue, must sometimes be investigated. It is important to explicitly look for the existence of HSDD when a man presents himself with another sexual condition. The effectiveness of treatment depends on how HSDD is successfully diagnosed and treated by the clinician.

The core issue for the proper diagnosis and classification of HSDD manifestations is an accurate medical history. All potential causes, including medication use and drug misuse, must be explored. Physical examination (including examination of the genitals and signs of gynaecomastia or galactorrhoea) and measurement of total serum testosterone, prolactin and thyroid function are required for generalized HSDD. It is important to examine relationship satisfaction and intimacy. Exploring sexual values (particularly conservative and restrictive attitudes towards sexuality) as well as feelings and cognition usually presented during sexual activity is essential. In circumstances where psychological factors play a central role in explaining HSDD, measuring these cognitive and emotional aspects is advisable [1, 10–12].

Clinical Management

Treatment of HSDD should be based on aetiology whenever possible. Typically a comprehensive, integrative biopsychosocial approach to the sexuality of both the male and the couple is required. Currently no pharmaceutical approach is commercially available and approved that can directly increase sexual desire. When hormonal disturbances are detected, adequate therapy can improve sexual desire. Remember, however, that maladaptive behaviour stemming from the HSDD (such as sleeping in separate bedrooms) should be corrected as well.

The removal or replacement of medication is not always feasible when drugs actually interfere with sexual desire, although it may solve the issue. In these cases the clinician should thoroughly assess the likelihood of modifying the current treatment or reducing it sufficiently. Watchful waiting, dose reduction, drug holidays, switching medication and use of add-on drugs are management techniques. While utilizing antidepressants, substitution of the antidepressant with another antidepressant with fewer sexual side effects (i.e., agomelatine, mirtazapine, bupropion, tianeptine, trazodone, vortioxetine, buspirone) is

favourable, but always after consultation with the prescriber.

Psychotherapy can be necessary if HSDD is specifically caused by a disturbance of the relational or intra-psychic variables. Psychological approaches to low desire, particularly in women, have been shown to be effective with sustained changes over time. There are, however, no randomized control studies specifically on the psychological treatment of HSDD in men. Experts suggest cognitive behavioural techniques because they combine both intra-psychic (i.e., sexual attitudes, cognitions, sexuality related emotions) and interpersonal aspects [13].

By exploring various erotic experiences, as well as focussing on sexual values and cognitive processes related to sexuality, it is possible to promote the recreational and pleasurable aspect of sexuality [14]. It is important to focus on improving communication between partners, which is often at the root of the issue. The patient and his partner should be referred for couple/relationship treatment when conflict and relationship distress are the cause of low sexual desire.

Erectile Dysfunction

Definition and Epidemiology

An erection is complex process with the needs for adequate function of nerves, arteries and veins. It involves physiological and psychological factors, the central nervous system, the peripheral nervous system, local factors within the erectile tissue (corpora cavernosa) or the penis itself, as well as hormonal and vascular components. The penile part of the process is just a single aspect of the erection process. Erections happen in response to touch, smell, auditory and visual stimuli that activate pathways in the brain. Information passes from the brain to the nerve centres at the base of the spine, where, during and after erections, primary nerve fibres bind to the muscles in the corpora cavernosa of the penis and control blood flow [1].

Many men experience some episodes of erectile problems during their lifetime. These erection problems are typically short and, in most cases, are linked to certain and unique life conditions, stressful issues and situations and an increased sympathetic tone with elevated catecholamine plasma concentrations (noradrenaline/adrenaline). These temporary erectile problems vanish in normal circumstances once the problem is solved and usually do not require consultation and assistance from a physician.

According to the DSM-5, ED is defined as the inability to achieve and/or maintain an erection that is satisfactory for the completion of sexual activity for a minimum duration of 6 months and the patient must experience the condition in all or almost all sexual activity situations and with marked distress [2].

Erectile dysfunction is one of the most common male sexual disorders. The prevalence of ED is age-dependent, with a sharp rise beyond the fifth decade. Some record a prevalence of up to 50% of men between 40 and 80 years of age [8]. The severity of ED is categorized with the International Index of Erectile Function (IIEF), using a scoring system from 1 to 30 in the Erection Function Domain of the IIEF. Erectile dysfunction is subdivided into mild (IIEF-EF score 17–25), moderate (IIEF-EF score 11–16) and severe (IIEF-EF score < 11), while an IIEF-EF score of 26–30 indicates normal erectile function [15].

Another method to categorize the severity of the erection is according to the hardness of the erection with the Erection Hardness Score (EHS) which is a single-item scoring for patient reported outcome. The IIEF and EHS are related to erection during intercourse. Recently the Masturbation Erection Index (MEI) has been validated for measuring erection quality during masturbation.

Pathophysiology

Broad evidence from the literature demonstrates that ED is substantially related to cardiovascular risk factors such as diabetes, hypertension, coronary artery disease, dyslipidaemia, atherosclerosis and metabolic syndrome in patients older than 40 years. There is substantially increased risk of cardiovascular risks/events in men with ED as compared with age-matched non-ED men and therefore the manifestation of ED should be considered a marker (warning sign) of cardiovascular disease, with a significant likelihood of a subsequent major cardiovascular event [16].

The severity of ED correlates with the severity of cardiovascular disease, as the same pathophysiology mechanism occurs in both penile vessels and heart vessels. According to the artery size theory, the smaller size of the penile vessels relative to the vessels of the heart causes ED to manifest first and could be accompanied in the next 2–3 years by a cardiovascular event.

Regarding ED caused by veno-occlusive dysfunction, also called cavernous insufficiency or venous leak, the pathophysiology of this disorder is not found in the veins themselves but in a decrease in the relaxant ability of the smooth muscle cells inside the cavernous bodies. Physiologically, the cavernous smooth muscle cells relax and extend and compress the veins that drain blood from the cavernous bodies against the tunica albuginea into the deep dorsal penile vein until erection happens. Arterial or venous anomalies can also be caused by surgery in the urogenital region and in the pelvis (radical prostatectomy and cystectomy). Perineum and pelvic region injuries can also cause irregular venous drainage of the penis.

Central and peripheral nervous system diseases can cause ED. Multiple sclerosis, spinal cord injury, Parkinson's disease and cerebrovascular disease are common central nervous system diseases. Peripheral nervous system disorders that can cause ED include peripheral polyneuropathy (e.g., induced by diabetes or excessive alcohol consumption), intervertebral disc prolapses or iatrogenic (surgical) pelvic nerve injury [16].

Androgens such as testosterone are essential for sexual desire and play an important role in maintaining and controlling the erectile capacity that affects the release and function of brain-level stimulating neurotransmitters and the release of nitric oxide (NO) caused by parasympathetic penile nerve fibres. In addition, elevated serum prolactin has a negative effect, especially on the sexual desire and erectile function of men.

Erectile dysfunction is associated with a variety of medications and recreational drugs. They either exert their adverse effects through central inhibitory neuroendocrine mechanisms and/or have an effect on hormone (testosterone/prolactin) metabolism. Erectile dysfunction is associated with antihypertensives, especially thiazides and non-selective beta-blockers, antidepressants/neuroleptics, antiarrhythmics, antiandrogens and inhibitors of 5-alpha reductase, oestrogens and recreational substances. Furthermore, it is important to mention that not only pelvic region operations are a risk for ED, but also radiation therapy as well [16].

Psychological variables, like physical factors, can predispose, cause or maintain ED. Factors that make someone vulnerable to the onset of ED are predisposing ones, but many of these may also have a maintenance role. Trigger factors can explain why at a certain situation or time the issue was initiated. Factors that are maintained are those that explain why the issue is still present. Patients usually want to know what triggered the issue.

At the predisposing level, studies have shown that in men with ED, neurotic personality traits are significantly more prevalent [17]. In addition, studies have shown that men with ED tend to report 'macho' beliefs which are demanding and unrealistic and make men more susceptible to ED. Example of such believes are: a man should be able to last all night, a man always wants and is prepared to have sex, a real man has sexual intercourse very often, and demanding beliefs about women such as a man who doesn't sexually satisfy a woman is a failure [18]. With respect to the maintenance factors, studies have shown that men with ED tend to interpret negative sexual events as a sign of failure and personal incompetence [19]. In addition, men with ED typically present thoughts about erection difficulties and failure anticipation and less erotic thoughts during sexual activity [20]. Depressed mood is strongly associated with sexual dysfunctions. Compared to sexually healthy men, ED patients report significantly more depression, disillusionment and anxiety and significantly less enjoyment and satisfaction during sexual activity [21].

A strong bidirectional association between ED and depression has been demonstrated. Population studies indicate that moderate to extreme depression can trigger ED and depressed mood can be triggered or aggravated by ED. In addition, treatment with antidepressants is also frequently associated with ED. Patients with ED will also have an anxiety disorder, although it is unknown what the primary disorder is in many cases. Poor clinical treatment results have been associated with the presence of anxiety symptoms in patients with arousal disorders.

Performance anxiety is a significant psychological cause of ED. Performance anxiety during sexual situations involves the interplay between cognitive, affective, behavioural and physiological responses. Any sexual stimulation that the man associates with his erectile ability or incapacity can cause performance anxiety. The negative emotions distract his attention from sexually pleasurable stimuli and experience and evoke excessive sympathetic arousal and contraction of the penile smooth muscle cells, which in their turn cause erectile failure. The increase of the sympathetic tone due to performance anxiety leads to an increase of both adrenaline and noradrenaline release in blood circulation (from the sympathetic nerves and from the adrenal glands), counteracting both the onset and the maintenance of the erection [16].

Relationship quality is a key factor affecting ED onset and maintenance. Men experiencing ED often report lower satisfaction with their relationship. One of the most common consequences of sexual dysfunction is relationship distress as the pressure of dealing with sexual difficulties can lead to a lack of confidence and closeness in the relationship and can motivate one or the other partner to pursue sexual pleasure outside of the relationship.

Contextual variables could be a significant cause of ED. They involve everyday stressors such as financial difficulties, unemployment, childrearing fatigue and the pressures of taking care of a sick parent or spouse. Environmental considerations such as spouses working in multiple shifts and not having adequate privacy also need to be considered.

Assessment

The diagnostic assessment involves individual evaluation and, whenever possible, evaluation of the couple. There is a need for comprehensive medical, sexual and psychosocial history. As noted previously in this chapter, attention should be paid to risk factors. Physical examination includes general screening for medical risk factors or comorbidities associated with ED, an assessment of secondary sexual characteristics and an assessment of the cardiovascular, neurological and genital systems with specific attention on the genitals. It is important to test the related hormones such as total testosterone and, in special indications, prolactin and thyroid-stimulating hormone (TSH). It should be considered normal to test routine laboratory parameters such as serum-cholesterol with LDL- and HDL-cholesterol and triglycerides, serum glucose and/or glycosylated haemoglobin (to evaluate diabetes regulation in diabetic patients). Specialized diagnostic tests are commonly available but have limited effect on the choice of treatment options and are necessary only in situations where there is possibility of a reversible type of ED [16].

Clinical Management

A detailed description of the findings with clear descriptions of the causes and underlying pathophysiology should be provided to patients. This stage should be used as an opportunity to inform patients on sexual function and well-being and to offer an adequate explanation of potential causes. It is important to appropriately clarify both psychogenic and organic factors associated with the onset and maintenance of ED. Available medical and psychological treatment methods must be addressed, even though a particular treatment approach is preferred by the patient. This is consistent with the fundamental concept of patient-centred medicine and collective decision-making.

Lifestyle modifications can be relevant in the prevention or reduction of the severity of ED when comorbidities are present. Evidence suggests that increasing exercise, reducing weight to achieve a body mass index of less than 30 kg/m^2 and quitting smoking can restore erectile function in men with mild to moderate ED [16].

Medical interventions. Type 5 phosphodiesterase inhibitors (PDE5is) are available as oral or sublingual medicines for the treatment of ED. For their activity, PDE5is need desire and sexual stimulation since they improve the normal sexual response by increasing the blood flow and muscle relaxation in the cavernous bodies. Actually, few compounds approved for ED are available in European countries. Sildenafil, vardenafil, tadalafil and avanafil are among the most prescribed. Despite the standard mechanism of action, the pharmacological features of the PDE5is are slightly different. All of them work within 30 minutes to 2 hours (depending on their pharmacokinetic profile), but the duration of action is different (Table 50.1).

Side effects are reported in about 10% of users. Headache, flushing and redness of the face, nasal congestion, indigestion, back pain or muscle aches and changes in vision such as blurredness, blue vision and increased susceptibility to light are the most common side effects.

In order to achieve a maximal response threshold, studies have shown that about one third of patients need six to eight doses and patients who attempt the drug only once or twice may be dissatisfied with the poor clinical effect and withdraw from therapy. The prescription of ED oral pharmacotherapy by a doctor who offers specific directions guarantees the medication is used properly by the patient and involves the partner when possible.

The PDE5is are usually successfully used on an on-demand basis (taken at least 1 hour before intercourse). One PDE5i, tadalafil 5 mg, was approved for once-a-day use, showing similar efficacy and safety as all other PDE5 inhibitors that are available on demand. Tadalafil can offer an interesting alternative on a daily basis as it removes the need to plan sexual activities and thus enables a spontaneous and natural sex life.

Intracavernosal injection therapy is with alprostadil (prostaglandin E1). Other medications, including the combination of phentolamine with either papaverine or a vasoactive intestinal polypeptide (VIP) plus phentolamine, are approved in some countries. Injection therapy is a safe and efficient second-line therapy for men with ED who do not respond to oral therapy or who have PDE5 contraindications such as nitrate or NO donor drugs. The key complication of priapism (unwanted persistent rigid erection lasting longer than 6 hours) can be prevented by medically monitored office visits for dose titration.

Intraurethral suppositories are an officially approved intraurethral medication and contain the same drug (aprostadil) used for intracavernosal injections. In studies the efficacy was inferior to that of intracavernosal injection therapy. The most common adverse effects are penile pain, urethral burning, dizziness and fainting. Candidates for both intracavernosal and intraurethral alprostadil therapy are typically unresponsive to oral drug therapy, mainly because of severe damage to the cavernous nerves, which is often the case after major pelvic surgery for cancer or in patients with severe neurogenic diseases such as polyneuropathy due to diabetes.

Table 50.1 Characteristics and pharmacokinetic of the most available PDE5is

Characteristic	PDE5 inhibitor			
	Avanafil	Sildenafil	Vardenafil	Tadalafil
T_{max} (range)	30–45 min	30–120 min	30–120 min	Not reported
T_{max} (median)	0.5–0.75 h	1 h	1 h	2 h
Effect of food on T_{max}	Delayed by 1.25 h	Delayed by 1 h	Delayed by 1 h	None
Plasma protein binding	99%	96%	95 %	94%
Half-life	6–17 h	3–5 h	4–5 h	17.5 h (mean)
Accumulation in plasma	None	Not reported	None	Not reported

A vacuum pump is a mechanical system which can be used to induce a fully rigid erection. It is a non-invasive procedure that can be used with oral drugs or other ED therapies alone or in combination. Because after vacuum-induced erections, the cavernous bodies are usually filled with low-oxygenated blood, the penis appears more bluish and feels cooler, which makes the erection feel unnatural. Therefore, the rates of vacuum devices' acceptance and long-term use are relatively poor.

A third-line medical care choice for men with severe ED is penile prosthesis. In patients with organic ED, penile implants are usually used when any other therapeutic choice has failed, which is common in patients with long-term diabetes. Often, in severely scarred penises after priapism, or sometimes even in penile curvature (Peyronie's disease), penile prosthesis remains the only alternative. Penile prostheses do not alter the feeling of the penis on the skin or the capacity of a man to achieve orgasm. A penile implant does not affect ejaculation. There is no way back after a penile prosthesis is implanted – that is, if an implant must be removed due to infection or failure and it is not replaced with a new unit, the penis remains non-functional with respect to the erection mechanism. In recent years there has been tremendous improvements in the quality of the implants and reduction in the prevalent of complications [16].

Psychosexual treatment. Psychosexual treatment consists of a variety of interventions, including traditional sex therapy, exercises (such as sensate focus, masturbation exercises, sexual stimulation techniques), cognitive behavioural interventions, interpersonal interventions, systemic interventions, mindfulness training, communication skills training and psychodynamic interventions. The choice of the appropriate interventions and their integration with medical interventions, such as PDE5is, depends on the patient and the couple's needs and wishes. Although medical treatments with PDE5 inhibitors can be used irrespective of the particular ethology of the problem, psychosexual interventions' focus on relationships issues, intimacy and sensitivity to the man and his partner's psychological problems contribute to significant satisfaction with treatment.

Documented research on the effectiveness of psychological therapies for sexual disorders show that psychological approaches are generally successful treatments for sexual dysfunction [22]. The efficacy of cognitive behavioural therapy has been confirmed by studies on ED. In this concept cognitive behavioural therapy uses sensate focus and cognitive restructuring as the primary methods of treatment. Munjack et al. found that, compared to the wait list control group, patients assigned to rational emotive therapy reported significantly more sexual intercourse attempts, higher rates of successful intercourse attempts and decreased sexual anxiety [23]. McCabe et al. indicated that, compared to a control group, men submitted to an internet-based cognitive behavioural intervention showed substantially higher improvements in erectile functioning and sexual relationship satisfaction [24].

Moreover, studies comparing single therapy to the combination of psychological therapy (including sensory focus and cognitive techniques) with drug therapy have shown the superiority of combined therapy. In addition, men in the drug-alone group demonstrated reduced sexual function over time while men in the mixed-treatment group retained improvements in most areas of sexual function.

Sensate focus is aimed at minimizing sexual performance anxiety and encouraging shifts in attention from self-monitoring (spectatoring) to sensual touch-related fun sensations. From non-demanding non-genital contact to genital and intercourse-oriented exercises, the technique uses incremental exposure to sexual activity. In the first step couples, excluding direct genital contact and intercourse, are allowed to participate in mutual touching and pleasurable stimulation. In the second step genital contact and caressing without orgasm are permitted while retaining the restriction on intercourse. The third stage allows intercourse without orgasm, while the fourth and final step allows intercourse with orgasm.

Cognitive restructuring in sex therapy helps to challenge dysfunctional sexual beliefs, shift the meaning attributed to negative sexual events and change the pattern of negative thoughts and emotions during sexual activity. The key elements of cognitive restructuring are: (1) the evaluation of the benefits and drawbacks of sexual beliefs, (2) the analysis of facts for and against beliefs, (3) testing the validity of thoughts in real-life contexts, (4) the development of alternative beliefs and (5) the implementation of alternative beliefs.

Mindfulness-based interventions have been used in the treatment of sexual dysfunction with positive results. Psychological efficacy has been demonstrated by mindfulness-based therapies across a wide variety of health issues, including chronic pain and psychological problems such as generalized anxiety disorder, eating disorders, ruminative feelings, negative affect and persistent depression. Recent studies have indicated a positive impact of mindfulness on the sexual well-being of women [25, 26] and a pilot study has confirmed its feasibility in men with ED [27]. Although these results are just preliminary, they seem promising.

Effective treatment includes the ability to synthesize interventions and adapt them to the patient and the couple's needs, as this may be a key factor for the effectiveness of ED therapy. The healthcare provider must determine the nature of the problem, the relationship and the issues leading to the generation and maintenance of ED.

Premature Ejaculation

Definitions and Epidemiology

Premature ejaculation (PE) has several different clinical forms, ranging from the complaint of a natural phenomenon to a syndrome of sexual dysfunction. Management should therefore be individualized. Premature ejaculation is a self-reported complaint that affects 20–30% of males. Depending on the patient's psychological and physical state, this subjective experience can vary from time to time. Due to diverse assessment modalities and a lack of agreement on its definition, the actual prevalence of PE can change widely from study to study. One of the most objective parameters used to describe PE seems to be the stopwatch-measured intra-vaginal ejaculation latency time (IELT), but loss of control during ejaculation with consequent interpersonal difficulties and distress is also an important diagnostic criterion [28].

According to the DSM-5, PE is defined as continuous or recurrent ejaculation with minimal sexual stimulation before, upon or shortly after penetration within approximately 1 minute of the beginning of sexual activity and before the individual wishes it. Symptoms of early ejaculation must have been present for at least 6 months and must be observed on all or nearly all occasions of sexual activity (approximately 75%) [2].

Most organizations and societies include in their definitions the elements of latency time to ejaculation, the control of ejaculation and the distress or

effect on interpersonal issues. The International Society of Sexual Medicine has implemented a new classification, introduced in 2007 by Waldinger [28, 29]. Two other variant forms were included in the new classification: 'natural variable PE' and 'premature-like ejaculatory dysfunction'. The presence of four different types of PE (lifelong, acquired, natural variable and premature-like ejaculatory dysfunction) indicates different underlying pathogenesis and suggests that, based on the patient's symptoms and expectations, the therapeutic approach should be individualized.

Pathophysiology

The specific aetiology of PE is still unclear, but there are many potential risk factors in its pathogenesis, including a number of biological and psychological factors. The pathogenesis of lifelong and acquired PE is associated with biological factors such as penile hypersensitivity, central serotonin neurotransmission disturbance, hyperthyroidism and local inflammation due to prostatitis. Waldinger et al. suggested that PE may result from dysfunction of the 5-hydroxytryptamine (5-HT) receptor. Waldinger hypothesized that 5-HT2 C receptor hyposensitivity and 5-HT1A receptor hypersensitivity are major neurobiological factors in PE [30].

Only part of the pathophysiology of lifelong and acquired PE can be explained by the role of serotonin disturbance in neurobiological ejaculation control. In addition, the presence of men identified as having the normal variable PE subtype or the premature-like subtype of ejaculatory dysfunction can demonstrate various underlying pathogeneses and indicate that individualized approaches should be used. Several psychological factors can affect sexual dysfunction and PE as well (e.g., anxiety, an early unpleasant sexual experience or violence or adverse family relationships). It is also stated that men with PE have reduced sexual self-confidence, difficulty in establishing relationships and distress about not satisfying their partners.

In natural variable PE men experience early ejaculation in situational or coincidental situations; the issue can be inconsistent and occur irregularly. With either a short or normal ejaculation time, they usually experience reduced ejaculation control. Men with premature-like ejaculatory dysfunction are concerned with an expected premature ejaculation or loss of ejaculation control, but the actual IELT is within the standard duration range or even longer.

Clinical Management

The choice of treatment is dictated by variations in the underlying pathophysiology and the aetiology of the four distinct types of PE. According to the condition and expectations of the patient, the management approach should be individualized. In the management plan the attitude of the partner and the sexual relationship of the couple should also be considered as this could maintain or intensify the dysfunction. Acquired PE treatment is etiologically specific and can include pharmacotherapy for ED in men with comorbid ED. Where psychogenic or relationship causes are present behavioural therapy is suggested, which is often better combined with PE pharmacotherapy in an integrated treatment program. Sexual methods that optimize arousal, should be educated, reassured and instructed. Another method used by many young men is masturbation before the anticipation of sexual intercourse.

Psychological counselling may facilitate the PE patient and his partner in enhancing their overall relationship, and pharmacotherapy may enhance the impact of psychological counselling or behavioural therapy. The principles of treatment are to learn to control ejaculation and to handle and overcome PE's potential impact on the man, partner and couple. The development of performance anxiety, reduced self-esteem, avoidance of sexual activity, frustration and anger of the partner and a substantial decline in the quality of the interpersonal relationship are all possible consequences of PE.

In cognitive behavioural therapy patients begin to understand their negative thinking patterns could lead to PE. They can learn cognitive restructuring – how to exchange negative thoughts for positive affirmations. In sex therapy patients learn to recognize the signs they are about to orgasm and then consider using a 'stop and start' technique where they stop moving during sex to help them relax. In long-term studies, this approach has been shown to be reliable but with lower effectiveness. Clinical studies as well as expert opinion [12] endorse the use of psychological interventions for PE (cognitive restructuring and therapeutic strategies such as stop, start, squeeze and sensory focus), but most outcome studies have so far been uncontrolled with small samples and minimal duration follow-up [31].

Many pharmacological compounds were used to prolong or delay the time of ejaculation; however, some had limited success or many side effects. The ejaculatory adverse effects of selective serotonin reuptake inhibitors (SSRIs), including delayed ejaculation and secondary anejaculation, make these drugs potentially useful in PE management. For PE patients clomipramine, fluoxetine, paroxetine, citalopram, escitalopram and sertraline seem to be effective off-label treatment options (see Table 50.2).

The American Urology Association has since 2004 recommended the use of topical lidocaine-prilocaine cream and serotonergic antidepressants (SSRIs) as a treatment of choice. None of these drugs, however, had Food and Drug Administration (FDA) or European Medicines Agency (EMA)–approved indications for PE treatment. Both clomipramine and SSRIs may delay ejaculation but can cause a decrease in libido and a moderate decrease in penile rigidity, which can negatively effect sexual satisfaction.

Dapoxetine was the first pharmacologic oral agent designed and approved (by both the FDA and the EMA) for the treatment of PE. Dapoxetine is a short-acting SSRI with a half-life of 60–80 minutes and a clearance rate of 95% after 24 hours. Dapoxetine is absorbed orally rapidly. The maximum plasma concentration is approximately 1–2 hours. The characteristics of rapid absorption and clearance have made this novel SSRI suitable for on-demand use. Nausea, dizziness, headache, diarrhea, sleepiness and insomnia are the most common side effects associated with the on-demand use of 30 mg or 60 mg dapoxetine. However, the majority of side effects were intermittent, mild in severity and tolerated by the patient.

During clinical trials orthostatic hypotension and syncope have been observed and should be a safety issue at the time of prescribing. The rate of syncope was 0.19% of participants receiving the first dose of dapoxetine; for subsequent doses, this was reduced to 0.08%. Dapoxetine safety reports showed no signs of mood swings, suicidality, or withdrawal syndrome following treatment, unlike current data on SSRIs. Furthermore, the dapoxetine trials were the first to show positive impact on the couple [29].

Topical anaesthetics have been used to treat PE patients for years. There are many commercial topical preparations, but most are indicated only for local analgesic purposes and not for treatment of PE. Most of these products consist of a cream, ointment, gel or spray formulation mixture of lidocaine and prilocaine and are intended for local anaesthesia. These PE products may cause numbness of the glans or may even cause ED at an excessive

Table 50.2 Dose, side effects and efficacy of drugs used in the management of premature ejaculation
IELT = intravaginal ejaculation latency time; PE = premature ejaculation; ED = erectile dysfunction; SSRI = selective serotonin reuptake inhibitor; PRN = *pro re nata*

Drug	Dose and usage	Side effects	Relative IELT increase
Dapoxetine (licensed SSRI)	30–60 mg PRN	Nausea, Diarrhea, Headache, Dizziness	2.5–3.0
Clomipramine (off-label)	12.5–50 mg PRN/Daily dose	Fatigue, Nausea, Dizziness, Dry mouth, Hypotension	4
SSRI (off-label)	Daily dose	Fatigue, nausea, Diarrhea, Yawing, ED, Libido loss	
Escitalopram	20–40 mg		2
Fluoxetine	20–40 mg		5
Fluvoxamine	25–50 mg		1.5
Paroxetine	10–40 mg		8
Sertraline	50–200 mg		5
Desensitizing agents	Smear PRN	Numbing of vagina, Irritation, ED	4–8
EMLA			
SS cream			
Tempe (PSD502)	Spray		
PDE5-I	PRN	Headache, Flushing, Nausea	
Vardenafil	10 mg		
Sildenafil	50–100 mg		
Tadalafil	10 mg		
Tramadol	50 mg PRN	Dizziness, Nausea, Addiction	3.6–7.0

dose. Well-designed clinical trials are warranted to address safety concerns about systemic side effects of lidocaine and the impact on the female partner of transvaginal absorption. To treat lifelong PE, a novel aerosolized lidocaine-prilocaine (2.5%) spray called PSD502 was recently developed. Nine natural herb extracts comprise another topical preparation called SS cream. The precise mechanism of action remains unclear [29].

Tramadol is a powerful analgesic that combines the activation of the opioid receptor and 5-hydroxytryptamine (5-HT) and noradrenaline reuptake inhibition. The mechanism of action of tramadol's non-opioid portion is mediated by inhibiting the reuptake of noradrenaline and 5-HT via alpha2-agonistic and serotoninergic activities. This characteristic, its short half-life (1.7 hours) and quick absorption have made tramadol a possible on-demand treatment for PE. Guidelines do not support the use of tramadol for the treatment of PE due to the lack of good efficacy and safety evidence from large-scale clinical trials and because of the risk of

addiction [29]. There are few publications about the use of PDE5is for the treatment of PE; PDE5is are recommended for patients with both PE and comorbid ED. However, clinical trials have not confirmed their use in PE patients without ED [29]. Using surgical procedures to treat PE is not supported by clinical trials and currently no guidelines recommend it.

Delayed Ejaculation

Definitions and Epidemiology

Usually delayed ejaculation is a self-reported diagnosis; there is no clear agreement about what constitutes a reasonable orgasm-attaining timeline. The DSM-5 and ICD-11 describe delayed ejaculation as belonging to a category of sexual dysfunctions usually characterized by a clinically relevant failure to sexually respond or experience sexual pleasure [1, 2]. To define a significant delay in or inability to achieve ejaculation, the term *delayed ejaculation* (DE) (also called retarded or inhibited ejaculation) has been used. The man experiences difficulty or inability to ejaculate despite the existence of sufficient sexual stimulation and the intention to ejaculate. The condition must persist for at least 6 months with no particular defined ejaculation latency duration. The disorder is only a problem for the patient or his partner if it causes severe distress. The diagnosis is made by self-report in most cases.

Delayed ejaculation is one of the least known, least common and least researched of all male sexual disorders. This disorder may be lifelong (primary) or acquired (secondary). It can also be global or situational. Available literature has shown that DE is associated with substantial reduction in health-related quality of life as well as self-esteem, anxiety and depression and has been linked to decreased sexual satisfaction and relationship dissatisfaction and discord.

The ejaculation process involves two clinically indistinguishable phases of emission and ejaculation, which usually require external genital stimulation (nocturnal emissions being the notable exception) from the pudendal nerves; efferent impulses migrate to the upper lumbar spinal sympathetic nuclei. Through the hypogastric nerve the impulses activate secretions and transport of sperm from the distal epididymis, vasa differentia, seminal vesicles and prostate to the prostatic urethra. Closure of the bladder neck and concomitant relaxation of the outer sphincter direct semen to the bulbous urethra, leading to emission.

The somatomotor efferent fibres of the pudendal nerve then cause the bulbocavernous muscle's subsequent rhythmic contractions, pushing the semen into a pressurized passage (the narrowed urethral lumen squeezed by the engorged cavernosa corpora) and releasing 2–5 mL of ejaculate. Since this action is involuntary, integrated autonomic and somatic actions are required for completion. The posteromedial bed nucleus of the stria terminalis, the posterodorsal medial amygdaloid nucleus, the posterodorsal preoptic nucleus and the parvicellular portion of the subparafascicular thalamus are the cerebral network that modulates and controls the final common output from all ejaculatory stimuli. The ejaculatory reflex has been suggested to be predominantly regulated by the central serotonergic and dopaminergic systems, with secondary functions being played by other neurotransmitters (e.g., nitric oxide, acetylcholine, oxytocin, adrenaline and gamma-aminobutyric acid (GABA)) [33].

It is estimated that the prevalence of DE is 1–4% of males. The true incidence of DE is not well known and there is no generally accepted accurate description of the disease. After the age of 50 years, the frequency of DE starts to increase. Compared to men younger than 59 years, men in their 80s experience twice as much trouble ejaculating [8]. Ejaculate volume is androgen-dependent and decreases with age; this decrease can result in a blunted orgasm experience in the elderly. I?n older men the age-related loss of fast-conducting peripheral sensory nerves, as well as with age-related reduction in sex steroid secretion, may be associated with the increased frequency of DE.

Pathophysiology

The assessment of this condition involves a focussed sexual and medical history, enquiries about the status of the partner and a physical examination that includes genitalia. In certain instances, in an attempt to achieve orgasm, there is a pattern of long-continued thrusting, which is sustained until the man becomes tired or experiences genital pain, thereby discontinuing his efforts. A persistent pattern of difficulty in ejaculating can lead a man to avoid sexual activity. Furthermore, some sexual partners may report feeling less sexually attractive due to this ejaculatory difficulty.

A history of injury or surgery is significant. In about 40% of patients with bilateral sympathectomy at the L2 level, ejaculatory dysfunction has been documented. High bilateral retroperitoneal lymphadenectomy may cause an even higher percentage of emission failures. Retrograde ejaculation can result from a dysfunction of the internal sphincter or bladder neck (e.g., post prostatectomy) following alpha-blocker therapy or autonomic neuropathy due to diabetes. It is mandatory to have a careful history of alcohol and illegal drug use. Delayed orgasm and anorgasmia were specifically associated with marijuana, methylenedioxy-N-methylamphetamine (MDMA or ecstasy) and alcohol consumption.

In a differential diagnosis the following groups of prescribed medications should be considered: alpha-adrenergic blockers (retrograde ejaculation), combined alpha- and beta-adrenergic blockers (inhibited ejaculation), sympathetic nerve blockers – guanethidine (ED and retrograde ejaculation) and tricyclic antidepressants (via increased serotonin-inhibited ejaculation). Clomipramine was reported to induce anorgasmia within days of starting treatment, which persisted with minimal tolerance over 5 months of clomipramine therapy. Monoamine oxidase inhibitors (via increased serotonin-inhibited ejaculation and decreased libido), SSRIs (via increased serotonin anorgasmia in 8–30%) and antipsychotics (mainly via increased prolactin and serotoninergic activity decrease libido and inhibit ejaculation) should also be considered [33, 34].

Psychological causes have been linked to primary suppressed male orgasm (e.g., a history of trauma, extreme guilt, a fear of pregnancy and ambivalence about children, or hostility towards a woman). In case of fear of pregnancy, the anejaculation is situational and often presents inability to ejaculate intravaginally. An increased frequency of DE can also be related to major depressive disorder.

Clinical Management

Laboratory tests attempt to identify abnormalities in the blood count, amount of glucose, level of hormones or function of the kidney. If a corrective aetiology is found therapy is aimed at correcting this disorder. Since it is poorly understood, DE is not easy to treat. The treatment for anejaculation is determined according to the cause of the problem and may include psychosexual or drug therapy or combined treatment for the patient and their spouse.

In case fertility is the reason for the clinical consultation, the infertility issue may need to be discussed first. If anejaculation alone is the reason for not having children and there is urgent request for fertility or in patients with spinal cord injury, penile vibratory stimulation (PVS) or electroejaculation (EEJ) can be applied. In PVS a vibrator is positioned against the penis and mechanical stimulation is given to induce ejaculation. Although PVS is a relatively secure and low-cost alternative, at least one intact segment of the lumbosacral spinal cord (above T10) is required. Electroejaculation may be effective in obtaining ejaculate of all forms of spinal cord injury. Usually EEJ is transrectally carried out in the lateral decubitus or dorsal lithotomy position. During stimulation antegrade ejaculation is captured and in case of retrograde ejaculation the semen is collected through post-procedural urine bladder catheterization. Measurements to prevent side effects mainly originating from autonomic dysreflexia should be applied [35]. With respect to fertility

issues, in cases of primary male anorgasmia, according to anecdotal report, an electro-vibrator applied at the lower surface of the glans penis can be an effective intervention [36].

In case of drug-induced anorgasmia, dose reduction, a drugs holiday or switching medications should be discussed. For antidepressant-induced inhibited male orgasm, consideration may be given to switching to or adding bupropion, mirtazapine or trazodone, which have fewer sexual side effects than do SSRIs [33]. Many agents of varying degrees of effectiveness have been reported as drug therapy for DE. Currently, the FDA and EMA have approved no drug to treat DE. Options include testosterone, cabergoline, bupropion, amantadine, cyproheptadine, imipramine, yohimbine, bethanechol and buspirone [33].

Many psychological aspects are correlated with DE. Despite having no difficulties in obtaining or maintaining erections, men with DE clearly indicate low levels of subjective sexual arousal and pleasure [34]. In addition, relative to sexually healthy men, these men report high levels of relationship distress, sexual dissatisfaction, anxiety about their sexual performance and lower frequencies of intercourse [37]. In addition, fear of impregnating the partner or transmitting sexually transmitted diseases and insufficient physical stimulation are common factors identified in men with DE [37]. Anger against the partner was also discovered in men with DE [38]. Historical factors may act as predisposing factors for DE, such as traumatic or negative past sexual experiences, negative cognitions about sex and strict or rigid religious or moral background and uncommon habits of masturbation [39].

Men suffering from DE will benefit from various psychological interventions, including sex education, goal-oriented anxiety reduction, improved and more genitally centred stimulation and sensate focus. A significant aspect of therapy is self-stimulation techniques that integrate fantasy, helping men to enhance sexual arousal and satisfaction. In addition, the reduction of demand or performance anxiety during sexual activity, which benefits from sensate focus exercises as well as cognitive restructuring, is an essential component of the treatment [39]. Couples or marital counselling can be suggested when serious relationship issues are present. There are few randomized controlled trail trials evaluating the effectiveness of current psychological treatments, but clinical and expert opinion endorse the use of this range of treatment approaches for DE [40].

References

1. Reisman Y, Porst H, Lowenstein L, Tripodi MF, Kirana PS (eds.). *The ESSM manual of sexual medicine*. Amsterdam: Medix, 2015.

2. American Psychiatric Association. *Diagnostic and statistical manual of mental disorders*. 5th edition. Washington, DC: American Psychiatric Association, 2013.

3. World Health Organization. *International statistical classification of diseases and related health problems*. 11th revision. Geneva: World Health Organization, 2018. https://icd.who.int/browse11/l-m/en.

4. Mitchell KR, Mercer CH, Ploubidis GB et al. Sexual function in Britain: Findings from the third National Survey of Sexual Attitudes and Lifestyles (NATSAL-3). *Lancet*. 2013;**382**:1817–29.

5. Reisman Y, Eardley I, Porst H. New developments in education and training in sexual medicine. *J Sex Med*. 2013;**10**(4):918–23. https://doi.org/10.1111/jsm .12140.

6. Seagraves KB, Segraves KRT. Hypoactive sexual desire disorder: Prevalence and comorbidity. *J Sex Marital Ther*. 1991;**17**:55–8.

7. Brotto LA. The DSM diagnostic criteria for hypoactive sexual desire disorder in men. *J Sex Med*. 2010;**7**:2015–30.

8. Lindau ST, Schumm LP, Laumann EO et al. A study of sexuality and health among older adults in the United States. *N Engl J Med*. 2007;**357**:762–74.

9. Gabrielson AT, Sartor RA, Hellstrom WJG. The impact of thyroid disease on sexual dysfunction in men and women. *Sex Med Rev*. 2019;**7**:57–7. https:// doi.org/10.1016/j.sxmr.2018.05.002.

10. Carvalho J, Nobre PJ. Predictors of men's sexual desire: The role of psychological, cognitive-emotional, relational, and medical factors. *J Sex Res*. 2011;**48**(2–3):254–62. https://doi.org/10.1080 /00224491003605475.

11. Carvalho J, Nobre PJ. Biopsychosocial determinants of men's sexual desire: Testing an integrative model. *J Sex Med*. 2011;**8**(2):754–63.

12. Nimbi FM, Tripodi F, Rossi R, Simonelli C. Expanding the analysis of psychosocial factors of sexual desire in men. *J Sex Med*. 2018;**15**(2):230–44. https://doi.org/10.1016/j.jsxm.2017.11.227.

13. Brotto L, Atallah S, Johnson-Agbakwu C et al. Psychological and interpersonal dimensions of sexual function and dysfunction. *J Sex Med*. 2016;**13**:538–71. http://dx.doi.org/10.1016/j.jsxm.2016.01.019.

14. Nobre PJ. Treatments for sexual dysfunctions. In Hoffman S (ed.). *Clinical psychology: A global perspective*. Hoboken, NJ: Wiley-Blackwell, 2017, pp. 225–41.

15. Rosen RC, Cappelleri JC, Smith MD et al. Development and evaluation of an abridged, 5-item version of the International Index of Erectile Function (IIEF-5) as a diagnostic tool for erectile dysfunction. *Int J Impot Res*. 1999;**11**:319–26.

16. Porst H. Erectile dysfunction. In Reisman Y, Porst H, Lowenstein L, Tripodi MF, Kirana PS (eds.). *The ESSM manual of sexual medicine*. Amsterdam: Medix, 2015, pp. 426–543.

17. Quinta-Gomes A, Nobre PJ. Personality traits and psychopathology on male sexual dysfunction: An empirical study. *J Sex Med*. 2011;**8**:461–9.

18. Nobre PJ, Pinto-Gouveia J. Dysfunctional sexual beliefs as vulnerability factors to sexual dysfunction. *J Sex Res*. 2006;**43**:68–75.

19. Nobre PJ. Psychological determinants of erectile dysfunction: Testing a cognitive-emotional model. *J Sex Med*. 2010;**7**:1429–37.

20. Nobre PJ, Pinto-Gouveia J. Differences in automatic thoughts presented during sexual activity between sexually functional and dysfunctional males and females. *J Cognit Therapy and Research*. 2008;**32**:37–49.

21. Nobre PJ, Pinto-Gouveia J. Emotions during sexual activity: Differences between sexually functional and dysfunctional men and women. *Archives of Sexual Behavior*. 2006;**35**:8–15.

22. Frühauf S, Gerger H, Schmidt HM et al. Efficacy of psychological interventions for sexual dysfunction: A systematic review and meta-analysis. *Archives of Sexual Behavior*. 2013;**42**(6):915–33. https://doi.org/ 10.1007/s10508-012-0062-0.

23. Munjack DJ, Schlaks A, Sanchez VC et al. Rational-emotive therapy in the treatment of erectile failure: An initial study. *J Sex and Marital Therapy*. 1984;**10**:170–5. https://doi.org/10.1080 /00926238408405942.

24. McCabe M, Price E, Piterman L, Lording D. Evaluation of an Internet-based psychological intervention for the treatment of erectile dysfunction. *Intern J Impot Research*. 2008;**20**:324–30. https://doi .org/10.1038/ijir.2008.3.

25. Brotto L, Basson R, Luria M. A mindfulness-based group psychoeducational intervention targeting sexual arousal disorder in women. *J Sex Med*. 2008;**5**:1646–59.

26. Brotto L, Heiman J. Mindfulness in sex therapy: Applications for women with sexual difficulties following gynaecologic cancer. *Sexual & Relationship Therapy*. 2007;**22**:3–11.

27. Bossio JA, Basson R, Driscoll M et al. Mindfulness-based group therapy for men with situational erectile dysfunction: A mixed-methods feasibility analysis and pilot study. *J Sex Med*. 2018;**15**(10):1478–90. https://doi.org/10.1016/j.jsxm.2018.08.013.

28. Waldinger MD. Premature ejaculation: Definition and drug treatment. *Drugs*. 2007;**67**:547–68.

29. Althof SE, McMahhon CG, Waldinger MD et al. An update of the International Society of Sexual Medicine's Guidelines for the Diagnosis and Treatment of Premature Ejaculation (PE). *Sex Med*. 2014;**2**(2):60–90.

30. Waldinger M. The neurobiological approach to premature ejaculation. *J Urol*. 1998;**168**:2359–67.

31. Berner M, Günzler C. Efficacy of psychosocial interventions in men and women with sexual dysfunctions: A systematic review of controlled clinical trials. Part 1. The efficacy of psychosocial interventions for male sexual dysfunction. *J Sex Med*. 2012;**9**:3089–3107.

32. Giuliano F. Neurophysiology of erection and ejaculation. *J Sex Med*. 2011;**8**:310–15.

33. Clayton A, Croft HA, Handiwala L. Antidepressants and sexual dysfunction: Mechanisms and clinical implications. *Post Med*. 2014;**126**:91–9.

34. Giuliano F, Clement P. Physiology of ejaculation: Emphasis on serotonergic control. *Eur Urol*. 2005;**48**:408–17. https://doi.org/10.1016/j.eururo.2005.05.017.

35. Sønksen J, Ohl DA. Penile vibratory stimulation and electroejaculation in the treatment of ejaculatory dysfunction. *Int J Androl*. 2002;**25**:324–32. https://doi.org/10.1046/j.1365-2605.2002.00378.x.

36. Jenkins LC, Mulhall JP. Delayed orgasm and anorgasmia. *Fertil Steril*. 2015;**104**(5):1082–8.

37. Rowland D, Van Diest S, Incrocci L, Slob AK. Psychosexual factors that differentiate men with inhibited ejaculation from men with no dysfunction or another sexual dysfunction. *J Sex Med*. 2005;**2**(3):383–9.

38. Perelman MA, Rowland DL. Retarded ejaculation. *World J Urology*. 2006;**24**:645–52.

39. Rowland D, Perelman M, Althof S et al. Self-reported premature ejaculation and aspects of sexual functioning and satisfaction. *J Sex Med*. 2004;**1**(2):225–32.

40. Wincze JP, Carey MP. *Sexual dysfunction: A guide for assessment and treatment*. 2nd edition. New York: Guilford Press. 2001.

Chapter

51

Life-Course Approach to Sexual Health

Johannes Bitzer

Introduction

Sexual Health

The World Health Organization (WHO) defines sexual health in a comprehensive way [1, 2]. It is a central aspect of being human throughout life that encompasses sex, gender identities and roles, sexual orientation, eroticism, pleasure, intimacy and reproduction. Sexuality is experienced and expressed in thoughts, fantasies, desires, beliefs, attitudes, values, behaviours, practices, roles and relationships. While sexuality can include all of these dimensions, not all of them are always experienced or expressed. Sexuality is influenced by the interaction of biological, psychological, social, economic, political, cultural, legal, historical, religious and spiritual factors.

Life-Cycle Approach to Sexual Health

A life-course approach considers an individual's entire progress throughout life to explain why certain outcomes result [3–6]. The outcomes depend on the interaction of multiple protective and risk factors throughout people's lives. These factors include biological (including genetics), behavioural and social factors which throughout life and across generations act independently, cumulatively and interactively to influence health outcomes.

Health is hereby understood as the result of a dynamic interaction between risks/stressors on one side and protective factors on the other side across an individual's lifetime. The life course itself is described as a sequence of stages:childhood, adolescence, adulthood, late adulthood, old age

Childhood

Risk Factors (Stressors) for Sexual Health

The risk factors can be divided into factors from outside the child having a possible negative impact on the development of sexual health [7–11].

Environment

A broken family can experience persistent aggression among parents, separation and violence. In war and conflict children and women are the first and most severely damaged victims with follow-up morbidity. Migration, with its insecurity and constantly changing and threatening environment, puts children at risk of developing physical and mental disease with impact on their later sexual life.

There are also destructive sexual norms with the negation, suppression and punishment regarding child sexuality and sexual expression which create insecurity, fear, feeling of guilt and so forth which hinder healthy sexual development. A lack of child protection with no laws protecting children against violence contributes to the problem, as does children working with the consequence that children cannot learn and develop but are exploited in the workforce.

Individual

Not having a loving interpersonal environment can create a basic feeling of insecurity about one's own worth and can create mistrust. If there is no response to the needs of the child, including bodily needs like hunger and pain, the feeling of basic safety is difficult to obtain, and children are subject to different forms of abuse [9, 10]. The central element of abuse is that the adult person uses the helplessness of the child and his/her power over the child to satisfy his or her needs and desires, ignoring or denying the needs of the child. This lack of empathy and resonance by the adult damages the building up of positive representations of the self of the child with regard to his or her own value and what is right or wrong.

Protective Factors (Resources)

Important resources allow the child to develop sexual health.

Environment

A peaceful environment, including absence of war, conflicts and violence, is a precondition for healthy development. Another important factor is healthy families, which are defined by an internal culture of respect for all members, including the respect for boundaries, the ability of the family to cope with differences in values and opinions, negotiation and conflict-resolution skills and a habit of supporting each other, thus creating an atmosphere of security and reliability.

A comprehensive sexuality education and violence-free school environment empowers children by giving them answers to the many questions they have, especially as they are now exposed to social media with very mixed messages regarding what sexuality is, what it means and how it works. Child protection through law is an important protective factor as well.

Individual

A loving environment, support and so forth provides the basis to a general feeling of being in a world which is understandable and can be trusted, including the perception of the child's body. The child gains some basic security and connectedness and is enabled to establish stable patterns of relationship with others and with his/her body.

Possible Consequences for Sexual Health

If the risk factors outweigh the protective factors, these children may develop different physical, mental and behavioural symptoms. Abuse of the child's body can lead to chronic pain syndromes in the genital region. Victims of violence and abuse are at higher risk to become perpetrators themselves and abuse their own children (see Chapter 52 on sexual violence). Another consequence may manifest itself in difficulties to establish a trustful intimate relationship because of insecurity and mistrust which was experienced at this early age.

Sexual and Reproductive Health Prevention and Care

Prevention is based on early detection of parents and children at risk (see also Chapter 56). Some countries now have different programmes like the National Society for the Prevention of Cruelty to Children's (NSPCC) Underwear Rule [8, 10], which provides parents the tools to talk with their children about personal boundaries and self-awareness so as to prevent abuse. Such efforts could be preventing a lifetime of personal and social cost.

The school plays a central role not only in educational attainment, but also in the social development of children. In different countries different initiatives and programmes exist to provide children education about health and specifically also about sexuality. Age-appropriate sexuality education is at the centre of this prevention (see also Chapter 6).

Contact with the healthcare system during regular check-ups allows paediatricians and general practitioners to be sensitive to signals of parent–child interactions which represent risks for the development of the child and also to signs indicating physical and sexual abuse.

Adolescence

Adolescence is a time of great change both physically and emotionally [12–18]. The body undergoes a process of maturation towards the adult body with development of the reproductive potential (maturation of the HHO and the HHT axis and other parts of the neuroendocrine system). This is accompanied by various psychosocial challenges like separation from the family of origin, living in a peer group, life in school, learning and achievement. Regarding sexual health, this is the time of having the first sexual experiences and building a sexual identity.

Risk Factors and Stressors

Risks and stressors can be in the social environment but also in individual development.

Environment

A hostile and negative family and cultural environment towards sexuality considering it as dangerous or sinful, with many prohibitions and warnings, can hinder the development of a sexual identity and can inhibit experiencing sexuality as a source of pleasure. This is often combined with a complete lack of sexuality education. Emotionally traumatic, humiliating experiences during the first sexual encounters make sex a bad experience which will be retained in memory. Sexual violence and peer group pressure are unfortunately frequent risks as well.

Another risk comes from the impact of social media soliciting new images and norms regarding body image and behaviours which again hinder adolescents from finding their own way. A special threat comes from sexual harassment via the Internet with possible long-standing implications. A very vulnerable group are adolescents with non-heterosexual orientation and gender dysphoria who suffer social discrimination and bullying because of differences in sexual preferences and orientation.

Individual

Unintended pregnancies with feelings of guilt and sadness in the context of termination of pregnancy or teenage pregnancies and early childbirth with interruption of the education and personal development can present serious developmental crises. The experience of having been infected via sexual intercourse and contracting a sexually transmitted infection (STI), including HIV, can change the inner concept of sexuality as something pleasurable to something dangerous and dirty. The same is true if the adolescent is exposed to sexual violence.

Protective Factors (Resources)

There are important protective factors in the environment and within the individual.

Environment

The main elements are a sexually friendly and open environment (family, peer group, society) as well as sexual and reproductive health education and appropriate integrated services.

Individual

Adolescence is the phase of building a sexual identity and a personal sexual script and what can be called sexual intelligence and the skills to interact with partners. The first intimate encounter is a moment of high expectation and vulnerability with pleasurable excitement and anxious self-observation. This experience can in some individuals act as a learning matrix providing self-confidence and openness.

Adolescent sexuality is conscious and unconscious, a cognitive and emotional process towards an adolescent's sexual identity, including sexual preferences, sexual orientation, and gender identity. Allowing this process means that the adolescent can find out who he/she is and what she/he wants and what she/he does not want.

The development of personal resilience is an important acquisition during adolescence [18]. Resilience describes the capacity of a person to cope with critical life events. It is based on the development of specific personality traits, including optimism,

self-confidence, problem-solving capacities, social skills of communicating with others and getting help from others and the capacity to make realistic plans and take steps to carry them out, as well as emotional regulation. These are important skills to live a self-determined sexual life.

Frequent Sexual Health Problems

If the risk factors outweigh the protective factors, these adolescents may develop different physical, mental and behavioural symptoms with an impact on their sexual health. One consequence can be high-risk behaviour based on an incapacity to control emotions and impulsive behaviour with increased risk of contracting STIs, occurrence of unintended pregnancies and exposure to violence and drugs [17]. Another consequence of negative sexual experiences can be the development of avoidance and ambivalence towards sexuality with loss of interest and/or orgasmic difficulties but also sexual pain due to medical reasons (pelvic inflammatory disease as a consequence of STIs) or due to psychological factors like anxiety and guilt.

As described earlier, lack of sexual education and problematic messages in the media can lead to body image dissatisfaction, alienation from one's own body and even body dysmorphic disorders with requests for repetitive operations. Social discrimination and bullying of members of the LGBTQ+ community can lead to sexual dysfunctions, depression and suicide.

Sexual and Reproductive Health Prevention and Care

Age-adapted sexual education in school is one of the most important tools of prevention (see related chapters) with national programmes focussing on this age group's needs. Adolescent-friendly sexual and reproductive health (SRH) services should integrate contraception, protection against STIs, sexual counselling, emergency care for victims of sexual violence in an environment of confidentiality and easy access tailored to the special needs of this age group, including HIV screening and prevention, integrated sexual healthcare services and screening for at-risk adolescents (behavioural, environmental, victimization).

There are different special target groups which are frequently underserved. One is adolescent girls with sexual pain. Many of these girls are insecure as to which degree having pain is a sign of weakness and not normal and therefore do not ask for help. These girls may suffer from untreated vulvovaginal disease, endometriosis, vaginismus, orgasmic difficulties or having no desire. Another vulnerable group is boys with premature ejaculation or small penis syndrome. A very important group are adolescent girls and boys with gender dysphoria, homosexuality, sexual preferences experienced as irritating and creating anxiety and victims of discrimination and violence.

Adulthood

This life phase is characterized by choosing and performing a job, stable relationship, marriage, pregnancy, postpartum and settling down [19–24]. One of the big psychosocial challenges is care for children and adolescents and at the same time care for the elderly members of a family.

Risks and Stressors

The life phase typical stressors can be differentiated again into environmental and individual categories.

Environment

Many studies have shown that poverty has a negative impact on sexual well-being due to constant concerns and anxiety related to lack of control and satisfaction of basic needs. In a society in which a person's identity is strongly related to work the loss of a job can impair self-esteem and increase insecurity and depressed mood with negative impact on sexual health. Another factor is chronic distress (allostatic overload) at the workplace and in the family.

Social media produce images and stories about an ecstatic sex life, creating expectations which are not fulfilled in a real-life setting. Although there is a sensitization in many countries regarding sexual harassment and different forms of sexual violence, there is still a high prevalence of no respect and transgression of limits. At the same time there is insecurity in individuals who are not sure whether their wishes and fantasies are normal and correspond to their moral standard and self-image.

Individual

On the individual level, in this life phase, gynaecological disorders with symptoms like dysmenorrhea, heavy or irregular bleeding and pain can have a negative impact. The unfulfilled wish for a child represents a life crisis in which life objectives and plans are questioned with destabilization of the mind and distress for the relationship, including sexual problems.

Pregnancy complications with anxiety and traumatic experiences can have an actual or long-standing impact on sexual health. The experience of the mother of loss of control, helplessness and herself and the baby being in danger are frequently overlooked in having the focus of care on healthy outcomes of mother and baby. Postpartum depression is frequently accompanied by loss of desire and other sexual dysfunctions. The menopausal transition is not a disease but is accompanied by physical and endocrine changes which may negatively impact sexual health. There are many psychosocial stressors, including separation, divorce, loss of loved ones and so forth.

Protective Factors

Environment

Socioeconomic stability provides a background for individuals to feel safe and protected and reduce the necessity to live in the *survival modus*, a status of alarm and distress. Medical and psychotherapeutic professionals and their societies provide material which is accessible on the Internet to diminish myths and misconceptions about love and sex.

Workplace conditions taking into account the sexual health needs of employees can protect women and men from destructive contacts and experiences, including taking into account special needs for example for menopausal women. Accessibility to medical and psychological services can provide counselling at early stages of sexual problems. One of the most important protective factors is a loving, trustful relationship with the partner and family.

Individual

Life satisfaction is the result of a person's subjective judgement about the fulfilment or non-fulfilment of needs and expectations in actual life. Satisfaction is thus the result of the match between the environment (outer reality) and subjective needs and wishes. Persons who have learnt to accept that not all wishes will be fulfilled and to be satisfied with less-perfect (not optimal but good enough) realities are less prone to frustration and subjectively experienced dysfunctions. The same is true regarding resilience, as a partially inborn, partially acquired personality trait which facilitate a person's adaptation to changes and capacity to cope with crisis.

Frequent Sexual Health Problems

Pregnancy and birth complications can become traumatic experiences with psychosocial consequences including sexual dysfunctions like low desire and sexual aversion. The postpartum period is a time with many endocrine and psychological changes (low oestrogen, becoming mother and father, from the dyadic relationship to the triad, etc.), which frequently manifest as differences in desire between partners and changing sexual needs and priorities (closeness versus passion, etc.).

In the context of diseases sexual health may be impaired by different pathways, including destruction of organs involved in the sexual response or the endocrine and autonomous regulation of the response, but also through consequences of medical and surgical therapies. The main malignant diseases having an impact on sexual health are cervical carcinoma, endometrial carcinoma, breast cancer and their treatments

In this life phase women enter the pre and perimenopause, which is characterized by irregular and sometimes heavy bleeding due to lack of progesterone and oestrogen fluctuations. Many women experience symptoms like hot flushes, sleeping problems and irritability which can negatively impact sexuality and may lead to low desire and arousal difficulties. Some women may develop the so-called urogenital syndrome of menopause with recurrent bladder infections and vulvovaginal atrophy which again can lead to sexual pain and avoidance of sexual activity.

Differences in values and needs as well as the possible disparities in personal development can lead to partner conflicts which may ultimately end in separation and divorce. This can become a traumatic experience with a long-lasting negative impact on sexual health and well-being.

Prevention and Care

The basic strategies are the same as described earlier. An important additional strategy specific to this life phase is to focus on the Integration of sexual medicine in the training of general practitioners and medical specialists. This integration of medical sexology is an important support to give patients with benign and malignant diseases access to help with benign and malignant gynaecological diseases.

The same is true in the field of obstetrical care where women in the postpartum period need caregivers to diagnose and help with the various affective disorders which may develop. Women need information and education about the impact of pregnancy and childbirth on sexual function during pregnancy care and at postpartum control visits by obstetricians.

Women and men have questions about sexuality during pregnancy. What is allowed? What is not allowed? How do feelings change? What is normal? An important pillar of prevention and care are menopause clinics in which women can find holistic and comprehensive care, including sexual healthcare. Midlife consultations for men, including assessment of cardiovascular risks and sexual dysfunction, should be considered.

Ageing

Various biological changes occur due to the ageing process of the body with diminution of functions like sight, hearing and memory [25–28]. Some of these changes can be accentuated by hormonal transitions like the menopause in women and the andropause in men. On the psychosocial level many other challenges occur like decline in professional performance and capacity, increased morbidity and loss of partners and friends.

Risks and Stressors

The sexual biography with the transition through the different previous phases like traumatic experiences can be a source of risk manifesting itself in later stages.

Environment

In many societies ageing increases the risk for poverty, discrimination, loneliness and isolation. Modern societies have a youth- and performance-oriented culture in which elderly persons may feel not at home or alienated. Being old is per se negative and should be avoided by rejuvenation, meaning the needs of the elderly regarding mobility, participation and integration are not met, including inequalities in healthcare.

Individual

Ageing as a general process includes changes in all organ systems, especially in the neurovascular and neuromuscular systems, with a possible negative effect on all phases of the human sexual response. There are many other risks and stressors to sexual health like the age-related increase in morbidity, including cardiovascular diseases, malignant diseases and neurological diseases with medications which impact sexual health.

As described earlier, women's reproductive phase ends with the menopause, which means that ageing is accompanied by the cessation of ovarian hormone production. This has various general health consequences (e.g., increased risk of osteoporosis), including sexual health in general and leading to various sexual dysfunctions in both sexes.

The ageing couple is confronted with a different dynamic of changes between the partners and also a change in needs and wishes of both, leading to relationship difficulties and conflicts with either excluding sexuality or involvement of a third party (unofficial or official).

Protective Factors

Taking into account the fact that many European societies have a demography in which the percentage of women and men over 65 is increasing and is higher than the percentage of children and young people, it is important to have a stronger focus on 'ageing well' as an aim of politics and health care

Environment

Safe economic conditions with no daily concern and stress regarding economic survival facilitate living a sexual life and being sexually active. Special living conditions for the elderly which respond to their physical but also their emotional and interpersonal needs include the elderly in community work and create contacts between the generations.

Individual

A healthy lifestyle, including nutrition, exercise, developing hobbies, continuous learning and creative activities are the mainstay of ageing well. Family support, shared interests and values with others provides the feeling of belonging to something greater than oneself. Individual resilience is based on optimism, adaptation to change, problem-solving capacity and life experience and personal growth with basic feelings about life of coherence and meaningfulness [29].

Frequent Sexual Health Problems

Different types of sexual dysfunctions may occur. There is an age-related statistical decline in sexual interest and desire, more in women, but also in men with a large variability among individuals, but at the same time individual sexual needs and interest can be lifelong. A large proportion of the ageing population is not distressed by this change, especially if both partners feel the same. Relationship distress can occur when there is a discrepancy of needs between the partners and this conflict of needs cannot be resolved.

Loss of desire and sexual interest may also develop as a consequence of the hormonal changes (decline in testosterone and oestrogen). Testosterone is linked to spontaneous desire in both sexes (in men more than in women). Oestrogen seems to enhance the pro-sexual effect of testosterone to the brain, having a psychotropic effect by itself.

Arousal disorder in this age group can be a consequence of vascular disease or drug treatment in both sexes. Erectile dysfunction is a frequent problem with age-related increases in incidence. It can be the first sign of a cardiovascular problem and should be evaluated.

Local oestrogen plays an important role in women in maintaining healthy and functional peripheral tissue (vulvovaginal region) and blood flow to the vagina. Pain during attempts to have intercourse can be the result of vulvovaginal atrophy in women due to the loss of oestrogen action. Other possible reasons include the lack of adequate stimulation to the partner, rare attempts to practise intercourse or practising intercourse to please the partner without wanting it.

Prevention and Care

Sexuality in the elderly population is still taboo in many societies and groups. There is a need for education and information by medical experts, including media work to normalize sexual needs and activities in this life phase without building up new norms but encouraging individual sexual expression.

The integration of sexual healthcare into general care for patients with cardiovascular, oncologic, neurologic and psychiatric diseases will help to include the elderly via their medical care. It is in these consultations that the healthcare provider can help elderly individuals or couples to talk about their sexual needs and wishes (belonging, intimacy, pleasure, reliability, closeness), look for resources (e.g., shared life history etc.), understand the limitations (morbidity, age), help them to redefine their sexuality and help those with limitations to reach rehabilitation of their sexual life in a realistic way (see also Chapter 46).

Summary

The life-course approach to sexual health takes into account the different needs, challenges and opportunities of women and men regarding their sexual health during childhood, adolescence, adulthood and ageing [30]. In each life phase risks and stressors from the environment and the individual can occur, but protective factors are also known. The interaction of stressors and resources contributes to the individual's sexual health. Sexual healthcare should, apart from those practices appropriate throughout life like the general sexual medicine interventions, try to adapt to the different age groups

References

1. World Health Organization. *Defining sexual health: Report of a technical consultation on sexual health.* 2002. Geneva: World Health Organization, 2006.

2. World Health Organization. *Sexual health and its linkages to reproductive health: An operational approach.* Geneva: World Health Organization, 2017. https://bit.ly/3HEG7KR.

3. Health matters: A life course approach. http://bit.ly/3JorAED.

4. World Health Organization. *The implications for training of embracing a life course approach to health.* Geneva: World Health Organization, 2000.

5. World Health Organization. *Health at key stages of life: The life-course approach to public health.* Updated edition. Copenhagen: WHO Regional Office for Europe, 2011. www.euro.who.int/__data/assets/pdf.

6. Bitzer J, Horne AW. A new aged has come: The redefinition of women's health care. *J Fam Plann Reprod Health Care.* 2012;**38**:68–9.

7. Every Woman Every Child. *Global strategy for women's, children's and adolescents' health: 2016–2030.* Geneva: Every Woman Every Child. 2015.

8. National Sexual Violence Resource Center. An overview of healthy childhood development. National Sexual Violence Resource Center 103. https://bit.ly/3jky4JX.

9. https://bit.ly/3YdLs1q.

10. World Health Organization. *Make every mother and child count.* Geneva: World Health Organization, 2005.

11. World Health Organization. *Global accelerated action for the health of adolescents (AA-HA!): Guidance to support country implementation.* Geneva: World Health Organization, 2017.

12. Bellis MA, Hughes K, Leckenby N et al. National household survey of adverse childhood experiences and their relationship with resilience to health-harming behaviours in England. *BMC Medicine.* 2014;**12**:72.

13. WHO recommendations on adolescent sexual and reproductive health and rights. http://bit.ly/3WTLVEX.

14. https://bit.ly/3HqqYvD.

15. UNFPA Adolescent sexual and reproductive health 2014. http://bit.ly/3HJ353I.

16. Sitnick SL, Brennan LM, Forbes E et al. Developmental pathways to sexual risk behavior in high-risk adolescent boys. *Pediatrics.* 2014;**133** (6):1038–45.

17. American Psychological Association. *The road to resilience.* Washington, DC: American Psychological Association, 2014.

18. Johnson CE. Sexual health during pregnancy and the postpartum (CME). *JSM.* 2011;**1**:1267–84.

19. Bitzer J, Platano G, Tschudin S et al. Sexual counseling for women in the context of physical disease. *J Sex Med.* 2007 Jan;**4**(1):29–37.

20. Royal College of Obstetricians and Gynaecologists. High quality women's health care: A proposal for change. 2011. https://bit.ly/40fSaWl.

21. WHO Europe. UNFPA: A life course approach to sexual and reproductive health. Entre Nous: The European Magazine for Sexual and Reproductive Health. No. 82–2015. www.euro.who.int/entrenous.

22. National Survey of Sexual Attitudes and Lifestyles (NATSAL-3). *Lancet.* 2013;**382**(9907):1807–16.

23. Public Health England. *Promoting the health and wellbeing of gay, bisexual and other men who have sex with men.* London: Public Health England, 2014.

24. Bretschneider J, McCoy N. Sexual interest and behaviour in healthy 80 to 102 year olds. *Arc. of sexual behavior.* 1988; **17**(2):109–29.

25. Linday ST, Schumm P, Laumann EO et al. A study of sexuality and health among older adults in the United States. *N Engl J Med.* 2007;**357**:762–71.

26. Bitzer J, Platano G, Tschudin S, Alder J. Sexual counseling in elderly couples. *J Sex Med.* 2008;**5**: 2027–43.

27. Joint Opinion Paper. 'Ageing and sexual health' by the European Board & College of Obstetrics and Gynaecology (EBCOG) and the European Menopause and Andropause Society (EMAS).

28. Rees M, Lambrinoudaki I, Bitzer J, Mahmood T. *Eur J Obstet Gynecol Reprod Biol.* 2018;**220**:132–4.

29. Antonovsky A. *Health, stress, and coping: New perspectives on mental and physical well-being.* San Francisco: Jossey-Bass, 1979.

30. United Nations. *Transforming our world: The 2030 agenda for sustainable development.* New York: United Nations, 2015.

Introduction

Sexual violence against women is one of the most important threats to women's sexual and reproductive health and rights [1]. In a broader perspective sexual violence against women can be viewed as part of gender-based violence which is defined by the United Nations (UN) as 'any act … that results in, or is likely to result in, physical, sexual, or mental harm or suffering to women, including threats of such acts, coercion or arbitrary deprivation of liberty, whether occurring in public or in private life' [2].

The World Health Organization (WHO) defines sexual violence as part of this broader concept – any sexual act, attempt to obtain a sexual act, unwanted sexual comments or advances, or acts against a person's sexuality using coercion by any person regardless of their relationship to the victim, in any setting [3].

This definition has three dimensions. One dimension refers to all types of behaviours which violate the self-defined limits and sexual integrity of a person, including what a person wants and does not want. The second dimension is coercion. Coercion can cover a whole spectrum of degrees of force: physical force, psychological intimidation, blackmail or other threats. It also includes the threat of physical harm or dismissal from or of not obtaining a job if the victim does not fulfil the aggressor's wishes. The situation is the same if the victim is unable to give consent – for instance, while drunk, drugged, asleep or mentally incapable of understanding the situation. The third dimension refers to the aggressor and the setting. It states that sexual violence can be exerted by everybody and in all walks of life and situations.

Sexual violence is frequently part of intimate partner violence. This refers to a behaviour by an intimate partner or ex-partner that causes physical, sexual or psychological harm, including physical aggression, sexual coercion, psychological abuse and controlling behaviours. As there is considerable overlap between sexual violence and intimate partner violence, both dimensions of violence against women should be viewed together because the combination is one of the most important threats to women's sexual and reproductive health in terms of prevalence and in terms of health consequences.

Prevalence

Population-level surveys based on reports from victims show an incredibly high prevalence of both intimate partner and sexual violence. In an analysis conducted by the WHO in 2013 together with the London School of Hygiene and Tropical Medicine and the South Africa Medical Research Council, existing data from more than 80 countries were analysed and it was found that worldwide:

- One in three, or 35%, of women have experienced physical and/or sexual violence.
- Almost one third (30%) of all women who have been in a relationship have experienced physical and/or sexual violence by their intimate partner [4, 5].

There seems to be a regional and economic difference in the prevalence: 23.2% in high-income countries, 24.6% in the WHO's Western Pacific region, 37% in the WHO's Eastern Mediterranean region and 37.7% in the WHO's South-East Asia region.

Globally as many as 38% of all murders of women (femicides) are committed by intimate partners [4, 5]. In addition to intimate partner violence, globally 7% of women report sexual assault by someone other than a partner, although data for non-partner sexual violence are more limited [4, 5].

Major Manifestations of Sexual Violence

A wide range of sexually violent acts can take place performed by different perpetrators and in a large variety of circumstances and settings [3]. Sexual violence thus can be viewed as a worldwide pandemic [1]. The following list provides definitions of these manifestations, the perpetrators and the circumstances [3, 5–10].

Rape

Rape is defined as physically forced or otherwise coerced penetration – even if slight – of the vulva or anus using a penis, other body parts or an object. The attempt to do so is known as attempted rape. The broader definition includes other forms of assault involving a sexual organ, including coerced contact between the mouth and penis, vulva or anus. The perpetrators can be husbands, partners within a dating relationship, strangers, even individuals or groups (gang rape). Rape can happen within marriage or dating relationship, at the workplace, at home, basically everywhere.

Unwanted Sexual Advances or Harassment, Including Demanding Sex in Return for Favours

The perpetrators can be family members, strangers, colleagues at work, teachers or healthcare professionals. These acts happen not only in any place where women meet other individuals in person, but more and more this happens on the Internet.

Sexual Abuse of Mentally or Physically Disabled People

This vulnerable group can become victim of abuse by caregivers, family members or strangers in unprotected places either in institutions or in public.

Sexual Abuse of Children

Children are helpless and depend on the respect and care of the adults around them. Unfortunately children can become victims of abuse not only by strangers but even more often by parents and relatives either at home or in public but hidden places. The abuse can be a direct physical assault but also via media and the Internet.

Forced Marriage or Cohabitation, Including the Marriage of Children

The perpetrators can be family members, community elders and others in the context of traditions, norms and customs.

Violent Acts against the Sexual Integrity of Women, Including Female Genital Mutilation and Obligatory Inspections for Virginity

These practices are performed by family members and community elderly and follow long-standing traditions, norms and customs.

Forced Prostitution and Trafficking of People for the Purpose of Sexual Exploitation

Family members like fathers, brothers or even mothers can give the daughter or sister away to individual or organized prostitution, which is often then in the context of human trafficking and organized crime.

Denial of the Right to Use Contraception or to Adopt other Measures to Protect against Sexually Transmitted Diseases; Forced Abortion

This can include prohibition of contraception to adolescents through family members, laws and national health policies.

Health Consequences

Impact on Women

Sexual violence by intimate partners or non-related persons can negatively affect women's physical, mental, sexual and reproductive health [11–16].

Harm to General Health and Well-Being

Sexual aggression in the context of a relationship or committed by strangers leads in almost half of the cases to injuries and may end in homicide or suicide. This can be followed by a lifelong handicap or chronic pain. The consequences may include functional somatic symptoms like headaches, back pain, abdominal pain, gastrointestinal disorders or musculoskeletal disorders.

Harm to Sexual and Reproductive Health

These consequences include unintended pregnancies, induced abortions, sexually transmitted infections (STIs), including HIV, infertility, chronic pelvic pain or damage to the vulva, vagina or pelvic floor with subsequent pain during sexual activity. The 2013 analysis found that women who had been physically or sexually abused were 1.5 times more likely to have an STI and, in some regions, HIV, compared to women who had not experienced partner violence. They are also twice as likely to have had an abortion [4].

Pregnancy is a high-risk period for being exposed to intimate partner violence in different forms (battering, rape, etc.). Behaviours can fluctuate between verbal aggression and physical and/or sexual violence. The consequences are dramatic for the pregnant woman and the unborn child (premature contractions, bleeding, growth retardation, postpartum depression etc.).

Harm to Mental Health

Exposure to sexual violence can lead to various mental health disorders:

- Major depression.
- Post-traumatic stress disorder.
- Phobic anxiety.
- General anxiety disorder.
- Sleep difficulties.
- Somatization disorder.
- Eating disorders.
- Drug and alcohol abuse.
- Sexual pain disorders or dysfunctions.

The 2013 analysis found that women who have experienced intimate partner violence were almost twice as likely to experience depression and problem drinking [4].

Impact on Children

Children who grow up in families where there is violence may suffer a range of behavioural and emotional disturbances. These can also be associated with perpetrating or experiencing violence later in life [16, 17]. Intimate partner violence has also been associated with higher rates of infant and child mortality and morbidity (through, for example, diarrhoeal disease or malnutrition) [18].

One of the tragic consequences of sexual violence, particularly during childhood, is that the victims are at increased risk of developing additions (smoking, drug or alcohol misuse), sexual behaviour with increased risk of contracting an STI, including HIV, and there is unfortunately an association with perpetration of violence (for males) and being a victim of violence (for females) later in life [16, 3, 5].

Social and Economic Costs

The social and economic costs of intimate partner and sexual violence are difficult to quantify in economic terms [19]. The social and economic costs for women are mediated through loss of working capacity, jobs, work and income. There is also social isolation of the victims (blaming the victims) and thus reduction in regular activities. Women may lose interest in caring for themselves and their children.

Causes and Contributing Factors

Multiple factors are associated with the occurrence of sexual violence against women [20–24].

Sociocultural Factors

Two major beliefs and narratives in a society and community contribute to the occurrence of sexual violence [20]. One is the belief that women as human beings have less value than men and therefore have a lower status than men in the community (inferiority hypothesis).

From this belief or social narrative norms and prescriptions derive:

- Women should respond to their husband's or partner's wishes including sexuality.
- Women are an object which is part of a man's or a father's property.

The other is the belief or narrative that women are basically immoral and dangerous. This is unfortunately part of a long-standing misogynist tradition reflected in the story of Eve and in the concept of Madonna versus the whore. Behind this misogyny a profound fear of men may be at work regarding women's reproductive and sexual power. From this concept other norms and prescriptions derive which also have deleterious effects.

- Women who do not obey should be punished and excluded.
- Virginity is a central value linked to the honour of fathers and brothers.
- Early child marriage.
- Female genital mutilation.

Couple and Individual Factors

The sociocultural norms and environment favour the development of individual life experiences which represent risk factors for sexual violence against women. There are general risk factors for victims and perpetrators alike. These are factors contributing to a lack of communication skills, conflict resolution, negotiation between partners regarding the needs and views and internalized representations of early interactions and learned behaviour. These factors are empirically linked to a lack of impulse control on the perpetrator's side and lack of self-assertion on the victim's side.

- Low education, poverty.
- A history of exposure to child maltreatment.
- Witnessing family violence.
- Harmful use of alcohol.
- Marital discord and dissatisfaction.
- Difficulties in communicating between partners.
- Males' controlling behaviours towards their partners [3].

Apart from the general risk factors studies have shown that there are specific risks to becoming a perpetrator:

- Beliefs in family honour and sexual purity.
- Ideologies of male sexual entitlement.
- Weak legal sanctions for sexual violence.
- Antisocial personality disorder [3].

The risks for a woman to become a victim include:

- Low levels of access to paid employment.
- Exposure to mothers being abused by a partner.
- Abuse during childhood.
- Attitudes which accept violence.
- Male privilege and women's subordinate status [3].

An important contributing factor is the concept of just and unjust violence. This means that women deserve punishment when they do not obey, argue back, do not have food ready on time or do not care enough for their children – in other words, when they do not behave according to the rules which define women as subordinate to or property of the male partner [5].

Times of Increased Risk

Situations of conflict, post conflict and displacement may exacerbate existing violence, such as by intimate partners, as well as non-partner sexual violence, and may also lead to new forms of violence against women.

How to Fight Sexual Violence against Women

The UN, the WHO and many other international and national institutions and societies dedicated to women's sexual and reproductive rights agree that only a multilevel strategy can improve the situation, taking into account the interdependence of socioeconomic and legal conditions, cultural beliefs and norms, healthcare system priorities and organizations, community rules, media messages, partner

dynamics, school systems, individual predispositions, early life experiences and learning possibilities [2, 3, 5, 7].

This pyramid approach goes from macro factors to micro factors and looks into interventions to reduce sexual violence against women. Starting from the top of the pyramid (the victim) to the base (law, economy, politics), the following tasks and field of interaction emerge.

Comprehensive Care for the Victim

This care is characterized by standards which should be followed and monitored [25]:

- Victims should get care in an appropriate setting by trained healthcare professionals.
- This means that healthcare professionals should get training in communication and detection of victims, including appropriate non-invasive asking about exposure. They should have supervision to help them maintain a non-judgemental attitude, empathic listening and client-centred counselling.
- Primary support should be provided with emergency contraception, STI and HIV prophylaxis and the assessment of the relevant facts.
- The service should ensure privacy and confidentiality [26, 27].
- The service should be integrated into existing healthcare services, including obstetrics and gynaecology, treatment of STIs, abortion services and so forth.
- The service should offer help to report the incident if the woman chooses.

Psychological Care and Support

Counselling, therapy and support group initiatives have proven helpful following sexual assaults, especially where there may be complicating factors related to the violence itself or to the process of recovery. There is some evidence that a brief cognitive behavioural programme administered shortly after assault can hasten the rate of improvement of psychological damage arising from trauma [28]. These centres provide or coordinate a wide range of services, including emergency medical care and medical follow-up, counselling, collecting forensic evidence of assault, legal support and community consultation and education [29].

Preventive Measures

There are again different levels on which primary and secondary preventive measures can be implemented [30–32].

Community Level

At the community level healthcare providers can promote communication and relationship skills within couples. Communities can reduce access to and harmful use of alcohol. Outreach has been a major part of the response to partner violence from non-governmental organizations. Outreach workers – often peer educators – visit victims of violence in their homes and communities. Non-governmental organizations frequently recruit and train peer workers from the ranks of former clients, themselves earlier victims of partner violence.

Prevention campaigns. Attempts to change public attitudes towards sexual violence using the media have included advertising on buildings (billboards), in public transport and on radio and television. Television has been used effectively in South Africa and Zimbabwe. In Zimbabwe the non-governmental organization Musasa has produced awareness-raising initiatives using theatre, public meetings and debates, as well as a television series where survivors of violence described their experiences.

Manuals, interagency activities. Other initiatives besides media campaigns have been used in many countries. The Sisterhood Is Global Institute in Montreal, Canada, for instance, has developed a manual suitable for Muslim communities aimed at raising awareness and stimulating debate on issues related to gender equality and violence against women and girls.

Community activism by men. These initiatives come from men who want to help men to reduce their use of violence. These groups offer group discussions, education campaigns and rallies, work with violent men, and lead workshops in schools, prisons and workplaces. Actions are frequently conducted in collaboration with women's organizations involved in preventing violence and providing services to abused women.

School-based programmes. Programmes in schools have two objectives [33]. One is to educate about gender-based violence and how to prevent it. The other is to raise awareness of the fact that a sexual relation between a teacher and a pupil is not a serious disciplinary offence and policies on sexual harassment in schools either do not exist or are not enforced. This creates an environment which contradicts what the educational programme is trying to transmit.

Programmes for perpetrators. Men who commit sexual violence very often deny both that they are responsible and that what they are doing is violent [34, 35]. The group work focusses on confronting them with victims and involving them in the care of victims, and on making them aware that they can choose their actions and therefore the public views them as responsible for their actions and they should as well [34]. One way of achieving this is for programmes that target male perpetrators of sexual violence to collaborate with support services for victims as well as with campaigns against sexual violence.

Health Sector Activities

Healthcare systems traditionally focus on diagnosis and treatment of disease and neglect public health issues [25]. This is especially true for women's sexual and reproductive health and rights (except for obstetrics, which is considered essential for a country's future). There are many tasks and challenges:

- Development of national plans and policies to address violence against women.
- Make violence against women a central issue of discussion in congresses and meetings and denounce it as a major health threat like cancer and cardiovascular disease.
- Provide comprehensive services, sensitize and train healthcare providers in responding to the medical and psychosocial needs of survivors.
- Prevent recurrence of violence through early identification of women and children who are experiencing violence and providing appropriate referral and support.
- Work with teachers and school programmes focussing on life skills, sexuality education and gender roles and norms.
- Make sexual violence an important part of the research agenda, initiating surveys and performing implementation research about interventions and their outcome.
- Fight myths and 'fake news' about sexual violence against women, including that only certain types of women are raped, women falsely report rape, when women say no to sex they actually mean yes, sex workers cannot be raped and a man cannot rape his wife. The truth is that all women are at risk of sexual violence and false reporting is very rare. On the contrary, there is not enough

reporting. A no is a no and many sex workers endure violent acts. Marriage does not protect against or justify rape.

Other myths about rape include that sex is the primary motivation for rape, rape is perpetrated by a stranger, rape involves a great deal of physical violence and the use of a weapon and it leaves obvious signs of injury and rape is reported immediately to the police. The truth is that sexual violence has a lot to do with feelings of power and dominance, occurs more often in the context of a relationship, can take all forms of unwanted transgressions and does not leave visible traces on the body but invisible traces on the mind. Unfortunately a high percentage of rape is not reported. Healthcare providers involved in sexual and reproductive healthcare should provide interviews and write papers for the media correcting these false beliefs.

Advocacy and Involvement in Politics

Politics is a field in which many healthcare professionals feel uncomfortable because it is not part of their specific professional training nor is it part of science. It is about action again on several levels.

Legal System, Laws

Many countries have laws which discriminate against women in the context of marriage, divorce and custody. The same is true for inheritance laws which leave women without any security outside marriage. The dowry in India is a symbol of the extremely negative value given to a female child improving women's access to paid employment.

Laws alone are of course not sufficient if they are not applied in a consistent and persistent manner. This means that all men and women working in the field of public security should be sensitized about the importance of sexual violence and provided with clear guidance on how to react, and that this field of criminal law application should be monitored regularly to see if women are protected following the law. This is especially true with laws against child marriage, female genital mutilation and sex strafficking.

Economy

It has been shown that one of the most important measures to prevent sexual violence is the access of women to paid employment, building the basis for independence and empowerment which will allow women to defend themselves against all sort of violence including sexual violence [3–5]. This is an ongoing fight against rules, customs, practices and false beliefs which discriminate against women on one hand and fight against the multimillion-dollar business of exploitation and economic injustice against women on the other.

Summary

Sexual violence is a pandemic with many manifestations caused by human behaviour which is determined by a myriad of individual, politico-legal, socioeconomic and cultural factors.

Many victims of sexual violence do not report the incidences because of shame and social discrimination. Victims need specialized services to treat the many health consequences of sexual violence and to ensure a safe and protective environment which facilitates reporting and eventual legal action and which ensures long-term follow-up and treatment if needed.

Prevention is a multilevel task for all healthcare professionals . It includes work in the education system and on the level of communities (sexual education), but also public and political involvement to create a safe environment for women at home and at work by ensuring implementation of laws and policies which protect women and which reduce this destructive pandemic.

References

1. Heise L, Pitanguy J, Germain A. *Violence against women: The hidden health burden*. Discussion Paper No. 255. Washington, DC: World Bank, 1994.

2. United Nations. *Declaration on the elimination of violence against women*. New York: United Nations, 1993.

3. http://bit.ly/3HqrJVv.

4. Global and regional estimates of violence against women. Prevalence and health effects of intimate partner violence and non-partner sexual violence. WHO, Department of Reproductive Health and Research, London School of Hygiene and Tropical Medicine, South African Medical Research Council WHO reference number: 9789241564625.

5. Krug EG, Dahlberg LL, Mercy JA, Zwi AB, Lozano R (eds.). *World report on violence and health*. Geneva: World Health Organization, 2002. https://bit.ly/3JwNB42.

6. Goodman LA. *No safe haven: Male violence against women at home, at work, and in the community*. Koss MP, Browne A (eds.). Washington, DC: American Psychological Association, 1994.

7. World Health Organization. *Violence against women: A priority health issue* (document WHO/FRH/WHD/97.8). Geneva: World Health Organization, 1997.

8. Migration Information Programme. *Trafficking in women to Italy for sexual exploitation.* Geneva: International Organization for Migration, 1996.

9. Barnard M. Violence and vulnerability: Conditions of work for streetworking prostitutes. *Sociology of Health and Illness* 1993;**15**:683–705.

10. Church S, Henderson M, Barnard M, Hart G. Violence by clients towards female prostitutes in different work settings: Questionnaire survey. *British Medical Journal* 2001;**322**:524–5.

11. Campbell JC. Health consequences of intimate partner violence. *Lancet* 2002;**359**(9314):1331–6.

12. Martin SL, Macy RJ, Young SK. Health and economic consequences of sexual violence. In White JW, Koss MP, Kazdin AE (eds.). *Violence against women and children. Vol. 1: Mapping the terrain.* Washington, DC: American Psychological Association, 2011, pp. 173–95.

13. Coker AL, Smith PH, Bethea L, King MR, McKeown RE. Physical health consequences of physical and psychological intimate partner violence. *Archives of Family Medicine* 2000;**9**:451–7.

14. Murphy C, Schei B, Myhr TL, Du Mont J. Abuse: A risk factor for low birth weight? A systematic review and meta-analysis. *Canadian Medical Association Journal* 2001;**164**(11):1567–72.

15. Creamer M, Burgess P, McFarlane AC. Posttraumatic stress disorder: Findings from the Australian National Survey of Mental Health and Well-Being. *Psychological Medicine* 2001;**31**:1237–47.

16. Follette V, Polusny MA, Bechtle AE, Naugle AE. Cumulative trauma: The impact of child sexual abuse, adult sexual assault, and spouse abuse. *Journal of Traumatic Stress* 1996;**9**:25–35.

17. McCloskey LA, Figueredo AJ, Koss MP. The effects of systemic family violence on children's mental health. *Child Development* 1995;**66**:1239–61.

18. Edleson JL. Children's witnessing of adult domestic violence. *Journal of Interpersonal Violence* 1999;**14**:839–70.

19. Byrne CA, Resnick HS, Kilpatrick DG, Best CL, Saunders BE. The socioeconomic impact of interpersonal violence on women. *Journal of Consulting and Clinical Psychology* 1999;**67**:362–6.

20. Bitzer J. The pandemic of violence against women: The latest chapter in the history of misogyny. *Eur J Contracept Reprod Health Care.* 2015; **20**(1):1–3.

21. Casey E, Masters T. Sexual violence risk and protective factors: A systematic review of the literature. Injury and Violence Prevention. 24 March 2017. https://bit.ly/3kTMEsi.

22. World Health Organization. *Putting women first: Ethical and safety recommendations for research on domestic violence against women* (document WHO/FCH/GWH/01.01). Geneva: World Health Organization, 2001.

23. Crowell N, Burgess AW. *Understanding violence against women.* Washington, DC: National Academy Press, 1996.

24. https://bit.ly/3HqIhwm.

25. World Health Organization. Global plan of action: Health systems address violence against women and girls WHO/RHR/16.13 © World Health Organization 2016. http://apps.who.int/gb/ebwha/pdf_files/WHA69/A69_9-en.pdf.

26. Carmody M, Carrington K. Preventing sexual violence? *Australian and New Zealand Journal of Criminology* 2000;**33**(3):341–61.

27. Foa EB, Hearst-Ikeda D, Perry KJ. Evaluation of a brief cognitive-behavioural program for the prevention of chronic PTSD in recent assault victims. *Journal of Consulting and Clinical Psychology.* 1995;**63**:948–55.

28. Du Mont J, MacDonald S, Badgley R. *An overview of the sexual assault care and treatment centres of Ontario.* Toronto: Ontario Network of Sexual Assault Care and Treatment Centres, 1997.

29. Toward a multi-level, ecological approach to the primary prevention of sexual assault prevention in peer and community contexts. *Trauma, Violence and Abuse* 2009;**10**(2):91–114.

30. Centers for Disease Control and Prevention. *A review of the sexual violence prevention portfolio at CDC's division of violence prevention, 2000–2010* (for internal use only). Atlanta, GA: Centers for Disease Control and Prevention,2012.

31. Davison L et al. *Reducing domestic violence: What works? Health services.* London: Policing and Crime Reduction Unit, Home Office, 2000.

32. Jaffe PG et al. An evaluation of a secondary school primary prevention program on violence in intimate relationships. *Violence and Victims.* 1992:7:129–46.

33. Kaufman M. Building a movement of men working to end violence against women. *Development* 2001;**44**:9–14.

34. Foshee VA et al. The Safe Dates program: One-year follow-up results. *American Journal of Public Health* 2000;**90**:1619–22.

Sexual and Reproductive Healthcare for LGBTI*

Johannes Bitzer

The Variety of Human Sexual Expression

Human sexuality is characterized by a large variety of sexual expression which comprises several dimensions [1–3]. The physical biological dimension is described as male, intersex or female. The mental dimension is called sexual orientation and expresses itself as heterosexual, homosexual or bisexual. The emotional dimension consists of affective orientation and is communicated through expressions like the mental dimension, meaning heterosexual, homosexual and bisexual. Both the emotional and mental dimensions describe a person's physical, romantic and/or emotional attraction towards other people which may or may not manifest itself in behaviour.

The dimension of sexual or gender identity describes a person's deeply felt internal and individual experience of gender with self-definitions like being a man, being a woman or being both (queer). The social dimension, defined as gender expression, is the way in which an individual outwardly presents their gender through dressing, speaking and social conduct. The expression of gender typically aligns with the socially constructed binary of masculine and feminine. The way an individual expresses their gender is not always indicative of their gender identity. These social manifestations can be described with the categories of femininity, androgyny and masculinity.

Different dimensions may have specific combinations which are described as cisgender, meaning the gender identity matches the assigned gender at birth versus transgender, meaning the gender identity differs from the gender assigned at birth. The category of non-binary/queer/fluid describes individuals not identifying with a male–female binary who may have a fluid or multifaceted gender identity. The most common combination of the different dimensions is the male and female sexual identity with a mental and emotional heterosexual orientation.

Other combinations find expression in a multitude of combinations, including non-heterosexual and non-heterosexual emotional orientation with variable behavioural manifestations. The descriptions come from self-definitions of sexual attraction and specific behaviours and are named lesbian, bisexual or queer.

This same variety of combinations is true regarding different expressions of gender. Transgender includes individuals in whom gender identity differs from sex assigned at birth (vs. cisgendered) but also individuals who are not exclusively masculine or feminine (genderqueer, non-binary, pangender), individuals refusing any gender (agender, gender neutral) and individuals with a third gender and cross dressers, independent of the underlying motive. In intersex individuals the binary classification of biological sex is not possible due to variations in chromosomal, gonadal, hormonal or genital sex, meaning they have their own intersex identity.

The LGBT (LGBTIQ*) Community

The described expressions beyond the male and female sexual identity with a mental and emotional heterosexual orientation are summarized under the umbrella term of LGBT (lesbian, gay, bisexual, trans) or the broader term LGBTIQ* (lesbian, gay, bisexual, trans, intersex, questioning, non-binary, asexual). They represent sexual and gender minorities and the rainbow flag is a symbol of these diversities.

Lesbian, Gay

Lesbian women and gay men are attracted to individuals of the same sex and/or gender identity as themselves. Transgender (sometimes shortened to 'trans') describes people with a wide range of identities, including transsexuals (people who identify as a third gender) and others whose appearance and characteristics are perceived as gender atypical and whose sense of their own gender is different to the sex they were assigned at birth. Trans women identify as women but were assigned as males when they were born. Trans men identify as men but were assigned female when they were born. Some transgender people seek surgery or take hormones to bring their body into alignment with their gender identity; others do not.

Queer is an umbrella term commonly used to define lesbian, gay, bi, trans and other people and institutions on the margins of mainstream culture. Queer can be a convenient, inclusive term but, depending on the user, it might still have a devaluating undertone. Intersex people are born with physical or biological sex characteristics (including sexual anatomy, reproductive organs and/or chromosomal patterns) that do not fit the traditional definitions of male or female.

These characteristics may be apparent at birth or emerge later in life, often at puberty. Intersex people may be subjected to gender assignment interventions at birth or in early life with the consent of parents though this practice is largely contested by intersex persons and has been the subject of a number of recommendations by human rights experts and bodies.

Prevalence

The prevalence of these sexual minorities is difficult to determine. Members of this community often do not disclose their orientation and gender identity. In addition the aforementioned definitions of the expressions vary and there is no standardized instrument of assessment like a structured interview or a questionnaire. The estimate is that the prevalence of non-heterosexual individuals is about 7% while the prevalence of identified trans individuals seems to be 0.5–1.3% [4].

The Specific Medical, Politico-legal and Sociocultural Threats to LGBTIQ* People

The way medicine dealt with this community shows the sociocultural biases which influence definitions of normal and abnormal, of health and disease. Homosexuality was considered a mental disorder until 1973 in the *Diagnostic and Statistical Manual of Mental Disorders* (DSM) and until 1992 in the International Classification of Diseases (ICD). In

ICD-10 is was listed as ego-dystonic sexual orientation (F66) and was not mentioned anymore in ICD-11.

Trans(gender) was mentioned in the ICD-10 as gender identity disorder (ICD-10) and transsexualism (F64) was also included. In the ICD-11 it is classified as gender incongruence in the chapter about conditions of sexual health, and in the DSM-5 it is called gender dysphoria (302). Inter(sex) is listed in the ICD 10/11 as disorders of sex development.

Regarding the politico-legal framework created with respect to this community. there is criminalization on one side and protection on the other. The criminalization of gay, lesbian, bisexual and transgender people remains in many countries in Africa, the Middle East and parts of Asia, including India, and leads to all forms of punishment, in some countries even to the death penalty. Fortunately these activities are legal in many countries – many European and some South American countries as well as the United States, Canada, Australia and South Africa have created protective laws. Laws are based on decisions by governments. The environment of the individual is, however, strongly influenced by sociocultural beliefs and values. This is an ongoing challenge to the health of the members of this community [5–8].

Health Risks

Gay and bisexual men and men who have sex with men have the same health risks as other men and heart disease and cancer are the leading causes of death. They have additionally higher risks in different categories [9–11]. An important increased risk is sexually transmitted infections (STIs). These men have higher rates of HIV and other sexually transmitted diseases (STDs). The prevalence of HIV among sexual partners of gay and bisexual men and men who have sex with men is 40 times that of sexual partners of heterosexual men. Several factors contribute to this increased risk. It is known that receptive anal sex is 18 times more risky for HIV acquisition than receptive vaginal sex. Gay and bisexual men and men who have sex with men on average have a greater number of sexual partners over their lifetimes. Another threat to the health of these men is the increased tobacco and drug use and prevalence of depression in this community.

Other health risks come from the social environment. In many societies there is still a high degree of homophobia with a stigma (negative and usually unfair beliefs). There is discrimination (unfairly treating a person or group of people differently), lack of access to culturally and orientation-appropriate medical and support services, heightened concerns about confidentiality, fear of losing employment and fear of talking about sexual practices or orientation.

Lesbian and bisexual women and women who have sex with men and women have the same health risks as other women. They are additionally affected by homophobia and stigma based on the same beliefs as mentioned in relation to gay and bisexual men and men who have sex with men. They experience discrimination and suffer a lack of access to culturally and orientation-appropriate medical and support services. This leads to heightened concerns about confidentiality, fear of losing employment and fear of talking about sexual practices or orientation.

Special Needs for the LGBT Community in Sexual and Reproductive Healthcare

Members of the LGBT community need comprehensive sexual and reproductive healthcare services with easy access which includes responses to their special needs, including contraception and mental healthcare.

Special Needs regarding Communication and Counselling

Taking into account that, for many LGBT individuals there is still a fear of disclosing their preferences and identities, the healthcare professional needs to create a safe, non-judgemental and confidential environment by practising patient-centred communication which comprises open questions, giving time to answer, encouraging the patient to tell their story and avoiding going directly to closed questions [11–13]. It is also important to practice an interactive dialogue in which the healthcare provider can respond to emotions and establish a trustful therapeutic relationship with the patient.

Another important issue is the use of gender-neutral language and asking patients – especially those who are gender nonconforming – which pronouns they prefer and trying to avoid words which have a binary content like girlfriend and boyfriend. This includes the capacity to structure the conversation around the different issues the healthcare provider would want to talk about with the patient,

including obtaining permission. 'Now I would like to talk about your sexual life. Is that okay?' [12, 13].

This chapter of sexual history taking can be structured around sexual activity in general (are you sexually active?), partners (do you have sex with men, women, both?), questions about protection against unwanted pregnancies (what type of contraception?) questions about protections against STIs and history of STIs and questions about sexual practices and well-being, including sexual dysfunction. Healthcare providers should invite their patients to raise any other concerns or questions regarding their sexual life. It is important to summarize and give feedback to allow questions for clarification.

Special Needs regarding Sexual Healthcare

Many LGBT individuals cannot easily and openly live the sexual life they would like to live [3, 7, 8, 11–14]. As mentioned earlier in this chapter, the main threats to their sexual health and well-being are the fear of social discrimination, loss of economic stability and social position and violence which frequently contributes to an increase in risky behaviour that exposes the individual not only to STIs, but also to sexual abuse and violence in a vicious circle.

These people need help from professionals who can practise patient-centred counselling but also provide easy access to STI detection and treatment along with sexual advice and counselling with respect to sexual dysfunctions (desire, arousal, orgasm, pain; see also Chapters 45 through 50 on STIs, sexual counselling and sexual dysfunctions, respectively). This is especially important for transgender patients who after gender assignment surgery feel very well in their body but may have difficulties with the function or their sexual organs like arousal difficulties and pain in the neovagina. Another important part of care which should be provided is care for victims of sexual violence. The principles of care are the same as for non-LGBTI* individuals.

Special Needs regarding Contraception

For contraceptive counselling and care healthcare providers need to proactively ask for the need of contraception and explain the underlying endocrine processes which may make it necessary [15–20]. The communication should be as described earlier in this chapter, in a respectful and non-judgemental way informing and educating about all methods.

Queer women eventually are confronted with barriers to contraceptive counselling. They may be considered by themselves and by healthcare providers as having no need for contraception, they may face difficulties navigating contraceptive use on top of managing queer identity and there may be negative judgement from within the queer community which could undermine contraceptive use. In addition less frequent penile–vaginal intercourse (PVI) can make more effective contraceptive methods feel like overkill; use of condoms, withdrawal and emergency contraception are more common and they may have the experience of being stigmatized by the healthcare system. Contraceptive facilitators for queer women can include information about health benefits with respect to different menstrual difficulties, skin problems and so forth.

Endocrinology

Trans and non-binary people who are taking gender-affirming hormone therapy may think they no longer need birth control. Hormone therapy alone will not protect trans and non-binary people from pregnancy, however. Periods stop for most trans men and non-binary people who were assigned female at birth (AFAB) after taking testosterone for a few months but ovulation may still occur even if they never have a period. For trans women and non-binary people who were assigned male at birth (AMAB) and are taking oestrogen the development of sperm in the testicles can still occur. Gender-affirming hormone therapy does generally decrease fertility, but it can not be relied on as a form of contraception. Regardless of gender identity, if two people are having unprotected PVI, pregnancy can occur. Unplanned pregnancies do happen. Bisexual- and lesbian-identified adolescents report unintended pregnancy rates significantly higher than do their heterosexual peers.

Contraception for the Transgender Man

A transgender man has reproductive potential if they have an intact uterus and ovaries and until menopause or surgical sterilization. Testosterone may not completely suppress ovarian function, leading to irregular bleeding. It is important to note there is still a risk of pregnancy despite a lack of menstruation. Use of a contraceptive is still necessary even with testosterone therapy.

Combined Hormonal Contraceptives

Oestrogen may or may not interfere with testosterone therapy and thus inhibit the desired androgen action on the body, but there is no medical contraindication.

There is, however, the risk of unwanted oestrogen-related side effects on the body and brain, resulting in female fat distribution and eventually in irritability and mood instability.

Progestin-Only Contraceptives

Progestin-only contraceptive methods do not interfere with testosterone use and they have the advantage of inducing amenorrhea in trans men who still have bleeding under testosterone therapy. There may also be an additional masculinizing effect (hair growth) due to the action of an androgenic progestin like levonorgestrel. Progestin-only injectable and long-acting reversible contraceptives – implants and intrauterine devices – facilitate compliance and have a high rate of amenorrhea (depot DMPA has highest rate).

Non-hormonal Contraceptives

Non-hormonal contraceptives have the advantage that they do not interfere with endocrine treatment. The copper IUD, which in women may lead to hypermenorrhea, is especially suitable for women who are already amenorrhoic following hormone treatment. External and internal condoms are in general less effective but, in the situation of reduced fertility, they present a rather effective method with the advantage of STI protection. Permanent surgical options are available for patients who do not want to get pregnant at all.

Contraceptives for Transgender Women

For trans women and non-binary people who were AMAB and are taking oestrogen the development of sperm in the testicles can still occur. The male condom is an effective contraceptive method with the advantage of protection against STIs, especially HIV. Permanent surgical options like orchidectomy and vasectomy are available for patients who do not want to get pregnant at all.

Summary

The members of the LGBTI* community represent the great variety of human sexual expression. As a minority they are still in many countries not integrated into healthcare and not included as equals in society. They do, however, have the same rights, including the right to access healthcare services which respond to their specific sexual and reproductive needs: prevention, detection and treatment of STIs and sexual violence; help with problems in sexual function and mental health and appropriate contraceptive counselling and care.

References

1. www.cdc.gov/lgbthealth/index.htm.

2. University of California – San Francisco Transgender Care Navigation Program. Terminology and definitions. 17 June 2016. https://transcare.ucsf.edu/guidelines/terminology.

3. World Health Organization. *Defining sexual health: Report of a technical consultation on sexual health 28–31 January 2002*. Geneva: World Health Organization, 2006. https://bit.ly/3wLdup2.

4. http://bit.ly/3jhsnfT.

5. www.ncbi.nlm.nih.gov/books/NBK64801.

6. https://internap.hrw.org/features/features/lgbt_laws.

7. https://bit.ly/3XPBinV.

8. World Health Organization. *WHO gender, equity and human rights*. Geneva: World Health Organization, 2016.

9. Blondeel K, Say L, Chou D et al. Evidence and knowledge gaps on the disease burden in sexual and gender minorities: A review of systematic reviews. *International Journal for Equity in Health*. 2016;15:16–24. https://bit.ly/3Hlwlfh.

10. United Nations. Ending violence and discrimination against lesbian, gay, bisexual, transgender and intersex people. 2015. https://bit.ly/3DvlH4J.

11. Campbell S. Sexual health needs and the LGBT community. *Nurs Stand*. 2013;**32**:35–8.

12. Pan American Health Organization and World Health Organization. Addressing the causes of disparities in health service access and utilization for lesbian, gay, bisexual and trans (LGBT) persons. 2013. www.who.int/hiv/pub/populations/lgbt_paper/en.

13. https://bit.ly/3jgZGzy.

14. www.cdc.gov/std/treatment/sexualhistory.pdf.

15. Amato P. Fertility options for transgender persons. University of California – San Francisco Transgender Care Navigation Program. 17 June 2016. https://transcare.ucsf.edu/guidelines/fertility.

16. Shah M. Birth control across the gender spectrum. Bedsider. 2017. http://bit.ly/3wL2fNo.

17. Boudreau D, Mukerjee R. Contraception care for transmasculine individuals on testosterone therapy. *J Midwifery Womens Health*. 2019;**64**(4):395–402.

18. Francis A, Jasani S, Bachmann G. Contraceptive challenges and the transgender individual. *Womens Midlife Health*. 2018;**4**:12.

19. Jones K, Wood M, Stephens L. Contraception choices for transgender males. *J Fam Plann Reprod Health Care*. 2017;**43**(3):239–40.

20. Higgins A, Carpenter E. et al. Sexual minority women and contraceptive use: Complex Pathways between sexual orientation and health outcomes. *Am J Public Health*. 2019;**109**(12):1680–6.

54 Indicators of Sexual and Reproductive Health and Their Relevance to Policy Development

Charlotte Gatenby, Sambit Mukhopadhyay

Introduction

Indicators are important within sexual and reproductive health (SRH) as they can be used to evaluate service quality, aid in the development of new policies and ensure resources are correctly allocated, according to the needs of the population. Indicators can help healthcare professionals to understand the health and behaviours of a population. Thus, they can be used to guide the development of robust, accessible and appropriate services and to highlight methods in which optimal SRH can be achieved.

What Is Sexual and Reproductive Health?

The World Health Organization's (WHO) working definition of sexual health is:

> a state of physical, emotional, mental and social well-being in relation to sexuality; it is not merely the absence of disease, dysfunction or infirmity. Sexual health requires a positive and respectful approach to sexuality and sexual relationships, as well as the possibility of having pleasurable and safe sexual experiences, free of coercion, discrimination and violence. For sexual health to be attained and maintained, the sexual rights of all persons must be respected, protected and fulfilled. [1]

Why Use Indicators within a Healthcare System?

Indicators are important within SRH as they can be used to identify where improvements are needed. They can provide evidence for greater investment in, for example, contraception services, where there are high rates of unplanned pregnancy. These rates can be compared and benchmarked against national data which can support service provision and development [2].

Quality assurance following implementation of these indicators can be measured using audits. An example is monitoring abortion rates after developing a contraception service to ensure effective access and appropriateness to the population. This can also include identification of serious untoward incidents in which harm has come as a result of service contact and reviewing of policies to ensure that, if errors were made in patient care, steps are taken to avoid repetition. Patient evaluation surveys are also of vital importance to ensure services are responsive to patients' needs and response to feedback is delivered appropriately and in a timely manner.

Quality-improvement projects are also beneficial indicators within SRH and often involve patient feedback, identification of problems and provision of solutions [2]. An example of this within SRH services is promotion of cost saving by prescribing drugs generically instead of by brand. A further quality-improvement idea could be improving awareness of contraception choices and availability. Auditing contraception prescriptions can help to assess their cost-effectiveness. Patient feedback and monitoring abortion rates (likely failure rates) could provide evidence for a service so as to increase training provision for healthcare professionals in alternative methods such as contraceptive implant fittings and intrauterine devices, thus improving health outcomes for women. This could be regarded as the development of a gold standard to demonstrate progress within SRH.

Why Are Indicators Required for Sexual and Reproductive Health?

Sexual and reproductive health is a topic that relates to a great number of individuals. Similarly to most disciplines of medicine, SRH needs are multifactorial, dependent on age, sexual orientation, gender and ethnicity. Needs will vary widely within these subcategories, depending on the person accessing these services, at that point in time. However, some needs are more basic and must be achieved in order to establish a foundation upon which to build more substantial SRH services [3]. These include high-quality information to enable users to make informed decisions and high-quality services through which they can access treatments and/or interventions if required. Provision of good sexual healthcare services provides access to treatment for ill health whilst also promoting the attainment and maintenance of good health [4].

Sexual and reproductive health is integral to overall health and well-being, and not solely within the reproductive phase of life. Therefore it is vital that this is accounted for and acknowledged within policy development. Sexual and reproductive health is often regarded negatively following negative outcomes such as sexually transmitted infections (STIs) and unplanned pregnancies; as a result, policy development is often largely focussed on prevention and treatment. However, if SRH is regarded as an essential part of well-being, it is likely that SRH outcomes would be improved, provided policies were developed to reflect this. Healthcare systems need to take a holistic approach to SRH and recognise the many barriers, both societal and at the service level, that may prevent patient access [5]. Health promotion is a key area of SRH. Provision of good SRH should include free and confidential advice and information and education on contraception, STIs, HIV and unplanned pregnancies [3].

What Are Some of the Consequences of Poor Sexual Health?

The consequences of poor sexual health are vast and wide-ranging:

- Unplanned pregnancies their potential sequelae, including reduced educational, social and economic opportunities.
- Termination of pregnancy (and consequences of abortion care if not accessible or legal).
- Sexual exploitation, coercion and abuse with potential associated psychological consequences.
- Sexually transmitted infections including HIV, hepatitis and their sequelae, including pelvic inflammatory disease and the increasing potential incidence of ectopic pregnancy and/or infertility.
- Genital cancers.

- Rapid repeat pregnancies and short inter-pregnancy intervals, resulting in increased poor feto-maternal outcomes [3, 7].

What Are the Indicators of Sexual and Reproductive Health?

In 2006 the WHO developed a guideline on SRH indicators with the aim to provide governments and service providers with a clear outline of where to focus financial investment in services (see Table 54.1). The document highlights how to measure success rates of these interventions so as to ensure SRH provision is adaptable and responsive to patients' needs.

These indicators are markers of health status and can help to determine appropriate service provision and resource availability. They were designed to enable the monitoring of service performance and to facilitate continued observation. The goals can be measured and, as a result, they can determine the level of progress countries, individual localities and regions have made [4]. Measurement of these goals can be obtained through monitoring (see Table 54.2):

- Prevalence of contraception use, STIs, infertility and female genital mutation.
- Rates and ratios of maternal mortality and the total fertility rate.
- Data regarding services and knowledge such as patient feedback and access to services.

Table 54.1 The World Health Organization Shortlist of Indicators for Global Monitoring of Reproductive Health [4]

1. Total fertility rate
2. Contraceptive prevalence
3. Maternal mortality ratio
4. Antenatal care coverage
5. Births attended by skilled health professional
6. Availability of basic essential obstetric care
7. Availability of comprehensive essential obstetric care
8. Perinatal mortality rate
9. Prevalence of low birth rate
10. Prevalence of positive syphilis serology in pregnant women
11. Prevalence of anaemia in women
12. Percentage of obstetric and gynaecological admissions owing to abortion
13. Reported prevalence of women with genital mutilation
14. Prevalence of infertility in women
15. Reported incidence of urethritis in men
16. Prevalence of Human immunodeficiency virus (HIV) in pregnant women
17. Knowledge of HIV-related preventive practices

Table 54.2 Key factors to include in comprehensive reproductive healthcare [4]

	Descriptor	Example
Counselling	Clinical service provision of contraception	Provision of contraception and educational tools to increase contraceptive knowledge in the aim to increase usage, if desired
'Safe motherhood'	Antenatal care, labour care plans, postnatal care and breastfeeding support	Encourage engagement with SRH services to ensure that pregnancies are planned and women are offered support from pre-conception to post-partum.
Gynaecological care	Prevention of, if possible, miscarriage, treatment of complications and access to safe abortion care, as permitted by law	Timely and appropriate management of these conditions
Prevention and treatment of sexually transmitted infections (STIs)	Education provision on transmission and methods to prevent transmission	Condom provision, voluntary STI screening, appropriate counselling services
Prevention and management of sexual violence	Encourage increased knowledge and awareness of SRH rights	Provide support to those at risk of gender based and sexual violence
Increase awareness of harmful traditional practices	Include social and cultural leaders in education strategies to demonstrate the negative health outcomes associated with certain practices.	Female genital mutilation (FGM)
Reproductive health programmes	Targeted approaches within SRH aimed specifically at certain groups within society	Adolescents, sex-workers, people living with HIV (PLHIV), postnatal contraception care, men who have sex with men (MSM)

Monitoring of Indicators of Sexual and Reproductive Health

Monitoring can be difficult, especially in resource-poor settings, resulting in delays in response to local need. Data collection is extremely important in order to document changes in service attendances. This is because, ultimately, ensuring services adapt to the changing needs of service users improves the longevity of patients and of the service itself [4].

To ensure services provide the most personalised, efficient healthcare for the local population, feedback of data in both forward and backward directions is crucial. This will ensure investment from governments and local health boards and investors can be targeted appropriately. This can be challenging, particularly with limited data. However, it will still highlight trends and can help to predict future investment needs. Individual cases such as perinatal or maternal deaths can also be reviewed within this subset of data so as to identify specific causes for this and lead to changes in healthcare delivery following local review. Nonetheless there can be negative

implications of this data collection. Some of these errors and their implications are presented in Table 54.3.

What Is Policy Development?

Policy development is a multifaceted process but, ultimately, its goal is to promote and improve the health of individuals and of wider society. Global health is an increasingly complex environment due to the emergence of new challenges to health as a result of globalization, ageing populations and increasing urbanization. These issues are multifactorial and do not solely relate to SRH; however, health policy development is crucial to improving SRH service provision and access [7, 8].

The WHO encourages governments to provide functional healthcare systems to deliver high-quality services to their populations [8]. However, this is a dynamic process requiring continued engagement and investment within services to reduce the gap between need, access and usage of services and maintaining this can be a great challenge [9].

Table 54.3 Typical errors in data collection and interpretation

Error	Implication
Low precision of sample	Reduced specificity of results
Reporting bias	From service users and data collectors potentially resulting in changes that are not reflective of the specific needs of the population
Non-response bias	The non-responders may be those in greatest need of a change in services but may find them inaccessible or afraid of the consequences of their actions through reporting
Data collection changes	Resulting in an inability to validate results
Confounding factors	Has the potential to disguise an association or falsely demonstrate an association resulting in action that again may not be responsive to the actual population needs
Changes in the organization and delivery of services	New management teams may cause delay to rapid responses to changes in services needs if they do not fully understand service users

Policymaking can be regarded as a feedback cycle requiring multiple stages in development and continuous review. It usually begins with pressure for change or identification of a problem. This pressure or problem will then be examined by a team of experts who will review the evidence, the available policy options and the impact of health with each option.

Throughout this process barriers to implementation will be highlighted and discussed with stakeholders. These can include non-governmental organizations (NGOs), not-for profit organisations, healthcare providers and service users. In response to consultation and feedback from this panel, policies will be revised and adapted and an implementation plan will be developed with planned or fixed dates for review and evaluation of the new interventions.

This is not always as simplistic as has been summarised but usually follows a similar cycle. Development and implementation may require years following the initial emergence of pressure for change or a new problem; however, the benefit of this cycle is its continued and ongoing review.

How Is This Relevant?

Sexual and reproductive health needs are continually changing and, as such, outcomes require review and re-evaluation in response to service users' needs. Therefore it is essential that policy development is up to date and adaptable, responding to the needs of society [8, 9].

A brief example of this is the result of the HIV/AIDS epidemic which emerged on a wide scale in the 1980s.

- Health indicators changed considerably when a previously unknown virus started to affect otherwise healthy individuals.

- In response to this research was conducted into gaining greater understanding of HIV.
- New policies were developed to increase awareness of the disease and routes of and methods to prevent transmission.
- Following increased investment and research, treatment courses were developed to prevent the progression of HIV to AIDS.
- There is still an ongoing public health demand for management of HIV/AIDS and there is still much work to be conducted with regards to worldwide rollout of HIV/AIDS prevention and treatment regimens.
- HIV is now a chronic yet manageable condition with multiple treatment options available if such treatment is accessible.
- This is a result of health policy development and educational strategies aimed to increase awareness of HIV/AIDS in an attempt to reduce its transmission.

In 2008 the 'Swiss statement' was released confirming that people living with human immunodeficiency virus (PLHIV) on antiretroviral medications with undetectable viral loads of less than 50 were unable to transmit HIV to their partners. HIV infection remains incurable for these patients; however, transmission can be prevented. The term now used is 'U = U' – undetectable = untransmissible [10]. Development of a third U in this phrase includes 'universal access', demonstrating the continued development, evaluation and adaptation of health policy within a sexual health context.

Conclusions

Sexual health indicators are extremely relevant to policy development and investment. They provide a basic framework to target investment on a large scale. Through use of individualised policy development within services, investment can be developed and focussed on those areas with the greatest need and help to provide a blueprint for development of effective and responsive SRH provision.

Bibliography

1. World Health Organization. Defining sexual health. 2006. http://bit.ly/3HLWTb6.

2. National Institute for Health and Care Excellence. Standards and indicators. 2021. www.nice.org.uk/standards-and-indicators.

3. GOV.UK. Sexual and reproductive health and HIV: Applying all our health. 2019. http://bit.ly/3l0VKmX.

4. World Health Organization. *Reproductive health indicators: Guidelines for their generation, interpretation and analysis for global monitoring.* 1st edition. Geneva: World Health Organization, 2006. https://bit.ly/3WR6iCG.

5. Hoskins A, Varney J. *Entre Nous: A life-course approach to sexual and reproductive health.* 1st edition. Copenhagen: World Health Organization and Entre Nous, 2015. https://bit.ly/3jkAx7g.

6. *FSRH clinical guideline: Contraception after pregnancy.* 2nd edition. Edinburgh: Faculty of Sexual and Reproductive Healthcare, 2017. http://bit.ly/40fOvI5.

7. Rowlands G, Dodson S, Leung A, Levin-Zamir D. Global health systems and policy development: Implications for health literacy research, theory and practice. *HTI.* 2017;**240**:359–91. https://pubmed.ncbi.nlm.nih.gov/28972529.

8. Schmets G, Kadandale S, Porignon D, Rajan D. *Strategizing national health in the 21st century: A handbook.* 1st edition. Geneva: World Health Organization, 2016. https://bit.ly/3WNtykJ.

9. Baicker K, Chandra A. Evidence-based health policy. *New England Journal of Medicine.* 2017;**377** (25):2413–15. https://bit.ly/3kTHvAu.

10. Bereczky T. U=U is a blessing, but only for patients with access to HIV treatment: An essay by Tamás Bereczky. *BMJ.* 2019;**366**:l5554. www.bmj.com/content/366/bmj.l5554.

Health Systems for Sexual and Reproductive Health

Charlotte Gatenby, Sambit Mukhopadhyay and Tahir A. Mahmood

Introduction

In this chapter the role of public health in relation to the World Health Organization's (WHO) sustainable development goals (SDGs) and their interface within sexual and reproductive health (SRH) are described [1].

Why Is Public Health Important within Provision of Sexual Reproductive Healthcare?

The WHO defines public health as 'the art and science of preventing disease, prolonging life and promoting health through the organized efforts of society' (Acheson, 1988) [2]. Public health plays an integral role within SRH service delivery. Increased access to and promotion of awareness of services can result in wide-ranging positive socio-economic impacts, reducing the increasing burden of ill health and health inequalities. However, many taboos are associated with SRH which can act as barriers to access due to fear of stigma and embarrassment from seeking advice or treatment. This potentially reduces patient access, resulting in poor health outcomes. Public health campaigns promoting SRH can address these issues, stimulating a change in how SRH is regarded, leading to greater engagement and investment within services [3].

Key Public Health Issues within Sexual Reproductive Health

One of the principal problems within SRH is unmet need. These unmet needs relate to access and provision of healthcare [4]. Despite changes and increasing public health strategies to target these unmet needs, the following groups remain the most affected yet often the most vulnerable groups within society:

- Adolescents.

- People with limited economic means and therefore independence.
- People living in rural areas or within the outskirts of large cities.
- People living with undiagnosed human immune-deficiency virus (PLHIV) or not on treatment regimes.
- People who have become internationally displaced [5, 6].

In 2015 the WHO developed 17 SDGs which it urges countries to achieve by 2030 (Table 55.1). The intention of the SDGs is to increase sustainable economic growth and reduce inequality whilst also developing projects to protect the planet and its resources for future generations [1, 6]. These SDGs address key issues within public health and provide a blueprint for organizations and governments to develop health strategies to enable them to challenge unmet needs and respond appropriately.

Sexual and Reproductive Health and the World Health Organization Sustainable Development Goals: How Can Public Health Improve Sexual and Reproductive Health Outcomes?

Although this may be subject to debate, of the 17 SDGs, those most relevant to SRH will be discussed in this chapter – SDGs 3, 4, 5 and 10.

Goal 3: Good Health and Well-Being

This is essential within SRH as it is often closely linked to sexual function, which is known to be a key component in quality of life [7]. It is rarely investigated within a public health context; however, the National Survey of Sexual Attitudes and Lifestyles (NATSAL) studies have aimed to challenge this through exploring wider determinants of health

Table 55.1 United Nations sustainable development goals, as developed in 2015 [1, 6]

Sustainable development goal:	Descriptor
Goal 1 – No poverty	End poverty in all its forms, everywhere.
Goal 2 – Zero hunger	End hunger; achieve food security and improved nutrition. Promote sustainable agriculture.
Goal 3 – Good health and well-being	Ensure health lives and promote well-being for all at all ages.
Goal 4 – Quality education	Ensure inclusive and equitable quality education and promote lifelong learning with opportunities for all.
Goal 5 – Gender equality	Empower all women and girls to achieve gender equality.
Goal 6 – Clean water and sanitation	Ensure the availability and sustainability of water and sanitation for all.
Goal 7 – Affordable and clean energy	Ensure access to energy which is affordable, reliable and sustainable.
Goal 8 – Decent work and economic growth	Promotion of sustainable, inclusive economic growth with provision of decent work for all.
Goal 9 – Industry, innovation and infrastructure	Build and promote inclusive and sustainable industrialization and encourage innovation to development resilient infrastructure.
Goal 10 – Reduced inequalities	Reduced inequalities both within countries and amongst others.
Goal 11 – Sustainable cities and communities	Develop cities and settlements to be inclusive, sustainable and safe.
Goal 12 – Responsible consumption and production	Ensure sustainable production and consumption.
Goal 13 – Climate action	Combat climate change and its impacts.
Goal 14 – Life below water	Conserve marine resources and. when developing them, do so sustainably.
Goal 15 – Life on land	Protect, promote and restore terrestrial ecosystems and combat deforestation, desertification and halt loss of biodiversity.
Goal 16 – Peace, justice and strong institutions	Provide access to justice for all through promotion of peaceful, inclusive societies in which development is sustainable and all levels are held accountable for their actions.
Goal 17 – Partnerships for the goals	Implement, sustain and strengthen the global partnership for sustainable development.

and the impact of sexual function. The third NATSAL study reported one in six patients felt their health had an impact on their sex lives, reporting reduced sexual satisfaction and activity during poor health [7, 8]. Thus, through improving overall health and well-being, we can improve sexual relationships, ensuring sex is an enjoyable experience for all involved.

The study also reported that those in better mental and physical health and with full-time employment with higher incomes were more likely to have sex more frequently. Sexual activity, in this instance, is related to health and well-being and financial prosperity. Sexual behaviour is hugely variable and heavily influenced by socio-economic and cultural factors, physiology and health status. Thus, monitoring trends in frequency of sex and sexual satisfaction can be a way of monitoring health and well-being, although this can be subject to recall bias [8].

Goal 4: Quality Education

Informed individuals are empowered individuals with an ability to advocate for themselves and others. Important determinants in SRH include access to education and individuals' knowledge of their own SRH and that of others. Sexual and reproductive health can be highlighted to all ages within society in a 'life course' approach and SRH education needs to begin with the delivery of age-appropriate, incremental SRH education within schooling systems [3, 9].

Sexually active patients need access to sexual health counselling and education. Through this they can develop greater understanding of safe sexual practices and awareness of the legal aspects of sex and relationships, and they can use this information to protect themselves from sexually transmitted infections (STIs) and unplanned pregnancies. Further, with greater awareness of the benefits of engagement with their own sexual health, this can increase access to screening and treatment for STIs and cervical cancer, termination of pregnancy services and, for those who have undergone female genital mutilation (FGM), access to care, counselling and safeguarding, if required, to protect other family members at risk [9].

Goal 5: Gender Equality

A cornerstone of international development is the improvement of gender equality. Through wider public health campaigns targeting increased awareness of the socio-economic benefits of female empowerment and education this can be achieved. In order to accomplish this, however, misconceptions in healthcare relating to contraception must be addressed and social norms need to be challenged as access to and provision of contraception improves women's lives [3].

There is an increasing gap between the age of first sexual contact and the age of conception (if desired) and contraception provides women with the ability to control fertility and, as a result, to gain financial and socio-economic independence and autonomy. Improved access to contraception, especially within the postnatal period to promote increased inter-pregnancy intervals and to reduce rapid repeat pregnancies, can result in improved fetal and maternal outcomes in future pregnancies (if desired) [10]. Delivery of postnatal contraception can be complicated by funding issues. However, this contact with healthcare providers provides an opportunity to discuss and potentially to provide women with methods of contraception. This enables women to control their fertility. Therefore, improved gender equality through increased education, access to contraception and judicial review will improve SRH [3].

Goal 10: Reduced Inequalities

Through improved awareness, service provision and delivery of SRH services inequalities within healthcare can be reduced. Provision can be made at the point of contact of educational materials relating to safer sex practices which have lower failure rates than user dependent methods [3]. The contraceptive options include barrier methods (condoms) and long-acting reversible contraception. In combination with this, improved education, promotion and awareness of healthy relationships, progress can be made to reduce health inequalities in SRH.

Further, improved access to and the decriminalization of abortion care will also help to reduce inequalities within countries and economic regions.

Regardless of the legalities, abortion practices happen worldwide, and decriminalizing them will reduce the sequelae of illegal, unregulated abortion care with its attendants facing risks of severe morbidity and mortality. Provision of safe and accessible abortion care with access to and understanding of contraception following a termination will reduce maternal deaths, provide women with reproductive choices and increase their overall health and well-being.

How Is Public Health Used within Sexual and Reproductive Health?

Primary Prevention

Increasing awareness of diseases through education is a fundamental process integral to public health [11]. Without education and awareness, primary prevention is difficult to achieve. An example of primary prevention within SRH is pre-exposure prophylaxis (PrEP) [12].

Pre-exposure prophylaxis has been developed as a method to prevent acquisition of HIV in HIV-negative patients at elevated risk. Patients identified as at increased risk have had regular condom-less sex (vaginal or anal) for at least the previous 6 months or have had ongoing condom-less sex in a non-exclusive relationship with an HIV-positive partner not on antiretroviral therapy (ART) or with a viral load of more than 200 copies/mL [12]. Pre-exposure prophylaxis has revolutionized the SRH of its users and reduced HIV transmission rates. It is widely accessible within the United Kingdom. Pre-exposure prophylaxis is a very good example of how public health campaigns have increased awareness of effective ways to control the spread of disease; prevention is more effective than long-term treatment [11].

Screening

Screening can be routine and regular, but it must always be voluntary. Promotion of screening as a part of a healthy lifestyle and awareness of treatment availability and access is essential. In order to test for disease there must be readily available access to a treatment, which must be offered to all patients attending following a positive result or partner notification [13].

Important statistical measures to be discussed in screening consultations are those relating to sensitivity and specificity. Testing for STIs is similar to hypothesis testing with the hypothesis being that the patient has an STI. The test result is dependent on the sensitivity and specificity of the STI screening test.

- Sensitivity involves identifying presence of the disease where true positive results represent patients with an STI testing positive and, importantly, false positive results represent patients without disease also testing positive.
- Specificity involves identifying absence of the disease where true negatives are patients without an STI having a negative test result, while false negatives are patients with an STI testing negative.
  - In hypothesis testing type 1 and type 2 errors can occur with test results.
- Type 1 errors are false positives. This indicates the test is not 100% sensitive and as such some patients will receive a positive test result when in fact they do not have the disease. This possibility must be explained to patients as such an error would cause a significant amount of undue distress.
- In type 2 errors false negatives arise whereby the test is not 100% specific and as such patients will receive a negative test result when in fact they do have an STI.

Once again this is equally important for both patient and clinician to be aware of in ensuring repeat testing can be considered, particularly in high-risk individuals.

Early Diagnosis

Early diagnosis with any disease can reduce long-term sequelae of the disease. Stigma in relation to testing and reluctance from healthcare professionals can act as a barrier to testing, especially for HIV. Through normalization of HIV testing into wider, routine practice, the discrimination associated with testing for HIV can be challenged.

The 2020 updates to the United Kingdom's HIV screening guidelines recommend testing be offered within all emergency departments in areas with high (> 2/1,000 and already undergoing venepuncture) or extremely high risk (> 5/1000, all attendees) of HIV seroprevalence within the community [14]. Screening should be completed with fourth-generation serology tests, 45 days following any unprotected sexual intercourse [14]. This has been introduced to increase early diagnosis so as to ensure HIV is treated at an earlier stage, improving health outcomes and reducing

onwards transmission risk and potential progression to AIDS.

Treatment

In HIV care advancements in treatment led to the 2011 'Swiss statement' determining that patients on treatment with undetectable viral loads (less than 50 in the United Kingdom) could continue within relationships without use of condoms as their undetectable viral load meant HIV was not transmissible. Undetectable viral load therefore means HIV is not transmissible, 'U = U' [14]. In relation to other STIs such as chlamydia, gonorrhoea and syphilis, treatments (see Table 55.2) are usually acceptable and accessible to patients, thus increasing uptake rates [15–19].

Another important tool in the long-term management of STIs is the test of cure (TOC). This is a repeat screening for infection following initial treatment to ensure the index patient is treated and thus does not continue the chain of infection. Timings related to TOC can be difficult to ascertain and the evidence base for this is under constant review (Table 55.2).

Partner Notification and Management

One of the most widely known roles of public health within SRH is the practice of partner notification or 'contact tracing' following confirmed diagnosis of an STI. If the index patient consents, they will provide details of their recent contacts, who will then be offered support and treatment [13].

The public health benefits include:

- Prevention of onwards transmission.
- Treatment for the index patient.
- Contacts of the index patient with an earlier diagnosis and linkage to care.
- STI screening for HIV, hepatitis B and vaccinations, if eligible.
- Education (if required).
- Prevention of long-term sequelae of untreated disease.

Surveillance and Data Monitoring

Surveillance and data monitoring provide an ability to monitor many factors within SRH. Examples include STI transmission, birth and termination rates. Surveillance can be an extremely useful tool in monitoring long-term patterns of health, noting changes and potential causes and associations which may be

Table 55.2 Summary outlining the most commonly reviewed sexually transmitted infections with information on diagnostic tests and treatments [15–19]

STI	Diagnosis method	First-line treatment advice for non-complicated infection, UK [1]	First-line treatment advice for non-complicated infection, EU	Test of cure
Chlamydia trachomatis	NAATs	Doxycycline 100 mg twice daily 7-day course	Doxycycline 100 mg twice a day for 7 days	• EU – Not routinely recommended but repeat testing 3–6 months after treatment if < 25 years • UK – Not routinely recommended for uncomplicated genital infection, as residual, nonviable chlamydial DNA can be detected by NAAT for 3–5 weeks after treatment
Neisseria gonorrhoeae	NAATs or culture	Antimicrobial susceptibility not known: • Ceftriaxone 1g intramuscularly, single dose Antimicrobial susceptibility known: • Ciprofloxacin 500 mg orally, single dose	Ceftriaxone 1 g intramuscularly, single dose in combination with azithromycin 2 g, single oral dose	Mandatory and recommended
Genital manifestation of Herpes Simplex Virus, (HSV) type 1 or type 2	HSV DNA detection by polymerase chain reaction (PCR)	Oral antivirals within 5 days of onset of episode	Oral antiviral drugs given within 5 days of onset of symptoms	n/a
Syphilis	PCR and serological testing	(Primary, secondary or early latent) Benzathine penicillin G 2.4 MU IM single dose	Benzathine penicillin G (BPG) 2.4 million units intramuscularly (IM) (one injection of 2.4 million units or 1.2 million units in each buttock) on day 1	UK – Recommended clinical and serological (RPR or VDRL) follow-up is at 3, 6 and 12 months, then if indicated, six monthly until VDRL/ RPR negative or serofas EU – Early syphilis, minimum clinical and serological (VDRL/ RPR) follow-up at 1 month and 3 months then at 6 and 12 months After treatment of early syphilis, the titre of a NTT taken at day 0 (e.g., VDRL and/or RPR) should decline by ≥ two dilution steps (≥ fourfold decrease in titre of antibodies) within 6 months

linked to these. These data can be used to ensure services adapt to the changing needs of society. In the United Kingdom termination of pregnancy is monitored through abortion notification forms sent to the chief medical officers of England and Wales. This provides a reliable source of data which can be used to lead investment and change in policy or education and the statistics are widely available online [11].

Indicators and Quality Assurance

Regular auditing and monitoring of services are required to ensure quality standards are maintained and can be compared against other services and across regions. This promotes good practice and ensures continuity of care. This can be achieved through audits, as mentioned previously, and through quality improvement projects in response to patient surveys and feedback. Auditing of data and rates of uptake for varying contraception methods or increased disease prevalence of STIs within certain areas or communities enables services to adapt and to develop public health strategies to target these areas, thus reducing outbreaks of disease and addressing health beliefs which, for example, may prevent patients from accessing certain methods of contraception [13].

Conclusions

Public health is of key importance within SRH strategy globally and continued investment in education and the life course approach is vital [9, 11]. As outlined within the 2015 WHO SDGs, it is essential that we address all determinants of health – environmental, social and economic [1, 6]. In order to achieve greater overall health and awareness of individual needs, SRH services must focus not only on mortality, morbidity and treatment of disease, but also on prevention through promotion of health and well-being at all phases within a patient's life. Thus the role of public health within SRH is one of empowerment and education.

References

1. THE 17 GOALS | Sustainable Development. Sdgs.un.org. 2015. https://sdgs.un.org/goals.

2. World Health Organization. *European action plan for strengthening public health capacities and services*. Malta: World Health Organization, 2012. https://bit.ly/3EC1Z7J.

3. World Health Organization. *Entre nous: Choices and planning*. 79th edition. Copenhagen: World Health Organization, 2013. https://bit.ly/3IrCg37.

4. Strong K, Noor A, Aponte J et al. Monitoring the status of selected health related sustainable development goals: Methods and projections to 2030. *Global Health Action*. 2020;**13**(1):1846903. www.tandfonline.com/doi/full/10.1080/16549716.2020.1846903.

5. Mitchell K, Mercer C, Ploubidis G et al. Sexual function in Britain: Findings from the third National Survey of Sexual Attitudes and Lifestyles (Natsal-3). *Lancet*. 2013;**382**(9907):1817–29.

6. Wellings K, Palmer M, Machiyama K, Slaymaker E. Changes in, and factors associated with, frequency of sex in Britain: Evidence from three National Surveys of Sexual Attitudes and Lifestyles (Natsal). *BMJ*. 2019;185–7. http://dx.doi.org/10.1136/bmj.l1525.

7. Hoskins A, Varney J. *Entre nous: A life-course approach to sexual and reproductive health*. 1st edition. Copenhagen: World Health Organization, 2015. https://bit.ly/3jkAx7g.

8. Faculty of Sexual and Reproductive Healthcare. *FSRH clinical guideline: Contraception after pregnancy*. 2nd edition. Edinburgh: Faculty of Sexual and Reproductive Healthcare, 2017. http://bit.ly/40fOvI5.

9. British HIV Association. *BHIVA/BASHH guidelines on the use of HIV pre-exposure prophylaxis*. 1st edition. London: British HIV Association, 2018. www.bashhguidelines.org/media/1189/prep-2018.pdf.

10. Palfreeman A, Sullivan A, Rayment M et al. British HIV Association/British Association for Sexual Health and HIV/British Infection Association adult HIV testing guidelines 2020. *HIV Medicine*. 2020;**21**(S6):1–26. https://bit.ly/3xR46kr.

11. Nwokolo N, Dragovic B, Patel S et al. 2015 UK national guideline for the management of infection with *Chlamydia trachomatis*. *International Journal of STD & AIDS*. 2015;**27**(4):251–67. www.bashhguidelines.org/media/1192/ct-2015.pdf.

12. Fifer H, Saunders J, Soni S, Sadiq S, FitzGerald M. 2018 UK national guideline for the management of infection with *Neisseria gonorrhoeae*. *International Journal of STD & AIDS*. 2019;**31**(1):4–15. www.bashhguidelines.org/media/1238/gc-2018.pdf.

13. Patel R, Green J, Clarke E et al. 2014 UK national guideline for the management of anogenital herpes. *International Journal of STD & AIDS*. 2015;**26**(11):763–76. www.bashhguidelines.org/media/1019/hsv_2014-ijstda.pdf.

14. Kingston M, French P, Higgins S et al. UK national guidelines on the management of syphilis 2015. *International Journal of STD & AIDS*. 2015;**27**(6):421–46. https://bit.ly/3Sqruif.

15. Lanjouw E, Ouburg S, de Vries H et al. 2015 European guideline on the management of *Chlamydia*

trachomatis infections. *International Journal of STD & AIDS.* 2015;27(5):333–48. https://bit.ly/3kkGoKp.

16. Unemo M, Ross J, Serwin A et al. 2020 European guideline for the diagnosis and treatment of gonorrhoea in adults. *International Journal of STD & AIDS.* 2020;095646242094912. https://bit.ly/3xPq1sb.

17. Patel R, Kennedy O, Clarke E et al. 2017 European guidelines for the management of genital herpes. *International Journal of STD & AIDS.* 2017;**28**

(14):1366–79. https://iusti.org/wp-content/uploads/2019/12/Herpes.pdf.

18. Janier M, Unemo M, Dupin N et al. 2020 European guideline on the management of syphilis. *Journal of the European Academy of Dermatology and Venereology.* 2020;**35**(3):574–88. https://bit.ly/3EzZjaR.

19. Quality statement 6: Partner notification | Sexual health | Quality standards | NICE. 2019. http://bit.ly/3EDeqjH.

Chapter

56

Prevention and Health Promotion in Sexual and Reproductive Health

Susan Brechin, Mark Steven, Helena Young

Introduction

Sexual and reproductive health (SRH) is an important part of overall health and well-being. Poor sexual health impacts health inequalities and inequalities themselves impact sexual health. Those in greatest need of medical care are often least likely to receive it [1]. Supporting everyone to achieve good SRH requires universal access to services and targeted provision for those at greatest risk of sexual ill health (unplanned pregnancy, sexually transmitted infections (STIs) and blood-borne viruses (BBVs)). Health improvement interventions at the individual, community or population level aim to effect change that will improve sexual health or prevent sexual ill health. Quality improvement (QI) methods can be used to support and evidence if change leads to improvements and can reduce variation in clinical practice. Health improvement initiatives and quality improvement examples in practice will be used to support understanding.

Background and Global Perspectives on Health Improvement

Health improvement (sometimes referred to as health promotion) is one of the three core functions of modern public health alongside health protection and population health. Health improvement is the practice of safeguarding or improving individual and collective health. It is a process where individuals or communities are supported by different health improvement interventions to control and improve their own health and well-being [2–5]. Sexual health improvement interventions focus on supporting people to reduce their risk of STIs, BBVs or unplanned pregnancy with a concentration on prevention (see Box 56.1).

Public policies have the potential to make a big impact on health systems and consequently the health of populations. Policies will influence and be influenced by local inequalities and national or global issues (war, famine or even global pandemics). Good health cannot be ensured by the health sector alone and therefore health improvement requires coordinated action by many different stakeholders (governments, health and social care, voluntary organizations, local authorities, industry and the media). The 17 United Nations sustainable development goals include 3 which are relevant to sexual health (good health and well-being, gender equality and reducing inequalities) [6].

Healthy societies prosper because population health is a stimulus for social, economic and personal development and quality of life. Policymakers are accountable for achieving this through political, economic, social, cultural and environmental policies. Health improvement interventions aim to make these conditions favourable through advocacy to achieve sexual health for all. Health improvement programmes should support people to take control of those things which determine health and to make well-informed choices (for example, choosing safer sex or participating in vaccination programmes). Everyone should have the same opportunity to achieve good sexual health and this may require targeted health improvement interventions to those at greatest risk of harm.

Concepts to Consider around Health Improvement

Some concepts which are important to be aware of when considering sexual health improvement interventions will be outlined briefly in what follows. The determinants of health (genetics, behaviour, environment, physical influences and social factors) influence individual health and so can have a significant impact on population health [7]. Health improvement interventions aim to change the determinants of health and interventions can be targeted towards individuals (behaviour, lifestyle), organizations or

Box 56.1 Examples of prevention in sexual and reproductive health

PREVENTION	OUTCOME
Sex & relationship education (SHRE)	Increases knowledge and capability of individual
Access to contraception	Reduce unplanned pregnancy by access to the most effective methods and emergency contraception locally
Asymptomatic testing	For sexually transmitted infection and blood-borne viruses, including testing individuals identified by partner notification as a contact of someone with infection. Early detection and treatment, reducing spread of infection, morbidity and mortality
Vaccination	Hepatitis B vaccination for at risk populations (men who have sex with men, people who inject drugs and people from areas where prevalence is high). Human papilloma virus vaccinations reduce cervical intraepithelial neoplasia (CIN) and genital warts.
Screening	Cervical screening supports early detection and treatment of CIN, reducing risk of cervical cancer. Routine STI testing in abortion care to reduce risk of post-abortion infection
Treatment as prevention	Hepatitis C treatment to reduce liver failure and malignancy and HIV to ensure virus is undetectable and untransmissable (U = U) HIV pre-exposure prophylaxis (PrEP) and post-exposure prophylaxis (PEP) reduces risk of new infection if started before unprotected sex in higher-risk groups (such as men who have sex with men or serodiscordant couples) and reduce risk of HIV acquisition after unprotected sex or needle-sticks.

governments (social, economic and environmental conditions).

Unconscious bias occurs when a judgement is taken about people based on personal experience, values, media or cultural stereotypes. This can have a detrimental effect on patient care and should always be considered when identifying appropriate health improvement interventions [8]. Stigma is discrimination against an identifiable group and is often directed towards people with STIs or having an abortion. It may cause fear or anger towards people and move focus away from reducing infection transmission (HIV prevention) or increasing access to contraception (teenage pregnancy). People may hide symptoms and not seek healthcare or avoid healthy behaviours. Health improvement interventions must take account of this diversity.

Bias and stigma can be barriers to rights-based reproductive healthcare which aims to support everyone having the right to decide if, when and how often they have children. All of this may influence the care provided to a woman having an abortion who is sad about her loss, to a 16-year-old who is continuing with her pregnancy, to a chaotic substance user who requests contraceptive implant removal to plan a pregnancy or when asking people about oral and anal sex.

Our approach to young people's sexual health often assumes that giving information on the risks and dangers of unprotected sex will in itself result in behaviour change. Health literacy goes beyond just giving information but should empower young people to negotiate condom use with partners, delay sex if not ready, access services to start more effective methods of contraception and use information to maintain good health. Health literacy is affected by gender with men more inclined to participate in higher-risk behaviours and less likely to seek medical advice when unwell or disclose symptoms [9, 10].

Models of behaviour change in sexual health recognise that the conditions for health and well-being, the ability to make what we as health practitioners would describe as good choices, are more nuanced and complex than people being given information alone [11]. Evidence-based programmes which use interventions tailored to the strengths and needs of young mothers, for example, have been shown to support children having the best start in life and supporting young women to believe in themselves and their ability to succeed [12].

Practising trauma-informed care looks to shift focus from 'What's wrong with you?' to 'What happened to you?', supporting a complete picture of a person's life situation (past and present) so effective health or social care interventions (holistic approach) can be introduced [13]. Trauma-informed care improves patient engagement, treatment adherence and health outcomes.

Health Improvement in Practice

Sexual health strategies pull together overarching aims which may include reducing unplanned pregnancy, reducing STI and BBV transmission and reducing avoidable deaths associated with BBV by prevention, early detection and treatment. How these are achieved will vary on population needs and demographics (for example, socioeconomic deprivation, race, gender). Summarising the health improvement interventions needed to achieve the aims visually can help teams to coordinate overall work plans in large programmes or small projects (see Figure 56.1). Health improvement is a process rather than an end point which enables people to take actions that will lead to change and works best when undertaken in partnership with people individually or at the group or community level [14]. Sexual health needs, risks and challenges inevitably change across a life course so health improvement interventions should be tailored accordingly [15].

Use of reliable data (for example, rates of abortion or prevalence of STIs) allows us to identify what type of health improvement interventions may be most likely to effect change and if this is needed at individual, community or population level. It also allows us to identify if the change led to an improvement. The change in health due to an intervention is a health outcome but may be difficult to measure. Outcomes (such as quality of life, morbidity or mortality) are better than inputs (number of tests, procedures or hospital beds) at identifying the interventions which led to the most improvement. Population data can be slow to show change. Quality improvement methods (outlined further later in this chapter) can provide evidence of change more quickly and at a smaller scale so ut can be used to implement change rapidly.

An outcome model for health improvement highlights three levels of outcomes [14]. At the highest level are health and social outcomes (quality of life,

> **Box 56.2** Three questions for health practitioners when considering outcomes model for health improvement [14]
>
> 1. What legislative and policy initiatives are likely to effect change that will improve health?
> 2. What cultural and group actions are likely to effect change that will improve health?
> 3. What individual and family actions and interventions are likely to effect change that will improve health?

morbidity and mortality). Intermediate health outcomes include things like healthy lifestyles, healthy environments and effective health services. Health improvement outcomes include health literacy, social influence and healthy public policies. In simple terms there are three questions for practitioners at these levels (see Box 56.2).

To reduce unplanned pregnancy we may choose to focus our interventions, for example, on women who have the highest rates of abortion (by age or living in areas of high deprivation). We may focus specifically on women aged under 20 years (teenagers) for whom a live birth has the potential to have an impact on their own educational attainment and cycles of intergenerational poverty. Targeting women with substance dependency who are at risk of poor pregnancy outcomes will require a different approach and different health improvement interventions. No single intervention is likely to be effective and a variety of health improvement interventions may be required at individual, group or community levels.

Quality Improvement in Practice

Quality improvement is a systematic approach to looking at efforts to improve patient care, support innovation, deliver continuous quality improvement, manage risk or reduce unwarranted variation in clinical practices (see Box 56.3) [16].

Driver diagrams used in QI work allow teams to organise, describe and test the interventions in health systems needed to effect change. An example looking at reducing teenage pregnancy is outlined (Figure 56.1) [17]. Driver diagrams are useful to track progress towards improvement for small projects or large programmes. The aim describes what better looks like, for

Box 56.3 Three key questions for the quality improvement model [16]

1. What are we trying to achieve?
2. How will we know the change is an improvement?
3. What change will make the improvement?

whom and by when, and should be SMART such as in Figure 56.1: specific to who is being targeted (women under age 25) and what is the change (reduction in all pregnancies including abortion, live birth, miscarriage, ectopic); measurable via national and other data; attainable; relevant to the multiagency team involved; and time-bound deliverable over the next 3 years. Primary drivers focus on key areas for change (process,

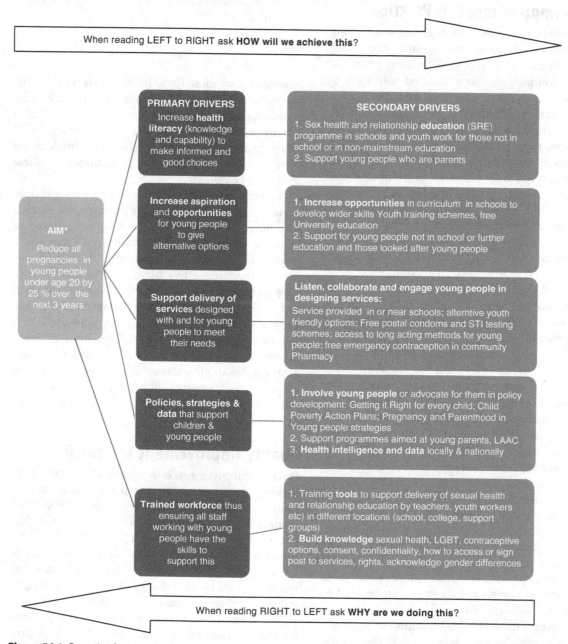

Figure 56.1 Example of a driver diagram to reduce pregnancies (includes abortion, live births, miscarriage and ectopic pregnancies) in young women under the age of 18 years (teenagers) [17]

A design process involves time spent discovering and defining issues before developing and delivering the solutions most likely to improve care. Few women with disadvantage (substance dependency, homelessness, offending behaviour) attend our drop-in sexual health clinics. These vulnerable women are at higher risk of sexual ill health and our aim was to make access easier to increase option for testing, treatment and prevention of unplanned pregnancy and STI including BBV. We engaged vulnerable women in informal workshops to explore barriers to accessing healthcare. Three key themes were identified: lack of knowledge; professionalism (feeling judged or justifying why need to be seen); accessibility (turned away, waiting too long). Changes to these areas are most likely to lead to improvement. After further joint work women came up with ACoRN (Access Care Respond to Needs) fast pass or code word. When used it highlights easily to staff a priority patient who will be seen without question, prioritised by the clinical team and given more time. Vulnerable women, previously reluctant to engage with health care services have used ACoRN to attended for the first time and it appeared to support women's' ability to access care (health literacy). Many have complex issues and a trauma informed approach supported a holistic approach. All women said they would not have attended if not for ACoRN, were happy with all aspects of care and would recommend the service to family or friends. We are now scaling up the ACoRN to different vulnerable groups to support access to mainstream sexual health services.

Figure 56.2 Example of health improvement work. Using a design approach to engage vulnerable women in designing good sexual health service access [24]

infrastructure, culture and people) and are broken down into secondary drivers which provide more detail on interventions. Testing a change helps to identify if the change resulted in an improvement to patient care and tools like Plan Do Study Act (PDSA) cycles can support this [16, 17].

All staff (administrative, domestic, nursing and medical) can be engaged in even basic QI work without formal training [18]. A few extra seconds spent now on a task may save time later, thus reducing frustration and increasing joy in work. Joy in work is linked to a positive environment, high-quality care and improved patient safety [19]. Safety is not just the absence of failures or adverse outcomes (Safety I) but the ability to make things go well and do more of this (Safety II) [20]. Appreciative inquiry is an approach to organizational change which focusses on strengths rather than on weaknesses and feedback from service users on what went well or badly and what is vital to support this [21].

Stakeholder engagement is important for any change project as this supports an understanding of problems and preferences from a patient's viewpoint. All stakeholders or service users (current patients, past and future patients and staff or other service providers who refer into your service, third-sector partners and other services) can support this process. Patient-engagement tools have been developed to support a consistent approach to public engagement to make improvements in care based on patient input and not only healthcare professionals' views [22]. Using the What Matters to You approach supports this to achieve better outcomes, build positive relationships, have more meaningful conversations, support shared decision making and have a personalised approach to care [23]. Design methods ensure time is taken to understand and define the problem before developing, testing and delivering change (Figure 56.2) [24].

Realistic medicine draws on the values and behaviours of staff and patients which allow for a good health care experience [25]. It encompasses shared decision-making and a personalised approach to care, reduces harm and waste, reduces unwanted variation, manages risk better and supports improvers and innovators. Supporting conversations to agree a care plan around what matters to people and how healthcare might realistically contribute to this is an essential tool in current healthcare.

References

1. Watt G. The inverse care law revisited: A continuing blot on the record of the National Health Service. *BJGP* 2018;**68**(677):562–3. https://doi.org/10.3399/bjgp18X699893.

2. McCracken K, Phillips DR. *Global health: An introduction to current and future trends*. London: Routledge, 2012.

3. Rayner G, Laing T. *Ecological public health: Reshaping the conditions for good health*. Abingdon: Routledge, 2012.

4. Dahlgren G, Whitehead M. *European strategies for tackling social inequities in health: Levelling up Part 2*. Liverpool: WHO Collaborating Centre for Policy Research on Social Determinants of Health University of Liverpool, reprinted 2007. https://bit.ly/3XSI6RE.

5. The World Health Organization Ottawa Charter adopted at an international conference on health promotion. The Move towards a New Public Health, 17–21 November 1986. Ottawa, Ontario, Canada. http://bit.ly/3wPBFTf.

6. United Nations. Sustainable development goals. https://bit.ly/3jhmS0L.

7. The Kings Fund. Broader determinants of health: Future trends. http://bit.ly/40ggxTS.

8. Fitzgerald C, Hurst S. Implicit bias in healthcare professionals: A systematic review. *BMC Med Ethics.* 2017;**18**(1):19. http://bit.ly/3Dp5oq3.

9. Oliffe J, Rossnagel E, Kelly M et al. *Men's health literacy: A review and recommendations.* Health Promotion International, 2019, pp. 1–15.

10. Kilfoyle KA, Vitko M, O'Conor R, Cooper Bailey S. Health literacy and women's reproductive health: A systematic review. *J. Womens Health.* 2016;**25** (12):1237–55.

11. De Vasconselos S, Toskin I, Cooper B et al. Behaviour change techniques in brief interventions to prevent HIV, STI and unintended pregnancies: A systematic review. *PLoS One.* 2018;**13**(9):e0204088. https://doi.org/10.1371 /journal.pone.0204088.

12. The family nurse partnership. https://fnp.nhs.uk/ about-us/the-programme.

13. Trauma informed care implementation resource center. http://bit.ly/3Yavrcj.

14. Nutbeam D. Health education and health promotion revisited. *Health Education Journal* 2019; **78**(6): 705–9.

15. Better care: A better future a new vision for sexual and reproductive health care in the UK. FSRH November 2015. www.fsrh.org.uk.

16. Langley G, Moen R, Nolan K et al. (eds.). *The improvement guide: A practical approach to enhancing organizational performance.* 2nd edition. San Francisco: Jossey-Bass.

17. NHS Lothian Quality. Better health, better care, better value. Resources tools for quality planning and implementation. https://qilothian .scot.nhs.uk.

18. Wadsworth D, Pilling R. 15 seconds 30 minutes: A social movement to reduce frustration and increase joy in work at NHS Bradford Teaching Hospitals. http://15s30m.co.uk.

19. Perlo J, Balik B, Swensen S et al. IHI framework for improving joy in work. IHI white paper. Cambridge, MA: Institute for Healthcare Improvement.

20. Hollnagel E, Wears R, Braithwaite J. From Safety-I to Safety-II: A white paper. Published simultaneously by the University of Southern Denmark, University of Florida, USA, and Macquarie University, Australia: The Resilient Health Care Net, 2015. https://bit.ly/3WTvAA2.

21. Care opinion: What's your story? 2005–20 Care Opinion CIC – Reg. no. 10824578. www .careopinion.org.uk.

22. National standards for community engagement. www .voicescotland.org.uk/support-materials.

23. What matters to you? www.whatmatterstoyou.scot.

24. Design Council. The double diamond: A universally accepted depiction of the design process. http://bit.ly /3jfI9Ie.

25. Realistic Medicine. Working together to provide the care that is right for you. www .realisticmedicine.scot.

Index

abortion
  background of, 239
  contraception after, 224
  as human right, 223
  medical, 239–40
  prevalence of, 223
  surgical, 233–8, 240–1
abortion access barriers, European
  abortion stigma, 12–13
  conscientious objection, 12
  practical, 11–12
  procedural, 10–11
abortion access, European
  barriers to, 10–13
  gestational restrictions, 10
  law databases, 10
  legislation liberalization, 10
  restrictive abortion laws, 34
  safety classification, 12
  signs of progress, 10
  World Abortion Laws Map, 10
abortion aftercare
  anti-D immunoglobulin
    administration, 243–4
  contraception, 244
  general principles, 243
abortion assessment
  abortion request, 223
  clinical investigations, 224
  counselling, 223–4
  examination, 224
  gestational age, 224
  history taking, 224
abortion complication management
  haemorrhage, 246
  incomplete abortion, 245–6
  infection risk, 246
  ongoing pregnancy, 245
  uterine perforation and rupture,
    246–7
abortion complications
  cervical trauma, 228
  haemorrhage, 227–8
  infection risk, 228
  retained products, 228
  uterine perforation, 227
  uterine rupture, 227
abortion methods
  choosing between, 226

medical abortion, 225–6, 229–31
  surgical abortion, 226
abortion risks
  mental health, 244
  unsafe abortion, 244–5
  venous thrombosis (VTE), 244
adenomycosis, 147–8
adolescence and sexual health
  life stage description, 334
  protective resources, 335
  risk consequences, 335
  risk factors, 334–5
  risk prevention, 335–6
adolescent contraceptive
    complications
  benefits, 209
  biological factors, 208
  combined hormonal contraception
    (CHC), 209–10
  condoms, male, 211
  copper intrauterine device
    (Cu-IUDs), 211
  depo medroxyprogesterone acetate
    (DMPA), 210
  efficacy of, 209
  fertility-awareness-based methods
    (FABM), 212
  health risks, 209
  levonorgestral-releasing IUDs, 211
  progestogen-only contraceptives
    (POCs), 210
  psychosocial factors, 208–9
  side effects, 209
adulthood and sexual health
  characteristics of, 336
  effect of separation/divorce, 336
  environmental factors, 336
  physical factors, 336
  protective resources, 336
  risk consequences, 337
  risk prevention, 337
*Advocating for Girls' and Women's
    Health and Human Rights*, 5
aerobic vaginitis
  defined, 271
  diagnosis, 271
  symptoms, 271
  treatment, 271–2
ageing process and sexual health

biological and psychological
    changes, 337
  environmental factors, 337
  physical factors, 337–8
  protective resources, 338
  risk consequences, 338
  risk prevention, 338
amenorrhoea
  lactational, 104
  progesterone-only pill (POP), 91
  progestogen-only contraceptives
    (POCs), 90
  progestogen-only implant, 92
  schizophrenia and contraceptives,
    176
anaemia, 54
anorexia nervosa and contraceptives,
  176
antenatal care
  defined, 3
  recommended interventions, 3
  WHO health model, 3–4
  world stats, 16
antibiotics, 135–7
anti-D immunoglobulin
    administration, 243–4
antiepileptic drugs (AEDs), 132–3
antifungals, 137
anti-phospholipid syndrome (APS)
  defined, 187
  pathophysiology, 187
antipsychotics, 133
antiretroviral drugs
  classes of, 167–8
  non-nucleotide reverse transcriptase
    inhibitors (NNRTIs), 168
  nucleotide reverse transcriptase
    inhibitors (NRTIs), 168
antiretroviral therapy (ART), 281–2
aprepitant, 137

bacterial vaginosis (BV)
  defined, 269
  diagnosis, 270–1
  symptoms, 269–70
  treatment, 271
bariatric surgery and contraception,
  83
Barker hypothesis, 50

barrier methods
  cervical cup, 103–4
  chronic kidney disease (CKD) and, 193
  dental dam, 103
  diabetes and, 197
  diaphragm, 103
  epilepsy and, 172
  female condoms, 103
  female physiology and, 103
  lupus autoimmune disease (LAD) and, 189
  male condoms, 102–3
  menopausal transition and, 215
  middle-aged women and, 213
  migraine headache and, 173
  multiple sclerosis (MS) and, 170
  non-hormonal reversible, 102–4
  schizophrenia and, 176
  transgender men, 350
basal body temperature (BBT), 100
behaviour change models (health and well-being), 366
benign breast disease, 146
benign ovarian tumours, 149–50
benign uterine disease and contraceptives
  adenomycosis, 147–8
  background of, 146–7
  endometrial hyperplasia, 148–9
  leiomyoma, 148
  polyps, 147
  uterine fibroids, 148
benzodiazepines, 134
biopsychosocial approach, defined, 38
bone density maintenance
  combined hormonal contraception (CHC) for, 80
  progestogen-only injectable, 93
breast cancer
  combined hormonal contraception (CHC) and, 83
  contraceptive complications, 140–1
breastfeeding
  combined hormonal contraception (CHC) and, 83
  postnatal support, 4
Bruce Quality of Care Framework, 73
bulimia nervosa and contraceptives, 176
bupropion, 133

calendar-based contraceptive methods
  calendar method, 99–100
  standard days method, 100
cancer and contraceptives
  background of, 140
  breast cancer, 83, 140–1
  cervical cancer, 40–1, 83, 142

colorectal cancer, 80, 142
combined hormonal contraception (CHC) and, 83
combined hormonal contraception (CHC) for, 80, 83
complication, 140–4
endometrial cancer, 80, 141–2
gastrointestinal cancer, 142–3
hepatocellular carcinoma, 143
Hodgkin lymphoma, 143–4
lung cancer, 144
non-Hodgkin lymphoma, 143–4
ovarian cancer, 80, 142
pancreatic cancer, 144
skin cancer, 143
summary, 144
thyroid cancer, 144
candida vulvo-vaginitis
  clinical presentation, 268–9
  diagnosis, 269
  frequency of, 268
  treatment, 269
cardiovascular diseases and contraceptives
  age and, 156
  combined hormonal contraception (CHC) and, 83
  diabetes, 156
  dyslipidaemia, 156
  hypertension, 156
  lupus, 156
  migraine headaches, 156
  obesity, 156
  smoking, 156
  surgery with immobilization, 157
  valvular heart disease, 156–7
catamenial epilepsy, 171
cerebral venous thrombosis (CVT) and contraception, 82
cervical cancer
  combined hormonal contraception (CHC) and, 83
  contraceptive complications, 142
  prevention approaches, 40
cervical cap, 128
cervical cup, 103–4
cervical intraepithelial neoplasia screening, 46–7
cervical secretions monitoring methods (CSMM), 100
cervical trauma, post-abortion, 228
cervix in contraception, 66–7
child marriage
  defined, 5
  forced marriage, 341
  health consequences from, 5
  as violation of human rights, 5
  world stats, 5
children
  sexual violence against, 341

sexual violence impact on, 342
children and sexual health
  environmental factors, 333
  inborn diseases, 333
  protective resources, 334
  risk consequences, 334
  risk prevention, 334
chlamydia, 47, 277–8
chronic distress prevention, 43–4
chronic kidney disease (CKD) and contraceptives
  background of, 192
  barrier methods, 193
  clinical recommendations, 194
  combined hormonal contraception (CHC), 192–3
  emergency contraception (EC), 194
  IUDs, 193
  progestogen-only contraceptives (POCs), 193
  sterilization, 193–4
cisgender, defined, 348
clinical screening, 46
cognitive behavioural therapy (CBT), 308
cognitive restructuring therapy, 324
coitus interruptus. see withdrawal
colorectal cancer
  combined hormonal contraception (CHC) for, 80
  contraceptive complications, 142
combined fertility indicator methods, 100
combined hormonal contraception (CHC)
  in adolescents, 209–10
  for disabled people, 179–180
  oestrogens used, 77
  mechanism of action, 77
  pharmacology, 77
  progestins used, 77–9
  transgender men, 350
combined hormonal contraception (CHC), adverse events
  harmless, 84
  serious, 83–4
combined hormonal contraception (CHC), clinical characteristics
  benefits, 79–80
  contraindications, 80
  efficacy of, 79
  use regimen, 79
combined hormonal contraception (CHC), key professional points
  checks before prescribing, 85
  history taking, 84–5
  missed pill rules, 85–6
  risk/benefit balance, 84
combined hormonal contraception (CHC), metabolic effects

carbohydrate metabolism, 79
coagulation system, 79
endocrine, 79
plasma lipids, 79
combined hormonal contraception
(CHC), risk factors
bariatric surgery, 83
breastfeeding, 83
cancer, 83
cerebral venous thrombosis (CVT),
82
chronic kidney disease (CKD),
192–3
depression and, 174
diabetes, 82
diabetes mellitus (DM), 198
epilepsy and, 171
hypertension, 82
ischemic stroke and, 82, 154
liver disease, 83
lupus and, 189–90
maternal age, 82
menopausal transition, 214–15
in middle-aged women, 212–13
migraine headaches, 172
mood changes, 123
multiple sclerosis and, 170
myocardial infarction (MI), 82, 154
obesity, 83
peripheral artery diseases, 154
schizophrenia and, 175
sexual side effects, 126–8
thyroid function and, 201–2
uterine bleeding and, 119–20
venous thrombosis (VTE), 80–2
combined oral contraceptives (COCs),
67
comprehensive life-course approach to
women's health, 35
comprehensive sexuality and
reproductive health education
(CSRE), 17–18, 23–4
conception prerequisites, 249–50
condoms, female
mechanics of, 103
transgender people, 350
condoms, male
in adolescents, 211
available contraceptive method, 219
available male contraceptive
method, 217
local barrier method, 128
overview, 102–3
transgender people, 350
conscientious objection, 12
contraception
access, denial to, 341
improvements in health-related
outcomes, 1
post-abortion, 224, 226–7

world need for, 1
contraception, combined hormonal
adverse events, 83–4
breastfeeding, 83
clinical characteristics, 79–84
oestrogens used, 77
key points, 84–6
mechanism of action, 77
metabolic effects, 79
pharmacology, 77
progestins used, 77–9
risk factors, 80–3
contraception, emergency
availability, 114
causes of failure, 115
copper intrauterine device
(Cu-IUD), 116
defined, 114
efficacy of, 114
European, 9–10
mechanism of action, 114
oral, 116
safety, 114–15
side effects, 115
starting contraceptives after, 115–16
contraception, failure rate, 73
contraception, hormonal
combined oral contraceptives
(COCs), 67
intra-vaginal rings, 68
levonorgestral-releasing IUDs, 68–9
patches, 67
progesterone receptor modulators
(PRM), 69
progestogens, 68
steroids, 68
contraception access, European
available methods, 9
Contraception Policy Atlas, 8–9
emergency contraception (EC), 9–10
stats, 9
usage rate, 8
contraception counselling, evidence-
based
Bruce Quality of Care Framework,
73
GATHER approach, 75
as human right, 71
principles of, 71–2
provider attitude effects, 72–3
contraception counselling,
intervention types
communication issues, 74
social inequities, 74–5
summary, 74
contraception endocrinology
cervix, 66–7
corpus luteum function interference,
65
endometrium, 66

fallopian tubes, 65–6
follicle development, 62
follicle rupture interference,
65
historical development, 61
hypothalamic-pituitary-ovarian
(HPO) axis, 61
implications, 65
ovarian and uterine cycles, 63
ovary, 64–5
Contraception Policy Atlas, 8–9
contraceptive complications
adolescent, 334
benign breast disease, 146
benign uterine disease, 146–9
cancer, 140–4
cardiovascular diseases, 155–7
chronic kidney disease (CKD),
192–4
diabetes, 196–9
disabled people, 179–181
drug–drug interactions, 131–8
eating disorders, 176
epilepsy, 170–2
herbal remedies, 137
HIV infection, 165–8
immunosuppressive disease,
183–5
ischemic stroke, 154
lupus autoimmune diseases (LAD),
187–90
major depression (MD), 174
menopausal transition, 214–15
metabolic disease, 159–62
microvascular disease, 154–5
middle-aged women, 212–14
migraine headache, 172–3
mood, 123–5
multiple sclerosis (MS), 170
myocardial infarction, 154
ovarian conditions, 149–52
peripheral artery diseases, 154
polycystic ovary syndrome (PCOS),
204–6
schizophrenia, 175–6
sexual side effects, 126–9
thyroid dysfunction, 200–2
uterine bleeding, 118–21
venous thromboembolism (VTE),
155
contraceptive vaccines, male,
220
contraceptives, female uterine bleeding
complication
frequency of, 115–16
management, 119
pathophysiology, 118–19
treatment options, 119–21
contraceptives, medical eligibility
criteria (MEC), 184, 188

contraceptives, non-hormonal
    reversible
  barrier methods, 102–4
  copper intrauterine device
      (Cu-IUDs), 104–5
  efficacy of, 98
  fertility-awareness-based methods
      (FABM), 97–102
  internet resources, 105–6
  lactational amenorrhea, 104
  methods, 97
  popularity of, 97
  spermicides, 104
contraceptives, progestogen-only
  amenorrhoea adverse event, 90
  benefits, 89
  characteristics, 88
  contraindications, 89
  delivery systems, 88
  efficacy of, 89
  formulations, 88
  hormonal intrauterine systems (IUSs),
      93–5
  indications, 89
  mode of action, 88
  progestogen-only implant, 91–2
  progestogen-only injectable, 92–3
  progestogen-only pill (POP), 90–1
  return to fertility, 89
  side effects, 90
  uterine spotting adverse event,
      89–90
copper intrauterine device (Cu-IUD).
    see also intrauterine device
  in adolescents, 211
  background of, 104
  chronic kidney disease (CKD),
      193
  complications, 105
  diabetes mellitus (DM), 197
  for disabled people, 179–181
  emergency contraception (EC),
      116
  epilepsy and, 172
  lupus and, 189
  menopausal transition, 215
  in middle-aged women, 213
  migraine headaches and, 173
  multiple sclerosis and, 170
  pain, 105
  placement, 104–5
  schizophrenia and, 175–6
  sexual side effects, 128
  transgender men, 350
corpus luteum function in
    contraception, 65
counselling provider attitude effects
  assessment difficulty, 72
  client bias, 72
  method-related biases, 72–3

cytolytic vaginosis
  diagnosis, 273
  treatment, 273

delayed ejaculation
  clinical management, 329
  defined, 327–8
  epidemiology, 328
  pathophysiology, 328–9
dental dam, 103
depo medroxyprogesterone acetate
      (DMPA)
  in adolescents, 210
  diabetes mellitus (DM), 198
  in middle-aged women, 213
depression and contraceptives
  combined hormonal contraception
      (CHC) and, 83–4, 174
  complications, 174
  major depression (MD), 174
  postpartum depression, 174
  progestogen-only contraceptives
      (POCs), 174
determinants of health, 365
developmental origin of health and
      disease (DOHaD)
  background of, 49–50
  epigenetic reprogramming and, 50
  evolutionary plasticity, 50
  fetal programming, 50
  inflammation and stress affecting, 50
  International Society for
      Developmental Origins of Health
      and Disease, 50
  sex-specific stress responses, 50
  summary, 50
diabetes and contraceptives
  barrier methods, 197
  classification, 196
  combined hormonal contraception
      (CHC), 198
  complications, 156
  contraception medical significance,
      196
  contraceptives summary, 197
  copper intrauterine device (Cu-
      IUD), 197
  emergency contraception (EC), 198
  fertility-awareness-based methods
      (FABM), 196
  levonorgestral-releasing IUDs, 198
  Medical Eligibility Criteria (MEC),
      196
  postnatal contraception, 198–9
  prevalence of, 196
  progestogen-only contraceptives
      (POCs), 198
  sterilization in women, 198
  type-1, 159–60
  type-2, 160, 161

diabetes mellitus (DM), defined, 196
diabetes mellitus (DM) types
  gestational diabetes mellitus, 196
  type 1 diabetes, 196
  type 2 diabetes, 196
diaphragm, 103
digitally assisted FABMs (d-FABMs),
      100–2
dilation and evacuation (D&E), 235
disabled people and contraceptives
  background of, 179–181
  combined hormonal contraception
      (CHC), 180
  comparison between, 180
  concept of disabilities, 180
  contraceptive consultation and
      examination, 180
  family planning consultation, 179
  five groups of disability, 179–181
  IUDs, 180
  progestogen-only contraceptives
      (POCs), 180
  treatment principles, 180
disabled people and sexual violence,
      341
dyslipidaemia, 156
doxycycline, 120–1
dyslipidaemia and contraceptives,
      161–2
dysmenorrhea, 79
dyspareunia
  assessment, 302
  defined, 300

eating disorders and contraception
  anorexia nervosa, 176
  background of, 176
  bulimia nervosa, 176
ectopic pregnancy, 112
education
  health literacy, 366
  public health sustainable
      development goals, 359–60
electric vacuum aspiration (EVA),
      233–4
emergency contraception (EC)
  availability, 114
  causes of failure, 115
  chronic kidney disease (CKD),
      194
  copper intrauterine device
      (Cu-IUD), 116
  defined, 114
  diabetes mellitus (DM), 198
  efficacy of, 114, 137–8
  European, 9–10
  lupus and, 190
  mechanism of action, 114
  Medical Eligibility Criteria (MEC),
      188

oral, 116
safety, 114–15
side effects, 115
starting contraceptives after, 115–16
endometrial cancer
combined hormonal contraception (CHC) for, 80
contraceptive complications, 141–2
endometrial hyperplasia, 148–9
endometriosis, 80
endometrium in contraception, 66
entry inhibitors, 168
epidemiological factors in public health policies for sexual and reproductive health
education, 30
environment, 30
health systems, 30
laws and norms, 30
special needs populations, 30
epilepsy and contraception
background of, 170–1
barrier methods, 172
catamenial, 171
combined hormonal contraception (CHC), 171
contraceptive summary, 171
IUDs, 172
progestogen-only contraceptives (POCs), 171
sterilization, 172
equality and public health, 360
erectile dysfunction
assessment, 322
definition and categorization, 321
pathophysiology, 321–2
erectile dysfunction clinical management
consultation pointers, 322–3
penile prosthesis, 324
pharmacological considerations, 323
vacuum pump, 324
erectile dysfunction psychosexual treatment
cognitive restructuring therapy, 324
mindfulness therapy, 324–5
overview, 324
sensate focus therapy, 324
oestrogen
in combined hormonal contraception, 77
and glucose metabolism, 159
and lipid metabolism, 161
and thyroid function, 200
uterine bleeding treatment, 120
ethinylestradiol (EE), 77, 131
Evaluation of Comprehensive Sexuality Education Programmes, 25
evolutionary plasticity, 50
exercise, lack of, 43–4

fallopian tubes in contraception, 65–6
family planning
disabled people, 179
as fundamental human right, 1
improvements in health-related outcomes, 1
world need for contraception, 1
female cognitive arousal disorder (FCAD), 295
female condoms, 103, 128
female genital mutilation (FGM)
defined, 4
forced sterilization, 17
as form of sexual violence, 341
health consequences from, 4
legislation banning, 5
overview, 17
as violation of human rights, 4
world stats, 4
female orgasmic disorder (FOD), 295
fertility-awareness-based methods (FABM)
in adolescents, 212
diabetes mellitus (DM), 196
lupus and, 188–9
menopausal transition, 215
in middle-aged women, 213–14
sexual side effects, 128–9
fetal alcohol syndrome, 56
fetal programming, 50
follicle rupture interference in contraception, 65
forced sterilization, 17

Gandarusa contraceptive pill, 220
gastrointestinal cancer contraceptive complications, 142–3
GATHER approach, 75
gay men, defined, 347
gender equality in public health, 360
gender expression, defined, 347
gender identity, defined, 347
gender-based violence. see also sexual violence
child marriage, 5
defined, 4
female genital mutilation (FGM), 4–5, 17
health consequences from, 4
legislation around, 4
public health and, 35
as violation of human rights, 17–18
world stats, 4
genetics and developmental origin of health and disease (DOHaD), 50
genital herpes, 274–5
genitourinary syndrome of menopause (GSM), 264
German Federal Centre for Health Promotion (BZgA), 25

gestational diabetes mellitus, 196
Global Abortion Policies Database (GAPD), 10
Global Communication Campaign for Women's Health, 5
glucose metabolism and contraceptives
familial type-2 diabetes, 161
polycystic ovarian syndrome (PCOS), 160–1
sex hormones and, 159–61
type-1 diabetes, 159–60
type-2 diabetes, 160
gonorrhoea, 47, 57, 276–7
good health and well-being in sexual and reproductive health
background of, 365
global perspectives, 365
importance of initiatives in, 365
good health and well-being in sexual and reproductive health concepts
behaviour change models, 366
determinants of health, 365
health literacy, 366
human rights-based reproductive health, 366
stigma, 366
trauma-informed care, 367
unconscious bias, 366
good health and well-being in sexual and reproductive health in clinical practice
intervention strategies overview, 367
outcome models, 367–9
quality improvement, 367–9
griseofulvin, 137

haemorrhage
medical abortion, 231
post-abortion, 227–8
surgical abortion, 236
health prevention approaches
biopsychosocial approach, 38
life-course approach, 38
health prevention targets
cervical cancer, 40
infertility, 42–3
lifestyle health risks, 43–4
pregnant mother and child morbidity, 43
sexual dysfunction, 41
sexual violence, 41–2
STIs and HIV, 39–40
unintended pregnancies, 38–9
hepatitis B, 282–3
hepatitis B vaccination, 57
hepatitis C, 282–3
hepatocellular carcinoma, 143
herbal remedies and contraception, 137
heterosexism, defined, 349

HIV
  antiretroviral therapy (ART), 281–2
  clinical presentation, 280
  definition and pathophysiology, 280
  diagnosis, 280
  early diagnosis public health
    important, 361
  LGBT+ sexual and reproductive
    health risks, 348
  pregnancy and, 282
  prevention approaches, 39–40
  public health and, 34–5
  screening, 47
  test interpretation, 280–1
  test of cure, 361
  testing indications, 281
  transmission, 280
  treatment goals, 282
  world knowledge stats, 2
HIV and contraceptives
  antiretroviral drugs, 167–8
  background of, 165
  disease progression influence, 165
  entry inhibitors, 168
  health risks, 166–7
  integrate strand transfer inhibitors,
    168
  pre-exposure prophylaxis (PrEP),
    168
  protease inhibitors, 168
  transmission risk, 166
HIV prevention
  PEP (post-exposure prophylaxis),
    282
  PrEP (pre-exposure prophylaxis),
    282
  safe sexual behaviour, 282
Hodgkin lymphoma, 143–4
homophobia, defined, 349
hormonal intrauterine systems (IUSs)
  adverse events, 94–5
  benefits, 94
  efficacy of, 93
  formulations, 93
  insertion, 93
  mode of action, 93
hormonal male contraception
  combination therapy, 221
  mechanisms of, 221
  MENT, 221
  monthly injections, 221
  weekly injections, 221
human papilloma virus (HPV), 47, 279
human rights-based reproductive
    health
  abortion access, 223
  contraception counselling, 71
  defined, 366
  family planning, 1
  family planning (WHO), 73

public health, 29
sexual and reproductive health
    (SRH), 8
UNFPA Operational Guidance for
    Comprehensive Sexuality
    Education: A Focus on Human
    Rights and Gender, 25
human sexuality features
  biopsychosocial phenomenon, 290
  changing with biology, 290
  continuum of spectrum, 290
  subjective, internal nature, 289–90
hypertension
  combined hormonal contraception
    (CHC) and, 82
  contraceptive complications, 156
hypoactive sexual desire disorder
    (HSDD), men
  assessment, 319–20
  clinical management, 320
  definition difficulty, 318
  lack of research on, 318
  pathophysiology, 319
  prevalence of, 318–19
  subtypes, 319
hypoactive sexual desire disorder
    (HSDD), women
  defined, 263, 295
  pathophysiology, 296
  risk factors, 296
hypothalamic-pituitary-ovarian
    (HPO) axis, 61
hypothyroidism, 201
hysterectomy. see sterilization in
    women
hysteroscopic sterilization, 111

immunosuppressive disease and
    contraceptives
  background of, 183
  contraceptive choices summary, 183
  hormonal contraceptives and, 185
  infection risk, 183
  pharmacological considerations,
    184–5
  practice guidelines, 185
  progestogen effects and VTE, 183–4
incomplete abortion, 245–6
indicators of sexual and reproductive
    health
  defined, 353
  guidelines, 354–5
  indicator requirements, 353–4
  key factors, 355
  monitoring, 355
  purpose of, 353
  risk consequences, 354
  WHO, 18–20
infertility
  causes of, 250

defined, 249
diagnostic criteria, 250–1
mental health impact, 252–4
physical health impact, 252
prevalence of, 249
prevention, 252
prevention approaches, 42–3
prognostic biomarkers, 251
sexual and reproductive threat, 16
treatment options, 251–2
integrate strand transfer inhibitors,
    168
international documents on sexual and
    reproductive health
  Evaluation of Comprehensive
    Sexuality Education Programmes,
    25
  International Technical Guidance on
    Sexuality Education, 25
  It's All One Curriculum, 25
  parts of, 25
  Standards for Sexuality Education,
    25
  UNFPA Operational Guidance for
    Comprehensive Sexuality
    Education: A Focus on Human
    Rights and Gender, 25
International Society for
    Developmental Origins of Health
    and Disease, 50
International Society for the Study of
    Vulvovaginal Disease (ISSVD),
    300–301
International technical guidance on
    sexuality education, 25
intersex people, defined, 348
intra-vaginal rings (contraceptive), 68
intrauterine device (IUDs). see also
    copper intrauterine device;
    levonorgestral-releasing IUDs
  background of, 104
  complications, 105
  emergency contraception (EC), 116
  mood change counselling, 125
  mood changes, 123
  pain, 105
  placement, 104–5
  post-abortion, 226
intrauterine devices (IUDs)
  for disabled people, 179–181
  multiple sclerosis and, 170
intra-vas device (IVD), 220
ischemic stroke
  combined hormonal contraception
    (CHC) and, 82
  migraine headaches, 172
ischemic stroke and contraceptives
  background of, 154
  combined hormonal contraception
    (CHC), 154

progestogen-only contraceptives (POCs), 154
isotretinoin, 137
It's All One Curriculum, 25

lactational amenorrhea, 104
lamotrigine, 133
laparoscopic sterilization, 110–11
laparotomy, 109–10
leiomyoma, 148
lesbian women, defined, 347
levonorgestral-releasing IUDs. *see also* intrauterine device
  in adolescents, 211
  chronic kidney disease (CKD), 193
  defined, 68–9
  diabetes mellitus (DM), 198
  for disabled people, 179–181
  epilepsy and, 172
  lupus and, 189
  menopausal transition, 215
  in middle-aged women, 213
  migraine headaches and, 173
  multiple sclerosis and, 170
LGBT+ contraception
  basics, 350
  counselling, 350
  transgender man, 350
LGBT+ sexual and reproductive healthcare
  clinical communication skills, 349–50
  definitions, 347–8
LGBT+ sexual and reproductive health risks
  health system, 349
  HIV and STDs, 348
  mental and societal, 349
life-course approach (sexual health)
  adolescence, 334–6
  adulthood, 336–8
  ageing process, 337–8
  children, 333–4
  defined, 38
  overview, 333
lifestyle health risks and prevention, 43–4
lipid metabolism and contraceptives
  dyslipidaemia, 161–2
  sex hormones and, 161
liver disease and contraception, 83
lung cancer, 144
lupus autoimmune disease (LAD) and contraceptives
  and arterial events, 156
  barrier methods, 189
  combined hormonal contraception (CHC), 189–90
  consultation tips, 190

copper intrauterine device (Cu-IUDs), 189
  emergency contraception (EC), 190
  fertility-awareness-based methods (FABM), 188–9
  levonorgestral-releasing IUDs, 189
  medical eligibility criteria for contraceptive use, 187–8
  medical significance of contraception, 187
  pathophysiology, 187
  progestogen-only contraceptives (POCs), 189
  for teratogenic medications, 190
  types of, 187

major depression (MD) and contraceptives
  clinical aspects, 174
  hormonal contraceptives, 174
  postpartum depression, 174
  symptoms, 174
male condoms, 102–3, 128
male contraception, general aspects
  available methods, 217
  pathophysiology, 217
  sperm production physiology, 217
male contraception, ideal
  hormonal approach, 219, 221
  non-hormonal approach, 219, 220
  pill usage, 217–19
male contraception, methods
  condoms, 219
  natural family planning, 219
  transgender people, 350
  vasectomy, 176, 217, 219–20
  withdrawal, 219
manual vacuum aspiration (MVA), 234–5
maternal and child morbidity prevention, 43
maternal healthcare
  antenatal care, 3–4
  defined, 3
  postnatal care, 4
  preconception counselling, 3
  world mortality stats, 3, 16
maternal mortality ratio
  childbirth and, 3
  world stats, 3
medical abortion. *see also* surgical abortion
  after 12 weeks, 230
  contraception after, 240
  defined, 229
  end of second trimester, 230
  infection risk, 231
  mifepristone and, 229
  misoprostol and, 229
  overview, 225–6

pain management, 230
  WHO medical abortion guidelines, 229
medical abortion 12–22 weeks, 239–40
medical abortion before 12 weeks
  efficacy of, 229
  follow-up, 229–30
  home treatment, 229
  mifepristone and, 229
  outcomes, 229
  overview, 239
medical abortion complications
  haemorrhage, 231
  uterine rupture, 231
medical abortion over 22 weeks, 240
melanoma, 143
menopausal transition and contraceptives
  background of, 214
  barrier methods, 215
  characteristics, 214
  combined hormonal contraception (CHC), 214–15
  copper intrauterine device (Cu-IUD), 215
  efficacy of, 214
  fertility-awareness-based methods (FABM), 215
  health risks, 214
  levonorgestral-releasing IUDs, 215
  progestogen-only implant, 215
  progestogen-only pill (POP), 215
  side effects, 214
menstruation and contraceptives, 97–9
MENT (7α-Methyl-19-nortesterone), 221
mental health and conception
  abortion risk, 244
  assessment, 56
  infertility impact on, 252–4
  psychotropic drug interactions with contraceptives, 133–4
mental health and sexual violence, 342
metabolic disease and contraceptives
  background of, 159
  glucose metabolism and, 159–61
  lipid metabolism and, 161–2
metformin, 205
microscopy for vaginal fluids, 48
microvascular disease, 154–5
middle-aged women and menopause, 214
middle-aged women and contraceptives
  barrier methods, 213
  biomedical factors, 212
  combined hormonal contraception (CHC), 212–13
  copper intrauterine device (Cu-IUD), 213

middle-aged women (cont.)
depo medroxyprogesterone acetate (DMPA), 213
efficacy of, 212
fertility-awareness-based methods (FABM), 213–14
health consequences from, 212
levonorgestral-releasing IUDs, 213
progestogen-only implant, 213
progestogen-only pill (POP), 213
psychosocial factors, 212
side effects, 212
mifepristone
medical abortion and, 116, 229
uterine bleeding treatment, 121
migraine headache and contraceptives
background of, 172
barrier methods, 173
combined hormonal contraception (CHC), 172
copper intrauterine device (Cu-IUD), 173
diagnostic criteria, 172
ischemic stroke risk, 172
levonorgestral-releasing IUDs, 173
progestogen-only contraceptives (POCs), 172–3
sterilization in women, 173
migraine headaches
combined hormonal contraception (CHC) and, 83
contraceptive complications, 156
mindfulness therapy, 324–5
minorities, sexual
comprehensive sexuality and reproductive health education (CSRE), 17–18
contraception counselling, 74–5
forced sterilization, 17
public health and, 34
misoprostol, 229
mood changes and contraceptives
defined, 123
aetiology, 124
factors affecting, 124
management, 125
pathophysiology, 123–4
psychoendocrine mechanisms, 124
studies, 123
multiple sclerosis (MS) and contraceptives
background of, 170
barrier methods, 170
combined hormonal contraception (CHC), 170
contraceptive summary, 171
IUDs, 170
progestogen-only contraceptives (POCs), 170

sterilization, 170
Mycoplasma genitalium, 47
myocardial infarction and contraceptives
background of, 154
combined hormonal contraception (CHC), 82, 154
progestogen-only contraceptives (POCs), 154

natural family planning (male), 219
non-Hodgkin lymphoma, 143–4
non-hormonal male contraceptives
contraceptive vaccines, 220
future plans for, 219
Gandarusa contraceptive pill, 220
intra-vas device (IVD), 220
reversible inhibition of sperm under guidance (RISUG), 220
ultrasound, 220
non-hormonal reversible contraceptives
copper intrauterine device (Cu-IUD), 104–5
efficacy of, 98
internet resources, 105–6
lactational amenorrhea, 104
methods, 97
popularity of, 97
spermicides, 104
non-hormonal reversible contraceptives, barrier methods
cervical cup, 103–4
dental dam, 103
diaphragm, 103
female condoms, 103
female physiology and, 103
male condoms, 102–3
non-hormonal reversible contraceptives, fertility-awareness -based methods (FABM)
background of, 97
basal body temperature (BBT), 100
biology of, 97–9
calendar-based methods, 99–100
cervical secretions monitoring methods (CSMM), 100
combined fertility indicator methods, 100
digitally assisted FABMs (d-FABMs), 100–2
non-nucleotide reverse transcriptase inhibitors (NNRTIs), 168
non-steroidal anti-inflammatory drugs (NSAIDs), 120
nucleic acid amplification tests (NAAT), 277
nucleotide reverse transcriptase inhibitors (NRTIs), 168
nutrition and conception

adult healthy diet principles (WHO), 53
anaemia, 54
child diet principles (WHO), 53
folic acid and vitamin B 12, 54
importance of, 53
nutrition-related health problems summary (WHO), 54–6

obesity
child, 51
combined hormonal contraception (CHC) and, 83
contraceptive complications, 156
and preconception health, 49
prevention approaches, 43–4
thyroid function and, 206
opioids, 135
oral contraceptives
mood changes, 124
post-abortion, 226–7
sexual side effects, 126–7
oral emergency contraception, 116
outcome model for health improvement levels
health and social, 367
health improvement, 367
intermediate health, 367
practitioner questions, 367
ovarian cancer
combined hormonal contraception (CHC) for, 80
contraceptive complications, 142
ovarian conditions and contraceptives
benign ovarian tumours, 149–50
ovarian endometriosis, 150–1
polycystic ovarian syndrome (PCOS), 151–2
ovarian cysts and contraceptives, 80
ovarian endocrinology, 64–5
ovarian endometriosis, 150–1

pain
defined, 301
dysfunctional, 312–13
inflammatory, 312
neuropathic, 312
nociceptive, 312
pain, female sexual. *see also* sexual dysfunction, women
assessment, 301–2
aetiology, 304
history taking, 304–6
physical conditions causing, 305
and sexual dysfunction, 301–6
specific disorders causing, 305
pain, female sexual, treatment
education, 307
goals of, 307

lifestyle changes, 307
overview, 306–7
pharmacological and surgical, 308–9
physical therapy, 307–8
psychotherapy, 308
patches (contraceptive), 67
pelvic inflammatory disease (PID), 278
penile prosthesis, 324
PEP (HIV post-exposure prophylaxis), 282
peripheral artery diseases and contraceptives
   background of, 154
   combined hormonal contraception (CHC), 154
   progestogen-only contraceptives (POCs), 154
pharmacological interactions and contraceptives
   antibiotics, 135–7
   antiepileptic drugs (AEDs), 132–3
   antifungals, 137
   aprepitant, 137
   background of, 131
   griseofulvin, 137
   isotretinoin, 137
   metabolism of steroid contraceptive hormones, 131
   opioids, 135
   psychotropic drugs, 133–4
   resorption of steroid contraceptive hormones, 131
polycystic ovarian syndrome (PCOS) and contraceptives, 160–1
   overview, 151–2
polycystic ovary syndrome (PCOS) and contraceptives
   background of, 204
   contraceptive options, 204–6
   pathophysiology, 204
   signs, symptoms, complications, 204
polyps, endometrial, 147
post-exposure prophylaxis (PEP), 168
postnatal care
   breastfeeding support, 4
   defined, 4
   recommended interventions, 4
postpartum depression and contraceptives, 174
preconception health care
   contraception counselling, 52
   data collection, 49
   defined, 52
   developmental origin of health and disease (DOHaD), 49–50
   evidence-based intervention, 53
   interventions not affecting progeny health, 50
   period of, 50

Preparing for Life Initiative (WHO), 52–3
   sexuality education guidelines, 53
preconception counselling
   defined, 3
   health promotion, 3
   risk assessment, 3
   targeted interventions, 3
pre-exposure prophylaxis (PrEP), 168, 360
premature ejaculation
   clinical management, 326
   defined, 325
   pathophysiology, 325
   pharmacological considerations, 326–7
   psychological therapy, 326
   surgery for, 327
PrEP (HIV pre-exposure prophylaxis), 282, 285
Preparing for Life Initiative (WHO), 52–3
primary prevention
   cervical cancer, 40
   defined, 38
   infertility, 42
   lifestyle health risks, 44
   pregnant mother and child morbidity, 43
   sexual dysfunction, 41
   sexual violence, 41–2
   STIs and HIV, 39
   unintended pregnancies, 38–9
progesterone receptor modulators (PRM), 69
progestins
   in combined hormonal contraception, 77–9
   and glucose metabolism, 159
   and lipid metabolism, 161
progestogen-only contraceptives (POCs)
   in adolescents, 210
   amenorrhoea adverse event, 90
   benefits, 89
   characteristics, 88
   chronic kidney disease (CKD), 193
   contraindications, 89
   delivery systems, 88
   depression and, 174
   efficacy of, 89
   epilepsy and, 171
   formulations, 88
   hormonal intrauterine systems (IUSs), 93–5
   indications, 89
   lupus and, 189
   migraine headaches and, 172–3
   mode of action, 88
   multiple sclerosis and, 170

progestogen-only implant, 91–2
progestogen-only injectable, 92–3
progestogen-only pill (POP), 90–1
return to fertility, 89
schizophrenia and, 175–6
sexual side effects, 127, 128
side effects, 90
transgender men, 350
uterine spotting adverse event, 89–90
in women with ischemic stroke, 154
in women with myocardial infarction (MI), 154
in women with peripheral artery diseases, 154
progestogen-only implant
   in adolescents, 211
   adverse events, 92
   benefits, 92
   diabetes mellitus (DM), 198
   efficacy of, 92
   formulations and release rate, 91
   insertion, 92
   menopausal transition, 215
   in middle-aged women, 213
   post-abortion, 226
   removal, 92
   risks, 92
progestogen-only injectable
   adverse events, 93
   benefits, 92–3
   for disabled people, 179–181
   formulations, 92
   post-abortion, 226
   risks, 93
progestogen-only pill (POP)
   amenorrhoea adverse event, 91
   benefits, 91
   diabetes mellitus (DM), 198
   for disabled people, 179–181
   dosages, 91
   efficacy of, 90–1
   formulations, 90
   menopausal transition, 215
   in middle-aged women, 213
   mode of action, 90
   side effects, 91
   starting instructions, 90
progestogens (contraceptive), 68
protease inhibitors, 168
public health
   background of, 28
   contested views on, 29
   human right, 29
   inequalities in, 28–9
   personal autonomy, 29
   social justice, 29
public health delivery
   comprehensive life-cycle approach to women's health, 35

public health delivery (cont.)
contraceptive methods, 33
gender-based violence, 35
migrant women barriers, 34
reducing abortion rate, 34
reducing teenage pregnancy, 33
restrictive abortion laws, 34
sexually transmitted infections
(STIs) and HIV, 34–5
target area identification, 33
workforce development, 35
public health indicators
defined, 353
guidelines, 354–5
indicator requirements, 353–4
key factors, 355
monitoring, 355
purpose of, 353
risk consequences, 354
public health instruments
environment, 31
finance, 32
governance, 32
health systems, 31–2
laws and norms, 31
performance monitoring, 32
public health policy challenge
epidemiological factors, 30–1
population status indicators, 30
public health policy development
defined, 355–6
relevance, 356
public health within sexual and
reproductive health
defined, 358
gender equality goal, 360
good health and well-being goal,
358–9, 365–9
quality education goal, 359–60
reduced inequalities goal, 360
sustainable development goals, 358
unmet needs issue, 358
public health within sexual and
reproductive health, uses in
early diagnosis, 361
primary prevention, 360
quality assurance indicators, 363
screening, 360–1
STI partner notification, 361
surveillance and data monitoring,
361–3

quality improvement model, 367–9
queer people, defined, 348

rape, 341
realistic medicine, 369
reproductive life plan
mental health, 56
nutrition, 53–6

substance abuse, 56
vaccines, 56–7
reversible inhibition of sperm under
guidance (RISUG), 220
Rhesus (Rh) alloimmunization, 236
rubella vaccination, 56

safe abortion access
barriers to, 2–3
European, 10
world stats, 3
schizophrenia and contraceptives
amenorrhea, 176
background of, 175
barrier methods, 176
clinician questions to ask, 175
combined hormonal contraception
(CHC), 175
copper intrauterine device (Cu-
IUD), 175–6
progestogen-only contraceptives
(POCs), 175–6
sterilization, 176
screening
cervical intraepithelial neoplasia,
46–7
clinical, 46
defined, 46
HPV vaccination assessment, 47
by microscopy of vaginal fluid, 48
public health within sexual and
reproductive health use, 360–1
STIs, 47
secondary prevention
cervical cancer, 40–1
defined, 38
infertility, 42
lifestyle health risks, 44
pregnant mother and child
morbidity, 43
sexual dysfunction, 41
sexual violence, 42
STIs and HIV, 39–40
unintended pregnancies, 39
selective serotonin reuptake inhibitors
(SSRIs), 133
sensate focus therapy, 324
sex hormones
drug–drug interactions and
contraception, 131
glucose metabolism and, 159–61
lipid metabolism and, 161
thyroid dysfunction, 200
sex hormones in women
biosynthesis and regulation, 256–8
the brain and, 258–9
genital tissues and, 262
lifespan changes, 259
production and action, 258
sexual motivation and, 261–2

sex hormones in women, female sexual
dysfunction (FSD)
genitourinary syndrome of
menopause (GSM), 264
hypoactive sexual desire disorder
(HSDD), 263
vulvo-vaginal atrophy, 264
sex hormones in women, physiologic
response
genital arousal and orgasm, 261
history of, 259–60
sexual desire, 260–1
sexual tipping point model, 260
sexual and reproductive health (SRH)
defined, 1, 15, 28, 353
family planning, 1
four dimensions of, 15
gender-based violence, 4–5
historical overview, 256
indicators, 18–20
integrating human rights into, 5
maternal healthcare, 3–4
safe abortion access, 2–3
scope of, 1
sexual education, 2
United Nations Agenda for
Sustainable Development Goals
(SDGs), 1
sexual and reproductive health (SRH),
empowerment
education, 5
legislative changes, 5
professional contraceptive
counselling, 71–2
social media, 5
sexual and reproductive health (SRH),
European
abortion access, 10–13
contraception access, 8–10
Evaluation of Comprehensive
Sexuality Education Programmes,
25
German Federal Centre for Health
Promotion (BZgA), 25
key human rights, 8
Standards for Sexuality Education,
25
sexual and reproductive health (SRH),
threat responses
H4+ initiative, 20
UNFPA, 20
WHO, 20
sexual and reproductive health (SRH),
threats to
gender-based violence, 17–18
genital organ diseases, 16
infertility, 16
malignant cycle of, 18
pregnancy, delivery, postpartum
pathologies, 16

sexual dysfunction, 17
sexually transmitted infections
    (STIs) and HIV, 16
unintended pregnancies, 16
unsafe abortion, 16–17
women bearing brunt of effects of,
    28
sexual behaviour, defined, 347
sexual contraceptive complications
    contraceptive methods, 127–9
    counselling, 129
    dimension levels, 126
    empirical studies, 126–7
sexual counselling consultation. see
    also sexual dysfunction
    addressing sexuality communication
        techniques, 291
    conditioning factors, 292–3
    conversation example, 291
    criteria, 290
    descriptive diagnosis, 291–2
    dysfunction diagnosis, 293
    need for, 289
    patient telling own story, 291
    shared decision-making, 293
    structured differentiation questions,
        291
    therapy objectives, 293
    treatment brainstorming, 293
sexual dysfunction. see also sexual
    counselling consultation;
        sexuality-related health problems
    defined, 17
    prevention approaches, 41
    substance/medication caused, 318
sexual dysfunction, men
    assessment factors, 317
    defined, 317
    delayed ejaculation, 327–9
    erectile dysfunction, 320–5
    evaluation, 318
    hypoactive sexual desire disorder
        (HSDD), 318–20
    male hypoactive sexual desire
        disorder, 318
    premature ejaculation, 325–6
    prevalence of, 317–18
sexual dysfunction, women. see also
        pain, female sexual
    assessment, 296–7
    defined, 294
    dyspareunia, 264, 300, 302
    epidemiology, 294
    female cognitive arousal disorder
        (FCAD), 295
    female genital arousal disorder
        (FGAD), 295
    female orgasmic disorder (FOD), 295
    general management principles, 297–8
    guidelines and classification, 294–5

hypoactive sexual desire disorder
    (HSDD), 295
non-organic vaginismus, 301
persistent genital arousal disorder/
    genito-pelvic dysesthesia (PGAD/
    GPD), 295
sexual aversion, 294
three-step interview algorithm,
    301–6
vaginismus, 301, 303–4
vulvodynia, 301, 302–3
sexual education
    defined, 2
    improvements in health-related
        outcomes, 2
    world need for, 2
sexual education, school
    comprehensive sexuality and
        reproductive health education
        (CSRE), 23–4
    as empowerment tool, 5
    historical development, 23
    international documents on, 24–6
    methods, 24
    topics in, 26
sexual health, defined, 333
sexual orientation, defined, 347
sexual tipping point model, 260
sexual violence. see also gender-based
        violence
    defined and dimensions, 340
    impact on children, 342
    and intimate partner violence, 340
    prevalence of, 340
    prevention approaches, 41–2
    social and economic costs, 342
sexual violence, advocacy
    economic, 345
    law enforcement, 345
    legal systems, 345
sexual violence, contributing factors
    risks to victim and perpetrator,
        342–3
    sociocultural, 342
    times of increased risk, 343
sexual violence, health consequences to
        women
    bodily harm, 341
    high-risk pregnancy, 342
    mental health, 342
    sexually transmitted infections
        (STIs), 341
sexual violence, interventions to
    reduce
    community prevention measures,
        344
    fight myths and fake news, 344–5
    healthcare systems, 344
    victim care, 343
sexual violence, manifestations

against children, 341
contraception denial, 341
against disabled people, 341
female genital mutilation (FGM),
    341
forced marriage, 341
forced prostitution, 341
rape, 341
unwanted advances, 341
sexuality education guidelines, 53
sexuality related health problems. see
    also sexual dysfunction
sexuality related health problems,
    classification
    Diagnostic and Statistical Manual of
        Mental Disorder (DSM-5), 317
    International Classification of
        Disease (ICD 10), 317
    prevalence studies, 317
sexually transmitted infections (STIs)
    chlamydia, 277–8
    defined, 274
    demographics, 274
    genital herpes, 274–5
    gonorrhoea, 276–7
    hepatitis B, 282–3
    hepatitis C, 282–3
    HIV, 280–2
    human papilloma virus (HPV), 279
    LGBT+ sexual and reproductive
        health risks, 348
    overview, 274
    partner notification in public health,
        361
    pelvic inflammatory disease (PID),
        278
    public health and, 34–5
    sexual violence and, 341
    syphilis, 283–5
    transmission, 274
    trichomonas vaginalis (TV), 275–6
skin cancer and contraceptives, 143
smoking
    lung cancer and contraceptive
        complications, 144
    during pregnancy, 56
    prevention approaches, 43–4
sperm production physiology, 217
spermicides, 104
St. John's wort, 137
standard days contraceptive method,
    100
Standards for Sexuality Education, 25
Staphylococcus aureus, 47
sterilization in men. see also vasectomy
    chronic kidney disease (CKD),
        193–4
    epilepsy and, 170
    multiple sclerosis and, 170
    post-abortion, 227

sterilization in men (cont.)
transgender people, 350
sterilization in women
causes of failure, 109
chronic kidney disease (CKD),
193–4
complications, 112
contraindications, 109
diabetes mellitus (DM), 198
effects of, 113
efficacy of, 109
epilepsy and, 170
migraine headaches and, 173
multiple sclerosis and, 170
post-abortion, 227
reversal of, 112–13
schizophrenia and, 176
timing, 109
transgender men, 350
sterilization in women, surgical
approaches
comparisons between, 110
hysteroscopic, 111
laparoscopic, 110–11
laparotomy, 109–10
steroids (contraceptive), 68
STI
prevention approaches, 39–40
screening, 47
stigma, 366
substance abuse
prevention approaches, 43–4
reproductive life plan, 56
superficial vein thrombosis (SVT), 155
surgical abortion. see also medical
abortion
under 14 weeks, 240–1
after 14 weeks, 241
choices, 233
contraception after, 241
overview, 226, 233
surgical abortion aftercare
bleeding pattern, 237
contraception, 237–8
surgical abortion methods
dilation and evacuation (D&E), 235
electric vacuum aspiration (EVA),
233–4
by gestational age, 233
manual vacuum aspiration (MVA),
234–5
vacuum aspiration, 233
surgical abortion procedural
considerations
analgesia, 235
cervical priming, 235
infection prevention, 235–6
VTE prophylaxis, 236
surgical abortion risks
adhesions, 237

cervical injury, 237
failed procedure, 237
haemorrhage, 236
infection, 237
retained products, 237
summary, 236
uterine perforation, 236–7
syphilis
background of, 283
diagnosis, 284
follow up, 285
pregnancy and, 284–5
screening, 47
testing for, 283–4
treatment, 284
type classification, 283
systemic lupus erythematosus (SLE)
combined hormonal contraception
(CHC), 189
contraceptive methods and MEC
scores, 188
defined, 187
pathophysiology, 187

tamoxifen, 121
teratogenic medication types for lupus,
190
tertiary prevention
cervical cancer, 41
defined, 38
infertility, 42–3
lifestyle health risks, 44
pregnant mother and child
morbidity, 43
sexual dysfunction, 41
sexual violence, 42
STIs and HIV, 40
unintended pregnancies, 39
tetanus vaccination, 56–7
thrombophilia, inherited, 155
thyroid dysfunction and
contraceptives
background of, 200
effects of hormonal contraceptives,
201–2
ovarian hormones, 200
thyroid dysfunction and
reproductive health, 200–1
tranexamic acid (TXA), 121
transgender men contraception
basics, 350
methods, 350
transgender people, defined, 347–8
transphobia, defined, 349
trauma-informed care, 367
trichomonas vaginalis (TV)
defined, 272
diagnosis, 272–3
as STI, 275–6
symptoms, 272

treatment, 273
tricyclic antidepressants (TCAs), 133
type 1 diabetes, defined, 196
type 2 diabetes, defined, 196

uliprital acetate
efficacy of, 137–8
uterine bleeding treatment, 121
ultrasound, 220
unconscious bias, 366
undernutrition, child, 51
UNFPA Operational Guidance for
Comprehensive Sexuality
Education: A Focus on Human
Rights and Gender, 20, 25
unintended pregnancies
emergency contraception (EC), 115
prevention approaches, 38–9
sexual and reproductive threat, 16
United Nations Agenda for Sustainable
Development Goals (SDGs), 1
unsafe abortion
abortion risk, 244–5
access in Europe, 10
defined, 3
global overview, 16–17
health complications, 3
prevention, 3
stigma around, 12–13
world stats, 3
uterine bleeding and contraceptives
combined hormonal contraception
(CHC) and, 119–20
comparison between, 121
frequency of, 115–16
management, 119
pathophysiology, 118–19
progestogen-only contraceptives
(POCs), 89–90, 120–1
uterine bleeding and contraceptives,
treatment
combined hormonal contraception
(CHC) and, 119–20
comparison between, 121
PALM-COEIN FIGO classification,
146–7
progestogen-only contraceptives
(POCs), 89–90, 120–1
uterine fibroids, 148
uterine perforation, 227, 236–7, 246–7
uterine rupture, 227, 231, 246–7

vaccination
hepatitis B, 57
HPV, 47, 57
rubella, 56
tetanus, 56–7
vacuum aspiration, 233
vaginismus
assessment, 303–4

defined, 301
testing for, 304
vaginitis screening, 47–8
valvular heart disease, 156–7
varicose vein, 155
vasectomy, 217, 219–20. see also
    sterilization in men
venous thromboembolism (VTE) and
    contraceptives
  background of, 155
  familial VTE history, 155
  inherited thrombophilia, 155
  personal VTE history, 155
  superficial vein thrombosis (SVT),
    155
  varicose vein, 155
venous thrombosis (VTE)
  abortion risk, 244
  combined hormonal contraception
    (CHC) and, 80–2
  and progestogen contraceptives in
    immunosuppressive disease, 184
  surgical abortion and, 236
vestbulectomy, 315
vestbuloplasty, 315
vestibulectomy, 309
vulva
  defined, 311–313
  International Society for the
    Study of Vulvovaginal Disease
    (ISSVD), 314

vulvar clinical exam
  additional tests, 311–314
  classification, 312
  eight most common
    histological patterns, 312–313
  special considerations, 312
  speculum examination, 314
  vulvoscopy, 314
vulvar disorders
  complexity of, 315–316
  history taking, 312
  psychological distress
    loop, 303
  vulvodynia, 311
  vulvologic counselling, 311–314
vulvodynia
  assessment, 302–3
  categorizations, 311
  defined, 301, 311
  epidemiology, 311
  factors affecting, 305
  symptoms, 313
vulvodynia diagnosis
  clinical examination, 313
  history taking, 313
  neuropathic pain, 313
  phenotype determination, 313–14
vulvodynia management
  counselling, 314–15
  medical/pharmacological treatment,
    315

physiotherapy, 315
  psychological therapy, 315
  surgical, 315
vulvodynia pathophysiology
  dysfunctional pain, 312–13
  inflammatory pain, 312
  neuropathic pain, 312
  nociceptive pain, 312
vulvoscopy, 312
vulvo-vaginitis
  aerobic vaginitis, 271–2
  bacterial vaginosis (BV), 269–71
  candida, 268–9
  cytolytic vaginosis, 273
  diagnosis, 267–8
  physiological changes, 267
  trichomonas vaginalis (TV),
    272–3

WELL! (Women Empowerment
    Learning Links), 5
withdrawal, 219
World Abortion Laws Map, 10
World Health Organization (WHO)
  European abortion stats, 10
  medical abortion guidelines,
    229
  public health sustainable
    development goals, 358–60
  sexual and reproductive health
    (SRH), threat responses, 20

Printed in the United States
by Baker & Taylor Publisher Services

defined, 301
testing for, 304
vaginitis screening, 47–8
valvular heart disease, 156–7
varicose vein, 155
vasectomy, 217, 219–20. *see also* sterilization in men
venous thromboembolism (VTE) and contraceptives
  background of, 155
  familial VTE history, 155
  inherited thrombophilia, 155
  personal VTE history, 155
  superficial vein thrombosis (SVT), 155
  varicose vein, 155
venous thrombosis (VTE)
  abortion risk, 244
  combined hormonal contraception (CHC) and, 80–2
  and progestogen contraceptives in immunosuppressive disease, 184
  surgical abortion and, 236
vestbulectomy, 315
vestbuloplasty, 315
vestibulectomy, 309
vulva
  defined, 311–313
  International Society for the Study of Vulvovaginal Disease (ISSVD), 314

vulvar clinical exam
  additional tests, 311–314
  classification, 312
  eight most common histological patterns, 312–313
  special considerations, 312
  speculum examination, 314
  vulvoscopy, 314
vulvar disorders
  complexity of, 315–316
  history taking, 312
  psychological distress loop, 303
  vulvodynia, 311
  vulvologic counselling, 311–314
vulvodynia
  assessment, 302–3
  categorizations, 311
  defined, 301, 311
  epidemiology, 311
  factors affecting, 305
  symptoms, 313
vulvodynia diagnosis
  clinical examination, 313
  history taking, 313
  neuropathic pain, 313
  phenotype determination, 313–14
vulvodynia management
  counselling, 314–15
  medical/pharmacological treatment, 315

physiotherapy, 315
psychological therapy, 315
surgical, 315
vulvodynia pathophysiology
  dysfunctional pain, 312–13
  inflammatory pain, 312
  neuropathic pain, 312
  nociceptive pain, 312
vulvoscopy, 312
vulvo-vaginitis
  aerobic vaginitis, 271–2
  bacterial vaginosis (BV), 269–71
  candida, 268–9
  cytolytic vaginosis, 273
  diagnosis, 267–8
  physiological changes, 267
  trichomonas vaginalis (TV), 272–3

WELL! (Women Empowerment Learning Links), 5
withdrawal, 219
World Abortion Laws Map, 10
World Health Organization (WHO)
  European abortion stats, 10
  medical abortion guidelines, 229
  public health sustainable development goals, 358–60
  sexual and reproductive health (SRH), threat responses, 20

Printed in the United States
by Baker & Taylor Publisher Services